I0056540

Essentials of Plastic and Reconstructive Surgery

Essentials of Plastic and Reconstructive Surgery

Edited by Adam Bachman

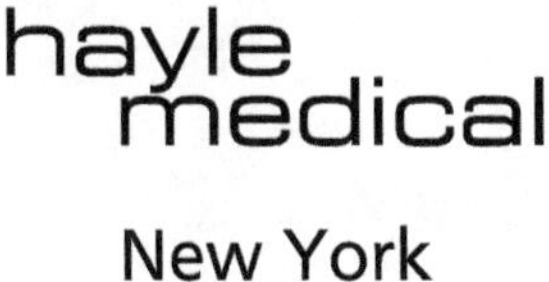

New York

Hayle Medical,
750 Third Avenue, 9th Floor,
New York, NY 10017, USA

Visit us on the World Wide Web at:
www.haylemedical.com

ISBN: 978-1-63241-432-8

The publisher's policy is to use permanent paper from mills that operate a sustainable forestry policy. Furthermore, the publisher ensures that the text paper and cover boards used have met acceptable environmental accreditation standards.

Printed in the United States of America.

Cataloging-in-Publication Data

Essentials of plastic and reconstructive surgery / edited by Adam Bachman.
p. cm.
Includes bibliographical references and index.
ISBN 978-1-63241-432-8
1. Surgery, Plastic. 2. Transplantation of organs, tissues, etc. 3. Tissue engineering. I. Bachman, Adam.
RD118 .E87 2017
617.95--dc23

Table of Contents

Preface

Plastic surgery refers to the surgical practice of reconstructing and restoring the human body. It is widely used in cosmetic surgery to beautify one's body. It is also applied in reconstructive surgery to restore the function and form of the affected body part, as well as in craniofacial surgery, microsurgery, burn treatment, etc. This book gives detailed information about plastic surgery and its applications and techniques. It includes thorough insights about its various sub-specialities. The book presents researches and studies performed by experts across the globe. Coherent flow of topics, student-friendly language and extensive use of examples make this text an invaluable source of knowledge. Students, researchers, experts, surgeons and all associated with plastic and reconstructive surgery will benefit alike from this book.

This book is a result of research of several months to collate the most relevant data in the field.

When I was approached with the idea of this book and the proposal to edit it, I was overwhelmed. It gave me an opportunity to reach out to all those who share a common interest with me in this field. I had 3 main parameters for editing this text:

1. Accuracy - The data and information provided in this book should be up-to-date and valuable to the readers.

2. Structure - The data must be presented in a structured format for easy understanding and better grasping of the readers.

3. Universal Approach - This book not only targets students but also experts and innovators in the field, thus my aim was to present topics which are of use to all.

Thus, it took me a couple of months to finish the editing of this book.

I would like to make a special mention of my publisher who considered me worthy of this opportunity and also supported me throughout the editing process. I would also like to thank the editing team at the back-end who extended their help whenever required.

Editor

1

Abnormal Interactions between Perifollicular Mast Cells and CD8+ T-Cells May Contribute to the Pathogenesis of Alopecia Areata

Marta Bertolini[1,2], Federica Zilio[1], Alfredo Rossi[3], Patrick Kleditzsch[4,9], Vladimir E. Emelianov[5,9], Amos Gilhar[6,7], Aviad Keren[6], Katja C. Meyer[1], Eddy Wang[8], Wolfgang Funk[9], Kevin McElwee[8], Ralf Paus[1,2,10]*

1 Department of Dermatology, University of Lübeck, Lübeck, Germany, **2** Department of Dermatology, University of Münster, Münster, Germany, **3** Department of Internal Medicine and Medical Specialties, University "La Sapienza", Rome, Italy, **4** Department of Gynaecology and Obstetrics, University of Rostock, Rostock, Germany, **5** Department of Pharmacology, Clinical Pharmacology and Biochemistry, Chuvash State University Medical School, Cheboksary, Russia, **6** Laboratory for Skin Research, Rappaport Faculty of Medicine, Technion–Israel Institute of Technology, Haifa, Israel, **7** Flieman Medical Center, Haifa, Israel, **8** Department of Dermatology and Skin Science, University of British Columbia, Vancouver, British Columbia, Canada, **9** Klinik Dr. Koslowski, Munich, Germany, **10** Institute for Inflammation and Repair, University of Manchester, Manchester, United Kingdom

Abstract

Alopecia areata (AA) is a CD8+ T-cell dependent autoimmune disease of the hair follicle (HF) in which the collapse of HF immune privilege (IP) plays a key role. Mast cells (MCs) are crucial immunomodulatory cells implicated in the regulation of T cell-dependent immunity, IP, and hair growth. Therefore, we explored the role of MCs in AA pathogenesis, focusing on MC interactions with CD8+ T-cells *in vivo,* in both human and mouse skin with AA lesions. Quantitative (immuno-)histomorphometry revealed that the number, degranulation and proliferation of perifollicular MCs are significantly increased in human AA lesions compared to healthy or non-lesional control skin, most prominently in subacute AA. In AA patients, perifollicular MCs showed decreased TGFβ1 and IL-10 but increased tryptase immunoreactivity, suggesting that MCs switch from an immuno-inhibitory to a pro-inflammatory phenotype. This concept was supported by a decreased number of IL-10+ and PD-L1+ MCs, while OX40L+, CD30L+, 4–1BBL+ or ICAM-1+ MCs were increased in AA. Lesional AA-HFs also displayed significantly more peri- and intrafollicular- CD8+ T-cells as well as more physical MC/CD8+ T-cell contacts than healthy or non-lesional human control skin. During the interaction with CD8+ T-cells, AA MCs prominently expressed MHC class I and OX40L, and sometimes 4–1BBL or ICAM-1, suggesting that MC may present autoantigens to CD8+ T-cells and/or co-stimulatory signals. Abnormal MC numbers, activities, and interactions with CD8+ T-cells were also seen in the grafted C3H/HeJ mouse model of AA and in a new humanized mouse model for AA. These phenomenological *in vivo* data suggest the novel AA pathobiology concept that perifollicular MCs are skewed towards pro-inflammatory activities that facilitate cross-talk with CD8+ T-cells in this disease, thus contributing to triggering HF-IP collapse in AA. If confirmed, MCs and their CD8+ T-cell interactions could become a promising new therapeutic target in the future management of AA.

Editor: Richard L. Eckert, University of Maryland School of Medicine, United States of America

Funding: This project was supported in part by a grant from DFG to RP and a PhD fellowship to MB (GRK1727/1) as well as by faculty funds to RP from the University of Manchester and by funds from the Associazione Associazione Nazionale Mediterranea Alopecia Areata funds to RP and MB. The funders had no role in study design, data collection and analysis, decision to publish, or preparation of the manuscript.

Competing Interests: The authors have declared that no competing interests exist.

* E-mail: ralf.paus@manchester.ac.uk

[9] These authors contributed equally to this work.

Introduction

Alopecia areata (AA), one of the most common human autoimmune disorders, represents a T-cell-dependent organ-specific autoimmune disease that is clinically characterized by sudden, mostly focal, hair loss [1,2]. The immunopathogenesis of AA and the relevant hair follicle (HF) autoantigen(s) remain to be clarified. However, transfer of CD8(+) cells alone induces localized AA-like hair loss in the C3H/HeJ mouse model [1,3], while CD8+ T-cell depletion abrogates AA onset in a rat model [4]. AA can be also induced by IL-2 stimulated NKG2D+/CD56+ immunocytes, many of which are CD8+, in human skin [5].

Growing (anagen) HFs exhibit relative immune privilege (IP) based on the suppression of MHC class I molecules and the over-expression of IP guardians like TGFβ1/2 [1,2,6–9]. The development of AA requires that the normal IP of growing HFs collapses, induced by excessive release of interferon-γ (IFNγ) for example [5,10,11] (for prevalent AA pathogenesis concepts, see [2]).

The perifollicular inflammatory cell infiltrate in lesional AA HFs contains lymphocytes (CD8+ and CD4+ T-cells), natural killer cells, some Langerhans cells and increased numbers of mature, histochemically detectable mast cells (MC) [12–18]. While T-cells, particularly CD8+ lymphocytes, have long been a focus of AA

Table 1. Experimental design and specific questions addressed.

Model	Question addressed	Investigated read-out parameters
Lesional and non-lesional skin from AA patients versus healthy skin	Do perifollicular MCs and their activities increase in AA?	Evaluation of MC number using c-Kit, TB and Ki-67/tryptase stainings. Evaluation of MC degranulation using TB and Ki-67/tryptase stainings. Evaluation of MC proliferation using Ki-67/tryptase, c-Kit/tryptase and Ki-67/c-Kit stainings.
	Do MCs switch to a pro-inflammatory phenotype in AA?	Evaluation of TGFβ1 and tryptase contents within MCs using TGFβ1/c-Kit and Ki-67/tryptase stainings. Evaluation of MC number positive for OX40L, CD30L, 4-1BBL, ICAM-1, IL-10 or PD-L1 using corresponding triple-staining.
	Do MCs interact with CD8+ T-cells in AA?	Evaluation of MC number in close contact with CD8+ T-cells using CD8/tryptase and CD8/c-Kit.
	Are the observed interactions between MCs and CD8+ T-cells likely to be pro-inflammatory or immuno-inhibitory?	Evaluation of MC number either degranulating or positive for OX40L, CD30L, 4-1BBL, ICAM-1, IL-10 or PD-L1 when in close contact with CD8+ T-cells using corresponding triple-staining.
Grafted C3H/HeJ mice [55,56]	Do perifollicular MCs and their activities increase in AA affected mice?	Evaluation of MC number using c-Kit/CD8 and mMCP6/CD8, stainings. Evaluation of MC degranulation using mMCP6/CD8 staining.
	Are MCs and MC-CD8+ T-cell interactions also abnormal in the C3H/HeJ AA mouse model?	Evaluation of MC number in close contact with CD8+ T-cells using mMCP6/CD8 and c-Kit/CD8 stainings.
Humanized-mouse model of AA [5,57]	Can key findings made in the skin of AA patients with respect to excessive MC number/activities and MC-CD8+ T-cell interactions be reproduced in experimentally induced AA-like lesions in previously healthy human skin?	Evaluation of MC number using c-Kit and tryptase/CD8, stainings. Evaluation of MC number degranulation using tryptase/CD8 staining. Evaluation of MC number in close contact with CD8+ T-cells using tryptase/CD8 staining.

research (e.g. [3–5,14,19–24], MCs have received much less attention (Background S1 in File S1).

While MCs have long been viewed as primary effector cells of innate immunity, more recent research has revealed that they also play a key role in connecting innate and adaptive immune responses [25–34]. In fact, MCs can even control antigen-specific CD8+ T-cell responses, namely in murine experimental auto-immune encephalitis (EAE) [35], another organ-specific auto-immune disease characterized by IP collapse. Consequently, the pathobiological contribution of MCs to autoimmune disorders such as type 1 diabetes and multiple sclerosis is attracting increasing attention [25,26,31,36–39].

This recent development made it compelling to further examine the enigmatic role of MCs in AA, whose number has been reported to be increased in lesional human AA skin by some authors [12,14–16]. Such a focus on MCs in AA was further encouraged by the fact that MCs are recognized hair growth modulators [40–44], and that the HF mesenchyme in humans and mice harbours resident MC progenitor cells, from which fully functional, mature skin MCs can differentiate *in loco* [45–47].

MCs are now appreciated to exert a dual immunoregulatory role [25–31,34,38,48]: Under physiological circumstances, MCs may be primarily immuno-inhibitory, thus contributing to the maintenance of IP and peripheral tolerance [27,31,34,37,48–53] and therefore, possibly, to the maintenance of HF-IP [2,53]. However, as MCs are primed to rapidly secrete proinflammatory 'danger' signals, their role can quickly convert into a tolerance-breaking, potentially autoimmunity-promoting one, such as during allograft rejection and EAE [25,26,31,38,39,48,52–54].

Given the recognized key role of CD8+ T-cells in AA pathogenesis [1–4,20], one main research challenge, therefore, is to characterize MC-CD8+ T-cell interactions in human AA pathobiology. However, for human MCs, one is currently restricted to phenomenological studies (see Discussion). In order to keep such analyses as instructive and clinically relevant as possible, we have combined the *in situ*-analysis of AA lesions in AA patients with the analysis of grafted C3H/HeJ AA mice [55,56] and of experimentally induced AA lesions in previously healthy human skin transplanted onto SCID mice [5,57]. In these independent, mutually complementary AA models, we have addressed the specific questions summarized in **Table 1**, using quantitative (immuno-)histomorphometry and triple-immunostaining techniques, as well as a range of relevant MC markers (Background S2 in File S1), so as to gauge skin MC function *in situ*.

Material and Methods

Human specimens

Human lesional and non-lesional scalp skin biopsies were obtained from 7 AA patients (n = 7, lesional skin, n = 4, non-lesional skin) after written patients' consent, and internal review board (Department of Internal Medicine, n. 11, 29-01-13) and

Table 2. Immunostainings.

Antigen(s)	Specimen	Antigen retrieval/fixation	1st detection system	2nd detection system	3rd detection system	Counter staining
C-Kit	Human	Sodium Citrate	ABC-HRP, DAB			Hematoxylin
Ki-67/tryptase	Human	Sodium Citrate	ABC-HRP, DAB	ABC-AP, SIGMAFAST		
C-Kit/tryptase	Human	Sodium Citrate	IF, FITC,	IF, Rho		DAPI
Ki-67/c-Kit	Human	Sodium Citrate	ABC-HRP, DAB	ABC-AP, SIGMAFAST		Hematoxylin
Ki-67/tryptase	Human	Sodium Citrate	IF, Rho	IF, FITC		DAPI
CD8/tryptase	Human, Hu-mouse	Sodium Citrate	ABC-HRP, DAB	ABC-AP, SIGMAFAST		Hematoxylin
TGFβ1/c-Kit	Human	Sodium Citrate	IF, Rho or IF, FITC	IF, FITC or IF, Rho		DAPI
TGFβ1	Human	Sodium Citrate	ABC-HRP, DAB			
OX40L/CD8/tryptase	Human	TRIS-EDTA	ABC-HRP, AEC	ABC-AP, Vector Blue	ABC-AP, SIGMAFAST	
CD30L/c-Kit/CD8	Human	Sodium Citrate	ABC-HRP, AEC	ABC-AP, Vector Blue	ABC-HRP, DAB	
4-1BBL/c-Kit/CD8	Human	Sodium Citrate	ABC-HRP, AEC	ABC-AP, Vector Blue	ABC-HRP, DAB	
ICAM-1/CD8/tryptase	Human	Sodium Citrate	ABC-HRP, AEC	ABC-AP, Vector Blue	ABC-AP, SIGMAFAST	
IL-10/c-Kit/CD8	Human	TRIS-EDTA	ABC-HRP, AEC	ABC-AP, Vector Blue	ABC-HRP, DAB	Methyl-green
PD-L1/c-Kit/CD8	Human	Sodium Citrate	ABC-HRP, AEC	ABC-AP, Vector Blue	ABC-HRP, DAB	
CD200/CD8/tryptase	Human	TRIS-EDTA	DAB	ABC-AP, Vector Blue	ABC-AP, SIGMAFAST	
C-kit	Hu-mouse	Sodium Citrate	ABC-AP, SIGMAFAST			Hematoxylin
C-Kit/CD8	Mouse	Acetone	ABC-HRP, AEC	ABC-AP, SIGMAFAST		Hematoxylin
mMCP6/CD8	Mouse	Acetone	Envision-HRP, AEC	ABC-HRP, DAB		Hematoxylin

List of all immunostainings which were performed and relevant details (For list of primary antibodies, see Table S1 in File S1).
ABC-AP: Avidin-biotin complex, alkaline phosphatase; ABC-HRP: Avidin-biotin complex, horseradish peroxidase; AEC: 3-amino-9-ethylcarbazole; DAB: 3,3′-diaminobenzidine, DAPI: diamidino-2-phenylindole, Envision-HRP: Envision- horseradish peroxidise; FITC: Fluorescein isothiocyanate; IF: immunofluorescence, SIGMAFAST™: Fast Red TR/Naphthol AS-MX tablets, Rho: Rhodamine.

ethic committee (n. 2973, 28-11-13) approvals, University "La Sapienza" of Rome.

An additional 23 human lesional scalp skin biopsies from AA patients were obtained from archival paraffin blocks (up to 10 years old) from biopsies that had been taken exclusively for diagnostic purposes from the Dermatopathology Paraffin Block Collection, Dept. of Dermatology University of Luebeck, after ethics committee approval (University of Luebeck, n. 13-007, 13-03-13). It was not possible to obtain the written consent as most patients were not traceable after such a long period. Consequently, anonymized use of these tissue blocks without formal written consent was approved by the ethics committee.

Clinically "healthy" frontotemporal human skin scalp samples obtained from 23 women without a record of AA (mean age: 55 years) undergoing cosmetic facelift surgery were used as controls after ethics committee approval (University of Luebeck, n. 06-109, 18-07-06) and written patient consent.

As positive control tissues for different immunostaining protocols, anonymized human tonsil and placenta tissue samples were obtained from the Dept. of Pathology, University of Luebeck, with ethics approval (n. 06-109, 20-01-2009), without the necessity of written patient consent.

All experiments were performed according to Helsinki guidelines.

Mice

Grafted C3H/HeJ AA model: 13 weeks-old female C3H/HeJ mice were purchased from The Jackson Laboratory, Bar Harbor, Maine USA and housed in the British Columbia University facility. The mice were transplanted with healthy hairy or alopecic skin isolated from older C3H/HeJ donors as previously described [55,56]. Most of the mice transplanted with alopecic lesions developed AA, here called AA mice (mAA), while a few mice failed to develop AA, here called failed-grafted mice (fAA). Mice transplanted with normal hairy skin did not develop AA, here called sham-grafted mice (mSH). For comparison non-transplanted mice were also used, here called normal mice (NM). After about one year, the mice were killed and the skin samples were collected from the mid to lower back close to the midline, avoiding the skin graft area, fixed in cryo-matrix and frozen in liquid

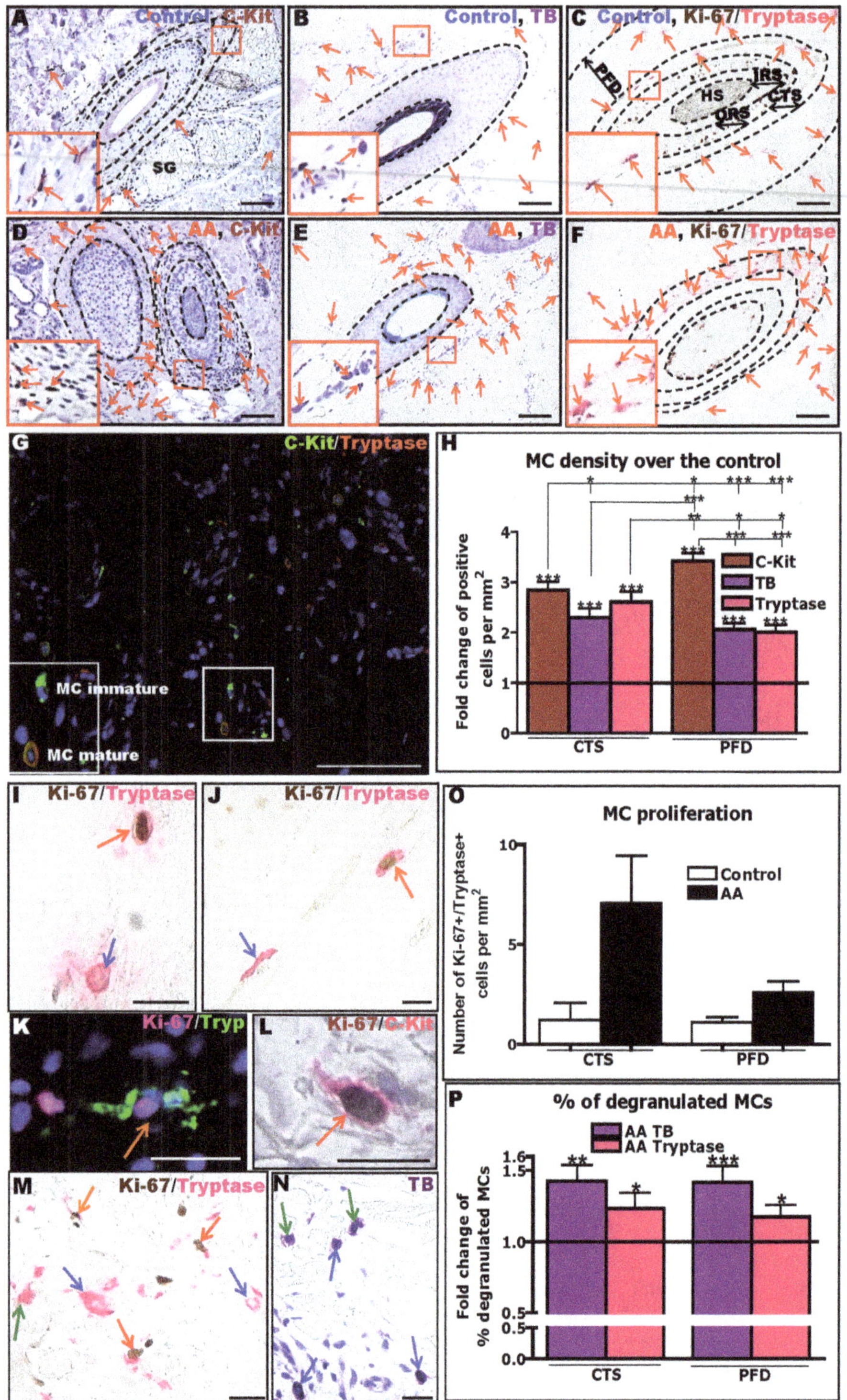

Figure 1. Human AA lesions show increased density, proliferation and degranulation of perifollicular MCs. The immunohistochemical identification and evaluation of MCs by c-Kit (A,D), TB (B,E) or Ki-67/tryptase (C,F) revealed a strong increase of MC numbers in AA (D–F) compared to control healthy (A–C) skin. Red arrows indicate MCs. C-Kit/tryptase double-IF shows immature c-Kit+ MCs (stained in green) and mature c-Kit+/tryptase+ MCs in AA skin (stained in green and red) (G). See inserted panels in the bottom left of each Figure for higher magnification views of the area highlighted in the small boxes. Reference area for the quantitative analysis using (immuno-)histomorphometry for cell counting in the connective tissue sheath (CTS) and perifollicular dermis (PFD). CTS+PFD represents the total area including the space demarcated up to 200 μm from the HF basement membrane (C,F). Fold change of MC density detected by c-Kit, TB and tryptase stainings (H). Black line indicates the control. Analysis derived from 69–81areas (HFs) of 11–17 AA patients and from 50–69 areas (HFs) of 5–7 healthy controls, ±SEM, *p≤0.05, **p≤0.01, ***p≤0.001, Mann-Whitney-U-Test or Student t-test (for c-Kit, TB and tryptase compared to respective controls and for comparing bars between CTS and PFD), Kruskal-Wallis test (p<0.0001) followed by Dunn's test (for comparing c-Kit, TB and tryptase within CTS and PFD). Identification of MCs by Ki-67/tryptase IHC (I,J,M), Ki-67/tryptase IF (K), Ki-67/c-Kit IHC (L) and TB (N) showing non-degranulating, non proliferating MCs (blue arrows), degranulating,

non-proliferating MCs (green arrows), non-degranulating MCs undergoing proliferation (red arrows) and proliferating degranulating MCs (orange arrows). Quantitative analysis of MC proliferation by Ki-67/tryptase IHC (O). Analysis derived from 81 areas (HFs) of 17 AA patients and 50 areas (HFs) of 7 healthy controls, ±SEM, Mann-Whitney-U-Test (ns). Quantitative analysis of MC degranulation by TB histochemistry and Ki-67/tryptase IHC (P). Black line indicates the control. Analysis derived from 69–81 areas (HFs) of 11–17 AA patients and 50–69 areas (HFs) of 5–7 healthy controls, ±SEM, *p≤0.05, **p≤0.05, ***p≤0.001 Mann-Whitney-U-Test (compare to control), Mann-Whitney test (TB compare to tryptase) (ns). Scale bars: 100 μm (A–G) and 20 μm (I–N) Connective tissue sheath (CTS), hair shaft (HS), inner root sheath (IRS), outer root sheath (ORS), perifollicular dermis (PFD), toluidine blue (TB), sebaceous gland (SG).

nitrogen (thus, "mAA" skin refers to new areas of alopecia arising apart from the engraftment site on the younger graft recipient mice). This experiment was performed following ethics approval by the University of British Columbia Animal Care Committee (n. A10-0166, 16-08-13). The skin samples were then shipped to the University of Lübeck for (immuno-)histomorphometry analysis.

Humanized AA mouse model: Paraffin sections of human skin were obtained from 6 C.B-17/IcrHsd-scid-bg mice (derived from 2 independent experiments) that had been transplanted with healthy human scalp skin and subsequently injected intradermally with allogeneic, IL-2 or PHA-treated, PBMCs from healthy donors enriched for NKG2D+/CD56+ cells (for details, see [5,57]. Mice that received an injection of IL-2-treated NKG2D+/CD56+ cell-enriched PBMCs clinically and histologically developed characteristic AA lesions in the transplanted, previously healthy hair-bearing human skin, while control mice receiving NKG2D+/CD56+-enriched cells cultured with PHA instead of IL-2 failed to develop AA in the human skin transplants. Human skin samples were obtained after informed patient consent and ethics approval (n. 919970072, 13-05-97) from the Flieman Medical Center and the Ministry of Health, Israel, and the study was performed in accordance with the Declaration of Helsinki Principles. Animal care and research protocols were in accordance with institutional guidelines and were approved by the Technion Institute Committee on Animal Use (n. IL-087-08-2011, 08-11).

Immunohistology

For detection of single antigens (for details see **Table 2**, Material and methods S3 and Table S1 in File S1), the skin sections were immunostained following established protocols [58,59] by using the avidin-biotin complex method and the corresponding chromogen. Similar protocols were used for each protein stained in double or triple-immunohistochemistry (IHC) in which we serially stained the sections for each protein (for details see **Table 2**, Material and methods S3 and Table S1 in File S1). To perform double- [60] and triple-immunofluorescence (IF) labelling, we used the appropriate primary antibody (Table S1 in File S1) and secondary antibodies conjugated to the correct fluorophore (**Table 2**). Each immunostaining protocol was also conducted with the appropriate positive and negative controls (Figure S1 in File S1), which confirmed both the sensitivity and specificity of the immunoreactivity (IR) patterns reported here.

Histochemistry

Mature MCs were also visualized histochemically with 1% toluidine blue (TB) as described [47,58].

Quantitative (immuno-)histomorphometry

The cell densities of MCs, CD8+ T-cells and MC-CD8+ T-cell interactions were evaluated in the HF connective tissue sheath (CTS) and the peri-follicular dermis (PFD) by (immuno-)histomorphometry. The total reference area (CTS+PFD) included all tissue within a distance of up to 200 μm from the HF basement membrane in a human skin section (**Figure 1C,F**). In murine skin, positive cells were counted in a perifollicular tissue area within 50 μm of the HF [58,61]. MCs with more than five granules located outside of the cell membrane were regarded as "degranulated" [43,47,58]. The staining intensity of TGFβ1 and tryptase of individual MCs was evaluated by quantitative analysis [58–59], using NIH image J software (National Institute of Health, Bethesda, Maryland).

Statistical analysis

All data were analyzed by Student's *t*- or Mann-Whitney-U- test when only two groups were compared, or by One Way-ANOVA or Kruskal-Wallis test followed by Bonferroni's or Dunn's multiple comparison tests, respectively, when more than two groups were analyzed, using GraphPad (GraphPad Prism version 4.00 for Windows; GraphPad Software, San Diego, CA, USA). Data are expressed as mean ±SEM; p values of <0.05 were regarded as significant.

Results

Human AA lesions show increased density, proliferation and degranulation of perifollicular MCs

First, we sought to resolve the controversy in the published literature on whether or not the number of MCs is increased in lesional AA skin [12,14–16,62]. Quantitative analysis of MC numbers in human AA skin by TB histochemistry and c-Kit and Ki-67/tryptase IHC, unequivocally revealed a significant increase in MC density in the HF mesenchyme (CTS) and in the surrounding perifollicular dermis (PFD) compared to both healthy control skin (**Figure 1A–F, H**) and non-lesional AA skin (Figure S2A in File S1). The variable absolute MC numbers, dependent on the MC detection method used (**Figure 1A–H**) (Resul S4 in File S1), are in line with the recognized presence of distinct MC subpopulations in human skin [47,63,64].

Next, we asked whether the increased MC number resulted from enhanced MC proliferation. Although quantitative Ki-67/tryptase double-IHC (**Figure 1I,J,M**) revealed a slightly higher number of proliferating mature MCs in both CTS and PFD in AA skin compared to healthy control skin, this did not reach significance (**Figure 1O**). Double-IHC for Ki-67+/c-Kit+ cells (**Figure 1L**) suggested a trend towards slightly increased MC proliferation in AA skin (Figure S2B in File S1). This raised the possibility that the substantial numeric increase of MCs in lesional AA skin not only results from increased intracutaneous proliferation of MCs, but also from increased proliferation and maturation of resident MC progenitor cells in human skin [45–47], and/or from an enhanced influx of MC progenitors from the circulation.

Quantitative analysis of TB histochemistry and tryptase IHC (**Figure 1I–K,M,N**) showed significantly more MC defined as "degranulated" in the CTS and PFD of AA skin than in healthy control skin (**Figure 1P**). Thus, AA lesions are associated with a greatly enhanced activation status of skin MCs *in situ*.

In order to assess whether MC numbers and granulation status are AA phase-dependent, AA patients were divided into three groups, based on their histological features [65] ("acute", "subacute" and "chronic" AA) and on clinical evaluation criteria

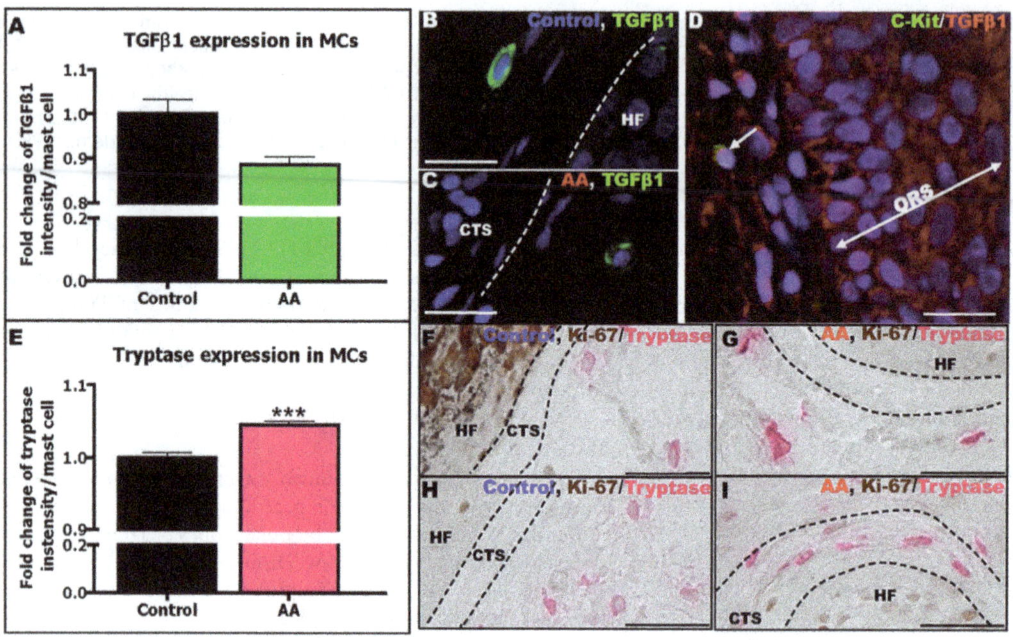

Figure 2. AA MCs contain less TGFβ1 and more tryptase compared to control MCs. Quantitative analysis of TGFβ1 IR in perifollicular MCs in AA patients compared to controls (A). Analysis derived from 272 MCs around 29 HFs of 10 AA patients and 175 MCs around 19 HFs of 2 healthy controls, ±SEM, Mann-Whitney-U-Test (ns). Representative pictures of TGFβ1+ MCs in human scalp skin of controls (B) and AA patients (C) stained by TGFβ1(green)/c-Kit(red) double-staining. Representative picture of TGFβ1(red)/c-Kit(green) double-staining (D). Quantitative analysis of tryptase IR in perifollicular MCs in AA patients compared to controls (E). Analysis derived from 272 MCs around 41 HFs of 14 AA patients and 182 MCs around 19 HFs of 2 healthy controls, ***$p \leq 0.001$, ±SEM, Mann-Whitney-U-Test. Representative pictures of tryptase+ MCs in human scalp skin of control (F,H) and AA patients (G,I) stained by Ki-67/tryptase double-staining. Scale bars: 20 μm (B–D) and 50 μm (F–I). Connective tissue sheath (CTS), hair follicle (HF), outer root sheath (ORS).

supplied by the attending dermatologist, using all three MC detection methods (c-Kit, TB, tryptase). This demonstrated a maximal increase of MC density in lesional PFD compared to healthy controls for the subacute AA group (Figure S3A-E in File S1 and data not shown), though significance was only reached when the number of c-Kit+ cells was analysed (Figure S3E in File S1).

MCs in AA skin are skewed towards a pro-inflammatory phenotype

Subsequently, we searched for phenotypic indications for changes in MC function *in situ*. MCs can release potent immunoinhibitors such as TGFβ1 [29,30,34,51,66–68], which is also one of the most important guardians of HF-IP [1,6–9,69]. Interestingly, TGFβ1 IR was lowered in the outer root sheath (ORS) of lesional AA-HFs (Result S5 and Figure S4A–C in File S1), consistent with compromised HF-IP [1,2,59,69]. Therefore, we examined whether the TGFβ1 expression in perifollicular MCs was also abnormal. Indeed, TGFβ1/c-Kit double-IF revealed that perifollicular MCs in lesional AA skin showed reduced TGFβ1 content compared to controls (**Figure 2A–D**). This suggests that the TGFβ-based immuno-inhibitory phenotype of perilesional MCs is attenuated in AA.

[LOOSESR]Tryptase is a pro-inflammatory, trypsin-like protease stored together with heparin within MCs and released upon degranulation [29,30,47,48,70–74]. Tryptase functions are mostly mediated by signalling via the PAR-2 receptor [70,71,73–75] and by activating other proteases such as collagenases [31,72]. Additional analyses showed that the MC content of tryptase was significantly up-regulated in perifollicular MCs in lesional AA skin compared to controls (**Figure 2E–I**). This further supports the concept that perifollicular MCs in AA switch from an immuno-inhibitory to a pro-inflammatory phenotype at some stage during AA pathogenesis.

The number of CD8+ T-cells that are in close contact with MCs is significantly increased in AA

In view of the accepted key role of CD8+ T-cells in AA pathogenesis [1–4,20] and the fact that MCs can activate CD8+ T-cells [25,26,29,30,35,76,77], we subsequently analyzed MC-CD8+ T-cell contacts in human AA. As expected from the literature [14,19,21,24,78,79], the number of CD8+ T-cells in the perifollicular mesenchyme was significantly higher in lesional compared to non-lesional AA (data not shown) and to healthy anagen HFs (Figure 3A–C).

Subsequent analyses provided the first evidence that MCs co-localize with CD8+ T-cells around the HF in AA skin significantly more frequently (**Figure 3B,D–J**) than in healthy control skin (**Figure 3A,D**) and non-lesional AA skin (data not shown). Moreover, during these interactions, almost 50% of MCs were found to be degranulated, as assessed by tryptase IHC (**Figure 3F,I,J**). These perifollicular MCs were strongly MHC class I-positive (Result S6 and Figure S5A–D in File S1) indicating their capacity to present autoantigens to cognate CD8+ T-cells.

MCs in lesional AA skin up-regulate co-stimulatory molecules for CD8+ T-cells

This led to the question how MCs and CD8+ T-cells may interact in AA. Since MCs can express many cell surface molecules that are either co-stimulatory or inhibitory for CD8+ T-cells (see

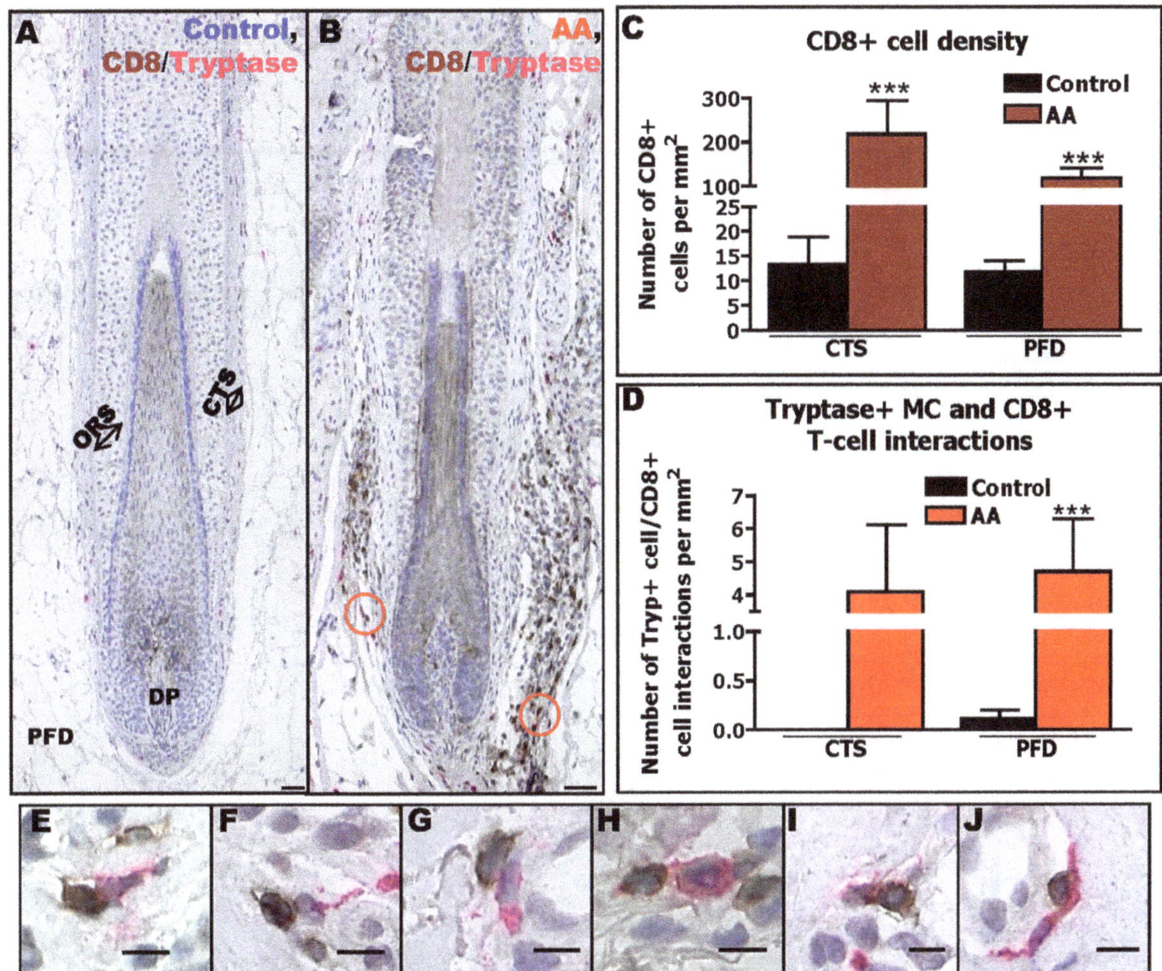

Figure 3. The number of perifollicular CD8+ T-cells and MC-CD8+ T-cell interactions are increased in AA. Immunohistochemical identification of tryptase+ MCs and CD8+ T-cells in human scalp skin of controls (A) and AA patients (B). Quantitative analysis of CD8+ T-cells (C) and of their interactions with tryptase+ MCs (D). Analysis derived from 56 areas (HFs) from 13 AA patients and 44 areas (HFs) of 7 healthy controls, $***p \leq 0.001$, ±SEM, p value was calculated by Mann-Whitney-U-Test. Non-degranulating MCs (E,G,H) and degranulating MCs (F,I,J) close to CD8+ T-cells Scale bars: 50 µm (A–B) and 10 µm (E–J). Connective tissue sheath (CTS), dermal papilla (DP), outer root sheath (ORS), perifollicular dermis (PFD).

e.g., [25,26,28–31,34,51]), MC-CD8+ T-cell interactions can be regulated and fine-tuned by multiple different signalling partners. As a first attempt towards dissecting these interactions *in situ*, we established triple-IHC for MCs, CD8+ T-cells and some of the best-characterized co-stimulatory molecules known to modulate MC-CD8+ T-cells interactions [25,26,28–31,76,77].

OX40L is a type II transmembrane soluble glycoprotein which activates OX40 during cell contact thereby stimulating CD8+ T-cell proliferation, survival, and cytokine production [76,77,80–85]. Quantitative (immuno-)histomorphometry showed that the total number of OX40L+ MCs was increased in lesional skin of AA patients (**Figure 4A–E,I–J**). In addition, the percentage of OX40L+ MCs among all tryptase+ MCs was significantly increased compared to non-lesional AA skin (**Figure 4I–K**). While most of the MCs interacting with CD8+ T-cells in all groups expressed OX40L, lesional AA showed a significant up-regulation of OX40L+ MCs that were in direct contact with CD8+ T-cells (**Figure 4G–H,L**).

Next, we also performed triple-IHC for CD30L, since its expression by MCs is up-regulated under pro-inflammatory conditions [86–88]; moreover, activated CD8+ T-cells can express CD30 which is implicated in the control of CD8+ T-cell proliferation and cytokine production [83,85,89–91]. **Figure 4M–S** shows that the total number and percentage of CD30L+ MCs was significantly up-regulated in lesional AA skin compared to healthy and non-lesional human skin (**Figure 4Q,S**). However, hardly any CD30L+ MCs were seen to be in contact with CD8+ T-cells (**Figure 4O,P**).

4–1BBL is expressed by activated MCs [35,76,92] and supports CD8+ T-cell survival/expansion after binding its receptor on activated T-cells [83,93–98]. Triple-IHC revealed that perifollicular 4–1BBL+ cells are exceptionally rare in healthy and non-lesional AA skin (**Figure 4W**). However, more 4–1BBL+ MCs were detectable in lesional AA skin, notably in a peribulbar location (**Figure 4T–U**), consistent with the typical peribulbar inflammatory infiltrate in AA [1,2,14,65], and occasionally also very close to CD8+ T-cells (**Figure 4T–V**).

ICAM-1 IR was also examined, since ICAM+ MC-derived exosomes can induce T lymphocyte proliferation and cytokine production [99,100]. Corresponding triple-IHC revealed a slight increase in the number of ICAM-1+ MCs in AA lesional skin

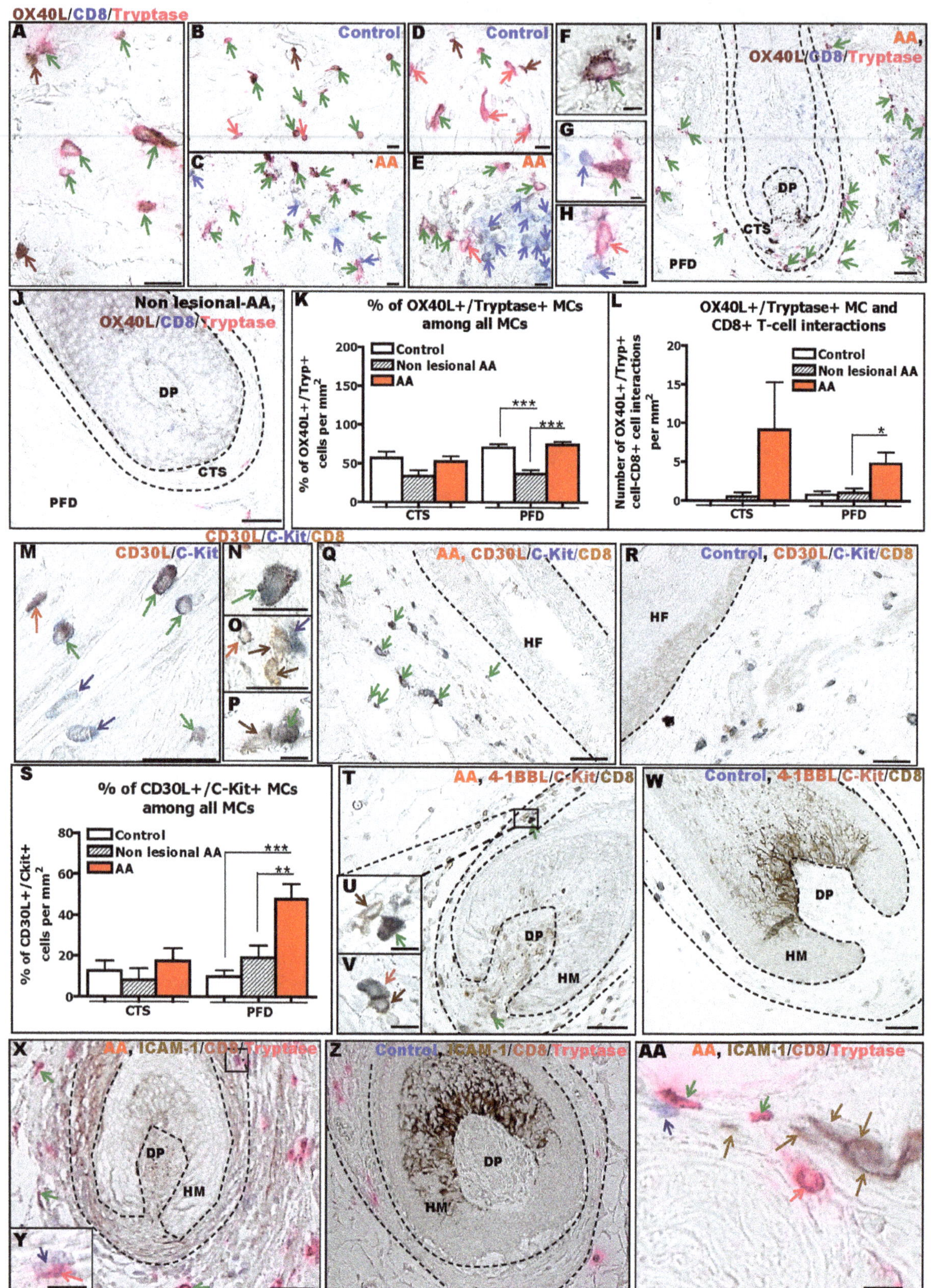

Figure 4. MCs in lesional AA skin up-regulate co-stimulatory molecules for CD8+ T-cells. Immunohistochemical identification of OX40L+/tryptase+ MCs, detected using OX40L/CD8/tryptase staining (A–E) and CD30L+/c-Kit+ MCs, detected using CD30L/c-Kit (M), showing the expression pattern of OX40L (A–E) and CD30L (M) within MCs, in human scalp skin of controls (A,B,D,M) and AA patients (C,E). Higher magnification of OX40L+/tryptase+ (F) and CD30L+/c-Kit+ (N) MCs. Representative pictures of OX40L+ (G) and OX40L− (H) (detected by tryptase) and CD30L− (O) and CD30L+

(P) (detected by c-Kit) MCs interacting with CD8+ T-cells. Immunohistochemical identification of OX40L+/tryptase+ (I,J) and CD30L+/c-Kit+ (Q,R) MCs and CD8+ T-cells in human HFs from lesional (I,Q), non-lesional (J) AA and healthy (R) skin. Brown cells are OX40L+ (A–J) or CD8+ (M–R) cells (brown arrows), blue cells are CD8+ (A–J) or c-Kit+ (M–R) cells (blue arrows), pink cells are tryptase+ cells (A–J) (pink arrows), red cells are CD30L+ cells (M–R) (red arrows), pink-brown cells are OX40L+/tryptase+ cells (A-J) and blue-red cells are CD30L+/c-Kit+ cells (M–R) (green arrows). Quantitative analysis of the % of OX40L+/tryptase+ MCs among all MCs (K), OX40L+/tryptase+ MCs interacting with CD8+ T-cells (L) and the % of CD30L+/c-Kit+ MCs among all MCs (S) in AA patients compared to controls. Analysis derived from 17–21 areas of 6–14 HFs of 6–7 healthy control and of 11–21 areas of 4–12 HFs of 3 AA patients for non-lesional skin and of 17–21 areas of 16–17 HFs of 7 AA patients for lesional skin. ±SEM ***$p \leq 0.001$, **$p \leq 0.01$, *$p \leq 0.05$ ±SEM, One-Way ANOVA or Kruskal-Wallis test followed respectively by Bonferroni's or Dunn's multiple comparison tests. Immunohistochemical identification of 4–1BBL+/c-Kit+ and 4-1BBL-/c-Kit+ MCs, detected using 4–1BBL/c-Kit/CD8 staining (T–W) and of ICAM-1+/tryptase+ and ICAM-1-/tryptase+ MCs, detected using ICAM-1/CD8/Tryptase staining (X-AA), around the HF bulb of AA patient (T,X) and control (W,Z). Representative pictures of 4–1BBL+/c-Kit+ (U), 4–1BBL-/c-Kit+ MCs (V), ICAM-1-/tryptase+ (Y) and ICAM-1+/tryptase+ (AA) MCs interacting with CD8+ T-cells. Brown cells are CD8+ (T–W) or ICAM-1+ (X-AA) cells (brown arrows), blue cells are c-Kit+ MCs (T–W) or CD8+ cells (X-AA) (blue arrows), red cells are 4–1BBL+ cells (T–W) (red arrows), pink cells are tryptase+ cells (X-AA) (pink arrows), blue-red cells are 4–1BBL+/c-Kit+ MCs (T–W) and pink-brown cells are ICAM-1+/tryptase+ MCs (X-AA) (green arrows). These stainings were observed in one section/subject of 6–8 healthy individuals and non-lesional skin from 4 AA patients and lesional skin from 11 AA patients. Scale bars: 20 µm (A–C, N–P,AA), 10 µm (D–E,U,V,Y), 5 µm (F–H), 50 µm (I–J,M,Q,R,T,W,X,Z). Connective tissue sheath (CTS), dermal papilla (DP), hair follicle (HF), hair matrix (HM), perifollicular dermis (PFD).

(**Figure 4X,Z**). Yet, only a few ICAM-1+ MCs were seen to be located in close proximity to CD8+ T-cells (**Figure 4AA**).

Collectively, these results further support the concept that MCs in AA are skewed towards pro-inflammatory activities and that the OX40/OX40L, and possibly also the 4-1BB/4–1BBL and/or ICAM-1/LFA-1 signalling pathways might be involved in regulating abnormal MC-CD8+ T-cell interactions in AA.

Immuno-inhibitory MCs appear to be defective in AA

We then asked whether immuno-inhibitory molecules are down-regulated on MCs in AA skin *in situ*, along with the reduced TGFβ1 expression of perifollicular MCs reported above (**Figure 2A–D**). First, IL-10 was assessed as MCs can regulate peripheral tolerance by releasing IL-10 [29,30,37,49,52,54,101], a predominantly immuno-inhibitory type II cytokine [102–104].

Interestingly, most of the cells expressing prominent IL-10 IR in healthy human skin were MCs, primarily in the in CTS and PFD (**Figure 5A**). However, the number of IL-10+ MCs was significantly decreased in lesional and non-lesional AA skin compared to healthy controls (**Figure 5A–D**), and the few IL-10+ MCs which remained visible in AA patients were localized only rarely in the perifollicular mesenchyme (i.e CTS or PFD) (**Figure 5B**). Moreover, IL-10 expression in individual MCs was decreased in AA skin compared to healthy controls (**Figure 5A,B**, see higher magnification insert). Generally, MCs that interacted with CD8+ T-cells did not express substantial IL-10 IR, neither in healthy nor in AA skin (**Figure 5E–H**).

PD-L1 is a type I transmembrane protein implicated in HF-IP [105]. It delivers an inhibitory signal through its receptor on T-cells (PD-1), inhibiting cytokine production and proliferation while stimulating T-cell death [106,107,108,109]. Here, we show the first evidence that primary human MCs can express varying levels of PD-L1 *in situ* in healthy human skin (**Figure 5I–L**), as has previously been shown for murine bone marrow derived-MCs [77]. In human healthy control skin, PD-L1+ MCs were rare (**Figure 5L**); their number appeared to be further reduced in lesional AA skin compared to healthy skin (**Figure 5L,M**). The number of PD-L1+ cells was too low to permit a quantitative analysis. Moreover, we could not detect any PD-L1+ MCs interacting with CD8+ T-cells in healthy or AA skin (data not shown).

The final functional MC marker we examined in this series of experiments was the important immuno-inhibitory "no danger-signal", CD200, which plays a key role in HF-IP maintenance [8,59,110] and whose receptor is expressed on T-cells [111]. However, in line with a previous report [112], we could find almost no CD200+ MCs, neither in healthy human skin nor in AA lesional skin (data not shown).

Taken together, our observation that MCs in healthy skin express classical immuno-inhibitory molecules supports the hypothesis that, physiologically, perifollicular MCs mainly have tolerance-promoting functions [53]. Furthermore, MC expression of immuno-inhibitory proteins was reduced in AA skin, particularly during their interactions with CD8+ T-cells. This underscores that MCs in AA are skewed towards pro-inflammatory activities and that MC-CD8+ T-cell interactions in AA are predominantly pro-inflammatory.

Pilot experiments that attempted to functionally probe MC-CD8+ T-cells interaction in organ-cultured intact human scalp HFs or skin *in vitro* were inconclusive due to methodological constraints that could not be overcome (see Result S7 in File S1 for details).

The number of MC-CD8+ T-cell contacts is also increased in C3H/HeJ mice affected by AA

Next we wished to probe whether abnormal MC-CD8+ T-cell interactions in human AA skin were also present in the C3H/HeJ mouse model for AA [55,56]. As shown in **Figure 6A–Q**, normal (NM), sham-grafted (mSH) and failed-grafted (fAA) mice showed only a few perifollicular MCs (detected by c-Kit (**Figure 6A–C**) and mouse MC protease (mMCP) 6 (**Figure 6I–K**)) and very few CD8+ T-cells (**Figure 6A–C,I–K**). In striking contrast, lesional skin of mice affected by AA (mAA) showed significantly more perifollicular (immature) c-Kit+ MCs (**Figure 6A–E**), increased MC degranulation (**Figure 6I–L,N,P**) and higher CD8+ T-cell numbers (**Figure 6A–D,F,I–L**) than control mice. This was accompanied by increased MC-CD8+ T cell interactions, both of c-Kit+ (**Figure 6G–H**) and of mMCP6+ MCs (**Figure 6O,Q**). However, the total number of mature, mMCP6+ skin MCs remained essentially unaltered between the groups (**Figure 6I–M**). These data from AA mice independently suggest that abnormal MC activities and MC-CD8+ T-cell interactions are a general feature of the AA phenotype across species.

MC-CD8+ T-cell interactions are also abnormal in experimentally induced human AA

During the course of these experiments, a novel humanized mouse model for AA research became available, in which healthy human scalp skin transplanted onto SCID mice is experimentally transformed into an AA phenotype [5,57].

Therefore, we asked whether abnormal MC-CD8+ T-cell interactions can also be seen in AA lesions in human scalp skin induced by IL-2-treated PBMCs from healthy donors that were enriched for NKG2D+/CD56+ cells.

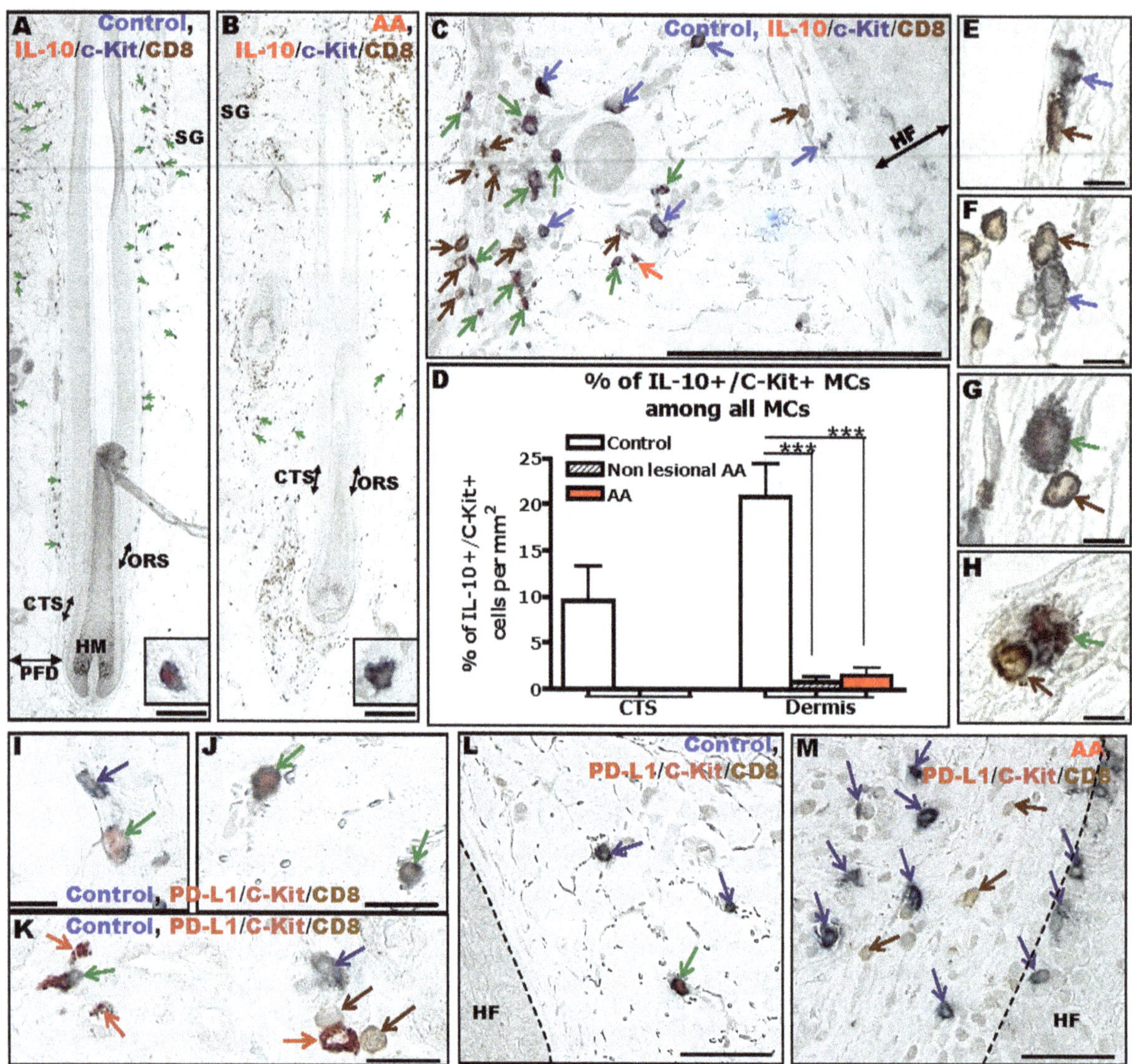

Figure 5. Immuno-inhibitory MCs and MC-CD8+ T-cell interactions appear to be down-regulated in AA. Immunohistochemical identification of c-Kit+/IL-10+ MCs and CD8+ T-cells in human scalp skin of controls (A) and AA patients (B), higher magnification of a single MCs in inserted panels. Higher magnification of IL-10/CD8/c-Kit triple IHC which shows c-Kit+ MCs (blue arrows), c-Kit+/IL-10+ MCs (green arrows), IL-10+ cells (red arrows) and CD8+ T-cells (brown arrows) (C). Quantitative analysis of IL-10+ MCs (detected by c-Kit) in AA patients compared to controls (D). Analysis derived from 20 areas of 11 HFs of 7 healthy controls and 14 areas of 5 HFs of 3 AA patients for non-lesional skin and 20 areas of 16 HFs of 7 AA patients for lesional skin, ***$p \leq 0.001$, ±SEM, Mann-Whitney-U-Test. Representative pictures of IL-10- (E,F) and IL-10+ (G,H) MCs (detected by c-Kit) interacting with CD8+ T-cells. Representative pictures showing low (I) and high (J) PD-L1 IR of human healthy skin MCs *in situ*. Immunohistochemical identification of PD-L1+/c-Kit+ MCs and CD8+ T-cells in human healthy skin (I-L) and AA patients (M). Brown arrows indicate CD8+ cells, blue arrows indicate c-Kit+ MCs, red arrows indicate PD-L1+ cells, green arrows indicate PD-L1+/c-Kit+ MCs. This staining was performed on one section/subject of 8 healthy individuals of non-lesional skin from 4 AA patients, and of lesional skin from 12 AA patients. Size bars: 200 µm (A–C), 50 µm (L,M), 20 µm (I,J) and 10 µm (E–H). Connective tissue sheath (CTS), hair follicle (HF), hair matrix (HM), outer root sheath (ORS), perifollicular dermis (PFD), sebaceous glands (SG).

Quantitative immunohistomorphometry confirmed that the experimentally induced AA lesions in transplanted human scalp skin show both more perifollicular CD8+ T-cells (**Figure 7B,E**), and more perifollicular MCs (**Figure 7B–D**) compared to human skin control transplants injected with PHA-treated PBMCs enriched for NKG2D+/CD56+ cells (**Figure 7A,C–E**). Moreover, the number of MCs in physical contact with CD8+ T-cells was higher in AA-like human skin lesions on SCID mice than in controls (**Figure 7A,B,F**). This further supports the hypothesis that abnormal MC-CD8+ T-cell interactions are functionally important for AA pathogenesis.

Discussion

The concept that MCs are involved in the pathogenesis of AA dates back several decades [12,14–16], but has still not been systematically followed-up. However, recent reports that antihistamines may be beneficial in at least some AA patients [113–115] underscore the practical clinical relevance of dissecting the contribution of MCs to AA pathogenesis. Our results essentially confirm and then significantly extend the previous literature (e.g. [12,14–16] (see Discussion S8 in File S1)) by focusing on MC

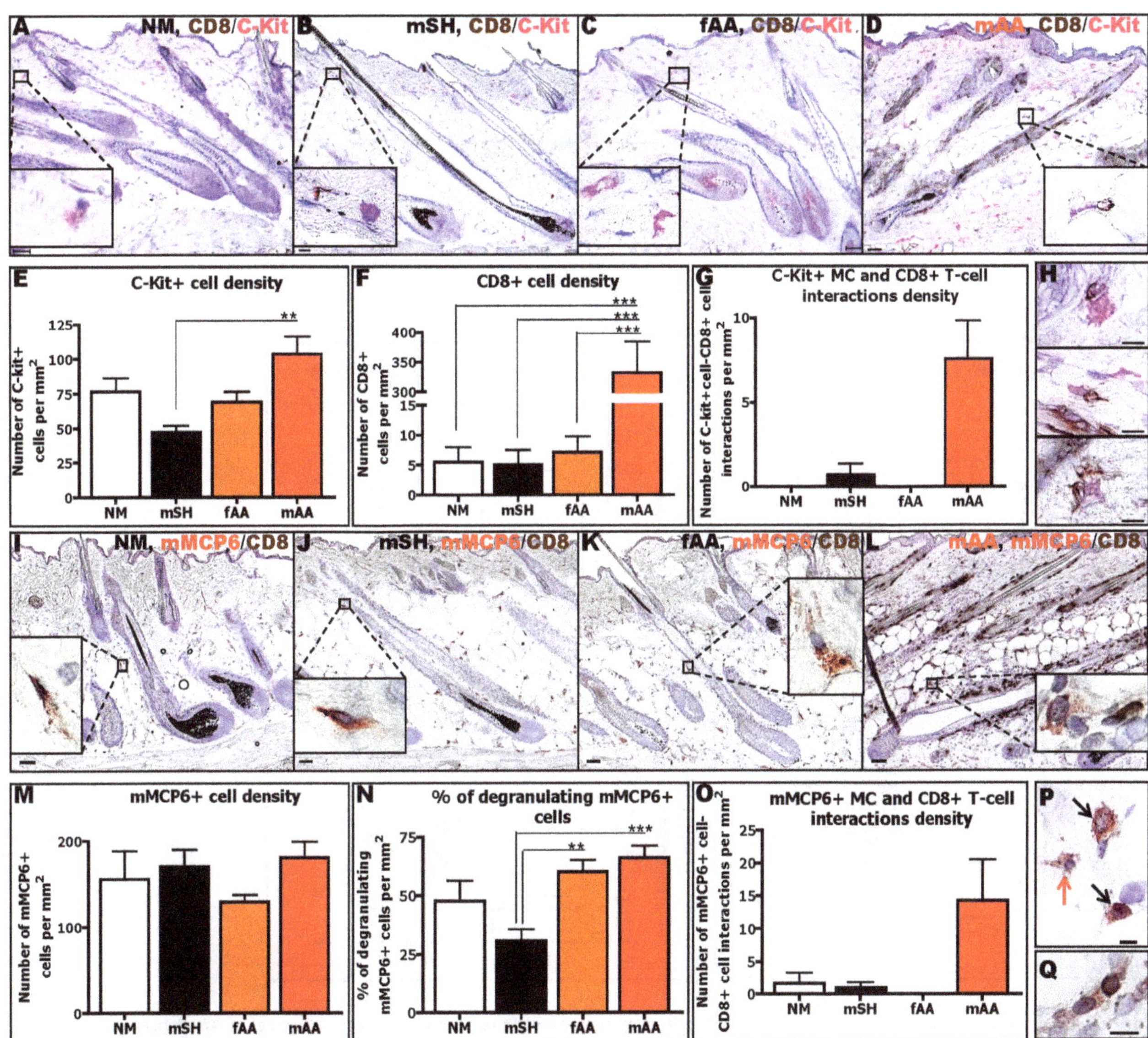

Figure 6. MC numbers, degranulation and interactions with CD8+ T-cells are increased in the C3H/HeJ-mouse-model of AA. Representative pictures of c-Kit/CD8 double-staining in normal (NM) (A), sham-grafted (mSH) (B), failed-grafted (fAA) (C) and AA (mAA) (D) mice. C-Kit+ MCs are labelled in pink while CD8+ T-cells are labelled in brown. Quantitative analysis of c-Kit+ (E), CD8+ T-cells (F) and c-Kit+ MC/CD8+ T-cell interactions (G) in mAA compared to NM, mSH and fAA control mice. Representative pictures of c-Kit+ MC-CD8+ T-cell interaction (H). Representative pictures of mMCP6/CD8 double-staining in normal (NM) (I), sham-grafted (mSH) (J), failed-grafted (fAA) (K) and AA (mAA) (L) mice. mMCP6+ MCs are labelled in red while CD8+ T-cells are labelled in brown. Quantitative analysis of mMCP6+ cells (M), % of degranulation (N) and mMCP6+ MC-CD8+ T-cell interactions (O) in mAA compared to NM, mSH, fAA control mice. Immunohistochemical identification of non-degranulating (black arrows) and degranulating (red arrow) of mMCP6+ MCs (P) and mMCP6+MC-CD8+ T-cell interaction (Q). Analysis derived from 6 HFs/mouse of 2–4 mice/group ±SEM, One-Way ANOVA or Kruskal-Wallis test followed by Bonferroni's test or Dunn's test (*p≤0.05, **p≤0.01, ***p≤0.001). Scale bars: 50 μm (A–D, M–L) and 10 μm (G,P,Q). AA mice (mAA), failed-grafted AA mice (fAA), normal mice (NM), sham-grafted mice (mSH).

interactions with CD8+ T-cells, the key immunocytes in AA pathogenesis [3–5,14,19–24].

We show that physical MC-CD8+ T-cell interactions, a fundamental prerequisite for CD8+ T-cell activation by MCs [35,77], are enhanced and abnormal in the perifollicular mesenchyme of lesional AA skin in a) AA patients, b) AA mice, and in c) healthy human skin experimentally transformed into lesional AA skin, i.e. in both spontaneous and induced AA and across two mammalian species.

Moreover, we demonstrate that MCs switch from a protective immuno-inhibitory to a pro-inflammatory phenotype (**Figure 8** and Table S2 in File S1). This may promote pathogenic CD8+ T-cell responses against HFs (Discussion S9 in File S1). We envision that this MC phenotype switch could enhance CD8+ T-cell secretion of IFNγ [35], the recognized key cytokine in AA pathogenesis [1,2,10,11]. Such a MC phenotype switch has already been reported in other autoimmune diseases [25,26,38,87]. IFNγ is expected to trigger two key events in AA pathogenesis [1,2]: the stimulation of premature HF regression (catagen) [116] and the induction of HF-IP collapse in humans and mice [11,117]. **Figure 8** summarizes the main phenotypic differences that distinguish, according to our results, MCs in

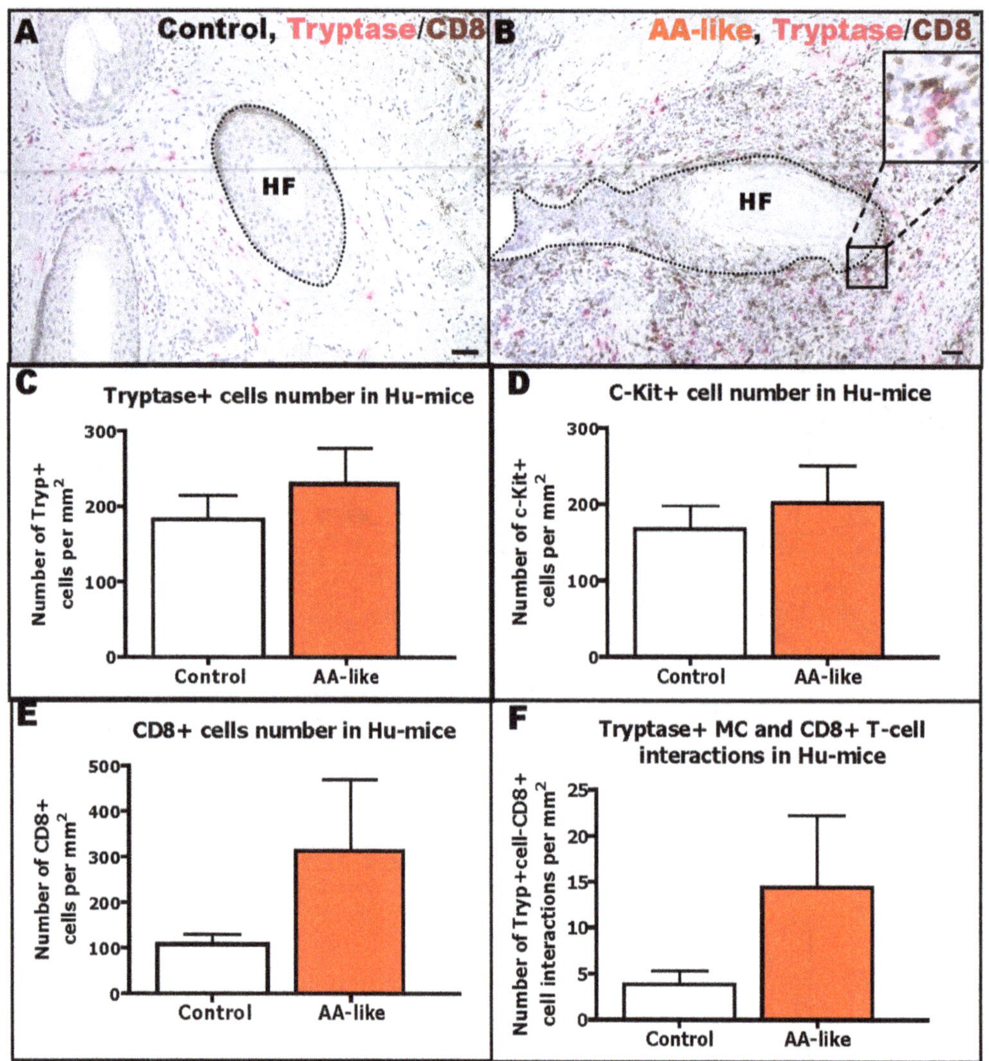

Figure 7. MC numbers and interactions with CD8+ T-cells are increased in the humanized-mouse model of AA. Representative pictures of tryptase/CD8 double-staining in control (A) and AA-like (B) mice. Tryptase+ MCs are labelled in pink while CD8+ cells are labelled in brown. Quantitative analysis of tryptase+ MCs (C), c-Kit+ MCs (D), CD8+ cells (E) and tryptase+ MC-CD8+ cell interactions (F) in AA-like mice compared to control mice. Analysis deriving from 1–6 areas (HFs)/mouse of 3 mice/group from 2 experiments, ±SEM, Student's t-test or Mann-Whitney-U-Test (ns). Scale bars: 50 μm.

healthy human skin from those in lesional AA skin, and develops a plausible hypothetical scenario how abnormal MC-CD8+ T-cell interactions may promote AA pathogenesis.

Methodologically, the major shortcoming of the current study is its exclusively observational nature, despite its rigorous quantitative approach as well as the use of triple-IHC techniques and mutually complementary AA models. Satisfactory functional experiments to definitely confirm or refute the basic hypothesis proposed here (**Figure 8**) can currently not be performed for the following reasons: 1) None of the routinely used MC-deficient or MC-overexpressing mouse models develop classic AA lesions. 2) It is not yet possible to selectively eliminate or exclusively modulate *only* MCs *in vivo* (mice) or in transplanted or organ-cultured human skin *without also* eliminating or damaging other cutaneous cell populations (e.g. c-Kit+ melanocytes and hair matrix keratinocytes, or FceR+ Langerhans cells). 3) Successful cross-breeding of mice that spontaneously develop AA-like lesions (C3H/HeJ mice) with MC-deficient mouse strains [118] has not yet been achieved by any group. 4) Frequently employed inhibitors of MC degranulation such as cromolyn or luteolyn are not effective for all MC subsets and/or are not MC-specific, as other cell populations, including CD8+ T-cells and sensory neurons and their axons, are also affected [119–122].

Therefore, the concept that abnormal MC-CD8+ T-cell interactions play a functionally important role in AA pathogenesis, remains hypothetical and the underlying mechanisms of action can only be regarded as speculative on the basis of our phenomenological evidence – until the methodological handicaps summarized above have been overcome. Since the management of AA in clinical medicine remains overall quite unsatisfactory [1,123] and in view of the psychoemotional stress this disease imposes on affected patients [124–126], it is a matter of urgency to develop more effective AA management strategies. Therefore, the phenomenological evidence presented here and the persuasive pathogenesis scenario deduced from it (**Figure 8**), are transla-

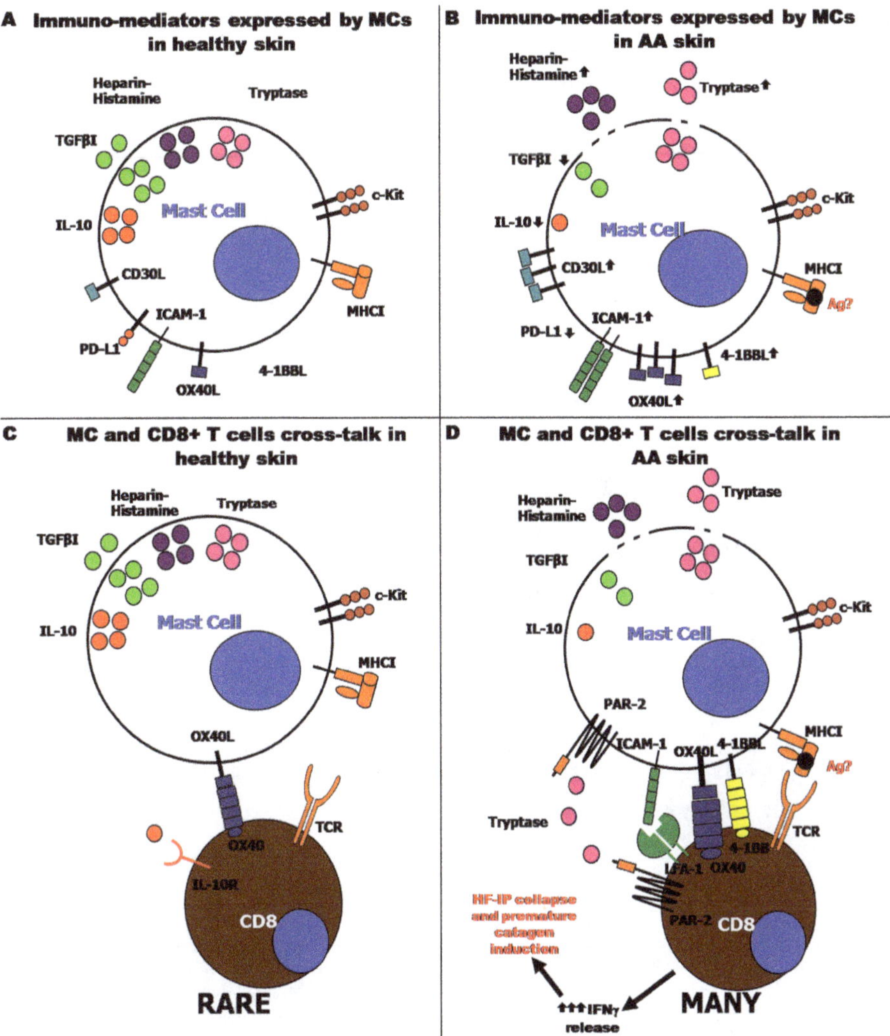

Figure 8. Schematic summary: MC immuno-phenotype and MC-CD8+ T-cell interactions in healthy compared to lesional AA skin. In human healthy skin, MCs are mostly non-degranulated and they express the SCF receptor, c-Kit, and MHCI molecules. Most of them express IL-10, TGFβ1 while only some express OX40L and PD-L1 and very few express CD30L and ICAM-1 (A). In lesional AA skin, the degranulation of MCs is increased (release of tryptase, heparin and histamine) and the expression of tryptase is increased, while the contents of TGFbeta1, IL-10 are decreased. Moreover, the numbers of OX40L+, CD30L+, 4-1BBL+ and ICAM-1+ MCs are up-regulated, while MCs positive for IL-10 and PD-L1 are down-regulated (B). In human healthy skin, rare MCs are found in close contact with CD8+ T-cells and most of them express OX40L. Therefore, we hypothesized that OX40/OX40L might mediate this interaction. Rarely, we found IL-10+ MCs interacting with CD8+ T-cells (C). In lesional AA skin, many MCs interact with CD8+ T-cells. During this cross-talk, most MCs express OX40L but instead, in some rare cases, 4-1BBL and ICAM-1 were expressed. These ligands might stimulate the activation and proliferation of CD8+ T-cells. Since MCs during the interaction are also degranulating, we hypothesize an activation of PAR-2 (tryptase receptor) on CD8+ T-cells. Finally, we suggest that MCs may operate as autoantigen-presenting cells (D). This schematic drawing was prepared using the Biomedical-PPT-Toolkit-Suite of Motifolio Inc., USA.

tionally important, since they help to identify novel candidate targets for future therapeutic intervention in AA.

Our findings predict that treatment regimens which promote an immuno-inhibitory phenotype and/or suppress the switch towards a pro-inflammatory MC phenotype, should down-regulate undesired CD8+ T-cell responses against human HFs. Our data suggest that it deserves to be tested in the two distinct AA mouse models employed here whether blocking OX40L/OX40 (e.g using oxelumab, which was first developed for the treatment of asthma [84,127]) or 4-1BB/4-1BBL interactions [96,128], or antagonizing PAR-2 [129,130] affects the development of AA lesions and/or hair regrowth. However, as these signalling molecules are broadly expressed on immunocytes, more specific therapies should be contemplated, including the use of bi-specific antibodies so as to selectively block MCs [120]. In any case, our study underscores that the therapeutic modulation of perifollicular MCs in human skin merits systematic exploration as a novel therapeutic strategy in the future management of AA.

Supporting Information

File S1 Background: S1–S2. Material and methods: S3. Result: S4–S7. Discussion: S8–S9. References. Figure S1. Positive controls for triple-immunostainings. Figure S2. MC density is significantly increased in lesional skin compared to non-lesional skin of AA patients and scalp skin from healthy subjects. The number of proliferating c-Kit+ MC is tendentially increased in AA lesional skin compared to control skin. Figure S3. The maximal increase of MC density is found in AA patients in subacute stage of the disease. Figure S4. TGFβ1 immunoreactivity is decreased in the HF ORS of AA patients. Figure S5. MHCI/CD8/Tryptase triple staining showing MHCI+ MCs in close contact with CD8+ T-cells. Table S1. Primary antibody. Table S2. Expression of pro-inflammatory and pro-inhibitory molecules and cytokines which are considered to be involved in the cross-talk between MCs and CD8+ T-cells in PFD of lesional AA skin compared to non-lesional AA and healthy skin.

Acknowledgments

We are grateful to Dr. Liat Samuelov and Dr. Akiko Arakawa for diagnostic assistance, and to Dr. Akiko Arakawa, Gerta Salamaj, Maria Paziuk, Inna Tokar, Nadine Dörwald, Heike Kraut and Gabriele Scheel for excellent technical support. We also thank Prof. Michael F. Gurish, Harvard Medical School, for kindly donating mMCP6 antibody. Our special gratitude goes to Prof. Rudi Manz, Lübeck, Germany and Prof. Roberto d'Ovidio, Bari, Italy, for excellent professional advice.

A minor part of the results presented here was used for the Master degree thesis of MB at the University of Padua, Italy, while the majority of the data shown here forms part of the PhD thesis of MB submitted to the University of Lübeck, Germany.

Author Contributions

Conceived and designed the experiments: MB RP. Performed the experiments: MB FZ PK VE EW AK. Analyzed the data: MB FZ PK VE. Wrote the paper: MB KCM RP. Provided lesional and non lesional skin form patients: AR. Provided skin samples of the humanized-mouse model: AG AK. Helped with writing the first draft of the manuscript, co-supervised an early stage of the project and edited the manuscript: KCM. Provided samples from C3H/HeJ mice: EW KM. Extensively edited the manuscript: KM. Provided skin from healthy human subjects and from a patient: WF.

References

1. Gilhar A, Etzioni A, Paus R (2012) Alopecia areata. N Engl J Med 366: 1515–1525.
2. McElwee KJ, Gilhar A, Tobin DJ, Ramot Y, Sundberg JP, et al. (2013) What causes alopecia areata?: Exp Dermatol 22: 609–626.
3. McElwee KJ, Freyschmidt-Paul P, Hoffmann R, Kissling S, Hummel S, et al. (2005) Transfer of CD8(+) cells induces localized hair loss whereas CD4(+)/CD25(−) cells promote systemic alopecia areata and CD4(+)/CD25(+) cells blockade disease onset in the C3H/HeJ mouse model. J Invest Dermatol 124:947–57.
4. McElwee KJ, Spiers EM, Oliver RF (1996) In vivo depletion of CD8+ T cells restores hair growth in the DEBR model for alopecia areata. Br J Dermatol 135: 211–217.
5. Gilhar A, Keren A, Shemer A, d'Ovidio R, Ullmann Y, et al. (2013) Autoimmune disease induction in a healthy human organ: a humanized mouse model of alopecia areata. J Invest Dermatol 133: 844–847.
6. Kang H, Wu WY, Lo BK, Yu M, Leung G, et al. (2010) Hair follicles from alopecia areata patients exhibit alterations in immune privilege-associated gene expression in advance of hair loss. J Invest Dermatol 130: 2677–2680.
7. Kinori M, Kloepper JE, Paus R (2011) Can the hair follicle become a model for studying selected aspects of human ocular immune privilege? Invest Ophthalmol Vis Sci 52: 4447–4458.
8. Meyer KC, Klatte JE, Dinh HV, Harries MJ, Reithmayer K, et al. (2008) Evidence that the bulge region is a site of relative immune privilege in human hair follicles. Br J Dermatol 159: 1077–1085.
9. Paus R, Nickoloff BJ, Ito T (2005) A 'hairy' privilege. Trends Immunol 26: 32–40.
10. Freyschmidt-Paul P, McElwee KJ, Hoffmann R, Sundberg JP, Vitacolonna M, et al. (2006) Interferon-gamma-deficient mice are resistant to the development of alopecia areata. Br J Dermatol 155: 515–521.
11. Ito T, Ito N, Bettermann A, Tokura Y, Takigawa M, et al. (2004) Collapse and restoration of MHC class-I-dependent immune privilege: exploiting the human hair follicle as a model. Am J Pathol 164: 623–634.
12. Baccaredda-Boy A, Giacometti A (1959) Clinical observations and experimental research on thyrotropin in pretibial limited myxodermia. Panminerva Med 1: 198–201.
13. Bodemer C, Peuchmaur M, Fraitaig S, Chatenoud L, Brousse N, et al. (2000) Role of cytotoxic T cells in chronic alopecia areata. J Invest Dermatol 114: 112–116.
14. Cetin ED, Savk E, Uslu M, Eskin M, Karul A (2009) Investigation of the inflammatory mechanisms in alopecia areata. Am J Dermatopathol 31: 53–60.
15. D'Ovidio R, Vena GA, Angelini G (1988) [Possible immunopathogenetic role of mastocytes in alopecia areata]. G Ital Dermatol Venereol 123: 569–570.
16. Finzi AF, Landi G (1964) [Action of the mast cell depletor 48/80 on skin temperature in alopecia areata]. Minerva Dermatol 39: 99–102.
17. Ito T, Ito N, Saatoff M, Hashizume H, Fukamizu H, et al. (2008) Maintenance of hair follicle immune privilege is linked to prevention of NK cell attack. J Invest Dermatol 128: 1196–1206.
18. Ranki A, Kianto U, Kanerva L, Tolvanen E, Johansson E (1984) Immunohistochemical and electron microscopic characterization of the cellular infiltrate in alopecia (areata, totalis, and universalis). J Invest Dermatol 83: 7–11.
19. Alli R, Nguyen P, Boyd K, Sundberg JP, Geiger TL (2012) A mouse model of clonal CD8+ T lymphocyte-mediated alopecia areata progressing to alopecia universalis. J Immunol 188: 477–486.
20. Gilhar A, Ullmann Y, Berkutzki T, Assy B, Kalish RS (1998) Autoimmune hair loss (alopecia areata) transferred by T lymphocytes to human scalp explants on SCID mice. J Clin Invest 101: 62–67.
21. Ito T, Bertolini M, Funakoshi A, Ito N, Takayama T, et al. (2013) Birth, life, and death of the MAGE3 hypothesis of alopecia areata pathobiology. J Dermatol Sci 72: 327–30.
22. Paus R, Slominski A, Czarnetzki BM (1993) Is alopecia areata an autoimmune-response against melanogenesis-related proteins, exposed by abnormal MHC class I expression in the anagen hair bulb? Yale J Biol Med 66: 541–554.
23. Petukhova L, Duvic M, Hordinsky M, Norris D, Price V, et al. (2010) Genome-wide association study in alopecia areata implicates both innate and adaptive immunity. Nature 466: 113–117.
24. Yano S, Nakamura K, Okochi H, Tamaki K (2002) Analysis of the expression of cutaneous lymphocyte-associated antigen on the peripheral blood and cutaneous lymphocytes of alopecia areata patients. Acta Derm Venereol 82: 82–85.
25. Brown MA, Hatfield JK (2012) Mast cells are important modifiers of autoimmune disease: With so much evidence, why is there still controversy? Front Immunol 3: 147.
26. Frenzel L, Hermine O (2013) Mast cells and inflammation. Joint Bone Spine 80: 141–145.
27. Frossi B, Gri G, Tripodo C, Pucillo C (2010) Exploring a regulatory role for mast cells: 'MCregs'? Trends Immunol 31: 97–102.
28. Galli SJ, Grimbaldeston M, Tsai M (2008) Immunomodulatory mast cells: negative, as well as positive, regulators of immunity. Nat Rev Immunol 8: 478–486.
29. Gri G, Frossi B, D'Inca F, Danelli L, Betto E, et al. (2012) Mast cell: an emerging partner in immune interaction. Front Immunol 3: 120.
30. Harvima IT, Nilsson G (2011) Mast cells as regulators of skin inflammation and immunity. Acta Derm Venereol 91: 644–650.
31. Sayed BA, Christy A, Quirion MR, Brown MA (2008) The master switch: the role of mast cells in autoimmunity and tolerance. Annu Rev Immunol 26: 705–739.
32. St John AL, Abraham SN (2013) Innate immunity and its regulation by mast cells. J Immunol 190: 4458–4463.
33. Tete S, Tripodi D, Rosati M, Conti F, Maccauro G, et al. (2012) Role of mast cells in innate and adaptive immunity. J Biol Regul Homeost Agents 26: 193–201.
34. Tsai M, Grimbaldeston M, Galli SJ (2011) Mast cells and immunoregulation/immunomodulation. Adv Exp Med Biol 716: 186–211.
35. Stelekati E, Bahri R, D'Orlando O, Orinska Z, Mittrucker HW, et al. (2009) Mast cell-mediated antigen presentation regulates CD8+ T cell effector functions. Immunity 31: 665–676.
36. Christy AL, Walker ME, Hessner MJ, Brown MA (2013) Mast cell activation and neutrophil recruitment promotes early and robust inflammation in the meninges in EAE. J Autoimmun 42: 50-61.
37. Gan PY, Summers SA, Ooi JD, O'Sullivan KM, Tan DS, et al. (2012) Mast cells contribute to peripheral tolerance and attenuate autoimmune vasculitis. J Am Soc Nephrol 23: 1955–1966.
38. Gilfillan AM, Beaven MA (2011) Regulation of mast cell responses in health and disease. Crit Rev Immunol 31: 475–529.
39. Walker ME, Hatfield JK, Brown MA (2012) New insights into the role of mast cells in autoimmunity: evidence for a common mechanism of action? Biochim Biophys Acta 1822: 57–65.
40. Botchkarev VA, Paus R, Czarnetzki BM, Kupriyanov VS, Gordon DS, et al. (1995) Hair cycle-dependent changes in mast cell histochemistry in murine skin. Arch Dermatol Res 287: 683–686.
41. Maurer M, Paus R, Czarnetzki BM (1995) Mast cells as modulators of hair follicle cycling. Exp Dermatol 4: 266–271.

42. Maurer M, Theoharides T, Granstein RD, Bischoff SC, Bienenstock J, et al. (2003) What is the physiological function of mast cells? Exp Dermatol 12: 886–910.
43. Paus R, Maurer M, Slominski A, Czarnetzki BM (1994) Mast cell involvement in murine hair growth. Dev Biol 163: 230–240.
44. Maurer M, Fischer E, Handjiski B, von Stebut E, Algermissen B, et al. (1997) Activated skin mast cells are involved in murine hair follicle regression (catagen). Lab Invest 77: 319–332.
45. Ito N, Sugawara K, Bodo E, Takigawa M, van Beek N, et al. (2010) Corticotropin-releasing hormone stimulates the in situ generation of mast cells from precursors in the human hair follicle mesenchyme. J Invest Dermatol 130: 995–1004.
46. Kumamoto T, Shalhevet D, Matsue H, Mummert ME, Ward BR, et al. (2003) Hair follicles serve as local reservoirs of skin mast cell precursors. Blood 102: 1654–1660.
47. Sugawara K, Biro T, Tsuruta D, Toth BI, Kromminga A, et al. (2012) Endocannabinoids limit excessive mast cell maturation and activation in human skin. J Allergy Clin Immunol 129: 726–738 e728.
48. Voehringer D (2013) Protective and pathological roles of mast cells and basophils. Nat Rev Immunol 13: 362–375.
49. Chan CY, St John AL, Abraham SN (2013) Mast cell interleukin-10 drives localized tolerance in chronic bladder infection. Immunity 38: 349–359.
50. de Vries VC, Pino-Lagos K, Elgueta R, Noelle RJ (2009) The enigmatic role of mast cells in dominant tolerance. Curr Opin Organ Transplant 14: 332–337.
51. Kalesnikoff J, Galli SJ (2011) Antiinflammatory and immunosuppressive functions of mast cells. Methods Mol Biol 677: 207–220.
52. Lu LF, Lind EF, Gondek DC, Bennett KA, Gleeson MW, et al. (2006) Mast cells are essential intermediaries in regulatory T-cell tolerance. Nature 442: 997–1002.
53. Waldmann H (2006) Immunology: protection and privilege. Nature 442: 987–988.
54. de Vries VC, Wasiuk A, Bennett KA, Benson MJ, Elgueta R, et al. (2009) Mast cell degranulation breaks peripheral tolerance. Am J Transplant 9: 2270–2280.
55. King LE Jr., McElwee KJ, Sundberg JP (2008) Alopecia areata. Curr Dir Autoimmun 10: 280–312.
56. Wang E, Chong K, Yu M, Akhoundsadegh N, Granville DJ, et al. (2013) Development of autoimmune hair loss disease alopecia areata is associated with cardiac dysfunction in C3H/HeJ mice. PLoS One 8: e62935.
57. Gilhar A, Keren A, Shemer A, Ullmann Y, Paus R (2013) Blocking potassium channels (Kv1.3): a new treatment option for alopecia areata? J Invest Dermatol 133: 2088–2091.
58. Bertolini M, Meyer KC, Slominski R, Kobayashi K, Ludwig RJ, et al. (2013) The immune system of mouse vibrissae follicles: cellular composition and indications of immune privilege. Exp Dermatol 22: 593–598.
59. Harries MJ, Meyer K, Chaudhry I, J EK, Poblet E, et al. (2013) Lichen planopilaris is characterized by immune privilege collapse of the hair follicle's epithelial stem cell niche. J Pathol 231: 236–247.
60. Ito N, Ito T, Kromminga A, Bettermann A, Takigawa M, et al. (2005) Human hair follicles display a functional equivalent of the hypothalamic-pituitary-adrenal axis and synthesize cortisol. FASEB J 19: 1332–1334.
61. Kloepper JE, Kawai K, Bertolini M, Kanekura T, Paus R (2013) Loss of gamma/delta T cells results in hair cycling defects. J Invest Dermatol 133: 1666–1669.
62. Spath U, Steigleder GK (1970) [Number of mast cells (MC) in Alopecia areata]. Z Haut Geschlechtskr 45: 435–436.
63. Algermissen B, Bauer F, Schadendorf D, Kropp JD, Czarnetzki BM (1994) Analysis of mast cell subpopulations (MCT, MCTC) in cutaneous inflammation using novel enzyme-histochemical staining techniques. Exp Dermatol 3: 290–297.
64. Buckley MG, McEuen AR, Walls AF (1999) The detection of mast cell subpopulations in formalin-fixed human tissues using a new monoclonal antibody specific for chymase. J Pathol 189: 138–143.
65. Whiting DA (2003) Histopathologic features of alopecia areata: a new look. Arch Dermatol 139: 1555–1559.
66. Aceves SS, Chen D, Newbury RO, Dohil R, Bastian JF, et al. (2010) Mast cells infiltrate the esophageal smooth muscle in patients with eosinophilic esophagitis, express TGF-beta1, and increase esophageal smooth muscle contraction. J Allergy Clin Immunol 126: 1198–1204 e1194.
67. Gordon JR, Galli SJ (1994) Promotion of mouse fibroblast collagen gene expression by mast cells stimulated via the Fc epsilon RI. Role for mast cell-derived transforming growth factor beta and tumor necrosis factor alpha. J Exp Med 180: 2027–2037.
68. Hugle T, Hogan V, White KE, van Laar JM (2011) Mast cells are a source of transforming growth factor beta in systemic sclerosis. Arthritis Rheum 63: 795–799.
69. Wahl SM, Wen J, Moutsopoulos N (2006) TGF-beta: a mobile purveyor of immune privilege. Immunol Rev 213: 213–227.
70. Hernandez-Hernandez L, Sanz C, Garcia-Solaesa V, Padron J, Garcia-Sanchez A, et al. (2012) Tryptase: genetic and functional considerations. Allergol Immunopathol (Madr) 40: 385–389.
71. Li Q, Jie Y, Wang C, Zhang Y, Guo H, et al. (2014) Tryptase compromises corneal epithelial barrier function. Cell Biochem Funct 32: 183–7.
72. Magarinos NJ, Bryant KJ, Fosang AJ, Adachi R, Stevens RL, et al. (2013) Mast cell-restricted, tetramer-forming tryptases induce aggrecanolysis in articular cartilage by activating matrix metalloproteinase-3 and -13 zymogens. J Immunol 191: 1404–1412.
73. Pejler G, Ronnberg E, Waern I, Wernersson S (2010) Mast cell proteases: multifaceted regulators of inflammatory disease. Blood 115: 4981–4990.
74. Shin K, Nigrovic PA, Crish J, Boilard E, McNeil HP, et al. (2009) Mast cells contribute to autoimmune inflammatory arthritis via their tryptase/heparin complexes. J Immunol 182: 647–656.
75. Zeng X, Zhang S, Xu L, Yang H, He S (2013) Activation of protease-activated receptor 2-mediated signaling by mast cell tryptase modulates cytokine production in primary cultured astrocytes. Mediators Inflamm 2013: 140812.
76. Kashiwakura J, Yokoi H, Saito H, Okayama Y (2004) T cell proliferation by direct cross-talk between OX40 ligand on human mast cells and OX40 on human T cells: comparison of gene expression profiles between human tonsillar and lung-cultured mast cells. J Immunol 173: 5247–5257.
77. Nakae S, Suto H, Iikura M, Kakurai M, Sedgwick JD, et al. (2006) Mast cells enhance T cell activation: importance of mast cell costimulatory molecules and secreted TNF. J Immunol 176: 2238–2248.
78. Nagai H, Oniki S, Oka M, Horikawa T, Nishigori C (2006) Induction of cellular immunity against hair follicle melanocyte causes alopecia. Arch Dermatol Res 298: 131–134.
79. Tsuboi H, Tanei R, Fujimura T, Ohta Y, Katsuoka K (1999) Characterization of infiltrating T cells in human scalp explants from alopecia areata to SCID nude mice: possible role of the disappearance of CD8+ T lymphocytes in the process of hair regrowth. J Dermatol 26: 797–802.
80. Croft M (2010) Control of immunity by the TNFR-related molecule OX40 (CD134). Annu Rev Immunol 28: 57–78.
81. Ilves T, Harvima IT (2013) OX40 ligand and OX40 are increased in atopic dermatitis lesions but do not correlate with clinical severity. J Eur Acad Dermatol Venereol 27: e197–205.
82. Ishii N, Takahashi T, Soroosh P, Sugamura K (2010) OX40-OX40 ligand interaction in T-cell-mediated immunity and immunopathology. Adv Immunol 105: 63–98.
83. Kober J, Leitner J, Klauser C, Woitek R, Majdic O, et al. (2008) The capacity of the TNF family members 4–1BBL, OX40L, CD70, GITRL, CD30L and LIGHT to costimulate human T cells. Eur J Immunol 38: 2678–2688.
84. Weinberg AD, Morris NP, Kovacsovics-Bankowski M, Urba WJ, Curti BD (2011) Science gone translational: the OX40 agonist story. Immunol Rev 244: 218–231.
85. Zhang Z, Sferra TJ, Eroglu Y (2013) T cell co-stimulatory molecules: a co-conspirator in the pathogenesis of eosinophilic esophagitis? Dig Dis Sci 58: 1497–1506.
86. Diaconu NC, Kaminska R, Naukkarinen A, Harvima RJ, Nilsson G, et al. (2007) Increase in CD30 ligand/CD153 and TNF-alpha expressing mast cells in basal cell carcinoma. Cancer Immunol Immunother 56: 1407–1415.
87. Fischer M, Harvima IT, Carvalho RF, Moller C, Naukkarinen A, et al. (2006) Mast cell CD30 ligand is upregulated in cutaneous inflammation and mediates degranulation-independent chemokine secretion. J Clin Invest 116: 2748–2756.
88. Molin D, Fischer M, Xiang Z, Larsson U, Harvima I, et al. (2001) Mast cells express functional CD30 ligand and are the predominant CD30L-positive cells in Hodgkin's disease. Br J Haematol 114: 616–623.
89. Cabrera CM, Urra JM, Carreno A, Zamorano J (2013) Differential expression of CD30 on CD3 T lymphocytes in patients with systemic lupus erythematosus. Scand J Immunol 78: 306–312.
90. Gruss HJ, Pinto A, Gloghini A, Wehnes E, Wright B, et al. (1996) CD30 ligand expression in nonmalignant and Hodgkin's disease-involved lymphoid tissues. Am J Pathol 149: 469–481.
91. Horie R, Watanabe T (1998) CD30: expression and function in health and disease. Semin Immunol 10: 457–470.
92. Sayama K, Diehn M, Matsuda K, Lunderius C, Tsai M, et al. (2002) Transcriptional response of human mast cells stimulated via the Fc(epsilon)RI and identification of mast cells as a source of IL-11. BMC Immunol 3: 5.
93. Chacon JA, Wu RC, Sukhumalchandra P, Molldrem JJ, Sarnaik A, et al. (2013) Co-stimulation through 4–1BB/CD137 improves the expansion and function of CD8(+) melanoma tumor-infiltrating lymphocytes for adoptive T-cell therapy. PLoS One 8: e60031.
94. Shao Z, Schwarz H (2011) CD137 ligand, a member of the tumor necrosis factor family, regulates immune responses via reverse signal transduction. J Leukoc Biol 89: 21–29.
95. Vinay DS, Kwon BS (2012) Immunotherapy of cancer with 4-1BB. Mol Cancer Ther 11: 1062–1070.
96. Wang C, Lin GH, McPherson AJ, Watts TH (2009) Immune regulation by 4–1BB and 4–1BBL: complexities and challenges. Immunol Rev 229: 192–215.
97. Watts TH (2005) TNF/TNFR family members in costimulation of T cell responses. Annu Rev Immunol 23: 23–68.
98. Wu C, Guo H, Wang Y, Gao Y, Zhu Z, et al. (2011) Extracellular domain of human 4–1BBL enhanced the function of cytotoxic T-lymphocyte induced by dendritic cell. Cell Immunol 271: 118–123.
99. Galli SJ, Nakae S, Tsai M (2005) Mast cells in the development of adaptive immune responses. Nat Immunol 6: 135–142.
100. Skokos D, Le Panse S, Villa I, Rousselle JC, Peronet R, et al. (2001) Mast cell-dependent B and T lymphocyte activation is mediated by the secretion of immunologically active exosomes. J Immunol 166: 868–876.

101. Chacon-Salinas R, Limon-Flores AY, Chavez-Blanco AD, Gonzalez-Estrada A, Ullrich SE (2011) Mast cell-derived IL-10 suppresses germinal center formation by affecting T follicular helper cell function. J Immunol 186: 25–31.
102. Groux H, Bigler M, de Vries JE, Roncarolo MG (1998) Inhibitory and stimulatory effects of IL-10 on human CD8+ T cells. J Immunol 160: 3188–3193.
103. Mosser DM, Zhang X (2008) Interleukin-10: new perspectives on an old cytokine. Immunol Rev 226: 205–218.
104. Soyer OU, Akdis M, Ring J, Behrendt H, Crameri R, et al. (2013) Mechanisms of peripheral tolerance to allergens. Allergy 68: 161–170.
105. Wang X, Marr AK, Breitkopf T, Leung G, Hao J, et al. (2014) Hair follicle mesenchyme-associated PD-L1 regulates T-Cell activation induced apoptosis: A potential mechanism of immune privilege. J Invest Dermatol. 134: 736–45.
106. Keir ME, Butte MJ, Freeman GJ, Sharpe AH (2008) PD-1 and its ligands in tolerance and immunity. Annu Rev Immunol 26: 677–704.
107. Podojil JR, Miller SD (2013) Targeting the B7 family of co-stimulatory molecules: successes and challenges. BioDrugs 27: 1–13.
108. Saresella M, Rainone V, Al-Daghri NM, Clerici M, Trabattoni D (2012) The PD-1/PD-L1 pathway in human pathology. Curr Mol Med 12: 259–267.
109. Wu YL, Liang J, Zhang W, Tanaka Y, Sugiyama H (2012) Immunotherapies: the blockade of inhibitory signals. Int J Biol Sci 8: 1420–1430.
110. Rosenblum MD, Yancey KB, Olasz EB, Truitt RL (2006) CD200, a "no danger" signal for hair follicles. J Dermatol Sci 41: 165–174.
111. Rygiel TP, Meyaard L (2012) CD200R signaling in tumor tolerance and inflammation: A tricky balance. Curr Opin Immunol 24: 233–238.
112. Cherwinski HM, Murphy CA, Joyce BL, Bigler ME, Song YS, et al. (2005) The CD200 receptor is a novel and potent regulator of murine and human mast cell function. J Immunol 174: 1348–1356.
113. Inui S, Nakajima T, Itami S (2007) Two cases of alopecia areata responsive to fexofenadine. J Dermatol 34: 852–854.
114. Ito T, Fujiyama T, Hashizume H, Tokura Y (2013) Antihistaminic drug olopatadine downmodulates T cell chemotaxis toward CXCL10 by reducing CXCR3 expression, F-actin polymerization and calcium influx in patients with alopecia areata. J Dermatol Sci 72: 68–71.
115. Ohyama M, Shimizu A, Tanaka K, Amagai M (2010) Experimental evaluation of ebastine, a second-generation anti-histamine, as a supportive medication for alopecia areata. J Dermatol Sci 58: 154–157.
116. Ito T, Ito N, Saathoff M, Bettermann A, Takigawa M, et al. (2005) Interferon-gamma is a potent inducer of catagen-like changes in cultured human anagen hair follicles. Br J Dermatol 152: 623–631.
117. Ruckert R, Hofmann U, van der Veen C, Bulfone-Paus S, Paus R (1998) MHC class I expression in murine skin: developmentally controlled and strikingly restricted intraepithelial expression during hair follicle morphogenesis and cycling, and response to cytokine treatment in vivo. J Invest Dermatol 111: 25–30.
118. Reber LL, Marichal T, Galli SJ (2012) New models for analyzing mast cell functions in vivo. Trends Immunol 33: 613–625.
119. Finn DF, Walsh JJ (2013) Twenty-first century mast cell stabilizers. Br J Pharmacol 170: 23–37.
120. Karra L, Berent-Maoz B, Ben-Zimra M, Levi-Schaffer F (2009) Are we ready to downregulate mast cells? Curr Opin Immunol 21: 708–714.
121. Theoharides TC, Kempuraj D, Iliopoulou BP (2007) Mast cells, T cells, and inhibition by luteolin: implications for the pathogenesis and treatment of multiple sclerosis. Adv Exp Med Biol 601: 423–430.
122. Vieira Dos Santos R, Magerl M, Martus P, Zuberbier T, Church MK, et al. (2010) Topical sodium cromoglicate relieves allergen- and histamine-induced dermal pruritus. Br J Dermatol 162: 674–676.
123. Harries MJ, Sun J, Paus R, King LE Jr. (2010) Management of alopecia areata. BMJ 341: c3671.
124. Gupta MA, Gupta AK, Watteel GN (1997) Stress and alopecia areata: a psychodermatologic study. Acta Derm Venereol 77: 296–298.
125. Matzer F, Egger JW, Kopera D (2011) Psychosocial stress and coping in alopecia areata: a questionnaire survey and qualitative study among 45 patients. Acta Derm Venereol 91: 318–327.
126. Paus R, Arck P (2009) Neuroendocrine perspectives in alopecia areata: does stress play a role? J Invest Dermatol 129: 1324–1326.
127. Catley MC, Coote J, Bari M, Tomlinson KL (2011) Monoclonal antibodies for the treatment of asthma. Pharmacol Ther 132: 333–351.
128. Gizinski AM, Fox DA, Sarkar S (2010) Pharmacotherapy: concepts of pathogenesis and emerging treatments. Co-stimulation and T cells as therapeutic targets. Best Pract Res Clin Rheumatol 24: 463–477.
129. Crilly A, Burns E, Nickdel MB, Lockhart JC, Perry ME, et al. (2012) PAR(2) expression in peripheral blood monocytes of patients with rheumatoid arthritis. Ann Rheum Dis 71: 1049–1054.
130. Michael ES, Kuliopulos A, Covic L, Steer ML, Perides G (2013) Pharmacological inhibition of PAR2 with the pepducin P2pal-18S protects mice against acute experimental biliary pancreatitis. Am J Physiol Gastrointest Liver Physiol 304: G516–526.

2

Insights from Computational Modeling in Inflammation and Acute Rejection in Limb Transplantation

Dolores Wolfram[1]*, Ravi Starzl[2], Hubert Hackl[3], Derek Barclay[4], Theresa Hautz[5], Bettina Zelger[6], Gerald Brandacher[7], W. P. Andrew Lee[7], Nadine Eberhart[1], Yoram Vodovotz[4], Johann Pratschke[5], Gerhard Pierer[1], Stefan Schneeberger[5,7]

1 Department of Plastic, Reconstructive and Aesthetic Surgery, Innsbruck Medical University, Innsbruck, Austria, **2** Language Technologies Institute, Carnegie Mellon University, Pittsburgh, Pennsylvania, United States of America, **3** Division of Bioinformatics, Biocenter, Innsbruck Medical University, Innsbruck, Austria, **4** Department of Immunology, University of Pittsburgh, Pittsburgh, Pennsylvania, United States of America, **5** Department of Visceral, Transplant and Thoracic Surgery, Innsbruck Medical University, Innsbruck, Austria, **6** Department of Pathology, Innsbruck Medical University, Innsbruck, Austria, **7** Department of Plastic and Reconstructive Surgery, Johns Hopkins University School of Medicine, Baltimore, Maryland, United States of America

Abstract

Acute skin rejection in vascularized composite allotransplantation (VCA) is the major obstacle for wider adoption in clinical practice. This study utilized computational modeling to identify biomarkers for diagnosis and targets for treatment of skin rejection. Protein levels of 14 inflammatory mediators in skin and muscle biopsies from syngeneic grafts [n = 10], allogeneic transplants without immunosuppression [n = 10] and allografts treated with tacrolimus [n = 10] were assessed by multiplexed analysis technology. Hierarchical Clustering Analysis, Principal Component Analysis, Random Forest Classification and Multinomial Logistic Regression models were used to segregate experimental groups. Based on Random Forest Classification, Multinomial Logistic Regression and Hierarchical Clustering Analysis models, IL-4, TNF-α and IL-12p70 were the best predictors of skin rejection and identified rejection well in advance of histopathological alterations. TNF-α and IL-12p70 were the best predictors of muscle rejection and also preceded histopathological alterations. Principal Component Analysis identified IL-1α, IL-18, IL-1β, and IL-4 as principal drivers of transplant rejection. Thus, inflammatory patterns associated with rejection are specific for the individual tissue and may be superior for early detection and targeted treatment of rejection.

Editor: Valquiria Bueno, UNIFESP Federal University of São Paulo, Brazil

Funding: Funding for this work was provided by the Armed Forces Institute for Advanced Regenerative Medicine Program (TATRC, DOD) Program, Department of Defense grant WX81XWH-07-1-0415, the Austrian Research Fund (Erwin Schrödinger Stipendium), the Austrian Society of Plastic and Reconstructive Surgery and the and the Pennsylvania Department of Health Commonwealth Universal Research Enhancement (CURE) program. The funders had no role in study design, data collection and analysis, decision to publish, or preparation of the manuscript.

Competing Interests: The authors have declared that no competing interests exist.

* E-mail: dolores.wolfram@i-med.ac.at

Introduction

Rejection in Vascular Composite Allotransplantation (VCA) is characterized by an inflammatory cell-mediated cytotoxic process, which progressively harms the epidermis and the junction between dermis and epidermis, unless reversed or prevented by immunosuppression. Understanding the immune signaling patterns of skin rejection would enable the development of targeted and local therapy with fewer side effects.

The current gold standard for the diagnosis of rejection is histological evaluation of tissue biopsies according to the BANFF 2007 working classification [1]. Assessing rejection by histology suffers from latency between initiation of tissue damage and diagnosis. Often, histological signs of skin rejection have been found in protocol biopsies despite absence of clinical signs of rejection. As stated previously by our group and others, the histopathological alterations associated with rejection are not specific, but rather similar to several common inflammatory dermatoses [2,3] or the result of an inflammatory trigger [4]. The differential diagnosis between skin rejection, infection and unspecific inflammation can be challenging in hand- and especially face transplantation. The conditions are similar in their appearance and may interfere with or trigger each other [5].

Traditional methods are of limited value for elucidation of how the immune/inflammatory response in the skin affects VCA through intricate signaling patterns and context-dependent behaviors. Advanced computational methods such as language technologies and machine learning offer significant advances in deciphering complex processes from other areas of science [6,7].

We hypothesized that mechanisms of rejection in VCA are tissue specific and can be detected in advance of gross histological damage by assessing leukocyte expression patterns with advanced computational tools. Based on our findings, promising diagnostic markers for skin and muscle rejection as well as possible targets for new therapeutic interventions in VCA have been identified.

Methods

Experimental design

All animal procedures, care, and housing were reviewed and approved by the Institutional Animal Care and Use Committee

(IACUC) of the University of Pittsburgh (protocol number: 0808858B-2), and followed the National Institutes of Health guidelines for the care and use of laboratory animals. A summary of the cohorts and the conditions they represent are presented in Table 1. Limb transplantations including skin, muscle, bone and vessels, were performed as per a standardized technique between eight- to ten-week-old male Brown-Norway (BN) and Lewis rats (LEW) weighing 200–250 g with (group 3) or without (group 1) immunosuppression and compared with untreated isografts (group 2) [8]. Animals were anesthetized with a combination of xylazine (Xylasol, 5 mg/kg) and ketamine (Ketavet, 100 mg/kg), injected intramuscularly.

Assessment of rejection

Animals were inspected daily for signs of rejection. Skin rejection was classified per appearance: Grade 0 – no signs of rejection; Grade I – erythema of the transplanted leg, Grade II – erythema and edema, Grade III – epidermolysis of the transplanted skin, Grade IV – mummification of the leg (limb necrosis). In untreated animals (allografts, ATC), rejection occurs after 3-4 days (Grade I rejection) and progresses to Grade IV rejection between day 9 and 11. Samples from allograft skin and muscle were collected at postoperative days (POD) 3, 5, 7, 9 and 11 in all three groups in a staggered fashion. To out rule an impact of the trauma an the readout of subsequent tissue samples, biopsies were taken from sites distant to another on days 3, 5, 7 and 11, or days 5, 9 and 11 (see Table 2). Since all animals showed mummification of the graft on POD 11 with super infection in some, samples from this time point were excluded from the study.

The size of each tissue biopsy per chosen time point was approximately 25×10 mm. This tissue sample was divided into 3 identical parts for further analyses. One biopsy part (piece) was fixed in 10% buffered formalin and processed routinely for hematoxilyn and eosin (H&E) staining. Sections were evaluated for lymphocytic infiltration, dermal/epidermal interphase reaction, dermal-epidermal separation and necrosis by a pathologist in a blinded fashion. The other biopsy parts were preserved in RNALater for protein analysis and RNA isolation.

Protein isolation and protein expression analysis

Proteins from skin and muscle samples were isolated using a disperser (T10, basic ULTRA-TURRAX, IKA, Germany) with 1 ml 1 x Cell Lysis Buffer (Cell Signaling, Danvers, USA) per sample on ice. Proteins were quantified after homogenizing using the BCA Protein Assay Kit according to the manufacturer's protocol.

Inflammatory mediator expression at the protein levels was measured using the Luminex inflammatory mediator bead set (RCYTO-80K-PMX-14-plex Milliplex Map Kit from Millipore, Billerica, MA) that included interferon (IFN)-γ, IL-1α, IL-1β, IL-2, IL-4, IL-5, IL-6, IL-10, IL-12p70, IL-18, monocyte chemotactic protein (MCP-1), GRO/KC, TNF-α, and granulocyte-macrophage colony stimulating factor (GM-CSF) in a Luminex 100 IS (Luminex Corporation, USA) and analyzed by xPonent 3.1 Rev.2 Software (Luminex Corporation, USA). Results for each of the 14 analytes were read in pg/ml and subsequently normalized to total mass of sample protein (pg inflammatory mediator/mg protein) by multiplying with 0.025 ml standard sample volume and dividing with 0.1 mg added total protein for each sample. Any analytes indicating a concentration above 20,000 pg/μl were excluded from analysis (NA) as being outside the linear range of the Luminex assay.

Table 1. Study groups and design.

Group (Name)	Animals per group	Donor	Recipient	Treatment	Samples per time point (POD 3,5,7,9)	Samples per animal	Tissue
1 (ATC)	10	BN	LEW	none	5	3	Skin & Muscle
2 (ISO)	10	LEW	LEW	none	5	3	Skin & Muscle
3 (TAC)	10	BN	LEW	Tacrolimus*	5	3	Skin & Muscle

* 1 mg/kg/day (for 11 days).

Table 2. Appearance (Grading for skin rejection: I–IV) of each allograft on POD 1–11.

Animals ID	POD (Postoperative Day)										
	1	2	3	4	5	6	7	8	9	10	11
ATC 1	0	0	0	I	**I**	II	II	III	**III**	IV	**IV**
ATC 2	0	0	0	I	**II**	II	III	III	**IV**	IV	**IV**
ATC 3	0	0	**0**	0	**I**	II	**III**	III	IV	IV	**IV**
ATC 4	0	0	**0**	0	**I**	II	**II**	III	IV	IV	**IV**
ATC 5*	0	0	**0**								
ATC 6	0	0	**0**	0	I	II	**II**	III	**III**	IV	**IV**
ATC 7	0	0	**0**	I	II	II	**III**	III	**IV**	IV	**IV**
ATC 8	0	0	0	I	**II**	II	**II**	III	IV	IV	**IV**
ATC 9	0	0	0	I	**II**	II	II	III	**IV**	IV	IV
ATC 10	0	0	**0**	I	I	II	**II**	III	III	IV	IV
ATC 11	0	0	0	I	**II**	II	II	III	**III**	IV	**IV**

*This animal died on POD 3 during the anesthesia. Bold numbers mark biopsy timepoints (skin and muscle) for each animal.

Statistical and computational analysis

Analyses were performed with the statistical framework R 2.13.1 using packages including *stats, nnet, multtest, MASS, beeswarm, randomForest.* The non-parametric Kruskal-Wallis test was used to compare mediator abundance among groups 1-3 (ATC, ISO, TAC) at POD 3/POD 5. The Wilcoxon rank-sum test was used to identify the tissue levels of those mediators whose levels varied significantly between animals exhibiting rejection (ATC) and animals treated with tacrolimus to prevent rejection (TAC) in the early postoperative phase (POD 3/POD 5), as well for selected inflammatory mediators at POD 3. All p-values were adjusted for multiple hypothesis testing based on the false discovery rate (FDR) [9].

The multivariate extension of the one-way analysis of variance (MANOVA) or the discriminant function analysis (based on the same formulation as MANOVA with inflammatory mediators as independent variables and the rejection group as dependent variable in the latter case) are used to determine the coefficients of the two orthogonal discriminant vectors (DV), which enable maximal separation of the groups. As a measure of contribution to these vectors for each mediator, the sum of the absolute values of the respective coefficients (loadings) were used and related to the overall sum. Pillai's trace statistic was used to test for the differences in the vectors of means. The mediators showing significant differences among the 3 groups and with >2.5% contribution to the DVs in both skin and muscle were subjected to multinomial (logistic) regression analyses. A model for skin and one model for muscle were selected based on minimal Akaike information criterion [AIC]. Classifier performance was assessed using a 8-fold cross validation procedure and visualized using confusion tables. Accuracy was defined as 1- misclassification rate and Welch's test was used to test the differences between the mean of the number of true predicted and the mean of the sum of the respective number of false predicted.

To assess similarity of inflammatory mediator levels among different time points and tissue types, complete-linkage hierarchical clustering was performed and visualized as heat map using Genesis [10] based on mean-centered log2-transformed profiles. For this analysis, the mean value for each group and mediator was used.

A Random Forest (RF) [11] approach was used for classification of the rejection group (ATC, ISO, TAC) including all time points. This method was also used to identify those mediators most important for classification or diagnosis. Classifier performances were assessed by confusion tables and the out-of-bag (OOB) error rate. Principal Component Analysis (PCA) was used to rank most variable (important) mediators and potential therapeutic target candidates [12]. PCA reduces a multidimensional dataset to a few principal components, which account for the most variability in the dataset. The underlying hypothesis is that a mediator which changes during a process is important to that process [12,13]. In this analysis, the data were combined from skin and muscle, mean centered, and variance scaled. Components sufficient to capture at least 70% of total data variance observed were included.

Results

Progression of rejection

Appearance. On postoperative day (POD) 3, none of the allografts (n = 10) showed signs of rejection, on POD 5, 50% of the allografts displayed Grade I rejection and 5 animals (50%) II rejection. On postoperative day 7, rejection Grade II was present in 7 animals (70%) and rejection Grade III in 3 animals (30%). On day 9, 4 animals displayed Grade III rejection and 6 animals

Grade IV. None of the syngeneic controls or tacrolimus treated animals showed any signs of skin rejection/inflammation (Table 2).

Histological evaluation of skin biopsies. Histological evaluation of allograft skin biopsies on day 3 showed no or minimal inflammatory infiltrates (Grade 0) in six animals and a mild perivascular infiltrate (Grade I) in one biopsy. No tacrolimus-treated animals showed any signs of rejection while a mild perivascular infiltration was seen in one of the syngeneic control animal. On POD 5, biopsies from allogeneic transplants displayed Grade I rejection in three animals, as well as a moderate to severe perivascular inflammation with or without mild epidermal and/or adnexal epidermal dyskeratosis or apoptosis (Grade II) in three animals. One biopsy taken from the allogeneic group showed a severe skin rejection (Grade III), with dense inflammation and epidermal involvement with epithelial apoptosis, dyskeratosis and keratinolysis on POD 5. No inflammatory response was observed in isografts on POD 5, but two out of five biopsies in the tacrolimus treated animals did show an inflammatory infiltrate. On POD 7, allogeneic animals showed Grade III rejection and, one skin biopsy taken from the isograft group and one from the tacrolimus group displayed a moderate inflammation corresponding with Grade I/II rejection. At the endpoint, all samples from allografts showed rejection Grade III and one biopsy (n = 5) taken from the isografts displayed the characteristics of Grade I rejection. Two out of five biopsies in the tacrolimus group showed a mild rejection (Grade I) and one biopsy was classified as Grade II rejection (Table 3 and Figure 1).

Histological evaluation of muscle biopsies. H&E stains from allograft muscle samples showed no or rare inflammatory cells on POD 3 in four biopsies and Grade I rejection in two biopsies. Muscle biopsies from syngeneic controls showed a mild infiltration in two biopsies, severe inflammation similar to rejection Grade II in one graft, and no inflammatory response at this time point in two animals. On POD 5, two biopsies from the allogeneic transplants were classified as Grade 0 rejection, three samples as Grade I and one muscle biopsy as Grade II rejection, four biopsies from the isografts showed no or rare inflammation and only one sample a mild inflammation.

On POD 7, all biopsies (n = 5) from allografts displayed Grade I rejection and only one biopsy from an isografts showed a mild muscle inflammation on both day 7 and 9. Allograft muscle biopsies on day 9 showed rejection Grade I (n = 1, Grade II (n = 2) or Grade III (n = 2). Tacrolimus treated animals did not show any signs of rejection except for one animal displaying mild inflammation in the muscle on POD 9 (Table 4 and Figure 1).

Significant differences of inflammatory mediator levels at early postoperative time points among the different transplant models

We examined the levels of 14 inflammatory analytes in skin and muscle biopsies of allogeneic, syngeneic and immunosuppressed hind limb transplants at different postoperative days (POD 3, 5, 7, and 9) with a focus on the early postoperative phase where no histological alterations were observed (POD 3 and 5, Figure 2 and Figure S2). Non-parametric univariate analysis of the inflammatory mediators from skin and muscle were performed. Five inflammatory mediators (GM-CSF, IL1-α, IL-4, IL-12p70, IL-5, TNF-α) were significantly different at least in one group (adjusted $p<0.05$; Kruskal-Wallis test [KW]) in both skin and muscle. IL-12p70 and TNF-α were highly significantly different in the allograft versus the tacrolimus-treated animals (adjusted $p<0.005$; Wilcoxon-rank sum test [WR]; Table 5).

In Figure 2, the levels of the concentrations of these inflammatory mediators at POD 3 of all three groups within skin

Table 3. Histological evaluation of skin biopsies from postoperative (POD) 3 to 9.

SKIN	POD 3				POD 5				POD 7				POD 9			
GRADE	0	I	II	III	0	I	II	III	0	I	II	III	0	I	II	III
ATC	6	1				3	3	1				6				5
ISO	3	1			4				4		1		4	1		
TAC	5				3	2			4	1			2	2	1	

Number of biopsies taken on each postoperative day (POD 3,5,7,9) in skin according to their histological grading (Grad 0-III) based on H&E staining.

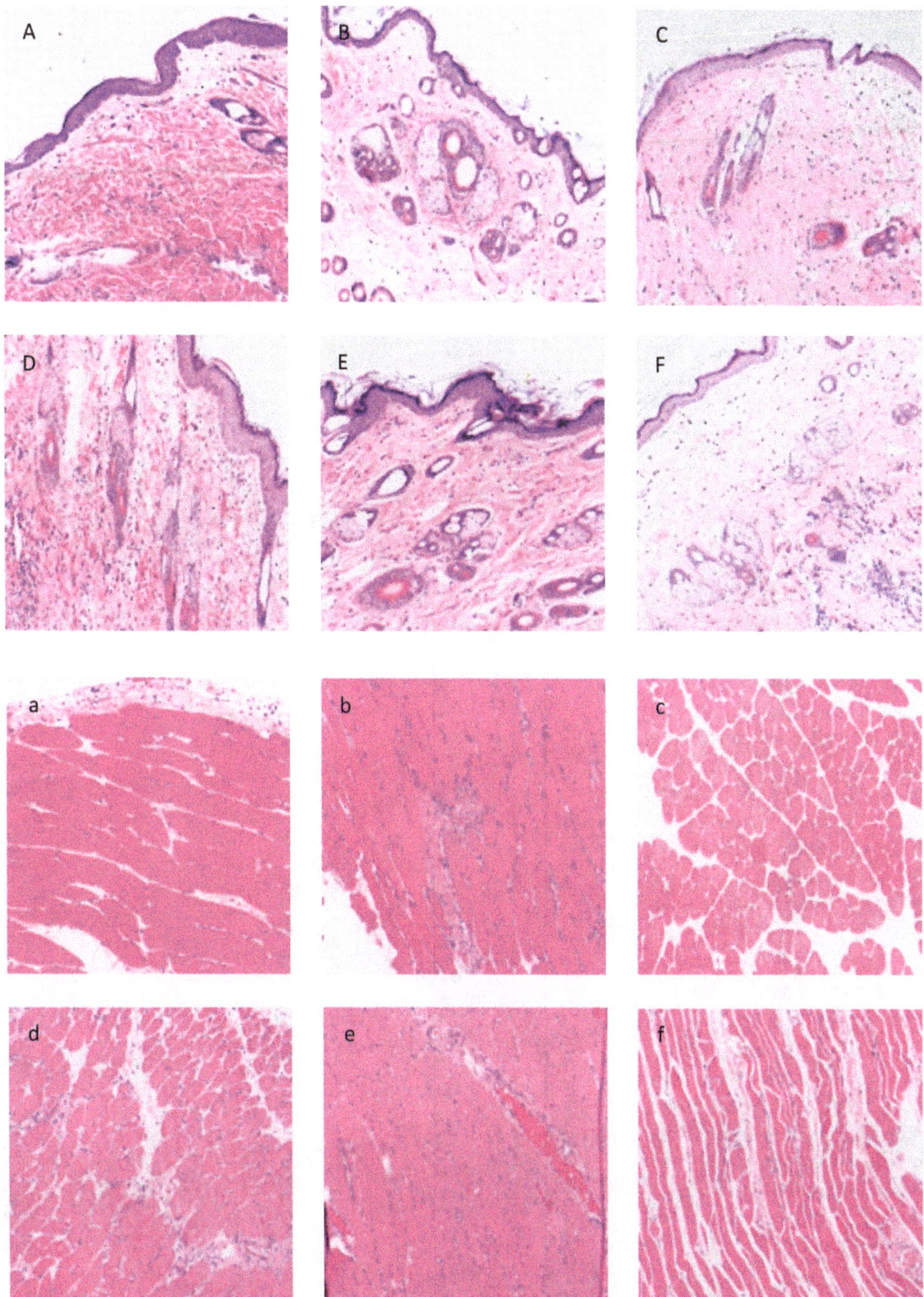

Figure 1. Histological evaluation of skin and muscle rejection in the early postoperative phase (POD 3 and 5). (A–C) Skin sample taken on POD 3 from an allograft without immunosuppression (A), from an isograft (B) and an allograft under TAC (C) showing no/rare inflammatory response (Grade 0 rejection). (D–F) Skin biopsies taken on POD 5 from a rejecting animal (D) displaying Grade 1 rejection, from an isograft (E) showing no/rare inflammatory response and a TAC treated allograft (F) characterized by a mild inflammatory response (Grade 0-I) in the deep dermis. (a–c) Muscle sample taken on POD 3 from an allograft without immunosuppression (a), from an isograft (b) and an allograft under TAC (c) showing no/rare inflammatory response (Grade 0 rejection). (d–f) Skin biopsies taken on POD 5 from a rejecting animal (d) displaying a mild inflammatory response (Grad 0-I rejection), from an isograft (E) and a TAC treated allograft (f) showing no/rare inflammatory response.

and muscle are depicted. Significantly higher concentrations of IL-12p70 in the skin from the allograft animals compared to the tacrolimus-treated animals (adjusted $p = 0.026$) as well as lower abundance of TNF-α in the allogeneic compared to the immunosuppressed transplants (adjusted $p = 0.026$) were detected. In muscle, numerical differences did not reach statistical significance (adjusted $p = 0.056$ in both cases).

For identification of inflammatory mediators with the highest predicting value, at early time points, multivariate analyses were performed. We fitted multivariate analysis of variance (MANOVA) models which resulted in $p = 8.9 \times 10^{-10}$ for skin and $p = 3.4 \times 10^{-5}$ for muscle from Pillai's trace statistic. Using these models, a functional discriminant analysis was performed. Mediators with the greatest absolute coefficients in the two resulting discriminant vectors might contribute most to the separation of groups (Table 5). The partition to the discrimination vectors for GM-CSF, IL-4, IL-12p70, IL-5, and TNF-α were > 2.5% in both tissues. We selected these inflammatory mediators as promising biomarkers candidates for further analyses.

Inflammatory mediators at early time points discern the procedure to which animals were subjected

A major goal of this study was to determine markers for early and accurate diagnosis of skin rejection in advance of major histological alterations. We applied several multivariate multinomial logistic regression models in skin and muscle samples for the classification of the three study groups at early postoperative time points (POD 3 and POD 5) using a combination of the selected inflammatory mediators (GM-CSF, IL-4, IL-12p70, IL-5, and TNF-α) as independent variables and study group as outcome. Based on the Akaike information criterion (AIC), which is a measure of the trade-off between the complexity of the model, i.e. number of variables, and the goodness of fit, optimal models for differentiation of the study groups could be found in skin rejection (based on IL-4, IL-12p70, and TNF-α: AIC = 16.0; residual deviance = 1.7×10^{-4}) and in muscle (based on IL-12p70 and TNF-α: AIC = 12.0; residual variance = 1.6×10^{-4}). The coefficients of the inflammatory mediators in the logistic regression models and classifier performance as assessed by 8-fold cross validation are detailed in Table 5. The prediction accuracy within skin was 87.1% and in muscle 100%, as derived from classification tables. A pairwise multivariate logistic regression analysis between the study groups (ATC vs. TAC, TAC vs. ISO, ISO vs. ATC) and applying a leave-one-out cross validation strategy resulted in an area under curve (AUC) from receiver operating characteristics (ROC) for skin of 0.5, 0.69, and 0.86 and for muscle of 1.0, 1.0, and 1.0, indicating a substantially better discrimination than by chance (AUC = 0.5) (Table 6).

Inflammatory mediator profiles are similar within each group

Hierarchical clustering was performed for all inflammatory mediators in the three experimental groups. Each row of the data matrix corresponds with one of the 14 inflammatory mediators, and each column corresponds with a group. The $\log_2$-transformed and mean-centered values (mean concentrations from each condition) are visualized as a heat map, with color codes shown in the color bar (Figure 3). The dendrogram on the x-axis shows the similarities among the samples. As expected, the rejection group (ATC skin and muscle samples), especially samples from later time points with pronounced histological changes, exhibit a completely different mediator clustering pattern vs. the control groups, with high abundance of IL-5, IL-18, IL-1β, MCP-1, IL-6, GRO-KC, and TNF-α. In TAC-treated animals, only IL-1α and TNF-α were highly abundant, whereas the expression of all other mediators assessed appeared suppressed.

The separation of the tacrolimus-treated group was also evident from the cluster analysis. Within sample cluster A (17 samples), 5.9% were from the tacrolimus and 94.1% were from study group ISO/ATC. In contrast, in cluster B (7 samples), 100% were from tacrolimus and 0% from the ISO/ATC groups. A Fisher's exact test ($p = 2.3 \times 10^{-5}$) suggested that the distribution between clusters A and B was not random. Profiles of MCP-1, IL-4, IL-1β, and IL-6 characterize rejecting grafts, whereas GM-CSF and IL-4 characterize isografts. This was also indicated by an absolute value of point-biserial correlation coefficient >0.6 comparing each group with the other groups. Interestingly, there appeared to be an

Table 4. Histological evaluation of muscle biopsies from postoperative (POD) 3 to 9.

MUSCLE	POD 3				POD 5				POD 7				POD 9			
GRADE	0	I	II	III	0	I	II	III	0	I	II	III	0	I	II	III
ATC	4	2			2	3	1			5				1	2	2
ISO	2	2	1		4	1			4	1			4	1		
TAC	5				5				5				4	1		

Number of biopsies taken on each postoperative day (POD 3,5,7,9) in muscle according to their histological grading (Grad 0-III) based on H&E grading. The first biopsy was taken from the lateral proximal part of the thigh, the second one from the lateral distal thigh, the third one from the ventral thigh and the last one from the medial part of the thigh.

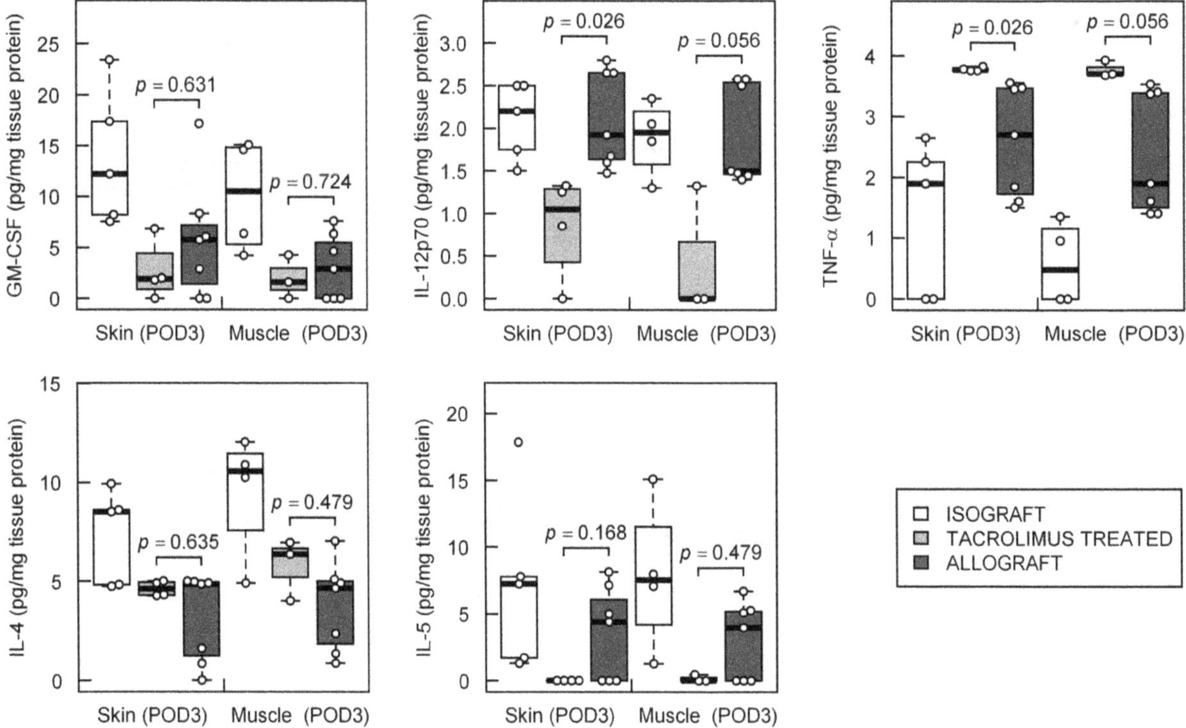

Figure 2. Distribution of inflammatory mediator levels at the earliest postoperative measurements (POD 3) in rat limb transplantation models. Adjusted p-values from Wilcoxon rank-sum test between the rejection group (ATC) vs. Tacrolimus treated group (TAC) for selected inflammatory mediators, which were tested to be included in a prediction model by multinomial logistic regression analysis, are presented.

Table 5. Statistical analysis for all 14 inflammatory mediator levels in skin and in muscle at early postoperative time points (combined group of POD 3 and POD 5).

	Skin POD 3/5			Muscle POD 3/5		
	p_{KW}	p_{WR}	Partition on DVs [%]	p_{KW}	p_{WR}	Partition on DVs [%]
GM-CSF	**0.0018**	0.3260	**4.26**	**0.0083**	0.6178	**2.60**
IL-1α	**0.0244**	1.0000	0.01	**0.0105**	0.0773	0.01
MCP-1	**0.0011**	**0.0026**	0.72	**0.0466**	0.3673	0.79
IL-4	**0.0040**	0.3421	**24.21**	**0.0194**	0.5312	**18.68**
IL-1β	0.2042	0.1577	0.10	0.8251	0.7577	0.09
IL-2	0.2042	0.2868	0.83	0.1779	0.5312	0.29
IL-6	0.1322	0.2824	0.27	0.5127	0.6178	0.29
IL-10	0.2777	0.2805	0.55	0.8251	0.8657	0.39
IL-12p70	**0.0019**	**0.0013**	**15.65**	**0.0030**	**0.0025**	**31.59**
IL-5	**0.0022**	**0.0123**	**4.85**	**0.0010**	0.2112	**5.03**
IFN-γ	0.2956	0.3729	**5.67**	0.2562	0.3619	1.90
IL-18	0.3462	0.2868	0.03	**0.0425**	0.7498	0.03
GRO-KC	**0.0040**	**0.0021**	0.27	0.5127	0.5312	0.11
TNF-α	**1.7×10^{-4}**	**0.0013**	**42.59**	**0.0001**	**0.0025**	**38.21**

Most promising inflammatory mediators for classification of rejection, based on early identification before histological manifestation of rejection is evident, are selected (p_{KW}<0.05 and *Partition on DVs* >1%, symbols in bold) and subjected to multinomial logistic regression analyses. For all measured inflammatory mediators adjusted p-values from Kruskal-Wallis test (KW) of overall equality between all 3 cohorts (ISO, TAC, ATC) and Wilcoxon rank-sum test (WR) for comparison between the rejection group (ATC) and the Tacrolimus treated group (TAC) as well as partition of each inflammatory mediator on the two discriminant vectors (DVs), which maximizes the separation between the 3 rejection groups, resulting from discriminant function analysis, are given.

Table 6. Results for multinomial logistic regression models in skin and muscle for classification of the rejection groups based inflammatory mediator/chemokine levels at early postoperative time points (POD 3/5) in rat transplantation models.

	Skin POD3/5			**Muscle POD3/5**		
ln(p(*TAC*)/p(*ATC*))	**-6.7-2.6*_IL4_-61.3*_IL12p70_+25.6*_TNFa_**			**-6.9-18.8*_IL12p70_+11.3*_TNFa_**		
ln(p(*ISO*)/p(*ATC*))	**-1094.8+112.6*_IL4_+250.4*_IL12p70_-28.6*_TNFa_**			**-10.0+25.1*_IL12p70_-27.0*_TNFa_**		
	ATC^{pred}	**TAC^{pred}**	**ISO^{pred}**	**ATC^{pred}**	**TAC^{pred}**	**ISO^{pred}**
ATC	12	0	1	13	0	0
TAC	0	8	0	0	7	0
ISO	3	0	7	0	0	9
	Accuracy = 87.1% $p = 0.020$			Accuracy = 100% $p = 0.031$		

Best prediction models for skin and muscle and their respective logistic prediction functions and classifier performance including confusion table (assessed by an 8-fold cross validation procedure) are summarized.

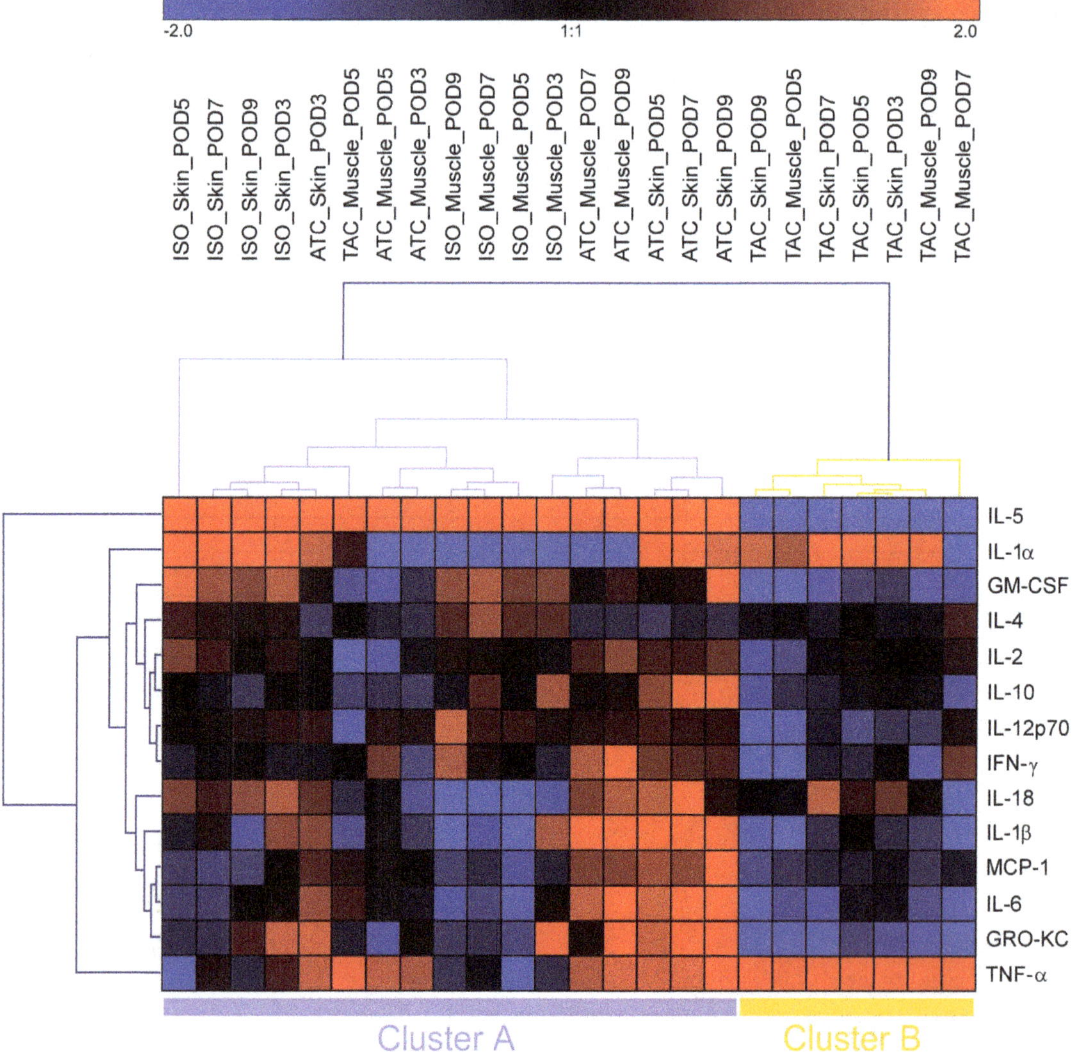

Figure 3. Similarity of sample groups and association between inflammatory mediators in rat limb transplantation models based on their profiles of mean levels in each condition. Heatmap as a result of complete linkage hierarchical clustering on log2-transformed and mean centered data. Log2-fold differences against the respective mean levels of each inflammatory mediator are color coded (red means higher inflammatory mediator levels and blue means lower inflammatory mediator levels than the mean levels of the respective inflammatory mediator according to the color scheme at the top). Dendrograms (trees) show similarity between different conditions and different inflammatory mediator profiles, respectively.

overlap in the expression pattern of the isografts and the rejecting animals for IL-5, IL-1α, IL-18, and GRO-KC.

Mediators relevant for classifications and progression of rejection

Random forest (RF) classification was performed for skin and muscle samples in all three cohorts at POD 3–9. The overall out-of-bag error rate was 6.7% for skin and 7.0% for muscle. The classification tables are shown in Figure 4. The importance of a variable in discriminating among study groups was demonstrated by ranked mean decrease accuracy as depicted in Figure 4. The mediator best capable of differentiating among experimental groups samples was MCP-1 in skin and TNF-α in muscle. Discriminant analysis suggested that the mediators best capable of discriminating among experimental groups in the early postoperative time points were GM-CSF, IL-4, IL-12p70, IL-5, and TNF-α; these mediators also appear within the seven top-ranked mediators in the RF analysis.

To identify inflammatory cytokines with high dynamic variability, we performed principal component analysis (PCA) on the combined mean-centered dataset including the whole postoperative time series over all study groups and tissues. The PCA scores of the first four principle components (explaining >70% of the variance) of all 14 cytokines were ranked based on the sum of the absolute PCA scores (loadings) of all 4 PCs (Figure 5). The top prioritized cytokines IL-1α, IL-18, IL-1β, and IL-4 might be promising candidates for new therapeutic regimens.

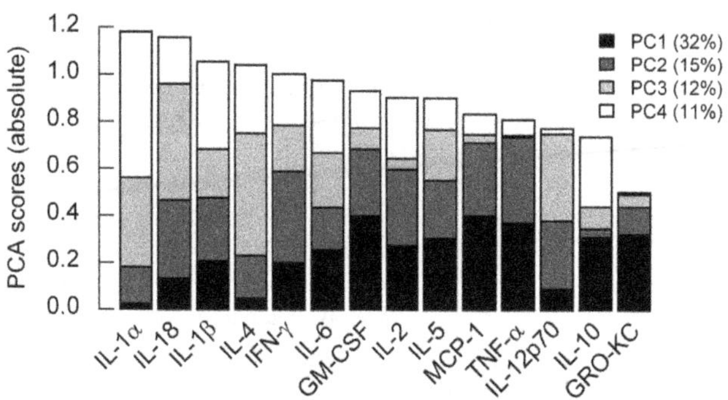

Figure 5. Most variable mediators identified by principal component analysis (PCA) suggesting new potential targets for therapeutic interventions to suppress limb transplant rejection. PCA scores (loadings) for the first four principal components (PCs), which represent more than 70% of information within the data, are displayed in a stacked bar plot for all inflammatory mediators (ranked by the overall PCA score of the 4 PCs).

Discussion

Experimental transplant rejection can be detected reliably in advance of the current clinical gold standard of histologic evaluation, using computational modeling that involves 14 inflammatory mediators in this model. These findings support the hypothesis that the immune signaling associated with rejection follows specific patterns of expression and is driven by different principal components than those associated with inflammation following syngeneic transplantation.

Detailed cellular and molecular assessment provides valuable insights into the role of the immune/inflammatory response in post-transplant pathophysiology [14,15]. Translation of these findings into biomarkers applied clinically, however, has been very limited. It remains a major challenge to reduce the complexity of dynamic biological systems to elements with diagnostic or therapeutic clinical value [16,17]. Data-driven investigations of genomic and proteomic studies in combination with mechanistic computational modeling based on measurements of circulating inflammatory mediators have given insight into the

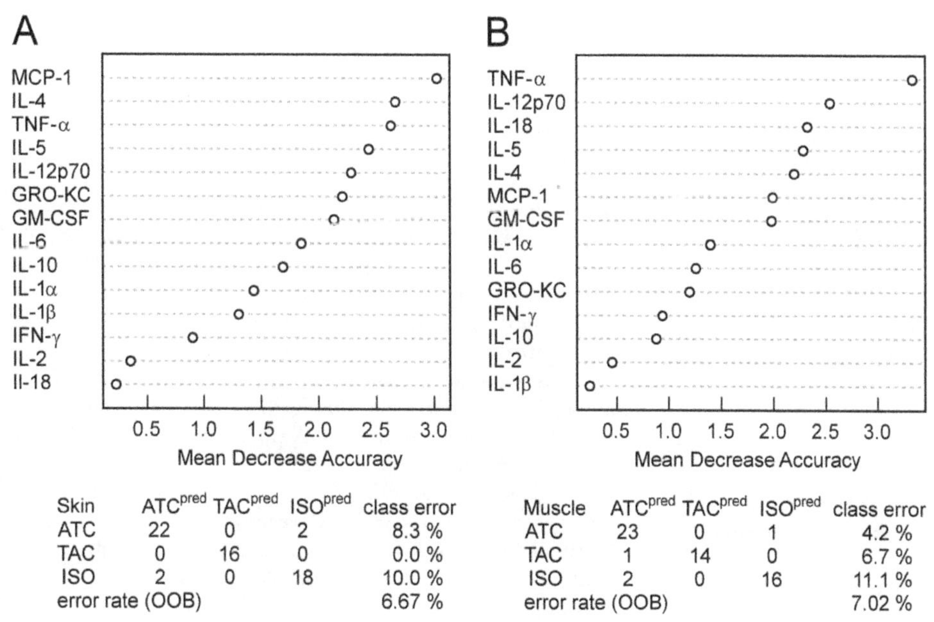

Skin	ATC^{pred}	TAC^{pred}	ISO^{pred}	class error
ATC	22	0	2	8.3 %
TAC	0	16	0	0.0 %
ISO	2	0	18	10.0 %
error rate (OOB)				6.67 %

Muscle	ATC^{pred}	TAC^{pred}	ISO^{pred}	class error
ATC	23	0	1	4.2 %
TAC	1	14	0	6.7 %
ISO	2	0	16	11.1 %
error rate (OOB)				7.02 %

Figure 4. Results from Random Forest classification of the different rejection groups (ISO, TAC, ATC) using over the whole time course (POD 3, POD 5, POD 7, POD 9) measured inflammatory mediators in skin (A) and muscle (B) samples of rat limb transplantation models. Most important mediators for the decision trees based classification approach are evident by ranked mean decrease accuracy. Performances of the classifiers are indicated by the confusion table and the out-of-bag (OOB) error rate.

pathophysiology of trauma, shock as well as organ transplantation [18–22].

Herein, we demonstrate that data-driven and expression pattern-oriented analyses of a high-content dataset can help to decipher the complexity of acute inflammation in VCA. In the present study, these advanced computational algorithms allowed to diagnose rejection in advance of gross histological damage. We suggest that measuring inflammatory mediators expressed in skin and muscle is clinically feasible in the setting of VCA since skin and muscle are more accessible as compared to solid organs. Isografts were compared to allografts and tacrolimus treated allografts in order to delineate between surgery/trauma/ischemia induced inflammation and allograft rejection. Tacrolimus treatment was sufficient to diminish rejection (but not completely eliminate the immune response).

In the samples analyzed in the present study, skin rejection was detected in advance of histological alterations based on the inflammatory mediators IL-4, IL-12p70 and TNF-α, with a prediction accuracy of >87%. In muscle rejection, IL-12p70 and TNF-α were identified as best and accurate classifiers. TNF-α, a canonical inflammatory mediator, is mainly produced by activated monocytes, macrophages, and T-cells, and exerts a direct effect on the proliferation, apoptosis, necrosis, differentiation, and function of virtually every cell type [23]. In the skin, mast cells appear to be the predominant source of preformed TNF-α, which can be released upon inflammatory stimuli [24]. TNF-α activates T-cells; increases the release of other inflammatory mediators; and induces neutrophil adherence, infiltration and the production of enzymes and reactive oxygen. These mechanisms are harmful to the allograft, and subsequently cause tissue injury as well as organ dysfunction [23]. Several studies have demonstrated increased TNF-α levels in the serum during episodes of rejection in liver, kidney and pancreas transplant recipients [25–27]. Interestingly, the increase in TNF-α levels occurred two days before clinical manifestation of rejection.

The production of IL-12 strongly promotes the development of IFN-γ producing helper T (TH)-cells. IL-12 may not only be essential for macrophage-mediated allograft rejection via induction of TH1 responses, but IL-12 may be involved in delaying rejection via induction of inducible nitric oxide synthase (iNOS) and indolamine 2,3 dioxygenase (IDO) [28]. This positive effect was shown in several skin or heart allograft models, as well as in the course of graft-versus-host disease (GVHD) [29–31].

Good performance of the multinomial logistic regression model, which models linear decision boundaries effectively, indicates that the patterns of inflammatory mediator expression in skin are fundamentally different in isograft and allograft skin tissue, and that this difference can be captured with reasonable performance by computationally efficient algorithms. Multinomial logistic regression performance for discrimination of rejection is even stronger and the consistency with which this distinction is made across a rather complex set of features implies a high level of biological significance. In other words, not only is the specific inflammatory mediator, but also the particular combination of mediators in the local inflammatory milieu seems to play a determinative role in the nature and progression of inflammation expressed.

The RF classification approach including more time points (POD 3-POD 9) achieves high levels of accuracy and continues to improve with the addition of variables. This finding implies that there are specific inflammatory mediator interactions that are relevant only under certain contexts [32], and that these interactions can be leveraged to identify potential targets for therapeutic intervention.

We hypothesized that mediators with time-dependent changes might be important in the different dynamic processes and describe principal drivers (principal components, PC), which could turn out as therapeutic targets. We were focusing on the first four PCs since they comprise more than 70% of the total variance. The four top-ranked mediators were IL-1α, IL-18, IL-1β, and IL-4 (Figure 5).

To discern the effect of the inflammatory mediators within each group, we performed the same PCA procedure for each group individually (Figure S1). The impact of IL12p70 already shown as potential early diagnostic marker for rejection was not as pronounced in the tacrolimus-treated animals as in the isograft and allograft study group. Interferon-γ and IL-4 had a high ranking in all groups (ISO, TAC, ATC) indicating a more unspecific effect in inflammation; In contrast, IL-1α and IL-18 exhibited an expression profile which indicates a possible key role in VCA rejection and makes these cytokines interesting candidates for therapeutic interventions.

Our studies identified IL-1α and IL-18 as possible candidates for the treatment of skin rejection. These inflammatory mediators share similarities regarding structure, receptor family, signal transduction pathways, and biological effects. Both inflammatory mediators are produced by monocytes/macrophages but also constitutively expressed by keratinocytes [33]. IL-1α plays an important role in sterile inflammation. During necrotic cell death, the IL-1α precursor is released [34] and binds to its receptor expressed on adjacent macrophages and epithelial cells, which in turn triggers a pro-inflammatory response characterized by an influx of neutrophils followed by macrophages [35,36]. IL-18, together with IL-2, IL-12, and IL-15, is a dominant IFN-γ inducing factor. Several human diseases, such as systemic lupus erythematosus, rheumatoid arthritis, Crohn's disease, psoriasis and graft-versus-host-disease are thought to be mediated in part by IL-18 [37]. Moreover, IL-18 stimulates ICAM-1 expression on monocytic cell lines, which is important for the recruitment of T-cells and other immune cells to the skin. Lymphocyte recruitment is known as a key mechanism in inflammatory skin disorders and [38,39]. Hautz et al. showed, that expression of ICAM-1 correlated closely with severity of skin rejection [8].

Based on our findings, IL-1α and IL-18 appear as interesting potential targets for intervention. Yuan J et al. already showed the efficacy of IL-1 receptor antagonist (IL-1ra) gene transfer treatment for acute corneal graft rejection in a rat model [40] The group demonstrated during acute rejection, that TGF-β1, RANTES and IL-1 levels were lower in the IL-1ra treatment group. Thus antagonizing the biological activitiy of IL-1 could effectively prolong graft survival. IL-ra, a specific inhibitor of both IL-1α and IL-β generically known as anakinra is clinically applied for the treatment of rheumatoid arthritis. IL-18-binding protein (IL-18BP), a specific inhibitor or IL-18 which neutralizes IL-18 bioactivity, was discovered during the search for soluble IL-18 receptors in humane urine [41]. A clinical preparation of human IL-18BP has been shown to be safe and effective in patients with RA or plaque psoriasis [42]. A soluble form of the IL-18 receptor accessory protein (sIL-18Rβ) has recently been identified as novel IL-18 inhibitor in collagen-induced arthritis in mice [43].

In summary, we herein provide information, which could help identifying a diagnostic profile and novel targets for treatment of skin rejection in VCA. The present study demonstrates that the application of advanced computational methods can be successfully applied in molecular assessment of skin rejection and provides novel insights into the inflammatory mediator communication patterns. The study remains observational in its nature and investigational trials are warranted in order to address the true functional value of the postulated treatment targets.

Supporting Information

Figure S1 Most variable (influential) mediators identified by principal component analysis (PCA) for each of the three study groups (ISO/TAC/ATC). PCA scores (loadings) for the first four principal components (PCs), which represent more than 75% of information, are displayed in a stacked bar plot for all inflammatory mediators (ranked by the overall PCA score of the 4 PCs) and a scatter plot of the first two PCs.

Figure S2 Distribution of inflammatory mediator levels (boxplots) at postoperative day 5 in rat limb transplantation models for selected inflammatory mediators. Adjusted p-values from Wilcoxon rank-sum test between the rejection group (ATC) versus Tacrolimus treated group (TAC) are provided.

Acknowledgments

We gratefully acknowledge the effort of Dr. Mario Cherubino and Dr. Yong Wang for performing a major part of hindlimb transplants. The help of Prof. Bernhard Zelger in preparing and evaluating histological sections and the editorial work by Mary Margreiter are also gratefully acknowledged.

Author Contributions

Conceived and designed the experiments: DW SS GB RS WAL YV. Performed the experiments: DW DB TH NE HH. Analyzed the data: DW HH RS TH NE BZ. Contributed reagents/materials/analysis tools: YV JP GP. Wrote the paper: DW HH SS.

References

1. Cendales LC, Kanitakis J, Schneeberger S, Burns C, Ruiz P, et al. (2008) The Banff 2007 working classification of skin-containing composite tissue allograft pathology. Am J Transplant 8: 1396–1400.
2. Kanitakis J, Jullien D, Nicolas JF, Frances C, Claudy A, et al. (2000) Sequential histological and immunohistochemical study of the skin of the first human hand allograft. Transplantation 69: 1380–1385.
3. Kanitakis J (2008) The challenge of dermatopathological diagnosis of composite tissue allograft rejection: a review. J Cutan Pathol 35: 738–744.
4. Schneeberger S, Gorantla VS, van Riet RP, Lanzetta M, Vereecken P, et al. (2008) Atypical acute rejection after hand transplantation. Am J Transplant 8: 688–696.
5. Hautz T, Wolfram D, Grahammer J, Starzl R, Krapf C, et al. (2012) Mechanisms and mediators of inflammation: potential models for skin rejection and targeted therapy in vascularized composite allotransplantation. Clin Dev Immunol: 1–9.
6. Tarca AL, Carey VJ, Chen XW, Romero R, Draghici S (2007) Machine learning and its applications to biology. PLoS Comput Biol 3: e116.
7. Coin L, Bateman A, Durbin R (2003) Enhanced protein domain discovery by using language modeling techniques from speech recognition. Proc Natl Acad Sci U S A 100: 4516–4520.
8. Hautz T, Zelger B, Grahammer J, Krapf C, Amberger A, et al. (2010) Molecular markers and targeted therapy of skin rejection in composite tissue allotransplantation. Am J Transplant 10: 1200–1209.
9. Benjamini Y, Hochberg Y (1995) Controlling the false discovery rate: A practical and powerful approach to multiple testing. J R Statist Soc B 57: 289–300.
10. Sturn A, Quackenbush J, Trajanoski Z (2002) Genesis: cluster analysis of microarray data. Bioinformatics 18: 207–208.
11. Breiman L (2001) Random Forests. Machine Learning 45: 5–32.
12. Mi Q, Constantine G, Ziraldo C, Solovyev A, Torres A, et al. (2011) A dynamic view of trauma/hemorrhage-induced inflammation in mice: principal drivers and networks. PLoS One 6: e19424.
13. Namas RA, Namas R, Lagoa C, Barclay D, Mi Q, et al. (2012) Hemoadsorption reprograms inflammation in experimental gram-negative septic peritonitis: insights from in vivo and in silico studies. Mol Med 18: 1366–1374.
14. Page EK, Dar WA, Knechtle SJ (2012) Biologics in organ transplantation. Transpl Int 25: 707–719.
15. Sarwal MM (2006) Chipping into the human genome: novel insights for transplantation. Immunol Rev 210: 138–155.
16. Vodovotz Y (2006) Deciphering the complexity of acute inflammation using mathematical models. Immunol Res 36: 237–245.
17. Mesarovic MD, Sreenath SN, Keene JD (2004) Search for organising principles: understanding in systems biology. Syst Biol (Stevenage) 1: 19–27.
18. Calvano SE, Xiao W, Richards DR, Felciano RM, Baker HV, et al. (2005) A network-based analysis of systemic inflammation in humans. Nature 437: 1032–1037.
19. Warren HS, Elson CM, Hayden DL, Schoenfeld DA, Cobb JP, et al. (2009) A genomic score prognostic of outcome in trauma patients. Mol Med 15: 220–227.
20. Chow CC, Clermont G, Kumar R, Lagoa C, Tawadrous Z, et al. (2005) The acute inflammatory response in diverse shock states. Shock 24: 74–84.
21. Bohra R, Klepacki J, Klawitter J, Thurman JM, Christians U (2013) Proteomics and metabolomics in renal transplantation-quo vadis? Transpl Int 26: 225–241.
22. Azhar N (2013) Analysis of serum inflammatory mediators identifies unique dynamic networks associated with death and spontaneous survival in pediatric acute liver failure.
23. Grenz A, Schenk M, Zipfel A, Viebahn R (2000) TNF-alpha and its receptors mediate graft rejection and loss after liver transplantation. Clin Chem Lab Med 38: 1183–1185.
24. Walsh LJ, Trinchieri G, Waldorf HA, Whitaker D, Murphy GF (1991) Human dermal mast cells contain and release tumor necrosis factor alpha, which induces endothelial leukocyte adhesion molecule 1. Proc Natl Acad Sci U S A 88: 4220–4224.
25. Imagawa DK, Millis JM, Olthoff KM, Derus LJ, Chia D, et al. (1990) The role of tumor necrosis factor in allograft rejection. I. Evidence that elevated levels of tumor necrosis factor-alpha predict rejection following orthotopic liver transplantation. Transplantation 50: 219–225.
26. Bubnova LN, Kabakov A, Serebrianaya N, Ketlinky S (1992) Interleukin-1 beta and tumor necrosis factor-alpha serum levels in renal allograft recipients. Transplant Proc 24: 2545.
27. Grewal HP, Kotb M, Salem A, el Din AB, Novak K, et al. (1993) Elevated tumor necrosis factor levels are predictive for pancreas allograft transplant rejection. Transplant Proc 25: 132–135.
28. Goriely S, Goldman M (2008) Interleukin-12 family members and the balance between rejection and tolerance. Curr Opin Organ Transplant 13: 4–9.
29. Piccotti JR, Chan SY, Goodman RE, Magram J, Eichwald EJ, et al. (1996) IL-12 antagonism induces T helper 2 responses, yet exacerbates cardiac allograft rejection. Evidence against a dominant protective role for T helper 2 cytokines in alloimmunity. J Immunol 157: 1951–1957.
30. Verma ND, Boyd R, Robinson C, Plain KM, Tran GT, et al. (2006) Interleukin-12p70 prolongs allograft survival by induction of interferon gamma and nitric oxide production. Transplantation 82: 1324–1333.
31. Dey BR, Yang YG, Szot GL, Pearson DA, Sykes M (1998) Interleukin-12 inhibits graft-versus-host disease through an Fas-mediated mechanism associated with alterations in donor T-cell activation and expansion. Blood 91: 3315–3322.
32. Nathan C, Sporn M (1991) Cytokines in context. J Cell Biol 113: 981–986.
33. Dinarello CA (1999) IL-18: A TH1-inducing, proinflammatory cytokine and new member of the IL-1 family. J Allergy Clin Immunol 103: 11–24.
34. Carmi Y, Voronov E, Dotan S, Lahat N, Rahat MA, et al. (2009) The role of macrophage-derived IL-1 in induction and maintenance of angiogenesis. J Immunol 183: 4705–4714.
35. Rider P, Carmi Y, Guttman O, Braiman A, Cohen I, et al. (2011) IL-1alpha and IL-1beta recruit different myeloid cells and promote different stages of sterile inflammation. J Immunol 187: 4835–4843.
36. van de Veerdonk FL, Netea MG (2013) New Insights in the Immunobiology of IL-1 Family Members. Front Immunol 4: 167.
37. Dinarello CA (2009) Immunological and inflammatory functions of the interleukin-1 family. Annu Rev Immunol 27: 519–550.
38. Robert C, Kupper TS (1999) Inflammatory skin diseases, T cells, and immune surveillance. N Engl J Med 341: 1817–1828.
39. Schon MP, Ludwig RJ (2005) Lymphocyte trafficking to inflamed skin—molecular mechanisms and implications for therapeutic target molecules. Expert Opin Ther Targets 9: 225–243.
40. Yuan J, Liu Y, Huang W, Zhou S, Ling S, et al. (2013) The experimental treatment of corneal graft rejection with the interleukin-1 receptor antagonist (IL-1ra) gene. PLoS One 8: e60714.
41. Novick D, Kim SH, Fantuzzi G, Reznikov LL, Dinarello CA, et al. (1999) Interleukin-18 binding protein: a novel modulator of the Th1 cytokine response. Immunity 10: 127–136.
42. Tak PP, Bacchi M, Bertolino M (2006) Pharmacokinetics of IL-18 binding protein in healthy volunteers and subjects with rheumatoid arthritis or plaque psoriasis. Eur J Drug Metab Pharmacokinet 31: 109–116.
43. Veenbergen S, Smeets R, Bennink M, Arntz O, Joosten L, et al. (2010) The natural soluble form of IL-18 receptor beta exacerbates collagen-induced arthritis via modulation of T-cell immune responses. Ann Rheum Dis 69: 276–283.

3

Evaluation of Anterior Cervical Reconstruction with Titanium Mesh Cages versus Nano-Hydroxyapatite/ Polyamide66 Cages after 1- or 2-Level Corpectomy for Multilevel Cervical Spondylotic Myelopathy

Yuan Zhang, Zhengxue Quan*, Zenghui Zhao, Xiaoji Luo, Ke Tang, Jie Li, Xu Zhou, Dianming Jiang

Department of Orthopedic Surgery, The First Affiliated Hospital of Chongqing Medical University, Chongqing, China

Abstract

Objective: To retrospectively compare the efficacy of the titanium mesh cage (TMC) and the nano-hydroxyapatite/ polyamide66 cage (n-HA/PA66 cage) for 1- or 2-level anterior cervical corpectomy and fusion (ACCF) to treat multilevel cervical spondylotic myelopathy (MCSM).

Methods: A total of 117 consecutive patients with MCSM who underwent 1- or 2-level ACCF using a TMC or an n-HA/PA66 cage were studied retrospectively at a mean follow-up of 45.28±12.83 months. The patients were divided into four groups according to the level of corpectomy (1- or 2-level corpectomy) and cage type used (TMC or n-HA/PA66 cage). Clinical and radiological parameters were used to evaluate outcomes.

Results: At the one-year follow-up, the fusion rate in the n-HA/PA66 group was higher, albeit non-significantly, than that in the TMC group for both 1- and 2-level ACCF, but the fusion rates of the procedures were almost equal at the final follow-up. The incidence of cage subsidence at the final follow-up was significantly higher in the TMC group than in the n-HA/PA66 group for the 1-level ACCF (24% vs. 4%, $p = 0.01$), and the difference was greater for the 2-level ACCF between the TMC group and the n-HA/PA66 group (38% vs. 5%, $p = 0.01$). Meanwhile, a much greater loss of fused height was observed in the TMC group compared with the n-HA/PA66 group for both the 1- and 2-level ACCF. All four groups demonstrated increases in C2-C7 Cobb angle and JOA scores and decreases in VAS at the final follow-up compared with preoperative values.

Conclusion: The lower incidence of cage subsidence, better maintenance of the height of the fused segment and similar excellent bony fusion indicate that the n-HA/PA66 cage may be a superior alternative to the TMC for cervical reconstruction after cervical corpectomy, in particular for 2-level ACCF.

Editor: Mohammed Shamji, Toronto Western Hospital, Canada

Funding: This research was supported by the National Natural Science Foundation of China (Grant No. 81272039). URL:http://www.nsfc.gov.cn. The funders had no role in study design, data collection and analysis, decision to publish, or preparation of the manuscript.

Competing Interests: The authors have declared that no competing interests exist.

* E-mail: quanzx18@126.com

Introduction

Several surgical techniques have been suggested for the treatment of multilevel cervical spondylotic myelopathy (MCSM). However, the optimal surgical procedure remains controversial [1,2,3,4]. Both anterior and posterior approaches have been reported with satisfactory clinical outcomes [5,6,7]. Full decompression of the spinal cord and stable reconstruction of cervical alignment are the two critical aims of this surgery [5]. Based on increased etiological data, recent reports have proposed that the compression of the spinal cord in MCSM most likely originates from anterior regions, such as cervical discs and osteophytes [8,9], suggesting that anterior procedures may be more reasonable for MCSM. Without the limitation of the disc levels, anterior cervical corpectomy and fusion (ACCF) is considered a favorable option compared with anterior cervical discectomy and fusion (ACDF) among the anterior techniques [10]. More importantly, ACCF can remove almost all pathologies that cause spinal cord compression, such as prolapsed discs, osteophytes and ossified posterior longitudinal ligament (OPLL) [11].

The reconstruction of the cervical spine is relatively important following corpectomy-mediated decompression. Using auto-grafts harvested from the iliac crest or fibula for fusion has been considered the "gold standard" for anterior cervical column reconstruction. Unfortunately, donor-site complications remain [12]. Allografts can be used to avoid the morbidity associated with autograft harvest, but this technique decreases the rate of arthrodesis and increases the rate of graft collapse [13]. Titanium mesh cages (TMCs) filled with local cancellous bone autografts have been used for decades for cervical reconstruction after corpectomy [9,14], with advantages including few donor-site complications, early biomechanical stabilization, a short operation duration and high fusion rates (range: 97%–100%); however, the inevitable complication of subsidence and other disadvantages, including stress shielding and radiopacity also occur [15,16,17,18,19]. The nano-hydroxyapatite/polyamide66 cage (nano-HA/PA66 cage) is a hollow cylinder manufactured of the n-HA/PA66 composite (Figure 1). The use of this cage filled with autograft has been reported for anterior cervical reconstruction in recent years, with satisfactory clinical outcomes [20,21]. Few studies have compared the outcomes of TMCs and n-HA/PA66 cages. The aim of the present study was to comparatively assess the clinical outcomes of TMCs vs. n-HA/PA66 cages for MCSM after 1- or 2-level corpectomy to provide a basis for selecting the appropriate method for reconstructing the cervical spine.

Materials and Methods

This study was approved by the Institutional Review Board of the First Affiliated Hospital of Chongqing Medical University, and all aspects of the study comply with the Declaration of Helsinki. The Institutional Review Board of the First Affiliated Hospital of Chongqing Medical University also waived the requirement for patient consent because this study was retrospective, the data were analyzed anonymously and patient care was not affected by the study. Between June 2006 and December 2010, a total of 117 consecutive patients (65 males and 52 females) who underwent ACCF for MCSM by a senior surgeon (QUAN) were evaluated retrospectively. All patients presented with myelopathy prior to the operation, and magnetic resonance images confirmed MCSM diagnoses. Patients with cervical trauma, infections, tumors, rheumatoid arthritis, congenital deformities, severe osteoporosis or previous cervical spine surgery were excluded from our study.

All patients underwent a 1- or 2-level corpectomy, based on the level of the lesion, followed by cervical reconstruction with a TMC (Medtronic Sofamor Danek, Memphis, TN, USA) or an n-HA/PA66 cage (Sichuan National Nanotechnology Co., Ltd., Chengdu, China). The n-HA/PA66 cages were designed and fabricated by the Institute of Materials Science and Technology, Sichuan University, and our department, and they have been approved for clinical use since 2005 by the State Drug and Food Administration of China. The n-HA/PA66 cages have an 8- to 14-mm outer diameter and a 3- to 8-mm inner diameter and are of appropriate length for clinical utilization; each cage has grooves at each end to increase the friction between the cage and vertebral endplates and several 2-mm holes in the wall of the cage [20,22]. We divided the patients into four groups based on the number of levels fused (1- or 2-level ACCF) and cage selection (TMC or n-HA/PA66 cage).

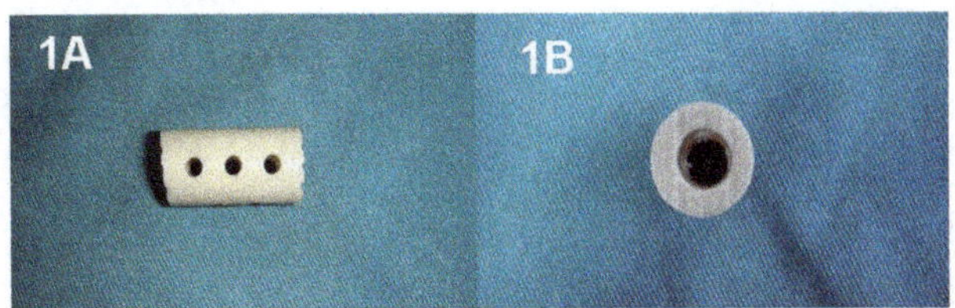

Figure 1. Photographs of lateral (1A) and superior (1B) views of the nano-hydroxyapatite/polyamide66 cage.

All surgeries were performed using a right-sided anterior cervical approach. After accurate exposure of the surgical region, a Caspar screw distraction was used for adequate distraction. Following the discectomy at the cephalic and caudal level of the lesion segment, 1- or 2-level corpectomies were performed using a Kerrison rongeur. Hypertrophic osteophytes and the posterior longitudinal ligament were removed in every case to ensure that the dura mater was widely exposed. The adjacent cartilage endplates were removed as fully as possible, and the bony endplates were preserved. An appropriately sized TMC or n-HA/PA66 cage was then prepared, filled with autogenous cancellous bone from the resected vertebra and then implanted into the intervertebral space after corpectomy using a titanium anterior cervical plate for internal fixation. All patients were instructed to wear a cervical collar for six weeks postoperatively.

The surgery time, blood loss and hospital stay were recorded. Clinical and radiological follow-ups were conducted immediately and at three months, six months and one year after surgery and then annually thereafter. The Japanese Orthopedic Association (JOA) score was used to assess neurologic status, and a 10-point visual analogue scale (VAS) was used to grade neck pain. The anteroposterior, neutral lateral and flexion/extension lateral cervical plain radiographs at preoperative, immediate postoperative, 1-year follow-up and the final follow-up were examined to assess radiologic parameters, including the height of the fused segment, the loss of height of the fused segment, cervical sagittal alignment and fusion status. The distance between the midpoint of the cephalic endplate and the caudal endplate of the fused segment was measured in millimeter (mm) and used as the height of the fused segment using Carestream software (Carestream Health, Inc. Toronto, Canada). Loss of height of the fused segment was defined as a reduction in height of the fused segment from the immediate postoperative period to follow-ups, and subsidence was defined as a loss of height of greater than 3 mm [23]. Cervical sagittal alignment was defined as the Cobb angle formed between the lower endplates of C2 and C7 on neutral lateral cervical plain film [24]. Bony fusion was defined as the trabeculation and bridging between the cage and adjacent endplates and the absence of motion between spinous processes upon flexion/extension in the fused segments. Three-dimensional computed tomography (3D-CT) scans were taken to further confirm the fusion status by observing the trabeculation between the autogenous cancellous graft and adjacent endplates [25].

Statistical analyses were performed using SPSS (version 16.0, SPSS Inc., Chicago, IL). Quantitative data are presented as the mean ± standard deviation. Repeated measures ANOVA was used for statistical analyses of differences in mean values, and the Chi-squared test was used for categorical data. The threshold for statistical significance was set to $p<0.05$.

Results

A total of 117 patients (65 males and 52 females) were included in this study, with a mean follow-up of 45.28±12.83 months (range: 25 to 70 months). Based on the number of corpectomies (1- or 2-level) and cage selection (TMC or n-HA/PA66 cage), the patients were divided into four groups. 52 patients underwent 1-level ACCF (Figure 2) and 19 patients underwent 2-level ACCF (Figure 3) with n-HA/PA66 cages. 25 patients underwent 1-level ACCF (Figure 4) and 21 patients underwent 2-level ACCF (Figure 5) with TMCs. The demographics of the patients are shown in Table 1. No significant differences were detected in gender, age, hospital stay, surgery time, blood loss or follow-up

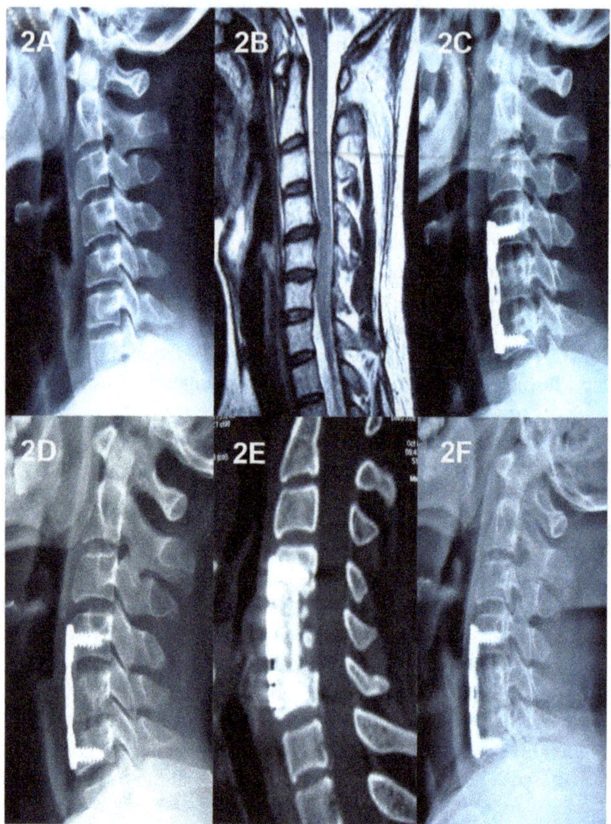

Figure 2. A 36-year-old male who underwent 1-level corpectomy with a nano-hydroxyapatite/polyamide66 cage used for cervical reconstruction. The preoperative cervical X-ray film (2A) and MRI scan (2B) show the spinal cord compression resulting from C4/5 and C5/6 disc herniations. The immediately postoperative lateral X-ray (2C) shows C5 corpectomy and the n-HA/PA66 cage used for reconstruction, and an obvious radiolucent gap can be observed between the cage and the endplates. The lateral X-ray film (2D) shows no obvious radiolucent gap, and the 3D-CT (2E) scan shows the autogenous bone granules filling the cage and achieving bony fusion with adjacent endplates at the 1-year follow-up. A lateral X-ray film (2F) at the final follow-up (four years and eight months) shows satisfying bony fusion and no obvious migration or subsidence.

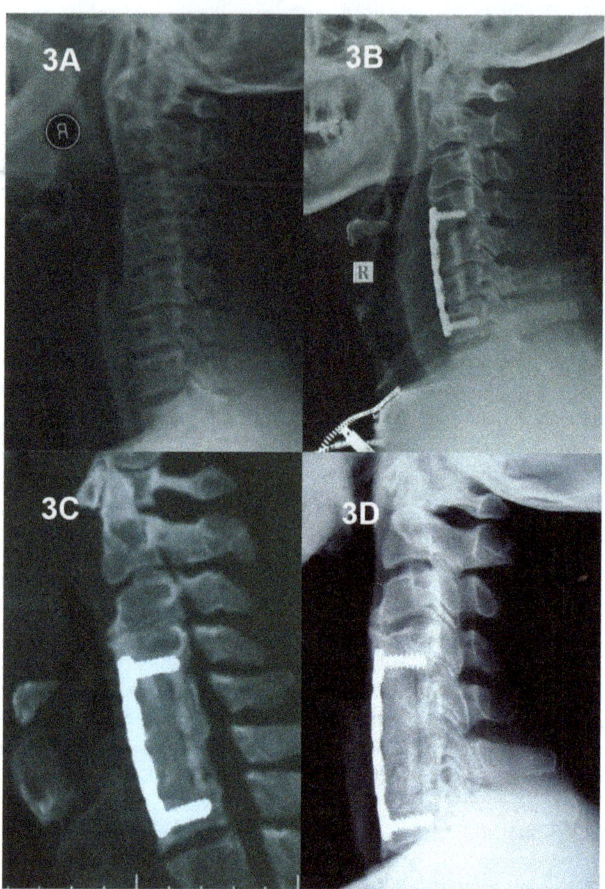

Figure 3. A 61-year-old male who underwent 2-level corpectomy with a nano-hydroxyapatite/polyamide66 cage used for cervical reconstruction. A preoperative cervical X-ray film (3A) shows a loss of cervical lordosis. The immediately postoperative lateral X-ray (3B) shows C5 and C6 corpectomy and the n-HA/PA66 cage used for reconstruction. The 3D-CT (3C) and lateral X-ray (3D) show obvious bony fusion and restoration of cervical alignment at the final follow-up (four years and four months).

(months) between the TMC group and the n-HA/PA66 group for either 1- or 2-level ACCF.

Radiological and clinical parameters are shown in Table 2. For 1-level ACCF, the mean height of the fused segment improved in the TMC group from 52.03±4.35 mm preoperatively to 59.52±4.36 mm immediately postoperative, and it improved from 53.55±6.20 mm to 61.84±6.86 mm in the n-HA/PA66 cage group. Similar results were observed for 2-level ACCF, with heights of 71.71±6.16 mm preoperatively improving to 80.04±6.00 mm immediately post-operative in the TMC group, whereas the heights were 70.30±8.08 mm in the n-HA/PA66 group preoperatively and improved to 77.28±7.56 mm immediately postoperative. Preoperative or immediately postoperative fused segment heights did not differ significantly for either 1- or 2-level ACCF between the TMC and n-HA/PA66 groups.

However, the loss in height of the fused segment in the TMC group was greater than that in the n-HA/PA66 group at the one-year follow-up (2.13±0.68 mm vs. 1.18±0.58 mm, $p<0.01$) and at the final follow-up (2.62±0.82 mm vs. 1.56±0.61 mm, $p<0.01$) for the 1-level ACCF, with similar results observed for 2-level ACCF (2.63±0.61 mm vs. 1.57±0.58 mm, $p<0.01$) at the one-year follow-up and (3.05±0.59 mm vs. 1.88±0.57 mm, $p<0.01$) at the final follow-up. The TMC group also showed a significantly greater rate of subsidence for 1-level ACCF than the n-HA/PA66 group at one year (16% vs. 2%; $p = 0.02$) and at the final follow-up (24% vs. 4%; $p = 0.01$). Furthermore, for 2-level ACCF, the TMC group suffered a more marked incidence of subsidence than the n-HA/PA66 group at one year (33% vs. 5%; $p = 0.03$) and at the final follow-up (38% vs. 5%; $p = 0.01$). The majority of cases with cage subsidence showed bony fusion at the final follow-up; moreover, no progression to neurological manifestations arose. No case with subsidence received revisional surgery. Bony fusions of the grafts were similar at the final follow-up, with 96% (24/25) of patients in the TMC group exhibiting them vs. 98% (51/52) in the n-HA/PA66 group for 1-level ACCF, whereas for 2-level ACCF, 95% (20/21) of patients developed bony fusions in the TMC group vs. 95% (18/19) in the n-HA/PA66 group. However, at the one-year follow-up, the TMC group exhibited a lower rate of bony fusion, although not statistically significant, than the n-HA/PA66 group (22/25 (88%) vs. 49/52 (94%) for 1-level ACCF; 16/21 (76%) vs. 17/19 (90%) for 2-level ACCF). No revisional surgery was required for patients who did not exhibit bony fusion at the

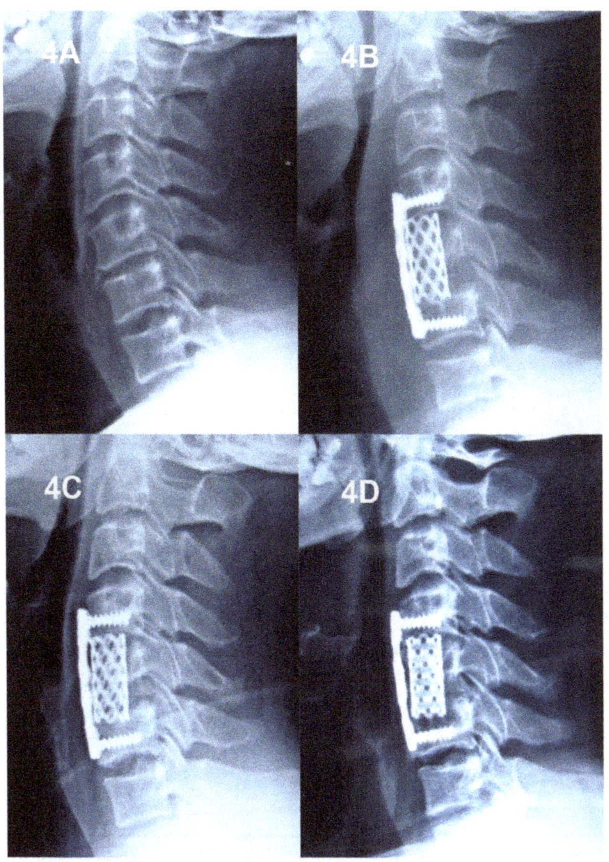

Figure 4. A 53-year-old male who underwent 1-level corpectomy with a titanium mesh cage used for cervical reconstruction. The preoperative cervical X-ray film (4A) and immediately postoperative lateral X-ray (4B) show C5 corpectomy and the titanium mesh cage used for reconstruction. The lateral X-ray one year postoperative (4C) and at the final follow-up (two years and six months; 4D) shows bony fusion between the graft and the adjacent endplates; nevertheless, marked cage subsidence was observed.

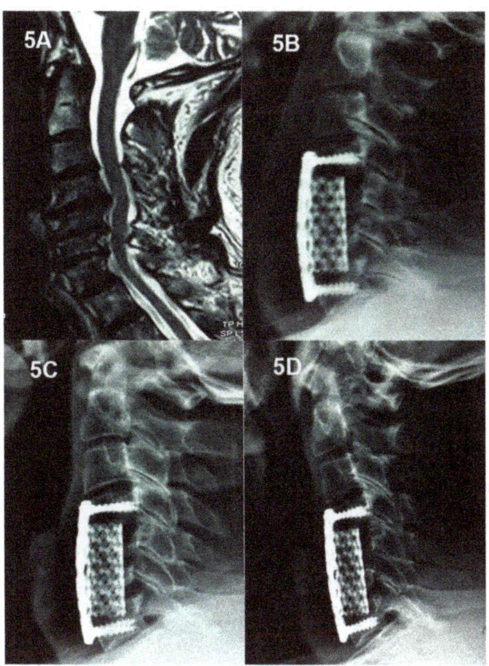

Figure 5. A 46-year-old male who underwent 2-level corpectomy with a titanium mesh cage used for cervical reconstruction. A cervical MRI scan (5A) shows multi-level disc herniations (C4/5, C5/6, C6/7) and oppression of the spinal cord. The immediately postoperative lateral X-ray (5B) shows C5 and C6 corpectomy and the titanium mesh cage used for reconstruction in which the cervical alignment was marginally restored. A lateral X-ray at the one-year follow-up (5C) shows subsidence. A lateral X-ray at the final follow-up (5D) shows increased subsidence and a loss of cervical alignment.

final follow-up because the anterior cervical plate and screws remained in position and the patients did not complain of discomfort. For all four groups, there was a slight improvement in the mean C2–C7 Cobb angle when preoperative values were compared with the final follow-up measurements. When preoperative or final follow-up postoperative measurements were compared, no significant differences were detected in Cobb angle between the TMC and n-HA/PA66 groups either for 1- or 2- level ACCF.

The preoperative JOA scores did not differ between the TMC and n-HA/PA66 groups regardless of the number of levels fused. At the final follow-up, JOA scores had improved significantly in all four groups. No significant differences were detected between the TMC and n-HA/PA66 groups for either 1-or 2-level ACCF at the final follow-up. The mean preoperative VAS score was similar between the two kinds of cage groups for both 1- and 2-level ACCF. However, at the last follow-up, the mean VAS score in the TMC group was higher, albeit insignificantly, than that of the n-HA/PA66 group (1.44 ± 1.08 vs. 1.17 ± 1.25 ($p = 0.42$) for 1-level ACCF; 2.33 ± 1.06 vs. 1.58 ± 1.12 ($p = 0.06$) for 2-level ACCF).

Discussion

In recent years, ACCF has been recognized as a reliable and effective procedure for the treatment of MCSM. The advantage of the direct decompression resulting from the resection of the object causing oppression of the spinal cord from the anterior column is supported by the many reports of successful clinical outcomes in treating MCSM [26,27]. In addition to decompression, reconstruction of the cervical spine is a critical procedure. TMC has been used widely for years. Packed with autogenous graft from the removed vertebra, this apparatus can provide early biomechanical stabilization of the anterior column, restoration and maintenance of the intervertebral height and cervical alignment and enlargement of the stenotic neural foramen and can avoid the potential complications caused by autogenous graft collection [28]. However, implant-related complications cannot be ignored. TMC subsidence, the typical hardware-related complication, has been reported to range from 0% to 30% [29]. Although the relevance of TMC subsidence remains controversial, the subsidence can have serious consequences, such as the buckling of the cervical ligamentum flavum, foraminal stenosis and re-compression of the cervical spinal cord and nerve roots [16,17,28,29].

The n-HA/PA66 is a composite made by infiltrating nano-HA into PA66; it mimics natural bone in that apatite is distributed within a collagen matrix. Thus, the composite possesses both the mechanical strength of HA and the elastic properties of PA66. A previous study documented that the n-HA/PA66 composite was safe and that its mechanical properties complement natural bone well [22]. The n-HA/PA66 cage is a biomimetic implant fabricated from n-HA/PA66 composite. This device has been

Table 1. Demographic and clinical data of patients.

Parameters	1-level ACCF		2-level ACCF	
	TMC	n-HA/PA66 cage	TMC	n-HA/PA66 cage
No.of patients (n)	25	52	21	19
Male/female (n)	11/14	29/23	13/8	12/7
Mean age (years)	55.04±11.09	56.56±12.13	57.81±11.50	57.00±10.95
Hospital stay (days)	16.04±3.67	14.90±3.73	16.76±4.04	15.42±2.39
Surgery time (minutes)	148.40±24.82	143.65±30.50	186.19±28.54	184.74±26.32
Blood loss (ml)	145.20±61.85	133.46±68.57	189.52±90.30	173.68±58.61
Follow-up (months)	49.80±13.06	44.06±13.60	43.42±12.18	44.74±10.33
Involved segments				
1-level corpectomy C4/C5/C6	6/16/3	7/36/9		
2-level corpectomy C4-C5/C5-C6			10/11	11/8

used for spinal reconstruction for several years, and considerable clinical results have been reported [20,21,30]. Our previous research showed a 94.3% bony fusion rate in 35 patients and a 2.9% subsidence rate with n-HA/PA66 cages in reconstructions following cervical corpectomy [20]. Yang et al. [30] reported using n-HA/PA66 cages for anterior reconstruction after thoracolumbar corpectomy in 51 patients and achieved a 90.2% bony fusion rate with a low incidence of cage subsidence. Yang et al. [21] achieved a 97% fusion rate and a 6% subsidence rate in 35 patients with n-HA/PA66 cages for single-level cervical corpectomy and fusion.

Subsidence was typically observed when TMC was used for cervical reconstruction after corpectomy. Daubs et al. [31]

Table 2. Radiographic and clinical outcomes in each group.

Parameter	1-level ACCF			2-level ACCF		
	TMC	n-HA/PA66 cage	P	TMC	n-HA/PA66 cage	P
Height of fused segments (mm)						
Pre-operation	52.03±4.35	53.55±6.20	0.29	71.71±6.16	70.30±8.08	0.52
Immediately post-op	59.52±4.36	61.84±6.86	0.11	80.04±6.00	77.28±7.56	0.21
Loss of height of fused segments (mm)						
One year follow-up	2.13±0.68	1.18±0.58	<0.01	2.63±0.61	1.57±0.58	<0.01
Last follow-up	2.62±0.82	1.56±0.61	<0.01	3.05±0.59	1.88±0.57	<0.01
Fusion rate						
One year follow-up	(22/25) 88%	(49/52) 94%	0.34	(16/21) 76%	(17/19) 90%	0.27
Last follow-up	(24/25) 96%	(51/52) 98%	0.59	(20/21) 95%	(18/19) 95%	0.44
Subsidence rate						
One year follow-up	(4/25)16%	(1/52) 2%	0.02	(7/21) 33%	(1/19) 5%	0.03
Last follow-up	(6/25) 24%	(2/52) 4%	0.01	(8/21) 38%	(1/19) 5%	0.01
C2-C7 Cobb angle (°)						
Pre-op	8.60±5.77	9.69±6.14	0.41	9.33±6.34	9.16±6.81	0.93
Immediately post-op	12.76±5.10	13.15±5.13	0.77	13.10±5.02	13.89±6.39	0.68
Last follow-up	9.96±5.29	10.98±5.20	0.44	9.81±5.81	12.16±6.18	0.23
JOA score (points)						
Pre-operation	12.24±2.18	12.17±2.26	0.87	11.10±2.53	11.63±1.86	0.42
Immediately post-op	14.40±1.63	14.75±1.37	0.41	13.48±2.23	14.26±1.33	0.23
Last follow-up	14.88±1.59	15.37±1.24	0.25	13.76±2.34	14.84±1.83	0.1
VAS of neck pain (points)						
Pre-operation	4.76±1.85	4.37±1.66	0.23	5.14±1.24	5.26±1.59	0.76
Immediately post-op	2.04±1.02	1.85±1.07	0.56	3.00±1.22	2.63±1.16	0.35
Last follow-up	1.44±1.08	1.17±1.25	0.42	2.33±1.06	1.58±1.12	0.06

described an early subsidence in 30% (7 of 27) of cases with ACCF. In our series, by the final follow-up, for 1-level ACCF, we observed that the n-HA/PA66 group exhibited a significantly lower rate of subsidence than the TMC group (4% vs. 24%; $p = 0.01$). Moreover, the difference in subsidence rates was much greater when compared for 2-level ACCF, we observed subsidence in 8 of 21 cases (38%) in the TMC group vs. 1 of 19 cases (5%) in the n-HA/PA66 group ($p = 0.01$). Increased patient age, severe osteoporosis, excessive endplate removal and intra-operative over-distraction have been demonstrated to be risk factors of TMC subsidence [17]. However, the metal attributes and the shape of the TMC are likely the most important factors. The sharp teeth at both ends of the TMC are beneficial to early stabilization by embedding the cage into adjacent endplates. Unfortunately, the contact interface between the TMC and endplates is small (we describe this pattern as a "point-to-surface contact"), and the intensity of pressure at the contact surface is so great that it may result in excessive insertion of the cage into the vertebra. In contrast, the n-HA/PA66 cage has a broader surface at both ends with which to contact the endplates. We describe this pattern as "surface-to-surface contact," and it distributes the loads on the interface and decreases incidences of cage subsidence. Unlike the sharp teeth that the TMC possesses, the n-HA/PA66 cage has grooves at the terminal faces that can increase the friction between the cage and endplates and that is sufficient to prevent cage migration. In our study, even in the case of 2-level ACCF, we did not observe n-HA/PA66 cage migration or extrusion.

Majd ME et al. [32] reported a fusion rate of 97% in cervical reconstructions with TMC, and a fusion rate of 100% was observed by Rieger et al. [33] using the same technique. In our study, for both 1- and 2-level ACCF, the fusion rates in the TMC group and the n-HA/PA66 group were almost equivalent at the final follow-up. However, the n-HA/PA66 group showed higher fusion rates, albeit insignificantly, than the TMC group at the 1-year follow-up (94% vs. 88% ($p = 0.34$) for 1-level ACCF; 90% vs. 76% ($p = 0.27$) for 2-level ACCF). Previous reports have demonstrated that the difference in fusion conditions was primarily due to the different elastic moduli between the two struts [20,22]. Compared with TMC, the n-HA/PA66 cage possesses an elastic modulus similar to that of the autogenous graft inside the cage [22,34]. As described by Wolff's law, bone grows in response to applied stress and is resorbed when mechanical stimulus is absent. Due to the appropriate elastic modulus, n-HA/PA66 cages may reduce stress shielding and promote fusion effectively. In addition, the n-HA/PA66 cage exhibits excellent biocompatibility and osteoconductive ability in vivo. Animal experiments demonstrated that when implanted, the cage can release Ca^{2+} and PO_4^{3-} from its surface, which gradually forms a crystal layer on the cage surface that bridges the graft and implant bed to provide a trestle for osteogenesis [35]. Moreover, the holes in the n-HA/PA66 cage wall may enable blood circulation between the implant bed and the autograft within the cage, which would aid in the growth of the bone graft. Previous studies have reported that subsidence occurs in up to 80% of patients during the early postoperative period prior to bony fusion [36]. In the present study, similar results were observed in all four groups, with the majority of height loss in the fused segment occurring during the 1st postoperative year and heights remaining almost identical to these levels at the final follow-up. Considering the reduced loss of fused segmental height and earlier bony fusion in the n-HA/PA66 group compared with the TMC group, the data indicate that the earlier bony fusion in the n-HA/PA66 group may contribute to the decrease in the loss of fused segmental height. However, the differences in present study are still insignificantly. In the future, larger samples and longer follow-ups should be required to demonstrate this conclusion.

Some studies have demonstrated that the number of corpectomy levels is a risk factor for TMC subsidence. The increase in ACCF levels may eventually cause not only a higher incidence of subsidence but also more severe subsidence when TMC cages are used [31,37]. We observed similar outcomes in our TMC groups. As a result of these published data, previous reports have suggested that 2-level ACCF using TMC cages may not be appropriate therapeutic options for treating MCSM. However, in this study, even for 2-level corpectomy, we observed that the amount of subsidence was much lower in the n-HA/PA66 group compared with the TMC group. Furthermore, we did not observe a high incidence of subsidence. These observations suggest that the n-HA/PA66 cage may provide greater stability than the TMC and may more effectively maintain fused segmental height. The data also indicate that the n-HA/PA66 cage may be a better therapeutic choice for 2-level ACCF.

With the utilization of TMC in cervical reconstruction after corpectomy, restoration of cervical alignment is possible [24]. In the present study, we employed the C2–C7 Cobb angle to evaluate cervical sagittal alignment, the preoperative Cobb angle were similar in four groups, and we observed an improvement in the Cobb angle at the final follow-up compared with preoperative values in all four groups, respectively. There were no significant differences in the Cobb angle at the final follow-up between the TMC and n-HA/PA66 groups in both the 1- and 2-level ACCF; however, we noted that the n-HA/PA66 groups showed little better improvements of C2–C7 Cobb angles. These differences may be due to the greater loss in segmental height when using TMC for cervical reconstructions.

The JOA and VAS scales were used to assess clinical efficacy in our study. We noted improvements in these two parameters in all four groups. At the final follow-up, the mean JOA score was similar between the TMC and n-HA/PA66 groups for both the 1- and 2-level ACCF. However, we observed that the patients in the TMC group presented with higher, albeit non-significant, VAS scores than those in the n-HA/PA66 group, particularly in the 2-level ACCF group. Previous studies [9,31,36,37] showed that subsidence was strongly correlated with neck pain. Although no significant difference was detected in this outcome in our study, these results nevertheless indicate that patients treated with n-HA/PA66 cage for ACCF may suffer less axial neck pain than patients treated with TMC. In our view, the increased loss in segmental height in the TMC group may underlie these differences, and we will pay close attention to this issue in future follow-ups.

Conclusion

This retrospective study demonstrated that both the TMC and n-HA/PA66 cage resulted in effective clinical and radiographic outcomes when used to treat MCSM with cervical reconstruction after corpectomy. However, with its optimized biomechanical characteristics and unique shape, the n-HA/PA66 cage achieves similar bony fusion rates but lower rates of subsidence. Furthermore, even in the case of 2-level ACCF, the n-HA/PA66 cage can maintain fused segment height better and lower incidences of subsidence compared with TMC. The n-HA/PA66 cage may be a better alternative for cervical reconstruction than TMC after corpectomy, particularly for 2-level ACCF.

Author Contributions

Conceived and designed the experiments: YZ ZQ. Performed the experiments: YZ ZQ XL ZZ DJ KT. Analyzed the data: YZ JL XZ ZZ. Contributed reagents/materials/analysis tools: ZQ DJ. Wrote the paper: YZ.

References

1. Lin Q, Zhou X, Wang X, Cao P, Tsai N, et al. (2012) A comparison of anterior cervical discectomy and corpectomy in patients with multilevel cervical spondylotic myelopathy. Eur Spine J 21: 474–481.
2. Song KJ, Lee KB, Song JH (2012) Efficacy of multilevel anterior cervical discectomy and fusion versus corpectomy and fusion for multilevel cervical spondylotic myelopathy: a minimum 5-year follow-up study. Eur Spine J 21: 1551–1557.
3. Edwards CC 2nd, Heller JG, Murakami H (2002) Corpectomy versus laminoplasty for multilevel cervical myelopathy: an independent matched-cohort analysis. Spine (Phila Pa 1976) 27: 1168–1175.
4. Tani T, Ushida T, Ishida K, Iai H, Noguchi T, et al. (2002) Relative safety of anterior microsurgical decompression versus laminoplasty for cervical myelopathy with a massive ossified posterior longitudinal ligament. Spine (Phila Pa 1976) 27: 2491–2498.
5. Lian XF, Xu JG, Zeng BF, Zhou W, Kong WQ, et al. (2010) Noncontiguous anterior decompression and fusion for multilevel cervical spondylotic myelopathy: a prospective randomized control clinical study. Eur Spine J 19: 713–719.
6. Herkowitz HN (1988) A comparison of anterior cervical fusion, cervical laminectomy, and cervical laminoplasty for the surgical management of multiple level spondylotic radiculopathy. Spine (Phila Pa 1976) 13: 774–780.
7. Matz PG, Anderson PA, Groff MW, Heary RF, Holly LT, et al. (2009) Cervical laminoplasty for the treatment of cervical degenerative myelopathy. J Neurosurg Spine 11: 157–169.
8. Lu J, Wu X, Li Y, Kong X (2008) Surgical results of anterior corpectomy in the aged patients.with cervical myelopathy. Eur Spine J 17: 129–135.
9. Dorai Z, Morgan H, Coimbra C (2003) Titanium cage reconstruction after cervical corpectomy. J Neurosurg Spine 99: 3–7.
10. Oh MC, Zhang HY, Park JY, Kim KS (2009) Two-level anterior cervical discectomy versus one-level corpectomy in cervical spondylotic myelopathy. Spine (Phila Pa 1976) 34: 692–696.
11. Hilibrand AS, Fye MA, Emery SE, Palumbo MA, Bohlman HH (2002) Increased rate of arthrodesis with strut grafting after multilevel anterior cervical decompression. Spine (Phila Pa 1976) 27: 146–151.
12. Wittenberg RH, Moeller J, Shea M, White AA 3rd, Hayes WC (1990) Compressive strength of autologous and allogenous bone grafts for thoracolumbar and cervical spine fusion. Spine (Phila Pa 1976) 15: 1073–1078.
13. Kotil K, Tari R (2011) Two level cervical corpectomy with iliac crest fusion and rigid plate fixation: a retrospective study with a three-year follow-up. Turk Neurosurg 21: 606–612.
14. Kinoshita A, Kataoka K, Taneda M (1999) Multilevel vertebral body replacement with a titanium mesh spacer for aneurysmal bone cyst: technical note. Minim Invasive Neurosurg 42: 156–158.
15. Yan D, Wang Z, Deng S, Li J, Soo C (2011) Anterior corpectomy and reconstruction with titanium mesh cage and dynamic cervical plate forcervical spondylotic myelopathy in elderly osteoporosis patients. Arch Orthop Trauma Surg 131:1369–1374.
16. Hee HT, Madj ME, Holt RT, Whitecloud TS 3rd, Pienkowski D (2003) Complications of multilevel cervical corpectomies and reconstruction with titanium cages and anterior plating. J Spinal Disord 16: 1–8.
17. Lim TH, Kwon H, Jeon CH, Kim JG, Sokolowski M, Natarajan R, et al. (2001) Effect of endplate conditions and bone mineral density on the compressive strength of the graft-endplate interface in anterior cervical spine fusion. Spine (Phila Pa 1976) 26: 951–956.
18. Lee SH, Sung JK (2008) Anterior cervical stabilization using a semi-constrained cervical plate and titanium. J Clin Neurosci 15: 1227–1234.
19. Ying Z, Xinwei W, Jing Z, Shengming X, Bitao L, et al. (2007) Cervical corpectomy with preserved posterior vertebral wall for cervical spondylotic myelopathy: a randomized control clinical study. Spine (Phila Pa 1976) 32: 1482–1487.
20. Zhao Z, Jiang D, Ou Y, Tang K, Luo X, et al. (2012) A hollow cylindrical nanohydroxyapatite/polyamide composite strut for cervical reconstruction after cervical corpectomy. J Clin Neurosci 19: 536–540.
21. Yang X, Chen Q, Liu L, Song Y, Kong Q, et al. (2013) Comparison of anterior cervical fusion by titanium mesh cage versus nano-hydroxyapatite/polyamide cage following single-level corpectomy. Int Orthop 37: 2421–2427.
22. Wang X, Li Y, Wei J, de Groot K (2002) Development of biomimetic nano-hydroxyapatite/poly(hexamethylene adipamide) composites. Biomaterials 23: 4787–4791.
23. Gercek E, Arlet V, Delisle J, Marchesi D (2003) Subsidence of stand-alone cervical cages in anterior interbody fusion: warning. Eur Spine J 12: 513–516.
24. Andaluz N, Zuccarello M, Kuntz C (2012) Long-term follow-up of cervical radiographic sagittal spinal alignment after 1- and 2-level cervical corpectomy for the treatment of spondylosis of the subaxial cervical spine causing radiculomyelopathy or myelopathy: a retrospective study. J Neurosurg Spine 16: 2–7.
25. Liu Y, Qi M, Chen H, Yang L, Wang X, et al. (2012) Comparative analysis of complications of different reconstructive techniques following anterior decompression for multilevel cervical spondylotic myelopathy. Eur Spine J 21: 2428–2435.
26. Kirkpatric JS, Levy JA, Carillo J, Moeini SR (1999) Reconstruction after multilevel corpectomy in the cervical spine. A sagittal plane biomechanical study. Spine (Phila Pa 1976) 24: 1186–1191.
27. Sevki K, Mehmet T, Ufuk T, Azmi H, Mercan S, et al. (2004) Results of surgical treatment for degenerative cervical myelopathy: anterior cervical corpectomy and stabilization. Spine (Phila Pa 1976) 29: 2493–2500.
28. Chibbaro S, Benvenuti L, Carnesecchi S, Marsella M, Pulera F, et al. (2006) Anterior cervical corpectomy for cervical spondylotic myelopathy: experience and surgical results in a series of 70 consecutive patients. J Clin Neurosci 13: 233–238.
29. Bilbao G, Duart M, Aurrecoechea JJ, Pomposo I, Igartua A, et al. (2010) Surgical results and complications in a series of 71 consecutive cervical spondylotic corpectomies. Acta Neurochir (Wien) 152: 1155–1163.
30. Yang X, Song Y, Liu L, Liu H, Zeng J, et al. (2012) Anterior reconstruction with nano-hydroxyapatite/polyamide-66 cage after thoracic and lumbar corpectomy. Orthopedics 35: e66–73.
31. Daubs MD (2005) Early failures following cervical corpectomy reconstruction with titanium mesh cages and anterior plating. Spine (Phila Pa 1976) 30: 1402–1406.
32. Majd ME, Vadhva M, Holt RT (1999) Anterior cervical reconstruction using titanium cages with anterior plating. Spine (Phila Pa 1976) 24: 1604–1610.
33. Rieger A, Holz C, Marx T, Sanchin L, Menzel M (2003) Vertebral autograft used as bone transplant for anterior cervical corpectomy: technical note. Neurosurgery 52: 449–453.
34. HuangM, Feng J, Wang J, Zhang X, Li Y, et al. (2003) Synthesis and characterization of nano-HA/PA66 composites. J Mater Sci Mater Med 14: 655–660.
35. Xu Q, Lu H, Zhang J, Li G, Deng Z, et al. (2010) Tissue engineering scaffold material of porous nanohydroxyapatite/polyamide66. Int J Nanomedicine 13: 331–5.
36. Fengbin Y, Jinhao M, Xinyuan L, Xinwei W, Yu C, et al. (2013) Evaluation of a new type of titanium mesh cage versus the traditional titanium mesh cage for single-level, anterior cervical corpectomy and fusion. Eur Spine J 22: 2891–2896.
37. Chen Y, Chen D, Guo Y, Wang X, Lu X, et al. (2008) Subsidence of titanium mesh cage: a study based on 300 cases. J Spinal Disord Tech 21:489–492.

4

Pure Laparoscopic and Robot-Assisted Laparoscopic Reconstructive Surgery in Congenital Megaureter: A Single Institution Experience

Weijun Fu[1*], Xu Zhang[1*], Xiaoyi Zhang[2], Peng Zhang[1], Jiangping Gao[1], Jun Dong[1], Guangfu Chen[1], Axiang Xu[1], Xin Ma[1], Hongzhao Li[1], Lixin Shi[1]

1 Department of Urology, PLA General Hospital/Medical school, Beijing, China, **2** Department of Urology, The Second Artillery General Hospital of PLA, Beijing, China

Abstract

To report our experience of pure laparoscopic and robot-assisted laparoscopic reconstructive surgery in congenital megaureter, seven patients (one bilateral) with symptomatic congenital megaureter underwent pure laparoscopic or robot-assisted laparoscopic surgery. The megaureter was exposed at the level of the blood vessel and was isolated to the bladder narrow area. Extreme ureter trim and submucosal tunnel encapsulation or papillary implantations and anti-reflux ureter bladder anastomosis were performed intraperitoneally by pure laparoscopic or robot-assisted laparoscopic surgery. The clinical data of seven patients after operation were analyzed, including the operation time, intraoperative complications, intraoperative bleeding volumes, postoperative complications, postoperative hospitalization time and pathological results. All of the patients were followed. The operation was successfully performed in seven patients. The mean operation times for pure laparoscopic surgery and robotic-assistant laparoscopic surgery were 175 (range: 150–220) and 187 (range: 170–205) min, respectively, and the mean operative blood loss volumes were 20 (range: 10–30) and 28.75 (range: 15–20) ml, respectively. There were no intraoperative complications. The postoperative drainage time was 5 (range: 4–6) and 5.75 (range: 5–6) d, respectively, and the indwelling catheter time was 6.33 (range: 4–8) d and 7 (range: 7–7) d, respectively. The postoperative hospitalization time was 7.67 (range: 7–8) d and 8 (range: 7–10) d, respectively. There was no obvious pain, no secondary bleeding and no urine leakage after the operation. Postoperative pathology reports revealed chronic urothelial mucosa inflammation. The follow-up results confirmed that all patients were relieved of their symptoms. Both pure laparoscopic and robot-assisted laparoscopic surgery using different anti-reflux ureter bladder anastomoses are safe and effective approaches in the minimally invasive treatment of congenital megaureter.

Editor: Lorna Marson, Centre for Inflammation Research, United Kingdom

Funding: This work was supported by the National High Technology Research and Development Program ("863"Program) of China (NO. 2012AA021100). The funder had no role in study design, data collection and analysis, decision to publish, or preparation of the manuscript.

Competing Interests: The authors have declared that no competing interests exist.

* E-mail: fuweijun68@hotmail.com (WF); xuzhang@foxmail.com (XZ)

These authors contributed equally to this work.

Introduction

Congenital megaureter is a rare adult urinary tract anomaly that is due to distal ureteral muscle abnormalities, the loss of peristalsis from the vesicoureteral connection and vesicoureteral obstruction. Therefore, excision of the diseased segment plus with reimplantation of the distal ureter is often required.[1] Traditionally, open ureteral reparation and reimplantation is the gold standard therapy for primary symptomatic obstructive megaureter. Within the past decade, however, laparoscopic surgery has become popular in urology and has resulted in improved outcomes compared with open surgery, even in reconstruction procedures.[2] Today, the Da Vinci robot-assisted laparoscopic surgery platform (Intuitive Surgical, Sunnyvale, CA), which is characterized by stereoscopic vision and a flexible operating arm, provides us with the distinct advantages of minimally invasive reconstruction of the urinary tract, particularly in intracorporeal reparation and suturing. Particularly, for lower urinary tract reconstruction surgery, which is likely to be delayed by the narrow pelvic space, the robot-assisted laparoscopic surgery platform can be advantageous.[3] Here, we present our experience in the treatment of primary symptomatic obstructive megaureter by intracorporeal ureteral reparation, suturing and different anti-reflux methods using traditional pure laparoscopic surgery and robot-assisted laparoscopic surgery. To the best of our knowledge, this is the first time that ureteroneocystostomy has been reported to be performed by pure robotic repair followed by different anti-reflux strategies with a reasonable follow-up time.

Materials and Methods

The study was reviewed and approved by an institutional review board (IRB) of the Chinese PLA Medical School. Written informed consent was obtained from all participants before the initiation of study procedures. The stored specimen and database analysis was approved by the IRB and ethics committee at Chinese PLA Medical School.

We retrospectively reviewed seven patients (one of these patients exhibited bilateral megaureters) undergoing traditional pure laparoscopic surgery or robot-assisted laparoscopic surgery for primary symptomatic obstructive megaureter from December 2009 to August 2013 at PLA General Hospital (Beijing, China) (**Table 1**). There were two male patients and five female patients with a mean age of 28.14 years. All patients were evaluated by urinalysis, urine culture and assays of serum urea and creatinine levels as well as by imaging with ultrasonography, intravenous urography, computed tomography and emission computer tomography (ECT) renography. All surgeries were performed by experienced surgeons. (**Figure 1**)

For traditional pure laparoscopic surgery, the patient was placed in a supine position. The primary 10-mm port for the camera was placed along the lower lip of the umbilicus in the midline, and 2 secondary ports (5 mm and 12 mm) were placed in the mid clavicular lines on either side 2 fingers lower than the camera port. An additional 5 port mm for the assistant was placed 2 cm above the iliac crest if necessary.

For robot-assisted laparoscopic surgery, a low dorsal lithotomy with a steep Trendelenburg position was used. Trocar placement was distributed to 5 points. A 12 mm port for the camera was placed three fingers superior to the umbilicus. Two 8-mm robotic ports for arm 1 and 2 were placed 8 cm lateral to umbilicus. A port for arm 3 was placed 8 cm contralaterally parallel to arm 1 or 2. An additional 12-mm port for the assistant was placed in the anterior axillary line 2 cm above the iliac crest on the ipsilateral surgical side of the ureter.

Monopolar scissors and bipolar grasping forceps were used to cut the Toldt line. The colon was reflected medially to expose the megaureter at the bifurcation of the common iliac vessels. The reproductive vessels were protected, and the megaureter was gently grasped with a latex band by robotic arm 3. The megaureter was isolated down to the distal ureteral stricture segment with attention to the preservation of the ureteral adventitia. The bladder was then filled with 150 ml normal saline and isolated fully along the Retzius space. The lateral top of the free bladder was fixed to the on psoas muscle by suturing, if necessary.

The ureter was partially amputated at the junction of the stricture and the dilated section of the ureter. To facilitated trimming and suturing, the ureter was drafted by a rubber belt or robot arm 3. The ureter was longitudinally sharply incised in a 3–4 cm extension over a 7-Fr plastic urethral catheter and, for heavy dilated in megaureter, intracorporeally tailored using a 4-zero absorbed polyglactin running suture. The ureteral stricture specimen was mobilized and excised for histopathological examination.

We applied two methods to achieve anti-reflux, submucosal tunnel reimplantation or ureteral nipple implantation according to the degree of dilated in megaureter of patients to avoid the post-operative stricture. For those seriously dilated megaureter we chose ureteral nipple implantation; however, for those slightly dilated megaureter we chose submucosal tunnel reimplantation. For submucosal tunnel reimplantation, the bladder was filled with normal saline and longitudinally opened in the posterolateral aspect to expose the mucosa of the bladder. A submucosal tunnel was created with blunt dissection at the lowest part of the bladder with a ratio of 5:1 between the tunnel length and the diameter of the ureteral orifice. The ureter was positioned through the submucosal tunnel and a mucosa-to-mucosa ureterovesical anastomosis was completed with 4-zero absorbed polyglactin interrupted sutures. During this procedure, a 7Fr double J stent was passed into the ureter and advanced to the renal pelvis, and its

Table 1. Patient general information.

Patient	Sex	Age	Magaureter Side	Method	Operating Time(min)	Bleeding (mL)	Follow-up Time (mo)	Result
1	F	24	Right	Laparoscopic	150	10	46	Relieved
2	M	20	Left	Laparoscopic	155	20	38	Relieved
3	F	37	Bilateral	Laparoscopic/Right	220	30	17	Relieved/Right
				Laparoscopic/Left				Relieved/Left
4	M	25	Left	Robot-assisted	190	20	3	Relieved
5	F	35	Left	Robot-assisted	170	15	57	Relieved
6	F	32	Left	Robot-assisted	205	30	4	Relieved
7	F	24	Left	Robot-assisted	185	50	3	Relieved

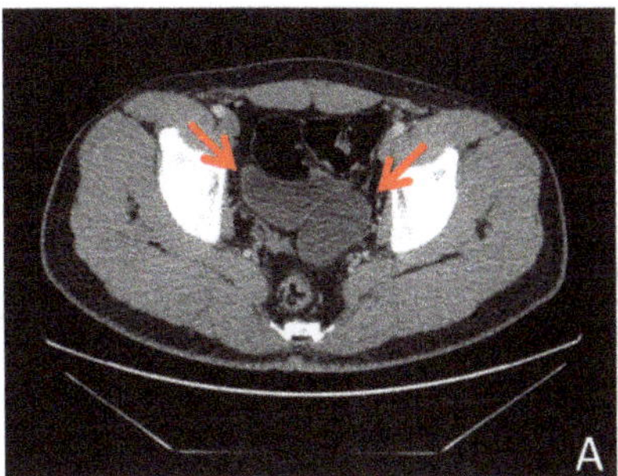
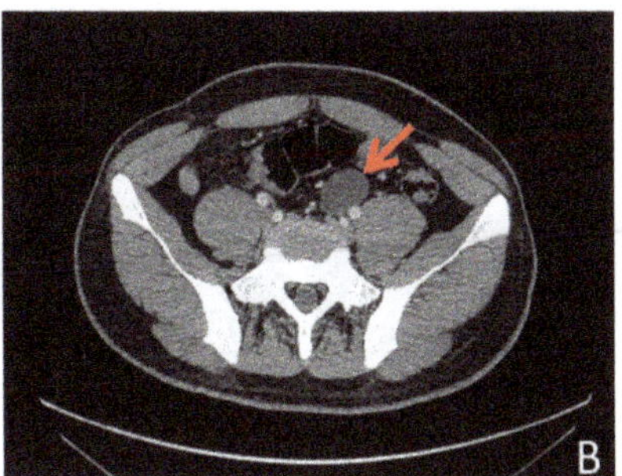

Figure 1. Preoperative CT scan of two patients. (A) The megaureter and bladder could be identified by CT scan. (B) The megaureter could be identified by CT scan.

distal end was fixed in the bladder. Subsequently, a running single layer suture with 2-zero polyglactin closed the bladder muscle. For this method, the ureter was covered with bladder detrusor muscle by suturing to form an anti-reflux submucosal tunnel (**Figure 2 A–C**).

For ureteral nipple implantation, the distal ureter was tailored and formed into a nipple structure. Subsequently, the bladder detrusor and mucosa were dissected laterally. At the position 6 o'clock to the anastomotic stoma, the bladder was sutured full-thickness with the seromuscular layer to the ureter at a distance of 1.5 cm to the end. Subsequently, a 7-Fr double J stent was indwelled. After the fixation at 12 o'clock position of the anastomotic stoma, an additional 4 interrupted sutures were performed bilaterally to complete the anastomosis (**Figure 2 D–F**, **Figure 3**).

A 14-Fr Nelaton drain was indwelled within the 5-mm port. Intravenous pyelography for the evaluation of residual obstruction and voiding cystourethrography for the evaluation of residual vesicoureteral reflux were performed postoperatively in all of the patients. Urinalysis, urine culture, assays of serum urea and creatinine levels and renal ultrasonography were also performed to evaluate renal function after the operation. The 7-Fr double J stent placed in operation was removed 4 weeks after operation by cystoscope.

Results

All of the operations were successfully completed. The mean operation time of pure laparoscopic surgery and robotic-assisted laparoscopic surgery were 175 (range: 150–220) min and 187 (range: 170–205) min, with an average intraoperative estimated blood loss of 20 (range: 10–30) ml and 28.75 (range: 15–20) ml, respectively. No major complications occurred during the two surgeries. Drainage times were 5 (range: 4–6) d and 5.75 (range: 5–6) d, respectively, and indwelling catheter times were 6.33 (range: 4–8) d and 7 (range: 7–7) d, respectively. The mean lengths of the postoperative hospital stay were 7.67 (range: 7–8) d and 8 (range: 7–10) d for the two groups, respectively. No significant postoperative pain, secondary bleeding, incontinence or other complications were observed after the operation. Histopathological reports for all of the patients revealed chronic inflammation of the urothelial mucosa (**Figure 4**). The double J ureteral stent was removed at 4 weeks after the operation.

The mean follow-up was 24 (range: 3–57) months. All patients experienced symptomatic relief. Follow-up ultrasonography and intravenous urography confirmed good drainage combined with a reduction of hydronephrosis. A statistically significant reduction was also achieved in the follow-up ureteral diameter compared with the preoperative ureteral diameter (**Figure 5**). The function of the salvaged kidney was preserved when compared with preoperative function. Nonobstructed clearance was also documented on diuretic renogram in all patients. The results retrograde cystogram also ensured that both of our two anti-reflux anastomses methods for reimplantation gained approving results. (Table 1).

Discussion

Congenital megaureter is caused by a short or absent intravesical ureter, congenital para-ureteric diverticulum or other derangements of the vesico-ureteric junction (VUJ). According to the international classification, congenital megaureter can be classified as obstructed, refluxing or unobstructed and unrefluxing.[1] Congenital megaureter is most frequently observed in males of 30–40 years old. Most patients report lower back pain, and 1/3 present with stones. For clinical treatment, surgery of megaureter tailoring plus ureteroneocystostomy is recommended.[4]

Patients with congenital megaureter can undergo a variety of surgical treatment, including endoincision with stent indwelling, trimmed or not trimmed VUJ anastomosis or nephroureterectomy, on the basis of the ureter state and residual renal function. In situations of competent renal function, one commonly used surgical approach is to remove the non-functioning ureter followed by distal ureter bladder anastomosis. With traditional technical limitations, the open space of the narrow pelvis must be exposed during surgery, which requires for a large abdominal incision. This approach leads to increased complications and delayed postoperative recovery.[5]

To reduce complications and shorten recovery time, minimally invasive surgery, including endoscopic incision and laparoscopic ureteral reimplantation, has been proposed in recent years. Although transurethral endoscopic laser or electronic ureteral resection provided good short-term results, further observation of its long-term effects are needed. [6,7] In recent years, laparoscopic ureteral reimplantation has been widely recommended in the treatment of congenital megaureter as a minimally invasive therapy. Pure laparoscopic reconstructive surgery requires extensive experience in laparoscopic surgery. Even for skilled surgeon, pure laparoscopic reconstructive surgery is a challenging technique.

The robot-assisted laparoscopic platform provides a new opportunity for complex urinary tract reconstruction surgery. The use of this approach in upper urinary tract reconstruction surgery has been widely reported and has proven to exhibit good

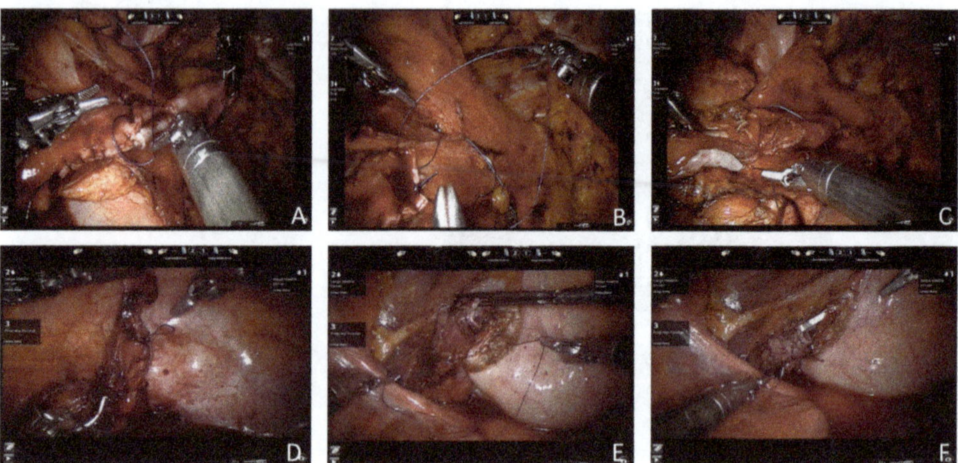

Figure 2. Robot-assisted laparoscopic surgery in congenital megaureter (A–C,submucosal tunnel reimplantation; D–E, direct ureteral nipple implantation). (A) The megaureter was intracorporeally tailored using a 4-zero absorbed polyglactin running suture. (B) The ureter was positioned through the submucosal tunnel and a mucosa-to-mucosa ureterovesical anastomosis was completed with 4-zero absorbed polyglactin interrupted sutures. (C) A running single layer suture with 2-zero polyglactin closed the bladder muscle. (D) The distal ureter was tailored and formed into a nipple. (E) The bladder was sutured full-thickness with the seromuscular layer to the ureter at a distance of 1.5 cm to the end at the 6 o'clock position to the anastomotic stoma. (F) After the fixation 4 interrupted sutures were made bilaterally to complete the anastomosis at the 12 o'clock position.

long-term results.[8] Robot-assisted laparoscopic ureteral reimplantation, vesico-ureteric anastomosis, psoas muscle fixation and bladder valvuloplasty have also been reported, which have provided us with new approaches to the minimally invasive treatment of distal ureteral reconstruction.[9,10] The robot-assisted surgery system has better dimensional vision and a more flexible operating arm and is therefore more suitable for narrow space reconstruction surgery.[11] In the lower urinary tract (lower ureter, the bladder and prostate) robot-assisted laparoscopic surgery, patients are placed in the low lithotomy position to facilitate the placement of the robot arm. Trocar placement for distal ureteral operations aims to provide the best operating space in the pelvic. During our surgery, robot arm 3 was used to hold the tissue dynamically. These alterations provide advantages by narrowing the necessary operating compared with pure laparoscopic surgeries.

In our single-institution study, we applied both pure laparoscopic and robot-assisted laparoscopic surgeries to patients with primary symptomatic obstructive megaureter. In both approaches, we tailored and sutured the megaureter intracorporeally to reduce the invasion of the ureter. In addition, we applied the vesico-ureteric anastomosis using two different methods, submucosal tunnel reimplantation or ureteral nipple implantation, to achieve an anti-reflux effect. To our knowledge, ureteral nipple implantation is not conventional according to the previous reports.

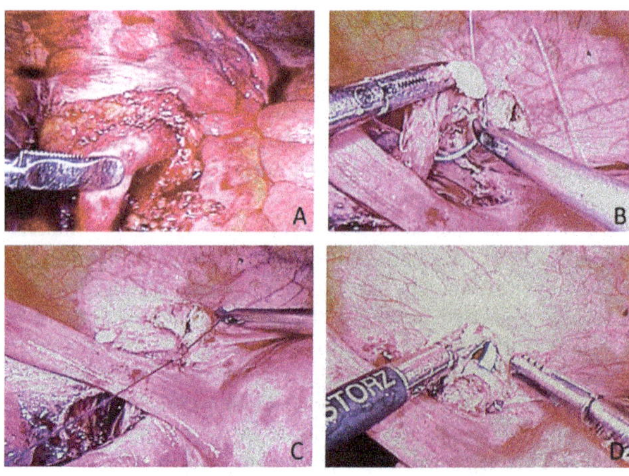

Figure 3. Pure laparoscopic surgery in congenital megaureter. (A) The megaureter was exposed at the bifurcation of the common iliac vessels. (B–C) The bladder was sutured full-thickness with the seromuscular layer to the ureter at a distance of 1.5 cm to the 6 o'clock position to the anastomotic stoma. (D) A 7-Fr double J stent was indwelled.

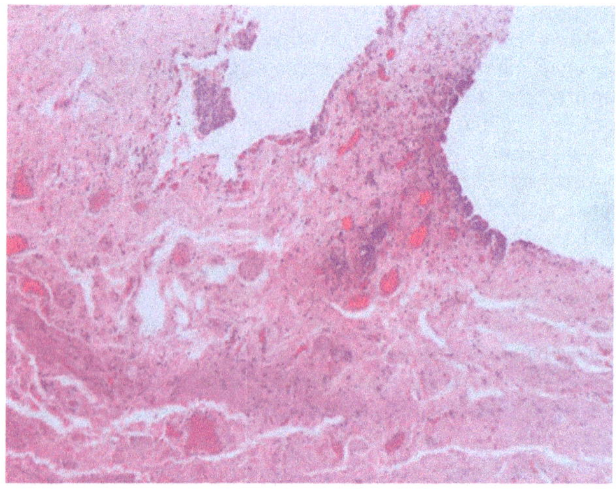

Figure 4. Histopathological reports for all the patients revealed chronic inflammation of the urothelial mucosa.

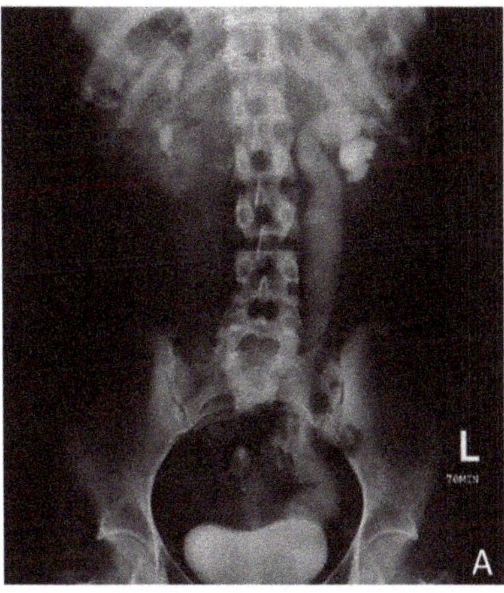

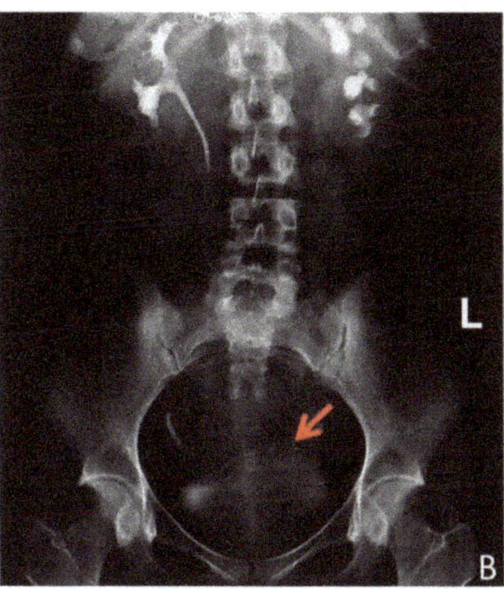

Figure 5. Preoperative and postoperative intravenous pyelography of one patient. (A) Preoperative intravenous pyelography of one megaureter patient. (B) Forty-months postoperative intravenous pyelography of one megaureter patient. The megaureter and hydronephrosis were relieved. The appearance of a filling defect due to the left nipple was identified.

[12,13] Al-Shukri and Alwan first reported direct nipple ureteroneocystostomy in patients with ureteral stricture.[14] Here, we approved several cases of ureteral nipple implantation, including pure laparoscopic and robot-assisted laparoscopic surgery. In both pure laparoscopic and robot-assisted laparoscopic surgery, we perform direct nipple ureteroneocystostomy by suturing the bladder full-thickness with the seromuscular layer of the ureter at a distance of 1.5 cm to the end at the 6 and 12 o'clock positions of the anastomotic stoma. Subsequently, 4 additional interrupted sutures are made bilaterally to complete the anastomosis. During this procedure, the double J stent is placed. According to the postoperative examinations, the anti-reflux effect of this strategy has demonstrated that it is a simple, safe and feasible means of vesico-ureteric anastomosis. In particular, the ureteral nipple implantation shortens the operative time.

These groups of patients in our center have been treated with pure laparoscopic surgery or robotic-assisted laparoscopic surgery. Both approaches have reasonable and similar operating times and blood loss, but robotic ureteroneocystostomy is easier and takes less time than pure laparoscopic ureteroneocystostomy. However, robotic surgery is new to China, and with the accumulation of experiences, the operation time will be shortened further in the future. There were no major complications occurred during or after the operations. The drainage time, indwelling catheter times and postoperative hospital stays were similar for both the pure laparoscopic and robot-assisted laparoscopic surgeries. According to our latest follow-up, all of the patients were symptomatically recovered. Hydronephrosis in 8 megaureters of 7 patients was relieved as confirmed by postoperative examinations. The results of the follow-up have demonstrated that the salvaged kidneys well drained and resolved of hydronephrosis, and their functions were preserved when compared with the preoperative examinations.

Conclusion

In summary, both pure laparoscopic and robot-assisted laparoscopic surgery for megaureter are technically feasible and safe. However, in our study, the number of cases is insufficient, and the follow-up time is short for some of the cases. More experience in robot-assisted laparoscopic surgery should be accumulated in future work. In the future, more clinical data are required to prove the convenience of robot-assisted laparoscopic surgery in complex genitourinary reconstructive operations.

Acknowledgments

The authors would like to thank Professors Xu Zhang (Department of Urology, PLA General Hospital) for his support, helpful advice and many valuable scientific discussions throughout the project.

Author Contributions

Conceived and designed the experiments: WJF XZ XYZ. Performed the experiments: WJF XZ XYZ PZ JPG JD GFC. Analyzed the data: AXX XM HZL LXS. Contributed reagents/materials/analysis tools: WJF XZ XYZ PZ JPG. Wrote the paper: WJF XZ XYZ PZ.

References

1. Shokeir AA, Nijman RJ (2000) Primary megaureter: current trends in diagnosis and treatment. BJU Int 86: 861–868.
2. Abraham GP, Das K, Ramaswami K, Siddaiah AT, George D, et al. (2012) Laparoscopic reconstruction for obstructive megaureter: single institution experience with short- and intermediate-term outcomes. J Endourol 26: 1187–1191.
3. Hemal AK, Nayyar R, Rao R (2009) Robotic repair of primary symptomatic obstructive megaureter with intracorporeal or extracorporeal ureteric tapering and ureteroneocystostomy. J Endourol 23: 2041–2046.
4. Hemal AK, Ansari MS, Doddamani D, Gupta NP (2003) Symptomatic and complicated adult and adolescent primary obstructive megaureter-indications for surgery: Analysis, outcome, and follow-up. Urology 61: 703–707.
5. Dorairajan LN, Hemal AK, Gupta NP, Wadhwa SN (1999) Primary obstructive megaureter in adults: need for an aggressive management strategy. Int Urol Nephrol 31: 633–641.
6. Bapat S, Bapat M, Kirpekar D (2000) Endoureterotomy for congenital primary obstructive megaureter: preliminary report. J Endourol 14: 263–267.
7. Biyani CS, Powell CS (2001) Congenital megaureter in adults: Endoscopic management with holmium: YAG laser - Preliminary experience. Journal of Endourology 15: 797–799.
8. Mufarrij PW, Woods M, Shah OD, Palese MA, Berger AD, et al. (2008) Robotic dismembered pyeloplasty: a 6-year, multi-institutional experience. J Urol 180: 1391–1396.
9. Patil NN, Mottrie A, Sundaram B, Patel VR (2008) Robotic-assisted laparoscopic ureteral reimplantation with psoas hitch: a multi-institutional, multinational evaluation. Urology 72: 47–50; discussion 50.

10. Thiel DD, Badger WJ, Winfield HN (2008) Robot-Assisted Laparoscopic Excision and Ureteroureterostomy for Congenital Midureteral Stricture. Journal of Endourology 22: 2667–2669.
11. Schimpf MO, Wagner JR (2009) Robot-Assisted Laparoscopic Distal Ureteral Surgery. Jsls-Journal of the Society of Laparoendoscopic Surgeons 13: 44–49.
12. Tatlisen A, Ekmekcioglu O (2005) Direct nipple ureteroneocystostomy in adults with primary obstructed megaureter. J Urol 173: 877–880.
13. Chung H, Jeong BC, Kim HH (2006) Laparoscopic ureteroneocystostomy with vesicopsoas hitch: nonrefluxing ureteral reimplantation using cystoscopy-assisted submucosal tunneling. J Endourol 20: 632–638.
14. Al-Shukri S, Alwan MH (1983) Bilharzial strictures of the lower third of the ureter: a critical review of 560 strictures. Br J Urol 55: 477–482.

5

Effect of Storage Temperature on Cultured Epidermal Cell Sheets Stored in Xenobiotic-Free Medium

Catherine Jackson[1,2]*, Peder Aabel[3,4], Jon R. Eidet[1], Edward B. Messelt[5], Torstein Lyberg[1], Magnus von Unge[3,4,6], Tor P. Utheim[1,5]

1 Department of Medical Biochemistry, Oslo University Hospital, Oslo, Norway, **2** University of Oslo, Oslo, Norway, **3** Ear, Nose and Throat Department, Division of Surgery, Akershus University Hospital, Lørenskog, Norway, **4** Institute of Clinical Medicine, University of Oslo, Oslo, Norway, **5** Department of Oral Biology, Faculty of Dentistry, University of Oslo, Oslo, Norway, **6** Centre for Clinical Research, LT Vastmanland, Uppsala University, Uppsala, Sweden

Abstract

Cultured epidermal cell sheets (CECS) are used in regenerative medicine in patients with burns, and have potential to treat limbal stem cell deficiency (LSCD), as demonstrated in animal models. Despite widespread use, short-term storage options for CECS are limited. Advantages of storage include: flexibility in scheduling surgery, reserve sheets for repeat operations, more opportunity for quality control, and improved transportation to allow wider distribution. Studies on storage of CECS have thus far focused on cryopreservation, whereas refrigeration is a convenient method commonly used for whole skin graft storage in burns clinics. It has been shown that preservation of viable cells using these methods is variable. This study evaluated the effect of different temperatures spanning 4°C to 37°C, on the cell viability, morphology, proliferation and metabolic status of CECS stored over a two week period in a xenobiotic-free system. Compared to non-stored control, best cell viability was obtained at 24°C (95.2±9.9%); reduced cell viability, at approximately 60%, was demonstrated at several of the temperatures (12°C, 28°C, 32°C and 37°C). Metabolic activity was significantly higher between 24°C and 37°C, where glucose, lactate, lactate/glucose ratios, and oxygen tension indicated increased activation of the glycolytic pathway under aerobic conditions. Preservation of morphology as shown by phase contrast and scanning electron micrographs was best at 12°C and 16°C. PCNA immunocytochemistry indicated that only 12°C and 20°C allowed maintenance of proliferative function at a similar level to non-stored control. In conclusion, results indicate that 12°C and 24°C merit further investigation as the prospective optimum temperature for short-term storage of cultured epidermal cell sheets.

Editor: Majlinda Lako, University of Newcastle upon Tyne, United Kingdom

Funding: Funding was provided by (1) South East Norway Regional Health Authority, Norway, grant number 2012074 (http://www.helse-sorost.no/omoss_/english_/) to CJ, and (2) University of Oslo, Norway. The funders had no role in study design, data collection and analysis, decision to publish, or preparation of the manuscript.

Competing Interests: The authors have declared that no competing interests exist.

* Email: catherinejoanjackson@gmail.com

Introduction

Preparation of cultured epithelial cell sheets (CECS) for clinical use requires a high level of expertise and specialized facilities. Tissue generation laboratories are subject to high safety and quality standards [1]. These conditions represent a barrier to the widespread use of CECS while demand is anticipated to increase as a result of research and clinical success [2]. Development of a reliable storage option for cultured cells would enable wider distribution from centralized laboratories to clinics worldwide [3]. In addition, a storage interval provides increased opportunity for quality control [4]. Current methods employed in the storage of epidermal cells include refrigeration of whole skin grafts and cryopreservation of cultured epithelial cell sheets (CECS). Poor viability (reduction to 50% within three days of storage), has been shown following refrigeration (4°C) of whole skin grafts in saline, which is the most common method of storage used in burns units according to a recent survey [5]. While some cryopreservation studies have shown relatively good cell viability [6], there are several examples of disintegration and unusable CECS architecture [7], as well as low cell viability using this method [8–10]. Moreover, it has been shown that cryopreserved skin must be used within two days upon thawing, as cell viability rapidly diminishes [11]. These disadvantages, coupled with the need for complicated freeze/thaw schedules and specialized equipment, makes reliable storage of CECS at above-freezing temperatures a promising alternative.

The treatment of large area burns and limbal stem cell deficiency (LSCD) are two applications that would especially benefit from the development of short-term storage by providing improved access and an extended interval for quality control. In the treatment of burns, a small biopsy taken from intact skin can be expanded to produce enough CECS to cover an adult body within three or four weeks [2]. Use of CECS is especially suitable when extensive injury does not allow the use of split-skin grafts. A reliable and convenient storage option would aid in flexible scheduling of surgery with respect to patient readiness, and provide reserve sheets for repeat operations within a certain interval, benefits that are particularly relevant to burns units when working with unstable patients [12].

LSCD is a painful disease caused by loss or damage to stem cells located at the periphery of the cornea, the limbus. Defects in the corneal epithelium and loss of vision may significantly reduce quality of life [13]. In 1997 Pellegrini *et al.* demonstrated that a small limbal biopsy taken from the patients' contralateral healthy eye could be cultured *in vitro* to provide an epithelial cell sheet for treatment of LSCD [14]. Almost 1000 cases of treatment using CECS have since been documented, with an overall success rate of approximately 75% [15].

With the goals of minimizing risk of damage to the healthy, or less damaged eye, and reducing exposure to immunosuppressive drugs, the use of an alternative autologous cell source holds great potential. Initial animal and human studies using alternative cell types have shown promising results. Examples include the use of cultured epidermal keratinocytes to treat damaged cornea in goat [15–17]. To date only cultured oral mucosa cells [18], cultured conjunctiva cells [19], and limbal cells [20] have been used successfully in the treatment of LSCD in humans. However, the abundance, ease of availability, low risk associated with harvest, and large expansion potential suggests that keratinocyte stem cells derived from a patient skin biopsy may be an ideal source of autologous cells in the treatment of LSCD [21].

The overall objective is therefore to establish optimal storage conditions for CECS to facilitate improved transplantation success and extend access to regenerative medicine. The purpose of this study was to first assess the effect of a range of above-freezing temperatures as an initial step towards achieving this objective.

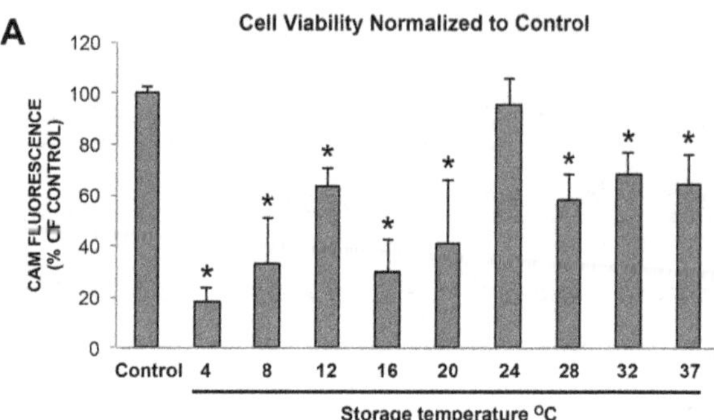

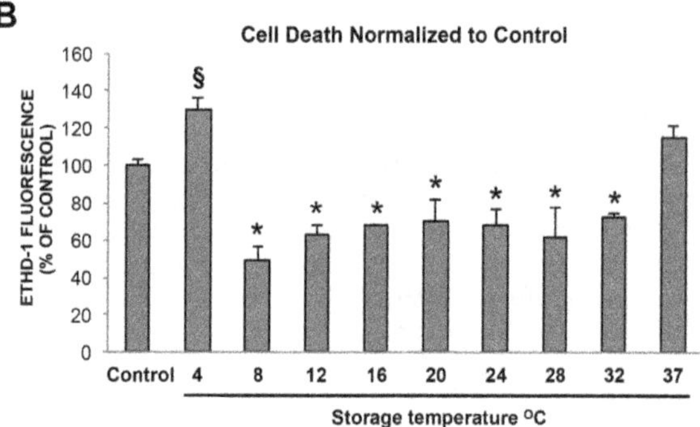

Figure 1. Cell viability and cell death after two weeks storage. (A) Cell viability (CAM fluorescence). Cell viability was clearly best maintained at 24°C with a value of 95.2 ± 9.91% compared to non-stored control cells (p = 0.984). All other temperatures had significantly reduced cell viability compared to non-stored control cells ($p < 0.001$). (B) Dead (EthD-1 fluorescence) values (n = 4). * = significantly lower compared to control ($p < 0.05$) § = significantly higher than control, ($p < 0.001$) (n = 4).

Materials and Methods

Supplies

Normal adult human epithelial keratinocytes (HEKa) and Keratinocyte Medium (KM) were obtained from ScienCell Research Laboratories (San Diego, CA). The provided cells originated from an 18 year old female undergoing breast-reduction surgery. Goat serum, trypsin-ethylenediaminetetraacetic acid (EDTA), 4-(2-hydroxyethyl)-1-piperazineethanesulfonic acid (HEPES), sodium bicarbonate, sodium azide, Tween-20, Triton X-100, gentamycin, bovine serum albumin (BSA), fetal bovine serum (FBS), 4', 6-diamidino-2-phenylindole (DAPI), were purchased from Sigma Aldrich (St Louis, MO). Nunclon Δ surface multidishes, glass coverslips, pipettes and other routine plastics were obtained from Thermo Fisher Scientific (Waltham, MA). Phosphate buffered saline (PBS) and minimum essential medium (MEM) were from Life Technologies (Carlsbad, CA).

Cell Culture

HEKa were seeded (5000 cells/cm^2) in serum-free KM (0.09 mM Calcium) on Nunclon Δ surface multidishes or glass coverslips. Cells were cultured in a 5% CO_2 incubator at 37°C for 5–7 days to obtain a confluent (90–100%) monolayer. Culture medium was changed every two days. To minimize confounding variation and to focus on temperature-associated differences, cells came from a single donor and were cultured on uncoated plastic, thereby limiting variation in the form of a biological substrate (e.g. amniotic membrane or fibrin).

Cell Storage

Following culture, each multidish was sealed and randomly selected for storage at one of nine different temperatures 4°C, 8°C, 12°C, 16°C, 20°C, 24°C, 28°C, 32°C and 37°C (n = 4 for each temperature). The standard deviation of the temperature in each storage container was ±0.4°C as demonstrated previously [22]. The storage medium consisted of MEM with 12.5 mM HEPES, 3.57 mM sodium bicarbonate and 50 μg/ml gentamycin. Cultured HEKa, not subjected to storage, served as controls. Cells were stored for 14 days in tightly sealed air-tight culture wells by means of Nunclon adhesive sheets. Following storage, MEM storage medium was replaced with KM, and cells were allowed to equilibrate in the 37°C incubator for 3 hours before all analyses in order to assess any potential damage incurred upon rewarming [23]. An extended storage period of 14 days was chosen to accentuate any temperature associated differences.

Assessment of Cell Viability

HEKa cells (n = 4) were incubated with calcein AM (CAM) (1:2000) which permeates the cell membrane and is hydrolyzed by live cells to yield green fluorescence, and ethidium homodimer-1(EthD-1) (1:1000) which permeates the membrane of dead cells, and labels nucleic acids to yield red fluorescence (Invitrogen Live/Dead Analysis Kit, Life Technologies, Grand Island, USA). Incubation was at room temperature for 45 minutes. Fluorescence was measured with a microplate fluorometer (Fluoroskan Ascent, Thermo Scientific, Waltham, MA) with the excitation/emission filter pairs 485/538 for CAM and 530/620 for EthD-1. Background fluorescence, measured in wells containing CAM and EthD-1 without cells, was subtracted from all values.

Metabolic Analysis

Metabolic readings taken from the storage medium were obtained directly upon removal of stored cells from storage at the nine different temperatures. Oxygen tension (pO_2), glucose, lactate, and pH values were measured using a Radiometer ABL

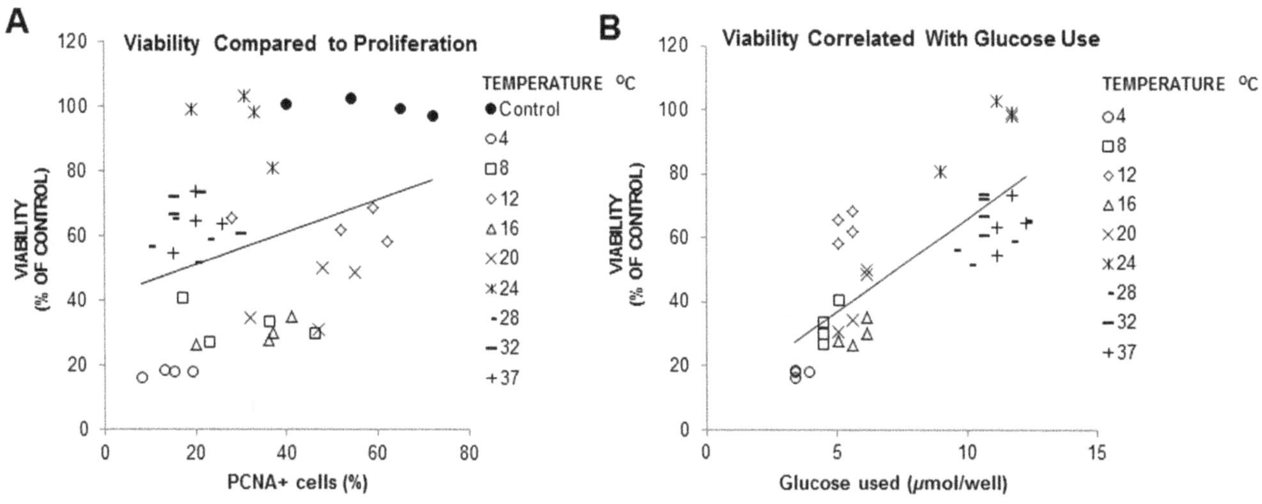

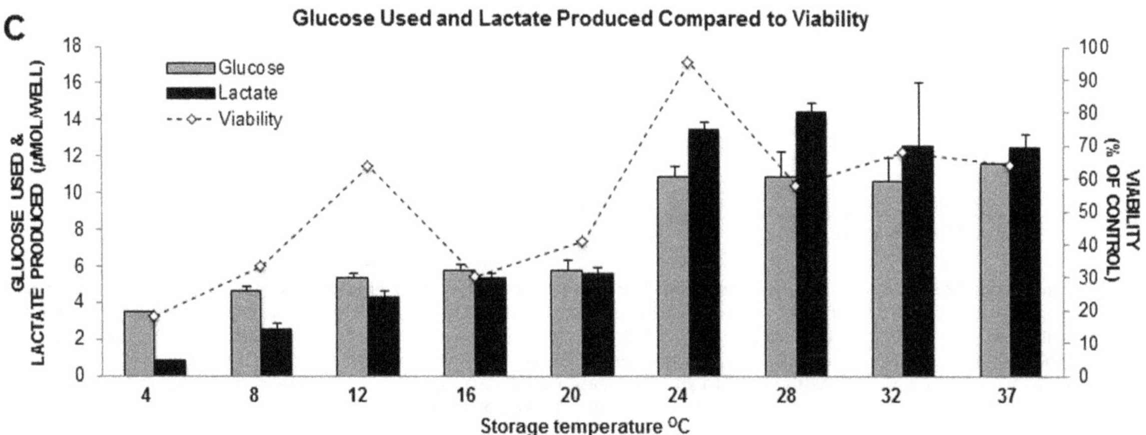

Figure 2. Cell viability comparison with PCNA, glucose use, and lactate production. (A) Correlation between cell viability and PCNA expression shows a distinct separation between high and low temperatures within the dataset ($r = 0.316$; $p < 0.05$). (B) Cell viability was also correlated with glucose use ($r = 0.782$; $p < 0.001$). (C) Cell viability compared to metabolic values by temperature. Values represent the average seen in n = 4 wells of a 12 well plate at each temperature.

700 blood gas machine (Bronshoj, Denmark). The analyzer was automatically calibrated following the manufacturer's protocol prior to analysis (Radiometer ABL 700 User Manual).

Light Microscopy

Light microscopy images were taken at 400X magnification, using a Leica DM IL LED microscope and Canon EOS 5D mark II camera (Canon, Oslo, Norway). Images were processed using Photoshop version CS6 extended software.

Scanning Electron Microscopy

HEKa cells cultured on glass coverslips were prepared for scanning electron microscopy (SEM) as previously described [24]. In brief, glutaraldehyde-fixed samples (n = 3) were dehydrated in increasing ethanol concentrations, then dried according to the critical point method (Polaron E3100 Critical Point Drier; Polaron Equipment Ltd., Watford, UK) with CO_2 as the transitional fluid. The specimens were attached to carbon stubs and coated with a 30 nm thick layer of platinum in a Polaron E5100 sputter coater before being photographed with an XL30 ESEM electron microscope (Philips, Amsterdam).

Immunocytochemistry

Cells cultured in Nunclon 24-well multidishes (n = 4) were rinsed in PBS, fixed in ice-cold 100% methanol, incubated at − 20°C for 7 minutes and washed with fresh PBS. Fixed cells were incubated in a 10% goat serum blocking buffer - 10% goat serum, 1% BSA, 0.1% Triton X-100, 0.05% Tween-20, 0.05% sodium azide in PBS, for 45 minutes at room temperature with gentle shaking. Cells were then incubated overnight at 4°C or at room temperature for 1 hour in a humidified chamber, with primary antibody to Proliferating Cell Nuclear Antigen (PCNA) (DAKO, Glostrup, Denmark) diluted in the same 10% goat serum blocking buffer. CY3-conjugated secondary antibodies were diluted in 0.2% PBS-Tween 20 with 1% BSA and incubated for one hour at room temperature. Addition of PBS in place of the primary antibody served as a negative control. The cells were rinsed three times in PBS before a wash containing 1 μg/mL DAPI to stain cell nuclei followed by a final wash with PBS. Using a magnification of ×200, random positions were selected for image capture using an inverted epi-fluorescence microscope (Nikon Eclipse Ti with a DS-Qi1 camera; Nikon Instruments, Tokyo, Japan). The exposure length and gain were kept constant. ImageJ software was used to process the images. The percentage and standard deviation of

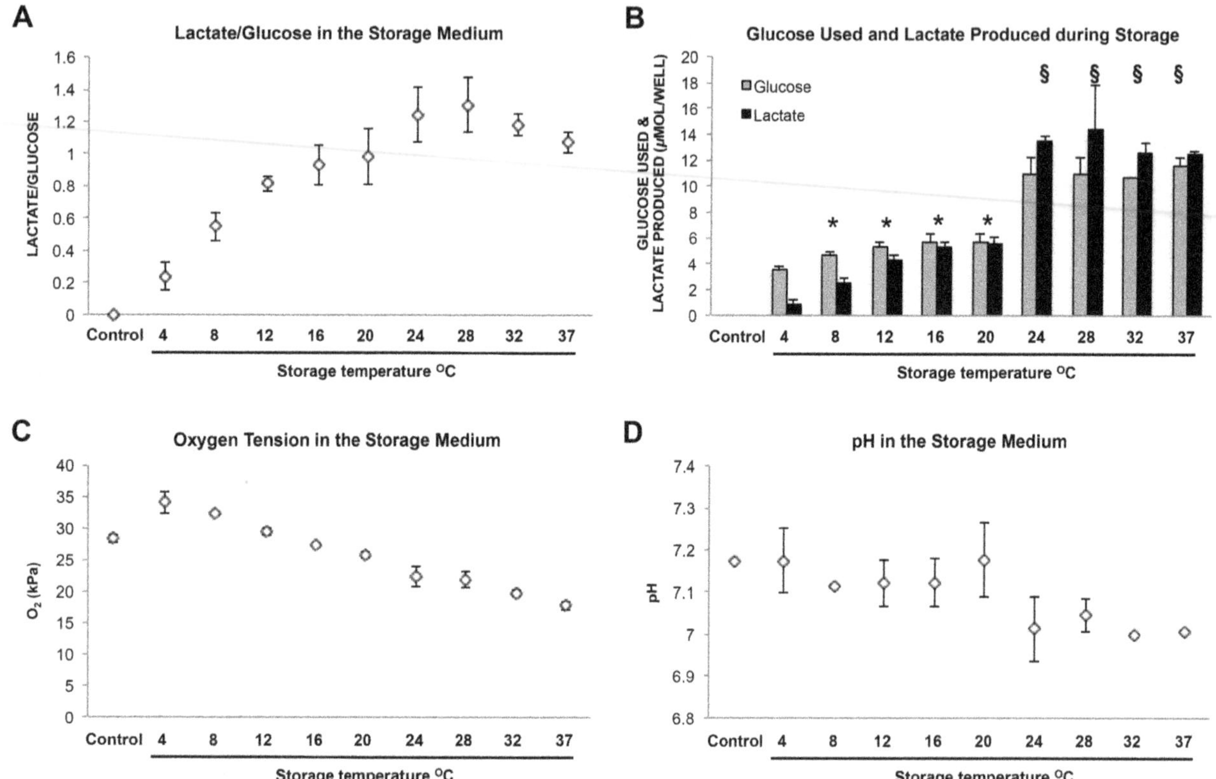

Figure 3. Metabolic measurements taken from the cell viability experiment after two weeks storage. (A) Lactate/glucose values increased with temperature (r = 0.927; $p < 0.001$ between 4°C and 28°C). (B) Glucose and lactate values were significantly grouped between 8°C and 20°C (* = significantly grouped - (glucose: $p > 0.05$; lactate: $p > 0.05$)) and values were approximately double between 24°C and 37°C (§ = significantly grouped - (glucose: $p > 0.05$; lactate: $p > 0.05$)). (C) Oxygen tension values were inversely correlated with temperature (r = - 0.939; $p < 0.001$). (D) pH fluctuated between pH 7.1 and pH 7.2 from 4°C to 20°C. Decreased pH fluctuating around pH 7.0 reflected higher lactate production between 24°C and 37°C. Values represent the average seen in n = 4 wells of a 12 well plate at each temperature.

positive staining was calculated based on an average calculated from counting ~100 cells from randomly selected positions in 4 wells.

Statistical Analysis

One-way ANOVA with Tukey's post hoc pair-wise comparisons (SPSS ver. 19.0) was used to compare the groups. Correlations were made using Pearson correlation. Data were expressed as mean ± standard deviation, and values were considered significant if $p<0.05$.

Results

Cell Viability and Cell Death Values

Calcein (CAM)/Ethidium Homodimer-1 (EthD-1) values reflect the relative live/dead numbers within the cell population remaining after removal of detached dead cells. Cell viability was clearly best maintained at 24°C with a value of 95.2±9.9% compared to non-stored control cells ($p = 0.984$) (Figure 1A). All other temperatures had significantly reduced cell viability compared to non-stored control cells ($p<0.001$). However, ~60% cell viability was conserved at 12°C, 28°C, 32°C, and 37°C. Cell viability was significantly correlated with PCNA expression ($r = 0.316$; $p<0.05$) (Figure 2A), and with glucose use ($r = 0.782$; $p<0.001$) (Figures 2B and 2C), throughout the temperature range.

Significantly higher cell death compared to the non-stored control was seen at 4°C ($p<0.001$) and there were also more dead cells at 37°C (Figure 1B). Cell death was significantly lower at all temperatures between 8°C and 32°C where values fluctuated at ~60% of the non-stored control cells ($p<0.001$ for all the groups). This may reflect detachment and removal of floating dead cells during storage and processing.

Metabolic Status

The metabolic status of cells stored in three different volumes (24-well, 12-well and 6-well plates) was assessed by measurements of glucose, lactate, pO_2 and pH in the media at the end of the storage period. The metabolic values taken from the cell viability experiment were investigated separately for correlation with cell viability results. Media without cells served as a control. The average glucose and lactate concentration in KM (used in cell culture before storage) was 5.04±0.32 mMol/L and 1.47±0.44 mMol/L respectively.

Glucose Use, Lactate Production, Oxygen Tension, and pH in the Cell Viability Experiment Group

The high lactate/glucose (L/G) ratios found at higher temperatures suggested that the glycolytic pathway accounted for a large part of energy production from glucose (at the highest, approximately 66% of glucose used was converted to lactate, given that the maximum possible L/G ratio is 2) (Figure 3A). The

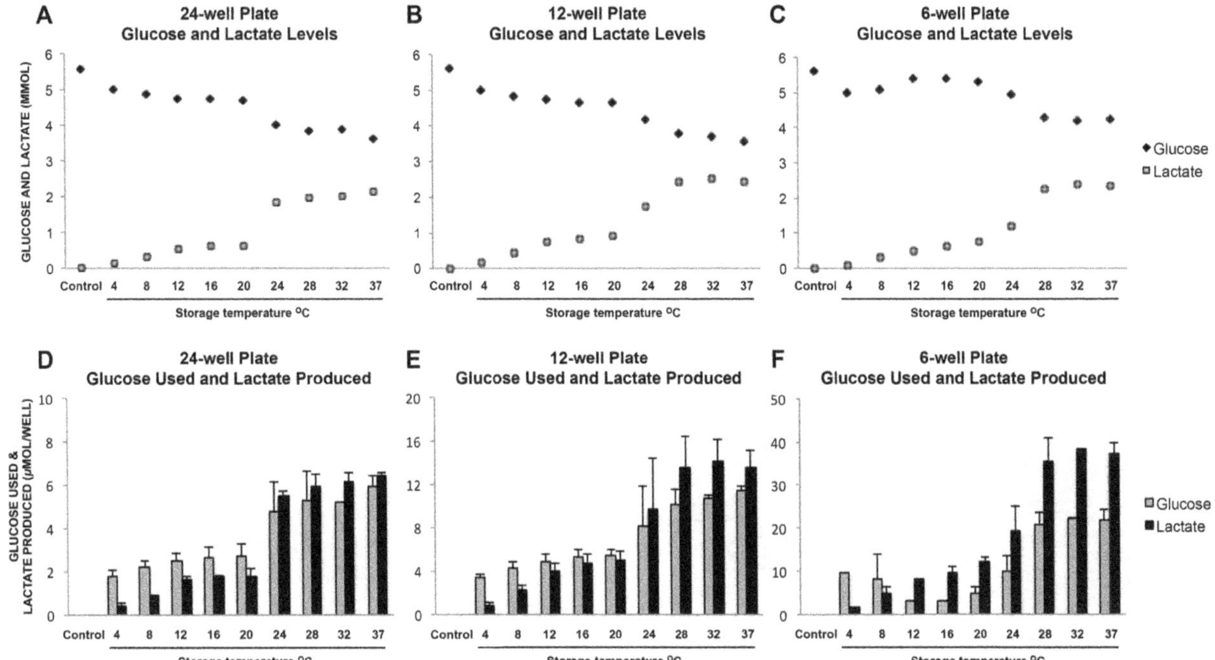

Figure 4. Metabolic measurements after two weeks storage showing different volumes. (A) (B) (C) Glucose and lactate concentration. (D) (E) (F) Glucose used and lactate produced (calculated from (A) (B) (C)). (A) and (D) 24 well plate volume 2mL, area 1.9 cm^2 (n = 3). (B) and (E) 12 well plate volume 5.6mL, area 3.5 cm^2 (n = 7). (C) and (F) 6 well plate volume 16 mL, area 9.6 cm^2 (n = 3).

strongest correlation between the L/G ratio and temperature was seen between 4°C and 28°C ($r = 0.927$; $p<0.001$). L/G ratio was lowest in the 4°C group (0.25±0.08), and the peak L/G value was seen after storage at 28°C (1.31±0.17). A lower L/G ratio relative to 28°C was seen at 32°C and 37°C (1.07±0.06) (Figure 3A).

Storage temperature effect on metabolic values could be bracketed into two distinct groups. The first group occurred between 8°C and 20°C where average glucose use was 5.36±0.42 µmol/well and average lactate production was 4.45±0.35 µmol/well (significantly similarly grouped (glucose: $p>0.05$; lactate: $p>0.05$)) (Figure 3B). A marked increase in metabolic activity was seen between 20°C and 24°C. The second group occurred between 24°C and 37°C, where both glucose use and lactate production were over twice that seen at lower temperatures; average glucose use was 11.03±0.80 µmol/well and average lactate production was 13.23±1.22 µmol/well (significantly similarly grouped (glucose: $p>0.05$; lactate: $p>0.05$)). Thus the highest glucose use and lactate production were seen at higher temperatures (Table S1, Figure 3B).

PO_2 values correlated inversely with increased temperature ($r = -0.939$; $p<0.001$), starting at 34.05 kPa (34% PO_2) at 4°C and decreasing steadily to 17.75 kPa (17.5% PO_2) at 37°C (Figure 3C). The control value was 28.35 KPa (28% PO_2), measured in the medium alone. The average in cell culture medium (KM) taken from cell cultures before storage was 22.75 kPa (22% PO_2). PO_2 was also inversely correlated with L/G ratio ($r = -0.808$; $p<0.010$) (data not shown).

KM in cell cultures before storage had an average pH of 7.47. During storage, small fluctuations ranging between pH 7.1 and pH 7.2 were seen from 4°C to 20°C and fluctuations around pH 7.0 were seen between 24°C and 37°C, reflecting the increase in lactate production at higher temperatures (Figure 3D).

Assessment of Metabolic Values in Volumes Used in Other Experimental Groups

The profile of glucose use and lactate production throughout the temperature range in other experimental volumes (24-well and 6-well) largely reflected the results described above in the cell viability experiment (12-well) (Figure 4A – F). Of note, no variation in metabolic values corresponding to storage volume was revealed.

Cell Morphology

HEKa cells were grown to confluence and had a characteristic cobblestone appearance before storage. Phase contrast micrographs were taken after exchanging storage media for KM and a 3 hour adjustment period in the 37°C incubator. Morphology most similar to control was observed at 12°C and 16°C, where cell-cell contact within epithelial sheets was well maintained (Figure 5A, D, and E). The presence of elongated filopodia, and an enlarged flattened appearance suggested more differentiation at temperatures above 16°C. In addition, dark granules were seen at the plasma membrane in some cells at 20°C and 24°C (Figure 5F and G). Changes in epithelial sheet morphology were also seen at temperatures above 16°C, with less distinct separation between adjacent cells. There was a tendency for cells to stream together at 28°C, 32°C and 37°C (Figure 5H - J). Clustered cells formed uneven islands at 32°C and 37°C (Figure 5H - J). Abnormally large intercellular space, indicative of cell shrinkage, was seen at 4°C and 8°C (Figure 5B).

Scanning electron microscopy (magnification: X2000) showed that cell-cell contact was similar to that of control cells at most temperatures in selected confluent areas (Figure 5K – T). Retention of individual cells with microvilli on the apical surface similar to the non-stored control was seen at all temperatures between 4°C and 24°C (Figure 5L – O).

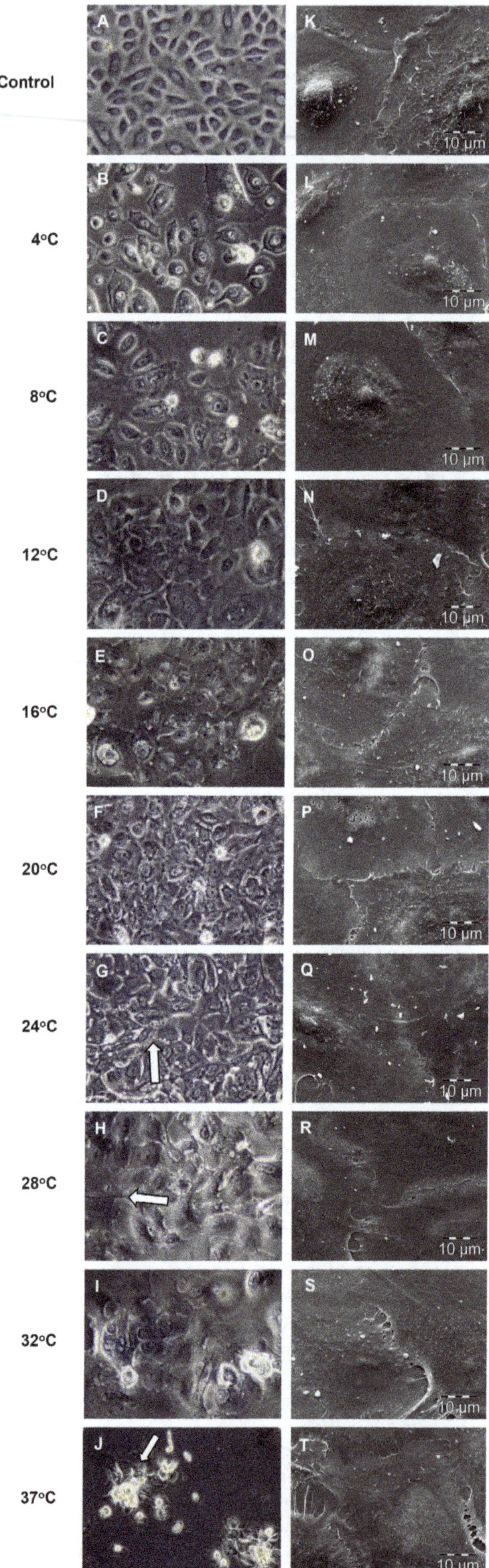

Figure 5. Morphology shown by phase contrast (X400) and SEM (X2000) micrographs. Morphology was most similar to non-stored control at 12°C and 16°C ((D) (E) (N) and (O)). Cell shrinkage was apparent at 4°C and 8°C ((B) and (C)); granulation (arrow (G)) and flattened cell morphology (arrow (H)) suggested more differentiation at higher temperatures ((F) - (J)). Cell clusters were seen at higher temperatures (arrow (J)). Representative SEM micrographs show preservation of cell-cell contact in selected areas ((L) – (T)) (n = 3).

Phenotype Analysis by Immunocytochemistry

The percentage of Proliferating Cell Nuclear Antigen (PCNA) positive cells is presented in graphical form to show comparison of expression between temperatures (Figure 6B). The percentage shown at 32°C and 37°C is an estimate, as counts were difficult to determine accurately due to clustering of cells. Since cell viability between temperatures varied significantly, and some dead cells were detached and lost during media change and fixation, it should be noted that values indicate the average percentage of remaining cells positive for the marker (n = 4). In control, PCNA was confined mostly to smaller cells that showed a very strong nuclear expression indicative of active proliferation (Figure 6A) [25]. Lowest expression was seen after storage at 4°C (Figure 6B). Expression was significantly reduced at all temperatures ($p<0.05$) except at 12°C (Figure 6B) and 20°C; significantly higher expression was seen at 12°C with 50±15% and 20°C with 46±10%, where values were comparable to the control value of 57±14% ($p = 0.983$ and 0.752, respectively). Fluorescence intensity began to weaken at 24°C (Figure 6A), and significantly lower expression compared to control was seen from 24°C to 37°C, at approximately 25% ($p<0.05$). Weak expression, confined to the center of aggregated cell clusters was characteristic of cells stored between 28°C and 37°C (Figure 6A).

Discussion

In the present study, the morphology, cell viability, phenotype and metabolic status following two weeks of xenobiotic-free storage of CECS were assessed. Glucose and lactate values in the storage media gave an indication of metabolic status and provided further evaluation of cell viability [26,27], whereas oxygen tension and pH measurements ensured storage conditions were within a physiologically relevant range.

Low cell viability values seen at 4°C and 8°C were corroborated by a high proportion of dead cells and low glucose consumption at these temperatures. In addition, phase contrast microscopy showed cell-cell contact was disrupted and cell shrinkage was apparent at 4°C and 8°C, indicative of apoptosis [28]. Retention of proliferative function was lowest at 4°C also confirming poor cell survival at this temperature. Low cell viability (~20%) seen at 4°C is in agreement with other studies that have shown cell viability ranging from ~20% to ~33% after storage at this temperature [5,12]. Rewarming after cold-storage has been shown to induce mitochondrial swelling and initiate apoptosis, which may account for the high cell death seen at 4°C [23,29]. Evidence of injury to epidermal cells associated with cold and re-warming seen at 4°C is particularly clinically relevant as refrigeration is the most common method of split skin graft storage and low cell viability may influence skin graft healing [5].

High cell viability at 24°C (~95%) shown here after 14 days of storage is contrary to that demonstrated in a study of pig skin at 25°C where cell viability declined to approximately 60% within one day [11]. Different storage conditions, inherent differences in cell function found between intact skin tissue and CECS, and species differences may explain the different results. Comparable

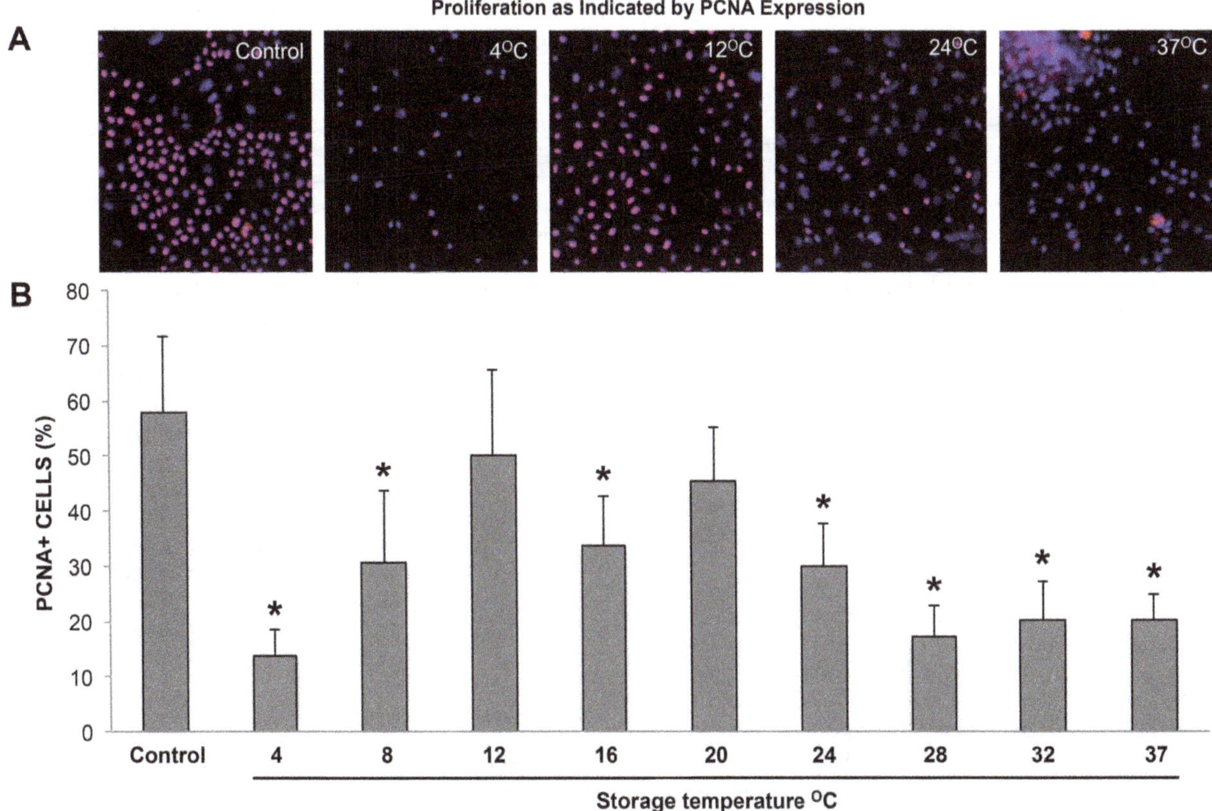

Figure 6. Proliferation as indicated by PCNA positive cells. (A) Representative images of PCNA staining (TRITC - red) combined with nuclear staining (DAPI – blue) showing 4°C, 12°C, 24°C and 37°C compared to non-stored control. Expression was significantly reduced at all temperatures (* = significantly reduced, $p < 0.05$) except at 12°C and 20°C (B); significantly higher PCNA expression was seen at 12°C with 50 ± 15% and 20°C with 46 ± 10%, where values were comparable to the control value of 57 ± 14% (p = 0.983 and 0.752, respectively).

cell viability has been demonstrated after storage of cultured limbal and conjunctival epithelial cells at 23°C for seven days [30,31]. A smaller peak in cell viability was seen at 12°C (~60%) which coincided with highest PCNA expression. A temperature study on storage of lung endothelial cells also reported similar results at 10°C [23]. The favorable conditions at 10°C were explained by minimal generation of catalytically available intracellular iron and reduced oxidative stress. Similarly, high proliferative capability was retained [23]. Higher cell viability, at approximately 60% or above, was shown in the present study at several temperatures (12°C, 24°C, 28°C, 32°C and 37°C), which is comparable to that reported in cultured epithelial autograft cryopreservation studies [27,32]. When combining PCNA results with cell viability, 12°C and 24°C appeared to be the most promising in terms of conservation of viable, proliferating cells following storage.

In accordance with other studies [33], cell viability as detected by CAM fluorescence was strongly correlated with glucose use. Exceptions were seen at 12°C and 24°C, where cell viability was higher, suggesting that conditions were especially favorable to efficient energy use. Optimum oxygen tension for keratinocyte growth has been shown at 18% O_2 [34] and lower (2% O_2) [35]. Therefore, the dampening effect of high oxygen tension may have contributed to the low cell viability found at 4°C (34% O_2), and the increase in cell viability and metabolic values seen between 24°C (22% O_2) and 37°C (17.5% O_2). In agreement with van't Hoff's principle stating that metabolic activity decreases by a factor of 1.5-2X for each 10°C drop in temperature, metabolic values (glucose use and lactate produced) at 28°C were on average twice that seen at 20°C [36]. However, the difference in metabolic activity between high and low temperatures did not decline in a continuous fashion; a sharp drop was seen below 24°C, accompanied by a notable decrease in the L/G ratio. From 20°C to 8°C, the decline in glucose use was more moderate, suggesting that epidermal cells may have an inbuilt adaptation to cooler temperatures below 24°C.

Lactate production was seen at all temperatures, despite sufficient oxygen to facilitate oxidative phosphorylation. This suggests that, at least in part, metabolic function was fulfilled through the use of the less efficient glycolytic pathway under aerobic conditions. The importance of glycolytic metabolism was particularly emphasized at high temperatures where L/G ratios were higher. In a comparable study, incubation of epidermal biopsies with or without oxygen resulted in no significant difference in lactate production [37]. Aerobic glycolysis, also known as the Warburg effect, has been described in cells with high energy requirements and proliferation rates [38], and it has been well documented that skin converts a high percentage of glucose to lactate [39]. Furthermore, oxidative phosphorylation has been found to be particularly dispensable in epidermal stem cells in favor of aerobic glycolysis [40]. Preference for use of the glycolytic pathway instead of oxidative phosphorylation may represent a defense mechanism against reactive oxygen species (ROS) generation, side-products of normal mitochondrial aerobic phosphorylation in situations of high-energy demand [41,42]. Thus the lactate production seen here confirms other findings showing the reliance of epidermal cells on glycolysis [37,39]. The distinct difference in metabolic values at high, compared to low, temperatures suggests a possible advantage of storage at temperatures below 20°C, due to a slower metabolic rate.

High L/G ratios were consistently seen at temperatures above 20°C regardless of storage volume. As the present study is the first to investigate the effect of storage temperature on the L/G ratio in CECS, direct comparisons were not possible. However, a high L/G ratio in CECS after 16 hours in a 37°C incubator following cryopreservation has been shown [9].This corroborates results shown here suggesting that glycolysis plays a fundamental role in serving energy needs even under aerobic conditions, especially at higher temperatures approximating normal skin temperature of 30°C [43], where normal metabolic rate may be expected.

Cell-cell and cell sheet architecture most resembling that of non-stored control cells was seen at 12°C and 16°C, whereas storage at temperatures above 20°C appeared to induce more differentiation [44]. Epidermal sheet disruption and rounded, uneven cell clusters, reminiscent of those seen in the disorganized epidermis of ΔNp63α-null mice were characteristic morphological features at 32°C and 37°C [45].

The number of viable cells remaining at the end of the storage period is a natural product of cell proliferation and cell turnover, therefore the contribution of cell proliferation to cell viability is of particular interest. In addition, continued proliferative function is especially relevant to cell sheet integration after surgery. PCNA staining varied widely throughout the temperature range indicating that storage temperature had a profound effect on proliferation. Cell viability was positively correlated with PCNA expression and trends below and above the best fit line between these two assessments indicated that proliferation played a more significant role in preservation of a viable cell population at lower temperatures, particularly at 12°C and 20°C. Conversely, weaker and lower PCNA expression was consistently seen at 24°C and temperatures above, despite generally higher cell viability and metabolic values. PCNA expression was mostly localized to smaller cells at every temperature. As small cell size is associated with stem cell character [46], increased differentiation at higher temperatures as indicated by increased occurrence of larger spreading cells and other morphological features, may have been responsible for lower PCNA expression.

The present study illustrates that temperature can have a profound effect on cell viability, morphology, and phenotype of CECS during storage. However, the use of cells from a single donor may be considered limiting. Factors that may affect extrapolation of these results include variation in donor cells as a consequence of systemic factors, such as donor health [47,48] and age [49]. Of note, studies comparing cell culture growth between donors have shown that the procurement and handling of starting material [47,49,50], as well as the health status of the individual donor [47,48], have a greater impact on cell growth when compared to the effect of age, supporting the use of cells from a young healthy donor in this study.

In conclusion, combined results suggest that the most extreme storage temperatures (4–8°C and 32–37°C) should be avoided for storage of CECS. Given the clear advantage of 24°C on cell viability, this may be the best temperature choice for the storage of cultured epidermal cells in preparation for surgery. Improved stability due to differentiation associated changes may have contributed to higher cell viability at this temperature. However, results at 12°C were particularly favorable in terms of maintenance of proliferative capacity and morphology of cultured cells after storage, while providing more than 60% cell viability. Metabolic values at 12°C suggest metabolism was dampened yet sufficient to allow slow cell growth, sustain intracellular homeostasis and a viable cell sheet population. Collectively, the data suggest that both 12°C and 24°C are strong candidates for storage of cultured epidermal cells that merit further investigation.

Supporting Information

Table S1 Values represent the average of n = 4 replicates for each temperature stored in a 12-well plate. Control values are those present in the storage medium on day 1.

Acknowledgments

Thanks to Rakibul Islam and Rima Maria Department of Medical Biochemistry, Oslo University Hospital, for their contribution in lab discussions and to Steinar Stoelen, Institute of Oral Biology, University of Oslo, for his help with SEM images.

Author Contributions

Conceived and designed the experiments: CJ TPU PA. Performed the experiments: CJ PA. Analyzed the data: CJ TPU PA JRE. Contributed reagents/materials/analysis tools: TPU TL EM MVU. Contributed to the writing of the manuscript: CJ TPU PA TL EM MVU JRE.

References

1. Barrandon Y, Grasset N, Zaffalon A, Gorostidi F, Claudinot S, et al. (2012) Capturing epidermal stemness for regenerative medicine. Semin Cell Dev Biol 23: 937–944.
2. Atiyeh BS, Costagliola M (2007) Cultured epithelial autograft (CEA) in burn treatment: three decades later. Burns 33: 405–413.
3. Ahmad S, Osei-Bempong C, Dana R, Jurkunas U (2010) The culture and transplantation of human limbal stem cells. J Cell Physiol 225: 15–19.
4. Utheim TP, Raeder S, Utheim OA, de la Paz M, Roald B, et al. (2009) Sterility control and long-term eye-bank storage of cultured human limbal epithelial cells for transplantation. Br J Ophthalmol 93: 980–983.
5. Knapik A, Kornmann K, Kerl K, Calcagni M, Contaldo C, et al. (2013) Practice of split-thickness skin graft storage and histological assessment of tissue quality. J Plast Reconstr Aesthet Surg 66: 827–834.
6. Udoh Y, Yanaga H, Tai Y, Kiyokawa K, Inoue Y (2000) Long-term viability of cryopreserved cultured epithelial grafts. Burns 26: 535–542.
7. Kito K, Kagami H, Kobayashi C, Ueda M, Terasaki H (2005) Effects of cryopreservation on histology and viability of cultured corneal epithelial cell sheets in rabbit. Cornea 24: 735–741.
8. Hibino Y, Hata K, Horie K, Torii S, Ueda M (1996) Structural changes and cell viability of cultured epithelium after freezing storage. J Craniomaxillofac Surg 24: 346–351.
9. Schiozer WA, Gemperli R, Muhlbauer W, Munhoz AM, Ferreira MC (2013) An outcome analysis and long-term viability of cryopreserved cultured epidermal allografts: assessment of the conservation of transplantable human skin allografts. Acta Cir Bras 28: 824–832.
10. Yeh HJ, Yao CL, Chen HI, Cheng HC, Hwang SM (2008) Cryopreservation of human limbal stem cells ex vivo expanded on amniotic membrane. Cornea 27: 327–333.
11. Ge L, Sun L, Chen J, Mao X, Kong Y, et al. (2010) The viability change of pigskin in vitro. Burns 36: 533–538.
12. Ghosh MM, Boyce SG, Freedlander E, MacNeil S (1995) A simple human dermal model for assessment of in vitro attachment efficiency of stored cultured epithelial autografts. J Burn Care Rehabil 16: 407–417.
13. Baylis O, Figueiredo F, Henein C, Lako M, Ahmad S (2011) 13 years of cultured limbal epithelial cell therapy: a review of the outcomes. J Cell Biochem 112: 993–1002.
14. Pellegrini G, Traverso CE, Franzi AT, Zingirian M, Cancedda R, et al. (1997) Long-term restoration of damaged corneal surfaces with autologous cultivated corneal epithelium. Lancet 349: 990–993.
15. Utheim TP (2013) Limbal epithelial cell therapy: past, present, and future. Methods Mol Biol 1014: 3–43.
16. Yang X, Qu L, Wang X, Zhao M, Li W, et al. (2007) Plasticity of epidermal adult stem cells derived from adult goat ear skin. Mol Reprod Dev 74: 386–396.
17. Yang X, Moldovan NI, Zhao Q, Mi S, Zhou Z, et al. (2008) Reconstruction of damaged cornea by autologous transplantation of epidermal adult stem cells. Mol Vis 14: 1064–1070.

18. Nishida K, Yamato M, Hayashida Y, Watanabe K, Yamamoto K, et al. (2004) Corneal reconstruction with tissue-engineered cell sheets composed of autologous oral mucosal epithelium. N Engl J Med 351: 1187–1196.
19. Ang LP, Tanioka H, Kawasaki S, Ang LP, Yamasaki K, et al. (2010) Cultivated human conjunctival epithelial transplantation for total limbal stem cell deficiency. Invest Ophthalmol Vis Sci 51: 758–764.
20. Rama P, Matuska S, Paganoni G, Spinelli A, De Luca M, et al. (2010) Limbal stem-cell therapy and long-term corneal regeneration. N Engl J Med 363: 147–155.
21. Green H, Kehinde O, Thomas J (1979) Growth of cultured human epidermal cells into multiple epithelia suitable for grafting. Proc Natl Acad Sci U S A 76: 5665–5668.
22. Pasovic L, Utheim TP, Maria R, Lyberg T, Messelt EB, et al. (2013) Optimization of Storage Temperature for Cultured ARPE-19 Cells. J Ophthalmol 2013: 216359.
23. Zieger MA, Gupta MP (2006) Endothelial cell preservation at 10 degrees C minimizes catalytic iron, oxidative stress, and cold-induced injury. Cell Transplant 15: 499–510.
24. Raeder S, Utheim TP, Utheim OA, Cai Y, Roald B, et al. (2007) Effect of limbal explant orientation on the histology, phenotype, ultrastructure and barrier function of cultured limbal epithelial cells. Acta OphthalmolScand 85: 377–386.
25. Roos G, Landberg G, Huff JP, Houghten R, Takasaki Y, et al. (1993) Analysis of the epitopes of proliferating cell nuclear antigen recognized by monoclonal antibodies. Lab Invest 68: 204–210.
26. Konstantinow A, Muhlbauer W, Hartinger A, von Donnersmarck GG (1991) Skin banking: a simple method for cryopreservation of split-thickness skin and cultured human epidermal keratinocytes. Ann Plast Surg 26: 89–97.
27. Pasch J, Schiefer A, Heschel I, Rau G (1999) Cryopreservation of keratinocytes in a monolayer. Cryobiology 39: 158–168.
28. Matylevitch NP, Schuschereba ST, Mata JR, Gilligan GR, Lawlor DF, et al. (1998) Apoptosis and accidental cell death in cultured human keratinocytes after thermal injury. Am J Pathol 153: 567–577.
29. Salahudeen AK, Huang H, Joshi M, Moore NA, Jenkins JK (2003) Involvement of the mitochondrial pathway in cold storage and rewarming-associated apoptosis of human renal proximal tubular cells. Am J Transplant 3: 273–280.
30. Utheim TP, Raeder S, Utheim OA, Cai Y, Roald B, et al. (2007) A novel method for preserving cultured limbal epithelial cells. Br J Ophthalmol 91: 797–800.
31. Eidet JR, Utheim OA, Raeder S, Dartt DA, Lyberg T, et al. (2012) Effects of serum-free storage on morphology, phenotype, and viability of ex vivo cultured human conjunctival epithelium. Exp Eye Res 94: 109–116.
32. Chen F, Zhang W, Wu W, Jin Y, Cen L, et al. (2011) Cryopreservation of tissue-engineered epithelial sheets in trehalose. Biomaterials 32: 8426–8435.
33. Bravo D, Rigley TH, Gibran N, Strong DM, Newman-Gage H (2000) Effect of storage and preservation methods on viability in transplantable human skin allografts. Burns 26: 367–378.
34. Horikoshi T, Balin AK, Carter DM (1986) Effect of oxygen on the growth of human epidermal keratinocytes. J Invest Dermatol 86: 424–427.
35. Kino-oka M, Agatahama Y, Haga Y, Inoie M, Taya M (2005) Long-term subculture of human keratinocytes under an anoxic condition. J Biosci Bioeng 100: 119–122.
36. Belzer FO, Southard JH (1988) Principles of solid-organ preservation by cold storage. Transplantation 45: 673–676.
37. Ronquist G, Andersson A, Bendsoe N, Falck B (2003) Human epidermal energy metabolism is functionally anaerobic. Exp Dermatol 12: 572–579.
38. Warburg O, Wind F, Negelein E (1927) The Metabolism of Tumors in the Body. J Gen Physiol 8: 519–530.
39. Halprin KM, Ohkawara A (1966) Lactate production and lactate dehydrogenase in the human epidermis. J Invest Dermatol 47: 222–229.
40. Baris OR, Klose A, Kloepper JE, Weiland D, Neuhaus JF, et al. (2011) The mitochondrial electron transport chain is dispensable for proliferation and differentiation of epidermal progenitor cells. Stem Cells 29: 1459–1468.
41. Balaban RS, Nemoto S, Finkel T (2005) Mitochondria, oxidants, and aging. Cell 120: 483–495.
42. Brand KA, Hermfisse U (1997) Aerobic glycolysis by proliferating cells: a protective strategy against reactive oxygen species. FASEB J 11: 388–395.
43. Smith AD, Crabtree DR, Bilzon JL, Walsh NP (2010) The validity of wireless iButtons and thermistors for human skin temperature measurement. Physiol Meas 31: 95–114.
44. Hennings H, Holbrook KA (1983) Calcium regulation of cell-cell contact and differentiation of epidermal cells in culture. An ultrastructural study. Exp Cell Res 143: 127–142.
45. Romano RA, Smalley K, Magraw C, Serna VA, Kurita T, et al. (2012) DeltaNp63 knockout mice reveal its indispensable role as a master regulator of epithelial development and differentiation. Development 139: 772–782.
46. Li J, Miao C, Guo W, Jia L, Zhou J, et al. (2008) Enrichment of putative human epidermal stem cells based on cell size and collagen type IV adhesiveness. Cell Res 18: 360–371.
47. Dragunova J, Kabat P, Koller J, Jarabinska V (2012) Experience gained during the long term cultivation of keratinocytes for treatment of burns patients. Cell Tissue Bank 13: 471–478.
48. Stoner ML, Wood FM (1996) Systemic factors influencing the growth of cultured epithelial autograft. Burns 22: 197–199.
49. Baylis O, Rooney P, Figueiredo F, Lako M, Ahmad S (2013) An investigation of donor and culture parameters which influence epithelial outgrowths from cultured human cadaveric limbal explants. J Cell Physiol 228: 1025–1030.
50. Zito-Abbad E, Borderie VM, Baudrimont M, Bourcier T, Laroche L, et al. (2006) Corneal epithelial cultures generated from organ-cultured limbal tissue: factors influencing epithelial cell growth. Curr Eye Res 31: 391–399.

6

Reconstruction of Beagle Hemi-Mandibular Defects with Allogenic Mandibular Scaffolds and Autologous Mesenchymal Stem Cells

ChangKui Liu[1,3]☙, XinYing Tan[1]☙, JinChao Luo[1], HuaWei Liu[1], Min Hu[1]*, Wen Yue[2]*

1 Department of stomatology, General Hospital of the PLA, Beijing, China, **2** Department of Stem Cell and Regenerative Medicine Lab, Beijing Institute of Transfusion Medicine, Beijing, China, **3** Department of Stomatology, The 451th hospital of the People's Libration Army, Xi'an, China

Abstract

Objective: Massive bone allografts are frequently used in orthopedic reconstructive surgery, but carry a high failure rate of approximately 25%. We tested whether treatment of graft with mesenchymal stem cells (MSCs) can increase the integration of massive allografts (hemi-mandible) in a large animal model.

Methods: Thirty beagle dogs received surgical left-sided hemi-mandibular defects, and then divided into two equal groups. Bony defects of the control group were reconstructed using allografts only. Those of the experimental group were reconstructed using allogenic mandibular scaffold-loaded autologous MSCs. Beagles from each group were killed at4 (n = 4), 12 (n = 4), 24 (n = 4) or 48 weeks (n = 3) postoperatively. CT and micro-CT scans, histological analyses and the bone mineral density (BMD) of transplants were used to evaluate defect reconstruction outcomes.

Results: Gross and CT examinations showed that the autologous bone grafts had healed in both groups. At 48 weeks, the allogenic mandibular scaffolds of the experimental group had been completely replaced by new bone, which has a smaller surface area to that of the original allogenic scaffold, whereas the scaffold in control dogs remained the same size as the original allogenic scaffold throughout. At 12 weeks, the BMD of the experimental group was significantly higher than the control group ($p<0.05$), and all micro-architectural parameters were significantly different between groups ($p<0.05$). Histological analyses showed almost all transplanted allogeneic bone was replaced by new bone, principally fibrous ossification, in the experimental group, which differed from the control group where little new bone formed.

Conclusions: Our study demonstrated the feasibility of MSC-loaded allogenic mandibular scaffolds for the reconstruction of hemi-mandibular defects. Further studies are needed to test whether these results can be surpassed by the use of allogenic mandibular scaffolds loaded with a combination of MSCs and osteoinductive growth factors.

Editor: Irina Kerkis, Instituto Butantan, Brazil

Funding: This work was Supported by the Beijing Municipal Commission of Science and Technology (D131100003013001) and Beijing Natural Science Foundation of China (7112124). The funders had no role in study design, data collection and analysis, decision to publish, or preparation of the manuscript.

Competing Interests: The authors have declared that no competing interests exist.

* Email: humin48@vip.163.com (MH); wenyue26@yahoo.com (WY)

☙ These authors contributed equally to this work.

Introduction

Mandibular defects can be caused by ablative surgery for oral and maxillofacial tumors, trauma, infection, or congenital deformities. The reconstruction of large mandibular defects is a highly challenging task for oral and maxillofacial surgeons. Despite the many reconstructive methods available, autologous grafts are considered to be the "gold standard" because of their advantages of osteogenesis, osteoinduction, and osteoconduction. The iliac crest is the most frequently chosen donor site because it provides easy access to good-quality cancellous autografts in appreciable numbers. However, harvesting autologous bone from the iliac crest lengthens the overall surgical procedure and is usually complicated by hematoma formation, pelvic instability, nerve injury, residual pain, and cosmetic disadvantages [1]. Also, the shape of the mandible reconstructed by autogenous bone grafts is poor. Hence, a better method for mandibular reconstruction is required [2].

As the number of bone banks has increased, so has the number of bone allografts used in reconstructive surgery to replace missing bone parts (e.g., critical size defects) [3]. Most massive allografts have long-term success, but 25% of reconstructions fail because of infection, fracture, or nonunion [4–6]. In humans, graft union at the host bone is a slow process. The effectiveness of this procedure is dependent upon the healing time and type of graft integration. The larger the amount of bone to be replaced, the more difficult is the integration. This process may involve only 20% of the graft over 5 years, as shown by studies on retrieved allografts [7]. The allograft is also far from being an "ideal" option for bone reconstruction because of the risk of triggering host immune responses and their lack of osteogenic capacity.

To overcome these shortcomings in bone grafts, scientists have attempted to develop a bone construct using the "traditional triad" of tissue engineering (including sufficient osteocompetent cell transfer), structured scaffolding (to maintain space and provide osteoconduction), and the application of miscellaneous growth factors (which can induce adjacent mesenchymal osteogenesis) [7]. The purpose of each component of these building blocks is to replicate the intrinsic properties of autograft reconstructions. However, the strength of scaffolds used in the engineering of bone tissue is not suitable to meet clinical requirements, and restoring the shape of the mandible is difficult.

Some scholars have suggested that the immunogenicity of freeze-dried bone allografts can be removed. Such allografts contain several osteoinductive growth factors (e.g., bone morphogenic proteins [BMPs)). Other non-collagenous proteins in the matrix support the formation of new bone. Allogeneic bone has a similar shape and biological properties. Freeze-dried allogenic bone can be used for scaffolds for bone engineering [8].

Human bone marrow contains stem cells that can differentiate. Mesenchymal stem cells (MSCs) have the potential for multilineage differentiation, and can differentiate into cells with an osteogenic phenotype. Several studies have shown that MSCs can promote osteogenesis in vivo [9–11]. These cells can propagate in vitro into the large numbers needed to promote regeneration of injured tissue. MSCs are currently being used in preclinical studies to regenerate bone in patients with massive bone defects.

Here, we employed a tissue-engineering approach to promote the reconstruction of hemi-mandibular defects using mandibular allografts as scaffolds and MSCs as seed cells. The aim of this study was to find out whether this approach can be conducted.

Materials and Methods

The study was authorized by the Ethics Committee of the General Hospital of the People's Liberation Army (PLA) Beijing China. Beagle dogs were cared for according to the guidelines set by the laboratory Animal Research Center of the General Hospital of the PLA. This study was conducted according to the National Institute of Health (NIH publication No. 85–23, revised 1985) Guideline for the Care and Use of Laboratory Animals.

Manufacture of freeze-dried allogenic mandibles

Mandibles were harvested from 2-year old beagle dogs. Soft tissues and the periosteum were removed and all teeth were extracted. Mandibles were split at the symphysis, and the parts in front of the first premolar were removed. Pores in the bone were then created using a 702-L straight fissure bur (width, 1 mm) at 1-mm intervals until the medullary bone was reached. This procedure was performed under abundant irrigation to allow MSC seeding and to facilitate angiogenesis. Subsequently, mandibles were immersed in 10% hydrogen peroxide for 24 hours at 38°C. The processed mandibles were then incubated in chloroform/methanol (1:1) for 1 hour at room temperature and then in 0.25% trypsin for 12 hours at 4°C. After this, mandibles were immersed in 0.5% sodium dodecyl sulfate for 6 hours at room temperature. Each processing procedure was followed by extensive washes with distilled water. Mandibles were then freeze-dried, packaged and finally sterilized by ^{60}Co gamma-ray irradiation ($20X10^3$ Gy), and stored at -70°C until implantation (Fig. 1).

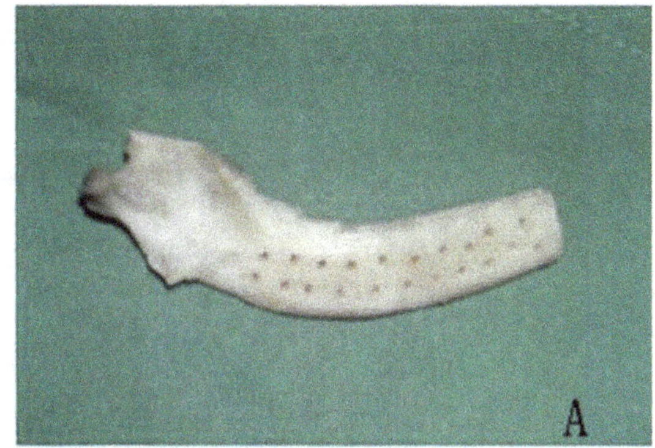

Figure 1. Manufacture of freeze-dried allogenic mandibles.

Isolation, cultivation and derivation of MSCs

General anesthesia was induced in beagle dogs using an intramuscular injection of xylazine hydrochloride (0.1 ml/kg). From each beagle, a 10-mL sample of bone marrow was aspirated from the posterior iliac crest under local anesthesia (5 ml lidocaine) (Fig. 2A). The sample was transferred to the clean room for cell isolation. The sample was then added to 50 mL of phosphate buffered saline (PBS; Clinimax, Bergisch Gladbach, Germany), loaded onto Lymphodex (Inno-Train, Kronberg, Germany), and centrifuged at 1,500 g for 20 min. Mononuclear cells were then collected and counted using a NucleoCounter NC-100 (ChemoMetec, Allerod, Denmark). The mononuclear cells were washed with PBS and plated at 1×10^6 cells/cm^2 in a culture flask with 15 mL alpha-modified minimum Eagle's medium (Gibco, Billings, MT, USA) supplemented with 100 IU/mL penicillin, 100 kg/mL streptomycin (Gibco), and 10% hyclone bovine serum (Thermo Scientific, Thermo Scientific, Waltham, MA, USA). Cultures were expanded through several successive subcultures until a sufficient number of mononuclear cells was achieved (Fig. 2B). Trypan blue staining was used to determine the number of viable cells. For transplantation, approximately 1×10^7 third-passage cells were suspended in 5 mL of normal saline and transferred to the operating room.

Injection of MSC-fibrin glue admixture

To load the cells, normal saline was removed from the suspension of MSCs, and the cells were resuspended in 5 mL fibrin glue. Pasteurized fibrin glue (Bolheal, Chemo-Sero-Therapeutic Research Institute, Kumamoto, Japan) was formed by mixing two separate solutions, A and B. Solutions A and B were mixed in a 4:1 (volume/volume) ratio. Briefly, normal saline was removed from the MSC suspension. The resulting pellet of cell was resuspended in solution A, which consisted of cells (1×10^7), fibrinogen (80 mg/mL), and fibrin-stabilizing factor XIII (75 units/mL) dissolved in 2.4 mL of plasmin inhibitor aprotinin (1000 kIE/mL). Solution B contained thrombin (250 units) dissolved in 0.6 ml of 40 μM $CaCl_2$. Solutions A and B [4:1 (volume/volume) ratio] were placed in the barrel of a sterilized 5-mL syringe and mixed by inverting the syringe repeatedly. The cell concentration in the admixture was approximately 3×10^6 cells/mL.

Experimental design and surgical procedure

Thirty healthy adult female beagles (1–2 year; 10.0±3.0 kg) were provided by the Laboratory Animal Center of the Chinese PLA General Hospital (Beijing, China). Surgical methods and animal care conformed to the principles of the Guide for the Care and Use of Laboratory Animals (NIH publication number 85–23, revised 1985). General anesthesia was induced with ketamine

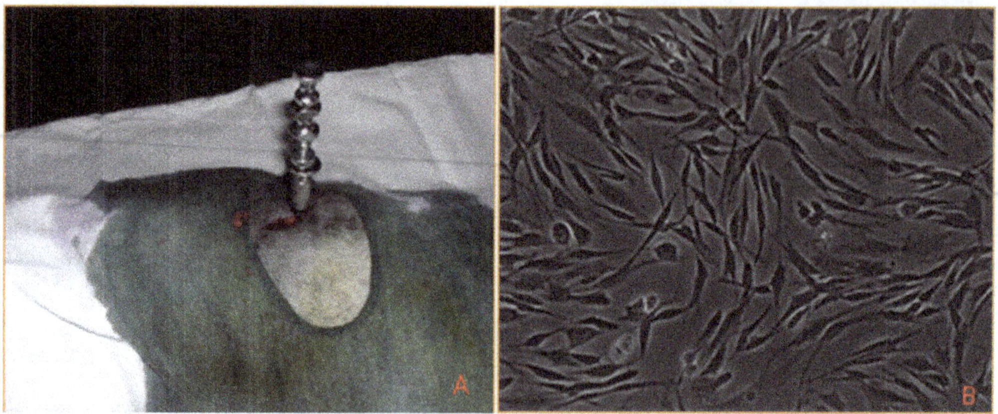

Figure 2. Preparation of the autologous grafts. A: Bone marrow was aspirated from the posterior iliac crest. B: MSCs.

hydrochloride (20 mg/kg, im or sc) and maintained with pentobarbital sodium (1–2%, iv). Beagles were prepared for the extraction of left mandibular teeth from the bicuspid tooth to the back molar (Fig. 3A). Three months after extraction, the wounds of the mucosal healed for the next segmental mandibulectomy (Fig. 3B).

All beagles were randomized into two groups: control and experimental. The anesthetized beagle was placed on the operating table in the left lateral position with their limbs in extension and the head aligned with the body and fixed on the left half-face. All surgical interventions were performed by the same surgeon (Changkui L). An incision of length 40–50 mm was made in the left mandible (a lower left paramandibular approach followed the mandible from the angle of the jaw to the chin). A subperiosteal dissection was made to lift a flap, which included skin, from the subcutaneous cellular tissue and mandibular periosteum. In the proximal zone, the mandibular insertion of the masseter and temporalis were separated to expose the outer cortex of the left mandible. Then, the internal cortex was dissected to the adherent gingival mucosa, medial pterygoid muscle, and the lateral pterygoid muscle. Finally, the condyle was dissected from the articular capsule and the inferior alveolar neurovascular

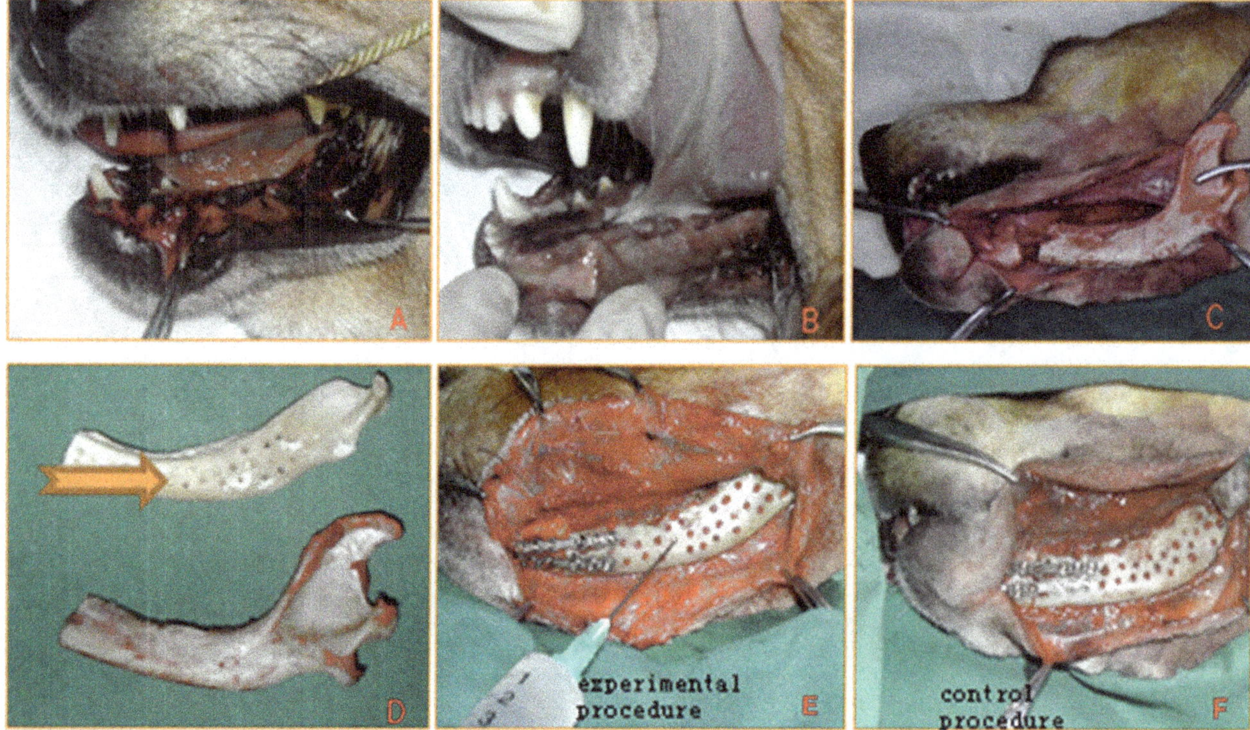

Figure 3. Experimental techniques. A: Extraction of left mandibular teeth. B: Three months after extraction. C: Hemi-mandibular bone was removed to establish a hemi-mandibular defect. D: The shape and size of the allogenic mandibular scaffold was matched (The arrow indicate the allogenic mandibular scaffold). E: In the experimental group, the hemi-mandibular defect was reconstructed using allogenic mandibular scaffold-loaded MSCs. F: In the control group, hemi-mandibular defects were reconstructed using allogenic mandibular scaffolds only.

bundle was ligated. Using a scroll saw, hemi-mandibular bone was removed from 1 cm of the posterior aspect of the mental foramen to establish a hemi-mandibular defect (Fig. 3C). The defect was replaced with a sterile freeze-dried allograft derived from previously sacrificed beagles and stored at −70°C. Two six-hole titanium plates (3.5-mm wide, 4.0-cm long; Beijing Gemma fly Medical Devices Co., Ltd.) were modeled to fix the graft (Fig. 3E, F). In the experimental group, the hemi-mandibular defect was reconstructed using allogenic mandibular scaffold-loaded autologous MSCs (Fig. 3E). In the control group, hemi-mandibular defects were reconstructed using allogenic mandibular scaffolds only (Fig. 3F). Postoperatively, all beagles were given penicillin (400,000 IU/kg/day, iv) and metronidazole (0.25 mg/day, iv) for 7 days, as required. Beagles were maintained on a soft diet for 12 weeks and subsequently on standard chow until sacrifice.

Clinical and CT examinations

The activities, responses, food intake, and would healing of surgical sites were observed in all animals. Bone regeneration of the meshes that carried allogenic mandibular scaffold-loaded autologous MSCs and allogenic mandibular scaffolds were examined during transplantation. At 4, 12, 24,and 48 weeks after implantation, four or three beagles of each group were killed by an intravenous overdose of sodium pentobarbitone.

CT scans were conducted before surgery and just after killing using a light-speed 32-slice system (120 kV; 80 mA; rotation time, 0.8 s; slice thickness, 0.2 mm; General Electric, Piscataway, NJ, USA). Three-dimensional reconstruction was conducted to observe the shape, erosion, and calcification of mandibles. Mandibles were excised for further analyses.

Evaluation of the BMD of mandibles

The BMD of the mandibles were evaluated by the 36-XR dual energy x-ray absorptiometry scan (Norland, USA). After scanning the image into the computer, the BDM of 3 × 3-mm size ROI areas were measured by appropriate software. Three times repeated measurements were recorded for each sample and the mean value was calculated (Fig. 4).

Micro-CT scanning

A micro-CT system was used to quantify the difference of the mandibles in the architecture of the cancellous bone. The prepared specimens of the micro-CT images were placed in a cylindrical cup filled with plastic foam padded to avoid any movement during the scanning procedure. The micro-CT images were obtained using a preclinical cone beam CT scanner (Healthcare Explore Locus SP, GE Medical Systems, Milwaukee, USA) of the Department of Orthopedics of Xijing Hospital. The Explore Locus is a CCD-based camera that acquires data by taking a number of planar images at a regular angular velocity. All adjustable angles were rotated from 180° to 360°. According to the scanning protocol, the images were acquired with the following parameters: (a) 80 kV as the X-ray tube voltage; (b) 80 μA as the anode current; (c) 3000 ms as the exposure time; (d) 1 × 1 as the binning combination; (e) 360° as the rotation angle and 0.4° as the angle increment; and (f) 21 μm as the scanning revolution rate. The micro-architecture of the trabeculae was automatically evaluated using the built-in program of the micro-CT with direct 3D morphometry to reconstruct the 3-D images that consist of an isotropic voxel with a cubic length of $21\mu m^3$.

A direct, model-independent method was used to quantify various architectural parameters. These parameters included the bone volume fraction (BV/TV), trabecular number (Tb.N), trabecular thickness (Tb.Th), and trabecular separation (Tb.Sp).

Histological analyses

Mandibular biopsy specimens taken during surgery were fixed in 10% neutral-buffered formalin. After dehydration, specimens were immersed in glycol methacrylate resin (Technovit 7200 VLC; Heraeus-Kulzer, Wehrheim, Germany). After solidification for 24 h, specimens were cut from the longitudinal section of mandibles. Tissues with allogenic mandibular scaffold-loaded autologous MSCs and allogenic mandibular scaffolds were separated for histological examination. Histological preparation was conducted as described previously[9]. Embedded samples were cut into thin sections (40×80 mm) and mounted on glass slides. Two ground sections from each specimen block (300-mm apart) were stained with hematoxylin and eosin (H&E).

Statistical analyses

Data from radiography and histology are the mean ± SEM and analyzed by one-way ANOVA. Differences between two groups among the six groups were assessed with the Student–Newman–Keuls test. $p<0.05$ was considered significant.

Results

Gross view and CT examinations

All beagles tolerated surgery and were able to eat a normal diet postoperatively. Two beagles from control group and one beagle from the experimental group were eliminated from the analyses because they developed postoperative wound infections.

The shape of the mandibles was observed by three-dimensional CT reconstruction and, after dissection, showed resorption of allogenic mandibular scaffolds in the experimental group at 4 weeks, but such resorption was not observed in the control group. At 12 weeks, new bone had formed in an irregular fashion on allogenic mandibular scaffolds in the experimental group. In the control group, new bone formation and scaffold absorption was not significant at 12 weeks. The shape of mandibles in the beagles of the two groups returned to almost normal at 48 weeks after surgery, but the pores were filled with new bone in the experimental group (Fig. 5).

Mandibular BMD

Twelve weeks after transplantation, the experimental group BMD was significantly higher than in the control group ($p<0.05$). With the progression of time, the BMD of the experimental group and the control group both increased, but at a significantly higher rate in the experimental group (Table 1).

Micro-CT findings

The mean, standard deviation and range for each of the micro-architectural parameters from the allogenic mandibular scaffolds of 30 beagles were tabulated, and the bone micro-architecture parameters of the allograft bone at 1cm of the proximal end were analyzed in 30 beagles in both the experimental and control groups (Table 2). The mean D-value of all micro-architectural parameters were significantly different between the groups ($p < 0.05$).

Histological findings

A small amount of trabecular bone growth towards allogenic bone was observed in the experimental group 4 weeks after surgery. Cortical allograft bone edges showed lacunar absorption, and a small amount of new bone was formed. The highest proportion of cells filling the allogenic mandibular scaffold were inflammatory (Fig. 6A). However, in the control group, allogeneic

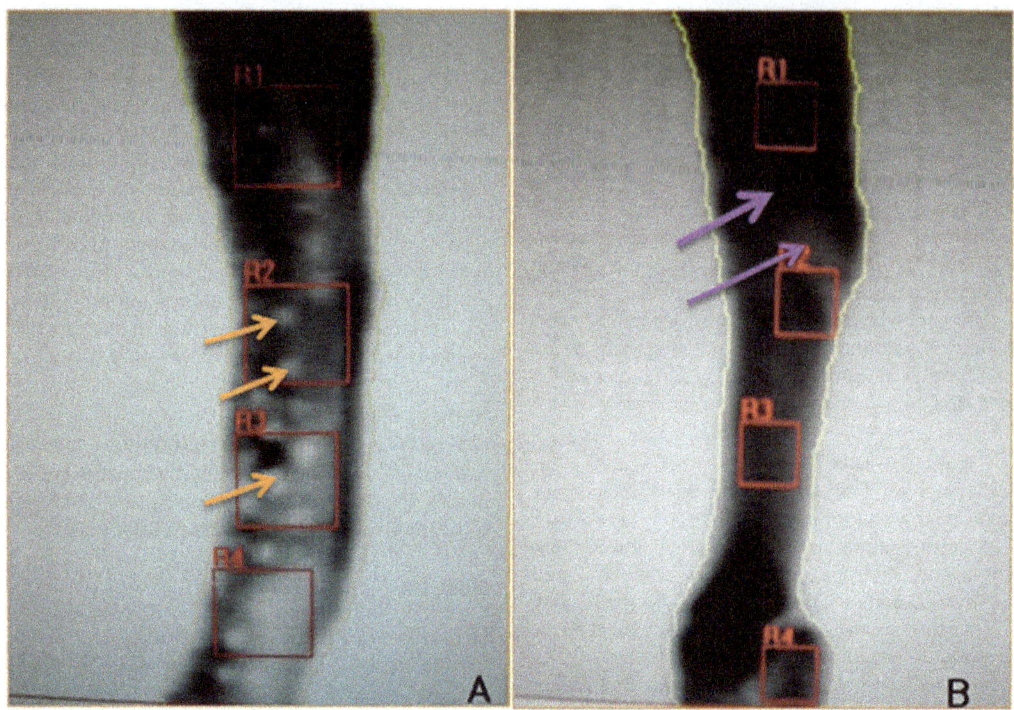

Figure 4. Evaluation of the BMD of mandibles. A: Evaluation of the BMD of control group mandible at 4 weeks after operation. The arrows indicate the pores still can be seen in the control group at this time. B:Evaluation of the BMD of experimental group mandible at 48 weeks after operation. The arrows indicate the pores were almost filled with new bone in the experimental group at this time.

bone edges showed less absorption, and virtually no new trabecular bone formed between autologous bone and allograft bone 1 month after surgery (Fig. 6D).

Twelve weeks after surgery, trabecular bone was observed to connect autologous and allograft bone in the experimental group scaffolds. Osteoblast progenitor cells and osteoblasts were observed to grow towards the inside of allogenic mandibular scaffolds at the edge of the allogeneic bone. Allogeneic bone was partially absorbed, the Haversian canal expanded, and fibrous tissues grew into allogenic mandibular scaffolds (Fig. 6B). Resorption of allogeneic bone was not clearly observed in the control group and there fewer fibrous tissues grew towards the inside of allogenic mandibular scaffolds than observed in the experimental group (Fig. 6E).

Forty-eight weeks after reconstruction, the new bone graft in the experimental group was smaller than the original, but almost all transplanted allogeneic bone was replaced by new bone, although most of it was fibrous tissues (Fig. 6C). Allogeneic bone was not absorbed in the control group, and it maintained its original shape. A small part of allogenic bone was replaced by new bone or fibrous tissues (Fig. 6F).

Discussion

This study demonstrated the successful reconstruction of beagle hemi-mandibular defects with allogenic mandibular scaffolds and autologous mesenchymal stem cells. The engineering of bone tissue requires three factors: scaffolds, seed cells, and growth factors. Studies have shown that bone induction is the main healing method after bone allografting. Bone induction is that allogenic bone in the form of scaffolds can induce stem cells surrounding the bone to be converted into osteoblasts and gradually result in osteogenesis. There are several advantages in using allogenic bone as scaffolds for the reconstruction of mandibular defects. These materials have structural similarities to host bone and are available in various shapes and sizes for mandibular defects. Also, as with autologous bone grafts, they can be incorporated into surrounding bone over time through "creeping substitution". Most importantly, obtaining allografts does not require killing host structures. Using an allogenic mandible as a scaffold for tissue engineering can be monitored with simple panoramic imaging as well as CT because of its similar density and porosity to natural bone.

Regarding seed cells, human bone marrow contains stem cells that can differentiate. Mesenchymal stem cells (MSCs) have the potential for multilineage differentiation, and can differentiate into cells with an osteogenic phenotype. Several studies have shown that MSCs can promote osteogenesis in vivo [9–11]. These cells can propagate in vitro into the large numbers needed to promote the regeneration of injured tissue.

The study has showed that the freeze-dried bone contain many growth factors such as BMP[12]. BMPs have unique osteoinductive proprieties. They act at an early stage and maintain both bone and cartilage formation, boosting the MSCs among cells with bone- and cartilage-forming capacity.

However, two factors influence the formation of bone tissue: the local milieu and the maintenance of stem cells in situ. Immunogenicity may be removed from freeze-dried bone allografts but cortical bone remains dense. This scenario is not conducive to permitting cells and nutrients to penetrate bone. Hence, we created many pores on the bone allograft scaffolds to permit the penetration of cells and nutrients. Fibrin glue was used in this study to maintain the position of the stem cells. Several studies have suggested that fibrin glue can be used for cell delivery because it is a biocompatible and biodegradable tissue adhesive

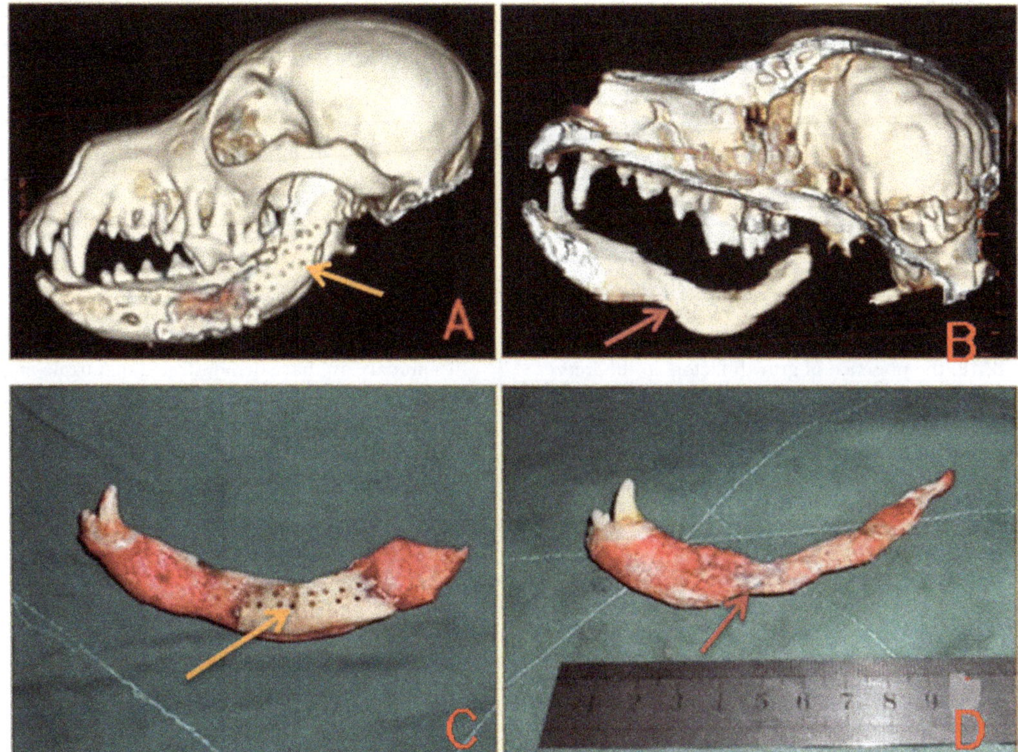

Figure 5. The shape of the mandibles was observed by gross inspection and three-dimensional CT reconstruction. A: The shape of the mandibles as observed by three-dimensional CT reconstruction showed no resorption of the allogenic mandibular scaffolds in the control group at 48 weeks. The arrow indicate the pores still can be seen in the control group at this time. B: Resorption was observed in the experimental group at 48 weeks. The arrow indicate the resorption. C: The pores still can be seen in the control group at 48 weeks. The arrow indicate the pores still can be seen in the control group at this time. D: The pores were filled with new bone in the experimental group at 48 weeks. The arrow indicate the resorption.

that stabilizes seeded cells and provides an equally distributed population of cells throughout the carrier. Authors have demonstrated that fibrin glue does not inhibit the proliferation of bone-marrow MSCs [13–15].

In this study, allogeneic bone began to absorb 1 month after transplantation in the experimental group. Absorption was significant 3 months after transplantation and new bone was formed at this time. The size of new bone was smaller than that of the original bone allograft scaffold, and almost all the bone allograft scaffold was replaced by new bone 1 year after transplantation. However, in the control group, the bone allograft was not absorbed 1 year after transplantation. The speed of the formation of new bone was slower than that observed in the experimental group. Approximately 30% of allogenic bone was replaced by new bone. It is possible that more dense bone was formed at the cortical bone, and therefore angiogenesis was slower.

Resorption of allogeneic bone in the experimental group was significantly greater (especially in the condyle), and formation of new bone faster, than that seen in the control group. These findings demonstrated that the mechanism of healing of bone allografts changed when bone marrow-derived MSCs were loaded onto the scaffolds. It is possible that the addition of cells with high osteoblastic potential could enhance the bone appositional phase from the early stages of remodeling. Nevertheless, investigation of the specific underlying mechanism merits further study.

However, histological analysis has shown that although almost all transplanted allogeneic bone was replaced by new bone in the experimental group, most of it was fibrous ossification. MSCs have the potential for multilineage differentiation into osteoblasts, chondrocytes, adipocytes, myocytes, cardiomyocytes, and neurons, amongst others. They can differentiate into osteoblasts in the presence of osteoinductive factors or an osteogenic environment. In this study, we used scaffolds and seed cells, and did not add

Table 1. The BMD of the experimental group and the control group (g/m^2, $x \pm s$).

	4 wk	12 wk	24 wk	48 wk
Experimental group	0.246±0.034	0.434±0.52	0.512±0.035	0.554±0.056
Control group	0.295±0.042	0.298±0.43	0.312±0.053	0.391±0.047
P-value	>0.05	<0.05	<0.05	<0.05

Table 2. Micro-architectural parameters of the experimental group and the control group (aggregate of all samples).

Parameters	Tb.N (/mm)	Tb.Th (mm)	Tb.Sp (mm)	BV/TV(%)
Experimental group	2.34±0.47	0.13±0.04	0.47±0.22	0.24±2.2
Control group	2.93±0.13	0.15±0.02	0.31±0.04	0.48±0.6
P-value	<0.05	<0.05	<0.05	<0.05

growth factors during the reconstruction of hemi-mandibular defects. Although the freeze-dried bone contain many growth factors such as BMP, the presence of growth factors in the freeze-dried bone was very limited. These limited growth factors could not have induced MSCs to differentiate into osteoblasts. It is possible reason that most of the "new bone" was fibrous ossification. In future studies, we will add growth factors such as BMP to assess whether more optimal results can be gained.

In summary, we have demonstrated that tissue-engineered bone could be created using bone allograft scaffold-loaded autologous marrow MSCs. MSCs accelerate the speed of absorption of bone allografts and ossification. The major drawback is infection, as two

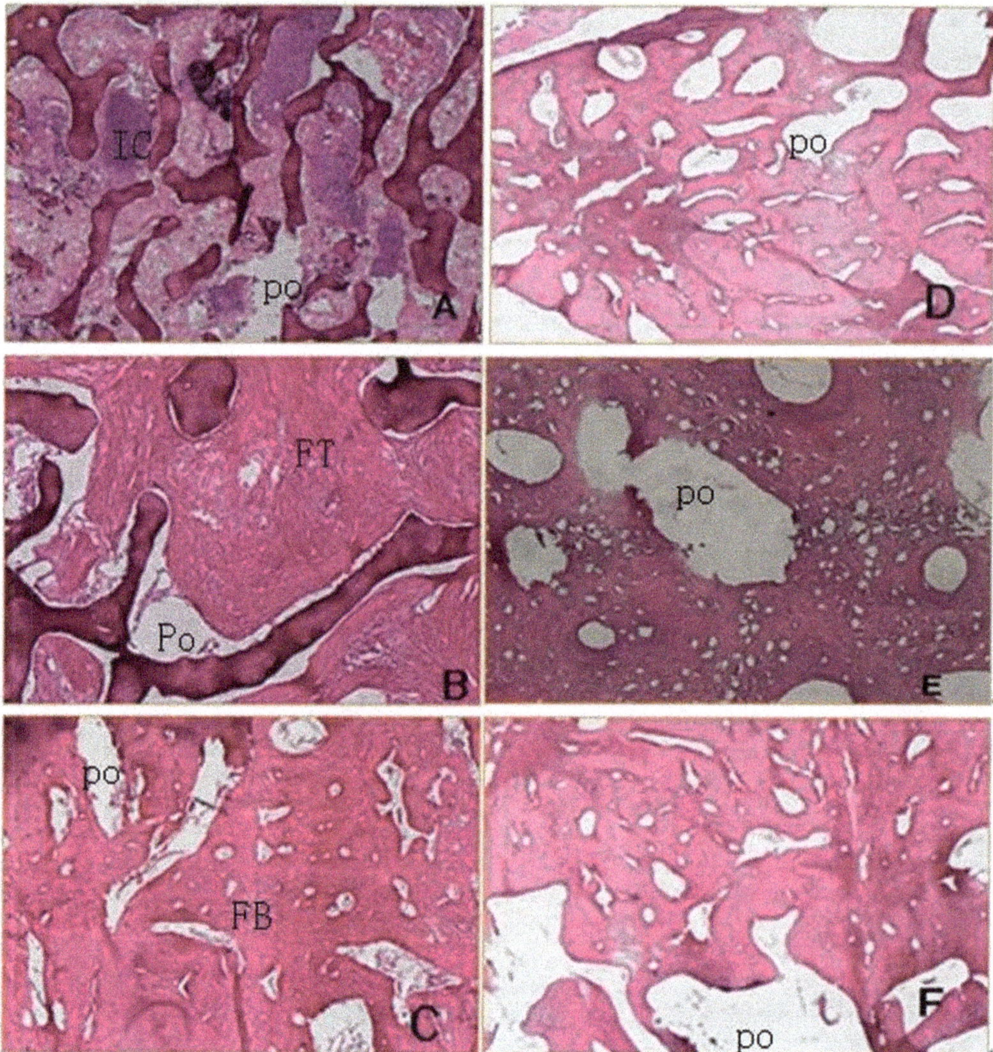

Figure 6. Histological analyses. A: Many inflammatory cells filled in the allogenic mandibular scaffold in the experimental group 4 weeks postoperatively. B: The pores were filled with fibrous tissue in the experimental group at 12 weeks after surgery. C: Most of the transplanted allogeneic bone was replaced by new bone (fibrous ossification) in the experimental group at 48weeks after the reconstruction. D: Allogeneic bone edges showed less absorption in the control group at 4 weeks after surgery. E: The pores could still be seen in the control group at 12 weeks after surgery. F: A small part of the allogenic bone graft was replaced by new bone in the control group at 48 weeks after reconstruction.(IC: inflammatory cell. Po: pore. FB: fibrous ossification. FT: fibrous tissue.)

beagles from control group and one beagle from experimental group had postoperative wound infections, and future studies will be needed to determine ways to reduce the rate of this complication.

Author Contributions

Conceived and designed the experiments: MH WY. Performed the experiments: CL XT. Analyzed the data: JL. Contributed reagents/materials/analysis tools: HL. Wrote the paper: CL.

References

1. Arrington ED, Smith WJ, Chambers HG, et al (1996) Complications of iliac crest bone graft harvesting. Clin Orthop 329:300–309.
2. Goh BT, Lee S, Tideman H, Stoelinga PJ (2008) Mandibular reconstruction in adults: a review. Int J Oral Maxillofac Surg37(7):597–605.
3. Donati D, Di Liddo M, Zavatta M, et al (2000) Massive bone allograft reconstruction in high-grade osteosarcoma. Clin Orthop377:186–94.
4. Caldora P, Donati D, Capanna R, et al (1995) Studio istomorfologico degli espianti di innesti omoplastici massivi: Risultati preliminari. Chir Org Mov 80:191–205.
5. Enneking WF, Campanacci DA (2001) Retrieved human allografts:A clinicopathological study. J Bone Joint Surg 83:971–86.
6. Enneking WF, Mindell ER (1991) Observations on massive retrieved human allografts. J Bone Joint Surg 73A:1123–42.
7. Street J, Winter D, Wang JH, et al (2000) Is human fracture hematoma inherently angiogenic? Clin Orthop 378:224–237.
8. Urist MR, Mikulski A, Lietze A (1979) Solubilized and insolubilized bone morphogenetic protein. Proc Natl Acad Sci USA76:1828–32.
9. Chen F, Chen S, Ding G (2002) Bone graft in the shape of human mandibular condyle reconstruction via seeding marrow-derived osteoblasts into porous coral in a nude mice model. J Oral Maxillofac Surg 60:1155–9.
10. Ueda M, Yamada Y, Ozawa R, et al (2005) Clinical case reports of injectable tissue-engineered bone for alveolar augmentation with simultaneous implant placement. Int J Periodontics Restorative Dent25:129.
11. Hasegawa N, Kawaguchi H, Hirachi A, et al (2006) Behavior of transplanted bone marrow-derived mesenchymal stem cells in periodontal defects. J Periodontol 77:1003.
12. Marshall R, Andrzej M, Arthur L (1979) Solubilized and insolubilized bone morphogenetic protein. Proc. Natl. Acad. Sci76(4):1828–1834.
13. Lee LT, Kwan PC, Chen YF, et al (2008) Comparison of the effectiveness of autologous fibrin glue and macroporous biphasic calcium phosphate as carriers in the osteogenesis process with or without mesenchymal stem cells. J Chin Med Assoc 71:66.
14. Ito K, Yamada Y, Naiki T, et al (2006) Simultaneous implant placement and bone regeneration around dental implants using tissue-engineered bone with fibrin glue, mesenchymal stem cells and platelet-rich plasma. Clin Oral Implants Res 17:579.
15. Isogai N, Landis WJ, Mori R, et al (2000) Experimental use of fibrin glue to induce site directed osteogenesis from cultured periosteal cells. Plast Reconstr Surg 105:953–963.

7

Effect of Topical Tranexamic Acid on Bleeding and Quality of Surgical Field during Functional Endoscopic Sinus Surgery in Patients with Chronic Rhinosinusitis: A Triple Blind Randomized Clinical Trial

Javaneh Jahanshahi[1], Farnaz Hashemian[1], Sara Pazira[1], Mohammad Hossein Bakhshaei[2], Farhad Farahani[1], Ruholah Abasi[1], Jalal Poorolajal[3]*

1 Department of Ear-Nose-Throat Surgery, School of Medicine, Hamadan University of Medical Sciences, Hamadan, Iran, **2** Department of Anesthesiology, School of Medicine, Hamadan University of Medical Sciences, Hamadan, Iran, **3** Modeling of Noncommunicable Diseases Research Center, Department of Epidemiology & Biostatistics, School of Public Health, Hamadan University of Medical Sciences, Hamadan, Iran

Abstract

Background: The effect of tranexamic acid (TXA) on bleeding and improvement of surgical field during functional endoscopic sinus surgery (FESS) is not clear yet. This study was conducted to answer this question.

Methods: This trial was conducted on 60 patients with chronic sinusitis at Beasat Hospital, Hamadan, Iran, from April to November 2013. Thirty patients in the intervention group received three pledgets soaked with TXA 5% and phenylephrine 0.5% for 10 minutes in each nasal cavity before surgery. Thirty patients in the control group received phenylephrine 0.5% with the same way. The amount of bleeding and the quality of surgical field were evaluated at 15, 30, and 45 minutes after the start of surgery using Boezaart grading.

Results: The quality of the surgical field in the intervention group compared to the control group was significantly better in the first quarter (P = 0.002) and the second quarter (P = 0.003) but not in the third quarter (P = 0.163). Furthermore, the amount of bleeding was much less during all periods in the intervention group than in the control group (P = 0.001).

Conclusion: Topical TXA can efficiently reduce bleeding and improve the surgical field in FESS in patients with rhinosinusitis. Based on these findings, topical TXA may be a useful method for providing a suitable surgical field during the first 30 minutes after use.

Trial Registration: Iranian Registry of Clinical Trials IRCT201212139014N15

Editor: Xiaoying Wang, Massachusetts General Hospital, United States of America

Funding: This study was funded by the Vice-chancellor of Research and Technology, Hamadan University of Medical Sciences. The funders had no role in study design, data collection and analysis, decision to publish, or preparation of the manuscript.

Competing Interests: The authors have declared that no competing interests exist.

* Email: poorolajal@umsha.ac.ir

Introduction

Bleeding during endoscopic sinus surgery is still a challenge for surgeons and anesthesiologists [1]. Although extensive blood loss is rare during endoscopic surgery, however, establishing a favorite surgical field is often difficult. The reason is that even slight bleeding may distort the view of the endoscope and increase the occurrence of complications, including blindness, diplopia, damage to the internal carotid artery, the longer duration of surgery, or even inconclusive surgery [2–4].

Many techniques have been proposed to improve the field of functional endoscopic sinus surgery (FESS). Bipolar diathermy, packing, local vasoconstrictors, and induced hypotension are the most commonly used techniques [3,5,6]. Diathermy can lead to local mucosal damage and delayed bleeding [3]. Using topical vasoconstrictions can lead to hemodynamic instability especially in patients with a history of hypertension or ischemic heart disease. Induction hypotension exposes the patients to more anesthetic drugs and hence a higher risk of potential side effects. However, neither of these methods guarantees a desirable surgical field with no bleeding. Therefore, investigators are working on more effective and safer methods to reduce bleeding and hence to improve the field of endoscopic sinus surgery [7].

Activation of fibrinolysis during and after surgery is a well-known phenomenon. Many mechanisms associated with coagulation disorders, such as surgical trauma, blood loss and consumption of coagulation factors and platelets, using crystalloid and colloid given during and after surgery, hypothermia, acidosis, foreign materials, and etc. [8,9]. In recent studies, systemic infusion of anti-fibrinlytic drugs have been used to reduce bleeding in various forms of surgery such as major orthopedic surgery, adeno-tonsillectomy, and endoscopic sinus surgery [7,10–12].

Tranexamic acid (TXA) is a synthetic antifibrinolytic agent that binds to the lysine binding sites of plasmin and plasminogen (13). Saturation of the binding sites causes separation of plasminogen from superficial fibrin and hence prevents fibrinolysis [13,14]. Any surgical procedure can cause a considerable tissue damage and hence trigger the release of enzymes, such as 'tissue plasminogen activator' that converts plasminogen to plasmin and activates fibrinolysis process. TXA can prevent fibrinolysis activity by inhibiting the activity of this enzyme [15].

Systemic infusion of TXA associated with several potential side effects such as nausea, vomiting, diarrhea, allergic dermatitis, dizziness, hypotension, seizures, impaired vision, achromatopsia (impaired color vision), and particularly thromboembolic events [16]. Several studies have been conducted on topical TXA in different types of surgery but no systemic absorption or side effects have been reported [13,17,18].

To date, limited trials have examined the effect of TXA on reduction of bleeding in FESS. There is no consensus on the efficacy of TXA and its effective dose in reducing bleeding [7,19–21]. This trial aimed to assess the effect of topical TXA on bleeding and improvement of surgical field during FESS in patients with chronic sinusitis with or without polyposis.

Materials and Methods

The protocol for this trial and supporting CONSORT checklist are available as supporting information; see Checklist S1 and Protocol S1.

This triple blind randomized clinical trial was conducted at Beasat Hospital, affiliated with Hamadan University of Medical Sciences, in the west of Iran, from April to November 2013. All patients were enrolled voluntarily and gave a written informed consent. The ethic committee of the university approved the consent procedure and the whole trial (D-P-9-35-16).

The eligible patients with chronic sinusitis with or without polyposis who referred to Ear-Nose-Throat clinic of Beasat Hospital were enrolled if they had the following criteria: (a) being candidate for FESS based on AAO-HNS criteria [22]; (b) age of 18 to 60 years; (c) hemoglobin >10 mg/dl; (d) normal clotting time (CT), bleeding time (BT), international normalized ratio (INR), prothrombin time (PT), Partial thromboplastin time (PTT). The patients with the following criteria were excluded from the trial: (a) having diathesis to hemorrhage such as hemophilia; (b) thrombosis; (c) acute or chronic renal failure; (d) using heparin during 48 hours before surgery; (e) using aspirin during fourteen days before surgery; (f) allergy to TXA; (g) cirrhosis; (h) chronic diseases such as hypertension, diabetes, and heart failure; (i) pregnancy; (j) color blind; (k) having a cardiac stent; (l) having a nasal tumor.

The patients in the intervention group received three pledgets soaked with TXA 5% and phenylephrine 0.5% for 10 minutes in each nasal cavity before surgery. The patients in the control group received three pads soaked with only phenylephrine 0.5% for 10 minutes in each nasal cavity before surgery. We did not use other topical agents during the course of sinus surgery to improve hemostasis.

The primary outcomes of interest were: (a) the quality of the surgical field at 15, 30, and 45 minutes after the start of surgery using Boezaart grading [23] with 0–5 scores; and (b) bleeding at 15, 30, and 45 minutes after the start of surgery using blood accumulated in the suction chamber after reducing the amount of normal saline used for washing and measurement of nasopharyngeal pack weight and converting the blood weight into ml. The secondary outcomes of interest included the potential side effects of the TXA such as: (a) nausea; (b) vomiting; (c) and impaired color vision 24 hours after surgery and three days later.

Before surgery, the paranasal sinus (PNS) CT scan was done for all patients and scoring was done [24]. In addition, for patients with polyposis, endoscopic grading was done [25]. The patients with polyposis received oral corticosteroid with the same type and dose for 10 days before surgery to reduce the inflammation of the polyposis and hence prevent massive bleeding.

Given the depth of anesthesia and anesthetic drugs on bleeding, all patients were treated under general anesthesia with the same method. For this purpose, the patients were monitored by electrocardiography and pulse oximetry. Patients' blood pressure was measured every three minutes. After premedication with fentanyl 0.1 ml/kg and midazolam 0.05–0.1 ml/kg, the induction of general anesthesia was done with lidocaine 0.5 mg/kg and propofol 2 mg/kg and atracurium 0.5 g/kg and then intubation was done with appropriate endotracheal tube. After head up position at level of 30 degrees, the patient was ready for surgery. All patients placed and maintained at the same position throughout the surgery. The general anesthesia was continued with O_2 and N_2O and infusion of propofol 1.5–4.5 mg/kg/hr to maintain the mean arterial pressure between 70 to 80 mmHg. Maintenance dose of atracurium was repeated every 20 minutes [26]. During surgery, ringer lactate was administered according to the amount of blood loss and the patient's weight. The quality of surgical field based on Boezaart grading was categorized (Table 1).

Alimian et al conducted a clinical trial and examined the effect of intravenous TXA on blood loss and the quality of the surgical field during endoscopic sinus surgery [7]. According the results of this trial, the bleeding score in the intervention and control groups was 14.3% and 42.9% respectively. Based on these results, we reached a sample of 30 for each group and a total sample of 60 at 95% significant levels and 80% statistical power.

The eligible patients were randomly assigned to the intervention and control groups using the balance block randomization method. For this purpose, we prepared six sheets of paper, writing on three sheets 'I' for 'Intervention' and on three 'C' for 'control'. The paper sheets were pooled, placed in a container, randomly drawn out one at a time for each patient without replacement until all six sheets were drawn. The six paper sheets were then placed back into the container and this action repeated until the sample size of 60 was reached. The allocation remained concealed during the study.

The random allocation was conducted by a resident of surgery, who was the coordinator of the trial group. Thus, the surgeon, who evaluated the effect of interventions, were not aware of the administered drugs. The statistical analyst was unaware of the trial groups either, until the data were analyzed and the labels were decoded. The patients were unconscious during the surgery and thus, they knew nothing about the type of intervention they received. Accordingly the trial was run as a triple blind design.

The *t*-test was used for analysis of continuous variables and the chi-square test and Fisher exact test for nominal variables. All statistical analyses were performed at a significance level of 0.05 using Stata software version 11 (StataCorp, College Station, TX, USA).

Results

Of 67 patients identified, 5 were ineligible, 2 declined to participate. The randomization was based on the remaining 60

Table 1. Boezaart grading for categorizing the quality of surgical field.

Grade	Description
0	No bleeding (cadaveric conditions)
1	Slight bleeding: no suctioning required
2	Slight bleeding: occasional suctioning required
3	Slight bleeding: frequent suctioning required, bleeding threatens surgical field a few seconds after suction is removed
4	Moderate bleeding: frequent suctioning required and bleeding threatens surgical field directly after suction is removed
5	Severe bleeding: constant suctioning required; bleeding appears faster than can be removed by suction; surgical field severely threatened and surgery usually not possible

patients, of whom 30 patients were randomly allocated to the intervention group (TXA plus phenylephrine) and 30 patients to the control group (phenylephrine alone). No patient was lost to follow-up thus the analysis was based on data from 60 patients (Figure 1).

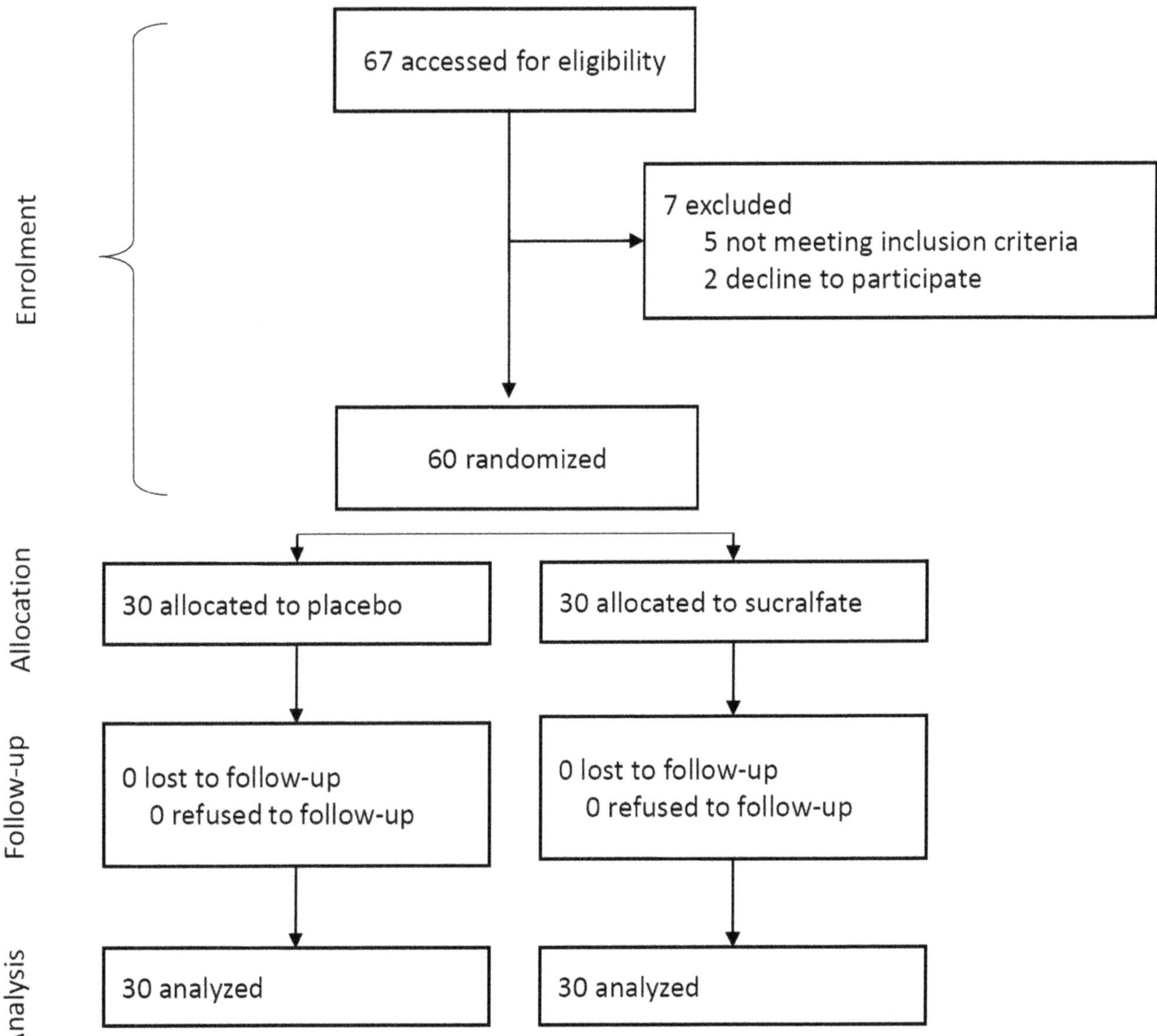

Figure 1. Flow diagram of the progress through the phases of the randomized trial of the two groups.

Table 2. Distribution of the characteristics of the study population by groups, intervention (tranexamic acid plus phenylephrine) versus control (phenylephrine alone).

	Intervention (n = 30)		Control (n = 30)		
Characteristics	**Number**	**Percent**	**Number**	**Percent**	***P* value**
Gender					0.292
Male	16	53.3	20	66.7	
Female	14	46.7	10	33.3	
Previous functional endoscopic sinus surgery					0.278
Yes	6	20.0	3	10.0	
No	24	80.0	27	90.0	
Polyposis					0.580
None	9	30.0	12	40.0	
Grade I	9	30.0	11	36.7	
Grade II	10	33.3	6	20.0	
Grade III	2	6.7	1	3.3	
Characteristics	**Mean**	**SD**	**Mean**	**SD**	***P* value**
Age (yr)	37.43	11.75	34.10	9.61	0.234
Duration of surgery (min)	114.00	37.93	102.73	25.36	0.182
Systolic blood pressure (mmHg)	100.27	7.48	102.83	7.90	0.201
Diastolic blood pressure (mmHg)	62.93	9.76	67.60	9.22	0.062
Heart rate (/min)	79.33	8.53	76.23	8.95	0.175
Mean arterial pressure (mmHg)	75.27	8.17	79.27	8.71	0.072
Total score (CT scan)	16.90	5.74	16.93	5.32	0.982
Hemoglobin (mg/dl)	14.33	1.65	14.36	1.52	0.955
Hematocrit (%)	44.13	0.70	43.69	4.17	0.667
Bleeding time (min)	2.00	0.49	1.84	0.55	0.242
Prothrombin time (s)	12.37	0.49	12.43	0.57	0.628
Partial thromboplastin time (s)	32.60	2.74	33.53	2.67	0.187
International normalization ratio	1.04	0.05	1.04	0.05	1.000
Platelet count (/mcl)	287166.70	95965.54	275633.30	67941.90	0.593

Thirty-six patients were males and 24 were females. The mean (SD) age of the patients was 35.77 (10.78) with a minimum and a maximum of 18 and 60 years respectively. The demographic and clinical characteristics of the intervention and control groups were similar with no statistically significant difference (Table 2).

The quality of surgical field based on Boezaart grading in the two groups at 15, 30 and 45 minutes after the start of surgery is given in Table 3. At 15 minutes after the start of surgery, the majority (76.7%) of the patients in the intervention group were in grade II whereas, at the same time, only 43.3% of the patients in the control group were in grade II. Furthermore, no patient in the intervention group was in grade IV while 13.3% of the patients in the control group were in grade IV ($P = 0.002$).

At 30 minutes after the start of surgery, the majority (70.0%) of the patients in the intervention group and only 26.7% of the patients in the control group were in grade II. The majority (53.3%) of the control group were in grade III ($P = 0.003$). At 45 minutes after the start of surgery, most (48.3%) of the patients in the intervention group were in grade II while most of the patients in the control group were in grade III, but the difference was not statically significant ($P = 0.163$).

The amount of bleeding in the intervention and control groups at 15, 30 and 45 minutes after the start of surgery is given in Table 4. The amount of bleeding during all periods was much higher in the control group than in the intervention group. The overall (whole time) amount of bleeding was on average 100.10 ml in the intervention group and 170.49 ml in the control group ($P = 0.001$).

Thirty-nine out of 60 patients had polyposis of different grades, 21 in the intervention group and 18 in the control group. The quality of the surgical field and amount of bleeding in the intervention and control groups was evaluated in patients with and without polyposis separately (Table 5 and 6). According to these results, in patients with or without polyposis, the quality of surgical field was much better in the intervention group than in the control group during all periods. However, there was no statistically significant difference between the two groups in patients with polyposis.

The potential side effects of TXA such as nausea, vomiting, and impaired color vision were evaluated 24 hours after surgery and three days later. But no side effect was reported.

Discussion

FESS is usually done for the treatment of patients with chronic sinonasal disease who do not respond to the conventional medical

Table 3. The effect of tranexamic acid plus phenylephrine versus phenylephrine alone on the quality of surgery field by duration of time after surgery based on Boezaart grading.

	Intervention (n = 30)		Control (n = 30)		
Quality of surgery field (grade)[a]	**Number**	**Percent**	**Number**	**Percent**	***P* value**
0–15 min					0.002
Grade I	3	10.0	0	0.0	
Grade II	23	76.7	13	43.3	
Grade III	4	13.3	13	43.3	
Grade IV	0	0.0	4	13.3	
16–30 min					0.003
Grade I	1	3.3	0	0.0	
Grade II	21	70.0	8	26.7	
Grade III	7	23.3	16	53.3	
Grade IV	1	3.3	6	20.0	
31–45 min					0.163
Grade I	1	3.5	0	0.0	
Grade II	14	48.3	7	24.1	
Grade III	11	37.9	17	58.6	
Grade IV	3	10.3	5	17.2	

[a]Grades of 0 and V were not seen.

treatment. Good visibility during FESS is necessary because nasal tiny anatomical structures, which are full of vessels, limit the nasal endoscopic access. In such situation, even a minor bleeding can lead the surgical procedure left unfinished [27].

Systemic infusion of antifibrinolytic drugs effectively reduces bleeding within and after surgery [7,11,12]. However, systemic infusion of fibrinolysis inhibitors can increase the tendency to thrombosis and thus the risk of thromboembolism. To avoid or at least reduce the risk of thromboembolism, topical TXA has been used in various surgical procedures [28]. TXA or trans-4-aminomethylcyclohexane carboxylic acid is a valuable antifibrinolytic agent that has been used for many years [29]. To date, many efforts have been made in the use of TXA to reduce bleeding and to improve the surgical field in FESS [7,19–21]. TXA is normally used intravenously. However, it is extensively used topically by several researchers in various kinds of surgical procedures. Nonetheless, yet there is no consensus on its effective dose [13,17,18,20,30].

The evidence showed that oral and intravenous TXA can reduce blood loss and improve surgical field [7,21]. To the best of our knowledge, two trials have been conducted to investigate the effect of topical TXA on bleeding and improvement of surgical field in FESS. Athanasiadis et al [19] designed a randomized controlled trial to examine the effect of topical epsilon-aminocaproic acid (EACA) and TXA on bleeding in the surgical field during FESS. In this study, 30 patients were randomized to receive either 2.5 g of EACA, 100 mg of TXA, or 1 g of TXA whereas the contralateral side received saline. They concluded that topical application of TXA could efficiently reduce bleeding and improve the surgical field. The results of this trial were consistent with our results.

Jabalameli et al [20] conducted a clinical trial on 56 patients to assess the effects of topical TXA on improving surgical field and hemostasis. In this trial, 26 patients received topical TXA and 30 patients received placebo. According to the results of this study, the amount of bleeding in the TXA group was less than the placebo group (174.0±10.6 vs 229.1±23.8 ml; $P<0.05$). Furthermore, the frequency of score 3 was 26% in TXA group and 70% in the placebo group (70%). They concluded that topical application of TXA can reduce intraoperative bleeding in FESS.

Table 4. The effect of tranexamic acid plus phenylephrine versus phenylephrine alone on the amount of bleeding by duration of time after surgery using ANOVA test.

	Intervention (n = 30)		Control 2 (n = 30)		
Amount of bleeding (ml)	**Mean**	**SD**	**Mean**	**SD**	***P* value[a]**
0–15 min	23.37	13.92	48.67	14.53	0.001
16–30 min	34.50	21.49	60.10	18.78	0.001
31–45 min	42.38	23.77	60.38	23.17	0.006
Total time	100.10	52.50	170.49	45.87	0.001

[a]Analysis of variance adjusted for polyposis and treatment-by-polyposis interaction (the interaction term was significant for no group).

Table 5. Effect of tranexamic acid plus phenylephrine versus phenylephrine alone on quality of surgery field by duration of time and with or without polyposis using Fisher exact test.

Quality of surgery field (grade)[a]	Without polyposis (n = 21)			With polyposis (n = 39)		
	Intervention	Control	*P* value	Intervention	Control	*P* value
0–15 min			0.010			0.085
Grade I	0	0		3	0	
Grade II	8	3		15	10	
Grade III	1	7		3	6	
Grade IV	0	2		0	2	
16–30 min			0.003			0.111
Grade I	0	0		1	0	
Grade II	8	2		13	6	
Grade III	1	8		6	8	
Grade IV	0	2		1	4	
31–45 min			0.014			0.951
Grade I	0	0		1	0	
Grade II	7	2		7	5	
Grade III	2	9		9	8	
Grade IV	0	1		3	4	

[a]Grades of 0 and V were not seen.

However, the way of drug prescription was not explained clearly. The effect of TXA was not examined in different periods of time after surgery either. Whereas in our study, we assessed the effect of TXA on bleeding and surgical field in different periods of time (15, 30, and 45 minutes) and indicated that the TXA had a significant effect on blood loss and improvement of surgical field at 15 and 30 minutes after the start of surgery but a non-significant effect thereafter. This may be attributed to the reduction in local concentration of TXA. Furthermore, we examined the effect of TXA on blood loss and quality of surgical field in patients with and without polyposis separately. We showed that TXA could provide an effective hemostasis and a suitable surgical field in patients without polyposis compared to control group. However, TXA had limited effect on bleeding and quality of surgical field in patients with polyposis. This may be either attributed to the hemorrhagic nature of polyposis which may overcome the hemostatic effect of TXA or it may be that the study was underpowered to show the difference in subgroups because the study did not have enough polyps patient to reach statistical significance. Furthermore, the total number of the patients with polyposis was 39; 21 of which were in the intervention group and 18 in the control group. That means the number of polyp patients and hence the risk of hemorrhage was higher in the intervention group than the control group. If the proportion of the polyposis was the same in the two groups, the difference between the two groups might become much greater and hence the statistical power of our study might become stronger. This issue favor our findings that topical TXA can efficiently reduce bleeding and improve the surgical field in FESS in patients with rhinosinusitis

The main limitation of this study was the small sample size. This might introduce random error in the results of subgroup analysis of patients with and without polyposis. Therefore, we suggest that randomized controlled trials are designed to examine the effect of TXA on bleeding and quality of surgical field in patients with and without polyposis separately. This would be an important area for a future adequately powered study for patients with polyps.

Conclusion

Topical TXA can efficiently reduce bleeding and improve the surgical field in FESS in patients with rhinosinusitis. Based on these findings, topical TXA may be a useful method for providing

Table 6. Effect of tranexamic acid plus phenylephrine versus phenylephrine alone on amount of bleeding by duration of time and with or without polyposis using Fisher exact test.

Amount of bleeding (mL) mean (SD)	Without polyposis (n = 21)			With polyposis (n = 39)		
	Intervention	Control	*P* value	Intervention	Control	*P* value
0–15 min	21.11 (6.49)	52.58 (11.12)	0.001	24.33 (16.15)	46.06 (16.19)	0.001
16–30 min	27.67 (16.44)	63.42 (20.60)	0.001	37.43 (23.05)	57.89 (17.73)	0.004
31–45 min	32.78 (16.19)	60.08 (17.91)	0.002	46.70 (25.67)	60.59 (26.82)	0.117
Total	81.56 (32.38)	176.08 (38.52)	0.001	108.45 (58.17)	166.53 (51.21)	0.003

a suitable surgical field during the first 30 minutes after use. However, additional trials should be conducted to explore TXA efficacy in different subgroups of the patients with or without polyposis.

Supporting Information

Protocol S1 Trial Protocol.

Checklist S1 CONSORT Checklist.

Acknowledgments

We would like to appreciate the Vic-chancellor of Research and Technology of Hamadan University of Medical Sciences for financial support of this work.

Author Contributions

Conceived and designed the experiments: JJ SP JP. Performed the experiments: JJ SP FF FH MHB RA JP. Analyzed the data: JJ SP JP. Contributed reagents/materials/analysis tools: JJ SP JP. Wrote the paper: JJ SP FF FH MHB RA JP.

References

1. Wormald PJ, Athanasiadis T, Rees G, Robinson S (2005) An evaluation of effect of pterygopalatine fossa injection with local anesthetic and adrenalin in the control of nasal bleeding during endoscopic sinus surgery. Am J Rhinol 19: 288–292.
2. Flint PW, Phelps T (2010) Cummings otolaryngology head & neck surgery. Philadelphia.
3. Wormald PJ (2005) Endoscopic sinus surgery: Anatomy,Three-Dimentional Reconstruction,and Surgical Technique. New York: Thieme.
4. Wormald PJ, van Renen G, Perks J, Jones JA, Langton-Hewer CD (2005) The effect of the total intravenous anesthesia compared with inhalational anesthesia on the surgical field during endoscopic sinus surgery. Am J Rhinol 19: 514–520.
5. Feldman M, Patel A (2009) Anesthesia for eye, ear, nose, and throat surgeryIn; In: Miller RD e, editor. New York: Churchill Livingstone.
6. Shaw CL, Dymock RB, Cowin A, Wormald PJ (2000) Effect of packing on nasal mucosa of sheep. J Laryngol Otol 114: 506–509.
7. Alimian M, Mohseni M (2011) The effect of intravenous tranexamic acid on blood loss and surgical field quality during endoscopic sinus surgery: a placebo-controlled clinical trial. J Clin Anesth 23: 611–615.
8. Fries D, Martini WZ (2010) Role of fibrinogen in trauma-induced coagulopathy. Br J Anaesth 105: 116–121.
9. Tanaka KA, Key NS, Levy JH (2009) Blood coagulation: hemostasis and thrombin regulation. Anesth Analg 108: 1433–1446.
10. Brum MR, Miura MS, Castro SF, Machado GM, Lima LH, et al. (2012) Tranexamic acid in adenotonsillectomy in children: a double-blind randomized clinical trial. Int J Pediatr Otorhinolaryngol 76: 1401–1405.
11. Crescenti A, Borghi G, Bignami E, Bertarelli G, Landoni G, et al. (2011) Intraoperative use of tranexamic acid to reduce transfusion rate in patients undergoing radical retropubic prostatectomy: double blind, randomised, placebo controlled trial. BMJ 343: d5701.
12. Ralley FE, Berta D, Binns V, Howard J, Naudie DD (2010) One intraoperative dose of tranexamic Acid for patients having primary hip or knee arthroplasty. Clin Orthop Relat Res 468: 1905–1911.
13. Bonis MD, Cavaliere F, Alessandrini F, Lapenna E, Santarelli F, et al. (2000) Topical use of tranexamic acid in coronary artery bypass operations: a double-blind, prospective, randomized, placebo-controlled study J Thorac Cardiovasc Surg 119: 575–580.
14. Longstaff C (1994) Studies on the mechanism of action of aprotinin and tranexamic acid as plasmin inhibitors and antifibrinolytic agents. Blood Coag Fibrinol 5: 537–542.
15. Katzung B (1995) Basic and clinical pharmacology. Norwalk: Appleton and Lange.
16. Food and Drug Administration (2011) Cyklokapron. 2896366 ed: FDA. pp.8.
17. Abrishami A, Chung F, Wong J (2009) Topical application of antifibrinolytic drugs for on-pump cardiac surgery: a systematic review and meta-analysis. Can J Anaesth 56: 202–212.
18. Tang YM, Chapman TW, Brooks P (2012) Use of tranexamic acid to reduce bleeding in burns surgery. J Plast Reconstr Aesthet Surg 65: 684–686.
19. Athanasiadis T, Beule AG, Wormald PJ (2007) Effects of topical antifibrinolytics in endoscopic sinus surgery: a pilot randomized controlled trial. Am J Rhinol 21: 737–742.
20. Jabalameli M, Zakeri K (2006) Evaluation of Topical Tranexamic Acid on Intraoperative Bleeding in Endoscopic Sinus Surgery. Iran J Med Sci 31: 221–223.
21. Yaniv E, Shvero J, Hadar T (2006) Hemostatic effect of tranexamic acid in elective nasal surgery. Am J Rhinol 20: 227–229.
22. Lau J, Zucker D, Engels EA, Balk E, Barza M, et al. (1999) Diagnosis and treatment of acute bacterial rhinosinusitis: summary. Bethesda: AHRQ Evidence Report Summaries.
23. Boezaart AP, van der Merwe J, Coetzee A (1995) Comparison of sodium nitroprusside- and esmolol-induced controlled hypotension for functional endoscopic sinus surgery. Can J Anaesth 42: 373–376.
24. Lund VJ, Kennedy DW (1997) International consensus report of the Rhinosinusitis Task Force. Otolaryngol Head Neck Surg 117: 35–40.
25. Lund VJ, Mackay IS (1993) Staging in rhinosinusitis. Rhinology 31: 183–184.
26. Ahn HJ, Chung SK, Dhong HJ, Kim HY, Ahn JH, et al. (2008) Comparison of surgical conditions during propofol or sevoflurane anaesthesia for endoscopic sinus surgery. Br J Anaesth 100: 50–54.
27. Lanza DC, Kennedy DW (2001) Endoscopic sinus surgery; Bailey BJ, editor. Philadelphia: lippincott Williams &Wilkins.
28. Dell'Amore A, Caroli G, Nizar A, Cassanelli N, Luciano G, et al. (2012) Can Topical Application of Tranexamic Acid Reduce Blood Loss in Thoracic Surgery? A Prospective Randomised Double Blind Investigation. Heart Lung Circ 21: 706–710.
29. Lundström J, Westin-Sjödahl G, Jönsson NÅ (2006) Synthesis of 14C-labelled tranexamic acid [trans-amino-(14C-methyl)-cyclohexane carboxylic acid]. J Labelled Comp Radiopharm 12: 307–310.
30. Kaewpradub P, Apipan B, Rummasak D (2011) Does tranexamic acid in an irrigating fluid reduce intraoperative blood loss in orthognathic surgery? a double-blind, randomized clinical trial. J Oral Maxillofac Surg 69: 186–189.

8

A Comparative Study of Four Types of Free Flaps from the Ipsilateral Extremity for Finger Reconstruction

Yujie Liu[1,2], Hongsheng Jiao[2], Xiang Ji[2], Chunlei Liu[2], Xiaopen Zhong[2], Hongxun Zhang[2], Xiaohen Ding[2], Xuecheng Cao[1]*

1 Department of Orthopedic and Traumatic Surgery, General Hospital of Jinan Military Command, Jinan, P. R. China, 2 The Hand Surgery Center of Chinese People's Liberation Army, The 401st Hospital of CPLA, Qingdao, P. R. China

Abstract

Aim: To compare the outcomes of finger reconstruction using arterialized venous flap (AVF), superficial palmar branch of the radial artery (SPBRA) flap, posterior interosseous perforator flap (PIPF), and ulnar artery perforator free (UAPF) flap harvested from the ipsilateral extremity.

Methods: We retrospectively reviewed the outcomes for 41 free flaps from the ipsilateral extremity in the reconstruction of finger defects in 41 patients with small/moderate skin defects, including 11 AVFs, 10 SPBRA flaps, 10 PIPFs, and 10 UAPF flaps. Standardized assessment of outcomes was performed, including duration of operation, objective sensory recovery, cold intolerance, time of returning to work, active total range of motion (ROM) of the injured fingers, and the cosmetic appearance of the donor/recipient sites.

Results: All flaps survived completely, and the follow-up duration was 13.5 months. The mean duration of the complete surgical procedure for AVFs was distinctly shorter than that of the other flaps ($p<0.05$). AVFs were employed to reconstruct skin defects and extensor tendon defects using a vascularized palmaris longus graft in 4 fingers. Digital blood supply was reestablished in 4 fingers by flow-through technique when using AVFs. Optimal sensory recovery was better with AVFs and SPBRA flaps as compared with UAPF flaps and PIPFs ($p<0.05$). No significant differences were noted in ROM or cold intolerance between the 4 groups. Optimal cosmetic satisfaction was noted for the recipient sites of AVFs and the donor sites of SPBRA flaps. The number of second-stage defatting operations required for AVFs was considerably lesser than that for the other flaps.

Conclusion: All 4 types of free flaps from the ipsilateral extremity are a practical choice in finger reconstruction for small/moderate-sized skin defects. AVFs play an important role in such operations due to the wider indications, and better sensory recovery and cosmetic appearance associated with this method.

Editor: Fabio Santanelli, di Pompeo d'Illasi, Sapienza, University of Rome, School of Medicine and Psychology, Italy

Funding: The authors have no support or funding to report.

Competing Interests: The authors have declared that no competing interests exist.

* Email: caoxchengjn@126.com

Introduction

The reconstruction of fingers with skin and soft tissue defects remains challenging. The optimal reconstructive treatment should be simple, reliable, cost effective, and provide pliable, sensitive, and cosmetically similar tissue that will allow adequate function [1]. Local and regional skin flaps, such as the palmar advancement flap [2], cross-finger flap [3], distally based homodigital island flaps [4], and pedicled perforator finger flaps [5,6], are excellent for rapid and easy reconstruction; however, they do involve certain drawbacks, such as limitations of flap advancement or coverage, poor sensation joint stiffness, large scars on donor and recipient digits, vulnerable venous return, and the potential for development of painful neuroma in the pedicle [3–6].

Although the concept of free tissue transfer to traumatized digits remains unpopular with many surgeons for high technique demand, a free flap of appropriate size may provide an ideal surgical solution, since it is associated with a shorter time of returning to work and satisfactory function and aesthetic appearance [7]. According to the "replace like with like" principle [8], free flaps used for the repair of the finger skin defects should ideally be obtained from the counterparts of the fingers–i.e., the toes. However, the markedly high rate of donor site morbidity is the main disadvantage of the free pulp flap [7,9,10]. Several types of distant free flaps are available for reconstructing finger injuries, such as the posterior auricular free flap [11] and the medial plantar artery perforator flap [12]. However, these procedures require two operative fields and complex anesthesia.

Four types of free flaps have been used in finger reconstruction from the ipsilateral extremity, including arterialized venous flap (AVF) [13], superficial palmar branch of the radial artery (SPBRA) flap [14], posterior interosseous perforator flap (PIPF) [15], and ulnar artery perforator free (UAPF) flap [16]. These flaps are characterized by the following features: (i) they need only one operative field and simple anesthesia involving a simple brachial block to the injured extremity, which is surgeon-friendly with a single tourniquet; (ii) low donor site morbidity, and without sacrificing the main vessels; (iii) allowing sensory recovery in the fingers due to the inclusion of a sensory nerve; and (iv) thin flap which can achieve better aesthetic appearance due to less subcutaneous fat [13–16].

However, in clinical practice, the selection of these flaps remains contentious since no study has investigated the differences in the clinical outcomes of these 4 free flaps. In this retrospective study, we compared and analyzed the outcomes in 41 patients with small/moderate skin defects who underwent finger reconstruction using AVF, SPBRA flap, PIPF, or UAPF flap.

Patients and methods

Patients

We included 41 patients admitted to our department from October 2006 to December 2012 in this retrospective analysis. Among these cases, finger reconstruction using AVFs was performed in 11 patients, while SPBRA flaps, PIPFs, or UAPF flaps were used for single finger injury in 10 patients. All the patients had sustained skin defects with the exposure of the deep structures, such as tendons, bones, or joints. All the patients were treated as emergencies within an average of 6 hours after injury (range, 2–10 h). The mechanisms of injury included crushing injury, degloving injury, and cutting injury (Table 1). Innervated flaps were employed in reconstruction only when all the finger pulps were damaged. Among the 41 fingers, 2 fingers for each flap type (n = 8) with finger pulp defects were constructed by a sensate flap. In other cases, nonsensate flaps were used.

Written informed consent was obtained from each patient prior to surgery and saved in the documentation department. The protocols used in this study were approved by the Ethics Committee of the 401st Hospital of Chinese People Liberation Army (Qingdao, China).

Methods

Cases were reviewed in terms of objective sensory recovery, cold intolerance, and time of returning to work. Sensory testing was undertaken using static two-point discrimination (s2PD), moving two-point discrimination (m2PD), and Semmes-Weinstein monofilament test (SWM test). The overall outcomes of the patients were assessed independently by the senior author (J.X.), who was blinded to the surgical procedure. Cold intolerance in the reconstructed digit was rated by the patients based on normal daily activity and graded as none, slight, moderate, or severe [17]. Patients' self-assessments for cosmetic appearance–mainly based on the appearance of the donor and recipient sites were carried out with a visual analog scale ranging from 0 (completely disappointed) to 10 (completely satisfied) and divided into 3 classes (good, 10–8; acceptable, 7–5; unacceptable, <5) [18,19].

Statistical analysis

The F-test was used to assess the homogeneity of variance of the demographic data for the 2 groups. Student's t-test was used to compare intergroup differences in the duration of operation and time of returning to work. The Wilcoxon signed-rank test was used to compare intergroup differences in cold intolerance, 2PD, and SWM tests. A p value <0.05 was considered to demonstrate statistically significant differences.

Table 1. Demographic data.

Group	Flaps (n)	Age	Sex	Sex	Injury mechanism			Finger		Extensor tendon defect	bilateral arteria digitalis defect
			Male	Female	CU	CR	DE	DF	Non-DF		
AVF group	11	31±7.2 (17–44)	7	4	4	4	3	6	5	4	4
SPBRA flap group	10	34±8.9 (19–42)	7	3	2	6	2	6	4	none	none
UAPF group	10	36±6.7 (16–45)	7	3	1	7	2	6	4	none	none
PIPF group	10	35±6.2 (17–42)	6	4	2	6	2	5	5	none	none

AVF: arterialized venous flap, SPBRA: superficial palmar branch of the radial artery flap, PIPF: posterior interosseous perforator flap, UAPF: ulnar artery perforator free flap, CR: crushing injury, DE: degloving injury, CU: cutting injury, DF, fingers of the dominant hand, non-DF, fingers of the non-dominant hand.

Table 2. General results.

Group	Flaps (n)	Flap size (mm)	Flap survival	Mean surgical duration (hour)	Time of returning to work (week)	Cold intolerance				Patients' self-assessments for cosmetic appearance		Mean of ROM (°)	Number of flaps needed for secondary surgery for defatting
						None	Slight	Moderate	Severe	Recipient Site	Donor Site		
AVF group	11	35×19	CS, 6 blister formation	3.4±1.2 (3.0–4.5)	12 (11–21)	2	5	2	2	good (9); acceptable (2)	good (4); acceptable (7)	208	none
SPBRA flap group	10	34×16	CS, 3 blister formation	4.9±1.7 * (4.1–6.5)	10 (7–15)	7	1	2	1	good (5); acceptable (5)	good (8); acceptable (2)	233	4
UAPF group	10	31×19	CS, 2 blister formation	5.1±1.3 * (4.5–6.1)	9 (6–15)	6	2	2	0	good (3); acceptable (7)	good (5); acceptable (5)	224	5
PIPF group	10	34×20	CS, 3 blister formation	4.8±1.8 * (4.0–6.7)	10 (7–16)	6	1	3	0	good (3); acceptable (7)	good (5); acceptable (5)	214	5

*, P<0.05, compared with the AVF group; AVF: arterialized venous flap, SPBRA: superficial palmar branch of the radial artery flap, PIPF: posterior interosseous perforator flap, UAPF: ulnar artery perforator free flap, CS: complete survival, ROM: range of motion. Surgical duration: from the induction of anesthesia until the patient was transferred from the operating room.

Table 3. Sensory evaluation results of 4 types of nonsensate flaps.

Group	Flaps (n)	s2PD	m2PD	SWM			
				NS (n)	DLT (n)	DPS (n)	LPS (n)
AVF group	9	7 (4–9)	6 (4–8)	3	3	2	1
SPBRA flap group	8	8 (6–9)	7 (5–9)	2	3	2	1
UAPF group	8	11 (7–14)*,#	12 (6–13) *,#	0	1	4	3
PIPF group	8	13 (8–16)*,#,†	11 (8–15) *,#	0	1	3	4

*, P<0.05, compared with the AVF group;
#, P<0.05, compared with the SPBRA group;
†, and P<0.05, compared with the UAPF group.
AVF: arterialized venous flap, SPBRA: superficial palmar branch of the radial artery, PIPF: posterior interosseous perforator flap, UAPF: ulnar artery perforator free flap, SWM: Semmes-Weinstein monofilament test, NS: normal sensation (filament level, 2.36–2.83), DLT: diminished light touch (filament level, 3.22–3.61), DPS: diminished protective touch (filament level, 3.84–4.31), LPS: loss of protective sensation (filament level, 4.56).

Table 4. Sensory evaluation results of 4 types of sensate flaps.

Group	Flaps (n)	s2PD	m2PD	SWM			
				NS (n)	DLT (n)	DPS (n)	LPS (n)
AVF group	2	5 5	5 4	1	1		
SPBRA flap group	2	6 5	6 5	1	1		
UAPF group	2	6 7	6 6	1	1		
PIPF group	2	7 8	6 7	1	1		

AVF: arterialized venous flap, SPBRA: superficial palmar branch of the radial artery, PIPF: posterior interosseous perforator flap, UAPF: ulnar artery perforator free flap, SWM: Semmes-Weinstein monofilament test, NS: normal sensation (filament level, 2.36–2.83), DLT: diminished light touch (filament level, 3.22–3.61), DPS: diminished protective touch (filament level, 3.84–4.31), LPS: loss of protective sensation (filament level, 4.56).

Surgical techniques

All the flaps were harvested from the forearm of the ipsilateral extremity under a brachial plexus nerve block. The surgery was performed using a pneumatic tourniquet. After thorough debridement, the recipient digital artery and nerve and the dorsal digital vein were identified and marked. All the flaps were tailored to a size 5–8 mm larger than the recipient site to alleviate possible postoperative swelling and edema.

Designing and harvesting the AVF. AVF elevation was performed as previously described [13]. Briefly, the flap was designed on the volar side of the forearm, which included 2 veins. The ratio of the afferent and efferent veins to be anastomosed was 1:1 or 1:2. The relatively smaller vein was used as the afferent vein, while the larger vein was used as the efferent vein. In total, 11 AVFs were harvested, among which 7 were allocated to type III (perfusion patterns: A-V-V, 1 through-valve and 6 against-valve), and 4 were allocated to type IV (perfusion patterns: A-V-A, 4 through-valve) according to Chen's classification [20]. The efferent vein was delivered to the dorsal anastomotic site through a loose subcutaneous tunnel. In 4 fingers, AVFs combined with a vascularized palmaris longus graft were employed to reconstruct extensor tendon defects simultaneously. In 4 other fingers, the digital blood supply was lost since the bilateral arteria digitalis vessels were severed. Digital blood supply was reestablished via the flow-through technique using the veins contained in AVF grafts. The anterior branch of the medial or lateral cutaneous nerve of the forearm was incorporated into the flap to create an innervated flap if necessary.

Designing and harvesting the SPBRA flap. The SPBRA flap was elevated as previously described [14]. Briefly, after the route of the flap and subcutaneous vein were marked, the SPBRA flap was designed over the volar aspect of the distal forearm according to the size of the finger defect. The flap was designed with an elliptical shape to facilitate donor site closure. The concomitant vein of the SPBRA flap and subcutaneous veins were preserved to facilitate subsequent venous return. The palmar cutaneous branch of the median nerve was incorporated into the flap to create an innervated flap if necessary.

Designing and harvesting the UAPF flap. The UAPF flap was raised as previously described [16,21]. In brief, the axis of the UAPF flap was the connecting line between the pisiform and the medial humeral epicondyle. The ulnar artery perforator arose from a branch of the ulnar artery, located approximately 40 mm proximal to the pisiform bone. The flap was designed according to the size of the defect. Then, an incision was made along the radial border of the flap. Once the perforator was identified, an incision was made for the ulnar border of the flap, and the flap was elevated. The accompanying vein and superficial vein in the flap were used for venous return. The terminal branch of the medial antebrachial cutaneous nerve was incorporated into the flap to create an innervated flap if necessary.

Designing and harvesting the PIPFs. PIPFs were designed as described previously after the perforator was preoperatively identified by Doppler examination [15]. The PIPF was elevated from the ulnar side to the radial side through the subcutaneous tissue plane. Once the perforator was identified, the intermuscular septum and a tiny ellipse of the deep fascial cuff were preserved around the posterior interosseous vessel. In some patients, the diameter of the accompanying vein was too narrow; therefore, the superficial vein was instead used for ensuring venous return. The posterior antebrachial cutaneous nerve was incorporated into the flap to create an innervated flap if necessary.

Upon the completion of flap grafting in the recipient sites, anastomoses of the blood vessels and/or nerves were performed

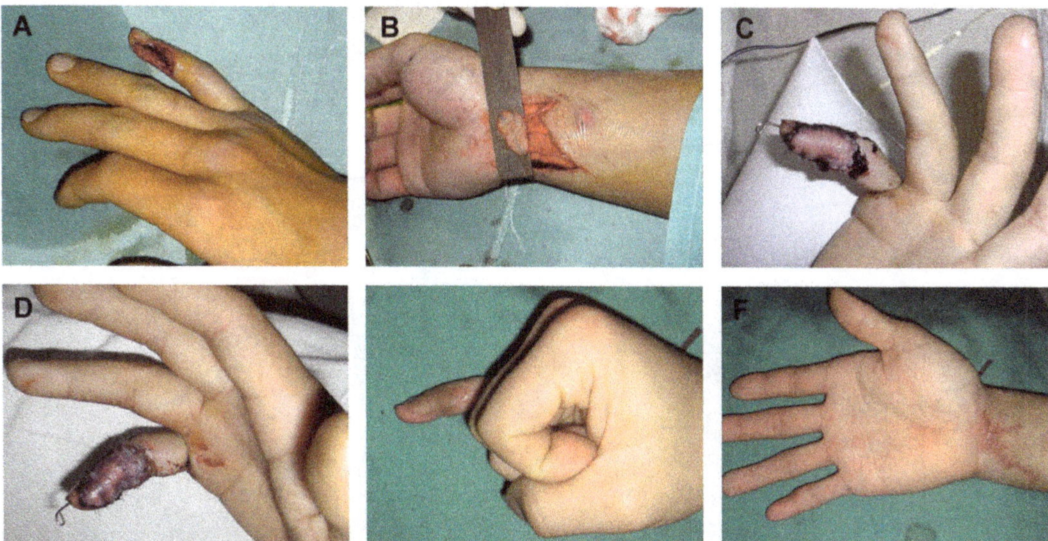

Figure 1. Finger reconstruction by AVF. Case 1: A 34-year-old man underwent finger reconstruction by AVF. (A) Preoperative defect of the little finger. (B) The design and elevation of the AVF. This flap contained 2 veins. The relatively smaller vein was used as the afferent vein, while the larger vein was used as the efferent vein. The perfusion pattern employed was the against-valve type. (C) The 4-day postoperative view shows good blood supply in the flap. (D) The 7-day postoperative view indicates the presence of blisters sporadically distributed over the flap, along with slight venous congestion. (E, F) The 10-month postoperative view shows that all the blisters subsided gradually without any special care. The flap completely survived, with excellent contour and texture. The patient's self-assessments for cosmetic appearance was good on recipient site (9 scores), acceptable on donor site (6 scores).

using an end-to-end method. Postoperatively, each flap was monitored hourly for 3 days. Each patient received oral aspirin (125 mg/day) and subcutaneously injected low-molecular-weight dextran (30 mL/day) for 7 days postoperatively. Further, a dorsal cast of plaster of Paris was used for immobilizing the injured limb for 1 week. Subsequently, an active and passive physical rehabilitation program was initiated to achieve the finger's maximal range of motion (ROM).

Results

All the patients included in the study were followed up for a mean duration of 13.5 months (9–18 months). The outcome was

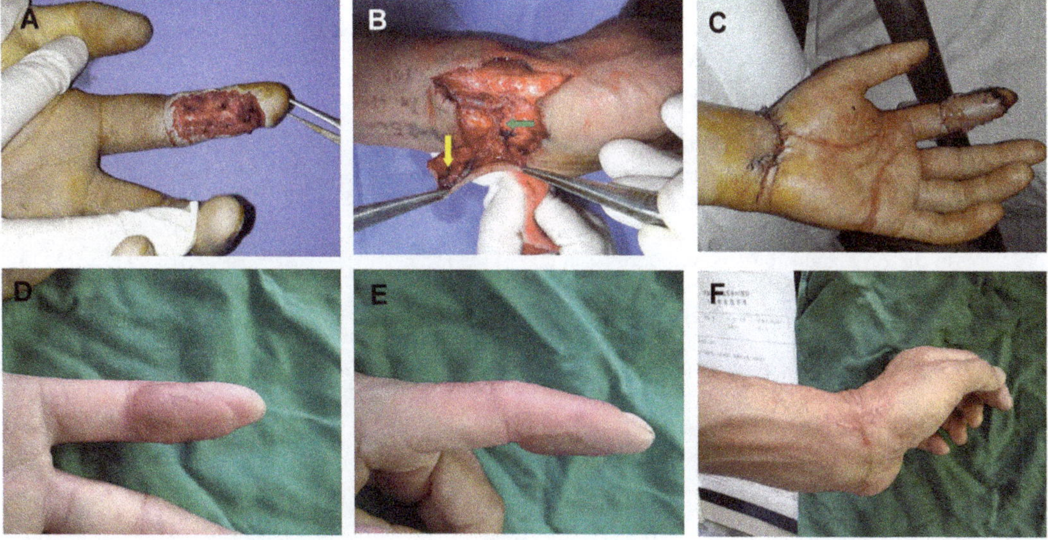

Figure 2. Finger reconstruction by using the SPBRA flap. Case 2: A 45-year-old man underwent finger reconstruction using the SPBRA flap. (A) Preoperative defect of the middle finger. (B) The elevation of the SPBRA flap. The green arrow indicates the SPBRA and its concomitant vein. The yellow arrow indicates a subcutaneous vein. The ratio of the artery and veins to be anastomosed was 1:2. (C) The 5-day postoperative view indicates the presence of blisters distributed over the flap. All the blisters subsided gradually without any special care. (D) The 10-month postoperative volar view. (E) The 10-month postoperative lateral view. (F) The 10-month postoperative donor site and wrist function view. The patient's self-assessments for cosmetic appearance was acceptable on recipient site (7 scores), good on donor site (9 scores).

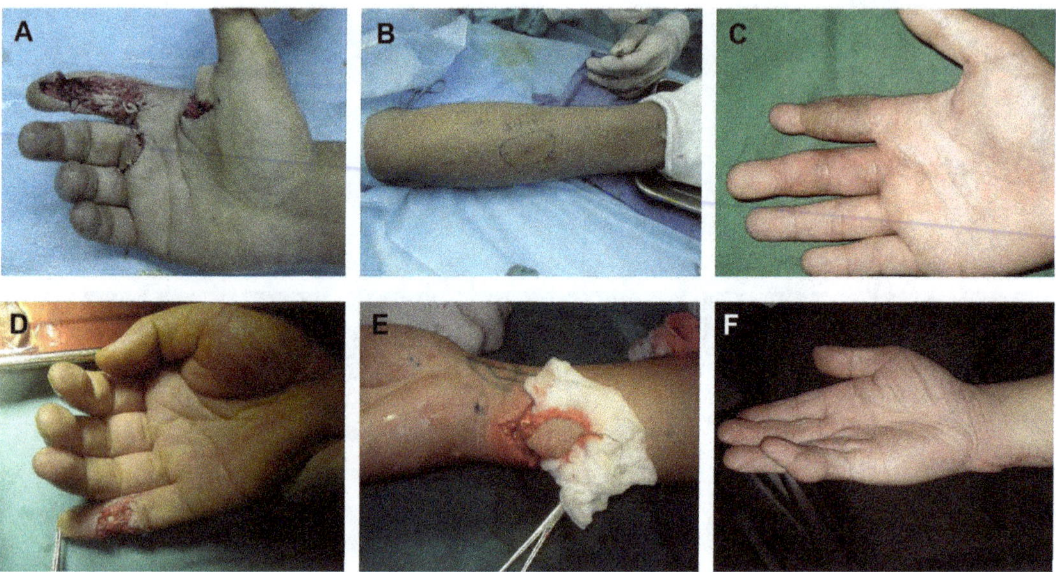

Figure 3. Finger reconstruction by using the PIPF and UAPF flap. Case 3: A 30-year-old man underwent finger reconstruction using the PIPF. (A) Preoperative defect of the index finger. The ulnaris digital artery was intact, whereas a defect of the radialis digital artery was noted. (B) The design of the flap, showing the perforator located at midpoint of Lister's tubercle and humerus epicondyle. The radialis digital artery was anastomosed with the posterior interosseous perforator. The diameter of the accompanying vein was too narrow; therefore, 2 superficial veins were used for ensuring venous return. (C) The 12-month postoperative view. This patient's self-assessments for cosmetic appearance was good on recipient site (8 scores). Case 4: A 42-year-old man underwent finger reconstruction using the UAPF flap. (D) Preoperative defect of the little finger. (E) The design and elevation of the flap, with the defected ulnar digital artery anastomosed with the ulnar artery perforator, which was located approximately 40 mm proximal to the pisiform bone. The accompanying vein and superficial vein were used for venous return. (F) The 15-month postoperative view. This patient's self-assessments for cosmetic appearance were acceptable on recipient site (6 scores).

recorded in each group and the details of complications have been provided in Table 2. The mean sizes of the AVF, SPBRA flap, UAPF flap, and PIPF were 35×19 mm, 34×16 mm, 31×19 mm, and 34×20 mm, respectively. All the flaps survived completely. All donor sites were closed primarily without dehiscence except for 4 flaps, including 2 UAPF flaps (measuring 5×3 cm and 5×3.5 cm) and 2 SPBRA flaps (measuring 5×3.2 cm and 4×2.6 cm). Full-thickness skin grafts were used to close these donor sites. The mean duration of the complete surgical procedure of AVF was 3.4±1.2 (3.0–4.5) h, which was distinctly shorter than that for the other flaps ($p<0.05$).

AVF grafts were more prone to blister formation as compared to the other graft types. In the AVF grafts, blister formation was observed in 6 flaps postoperatively (6/11), but only in 2–3 flaps from each of the other groups. All the blisters subsided gradually with no special care. In the AVF grafts, blisters were formed in a retrograde perfusion pattern in 1 flap, while in the other 5 flaps, they were formed in an antegrade perfusion pattern.

Almost full ROM was obtained in all the reconstructed fingers. The mean ROM was 198° in the 4 fingers where the vascularized palmaris longus tendon graft was used with AVF. Two fingers using AVFs showed moderate cold intolerance, while the 2 patients in whom the bilateral arteria digitalis were damaged demonstrated severe intolerance. No significant differences were noted in ROM or cold intolerance between the 4 groups ($p>0.05$).

The results of the sensory evaluation of the 4 types of nonsensate flaps are shown in Table 3. In the 33 grafts with nonsensate flap, good sensory recovery was obtained in the patients who received AVF and SPBRA flaps, with s2PD of 7 mm (4–9 mm) and 8 mm (6–9 mm), respectively (Table 3). However, poor sensation was recorded for the fingers reconstructed using UAPF flaps and PIPF, with s2PD of 11 mm (7–14 mm) and 13 mm (8–16 mm), respectively. With regard to SWM, a higher percentage of normal sensation (filament level, 2.36–2.83) was noted in the grafts with AVF (3/9, 33.3%) and SPBRA flap (2/8, 25%). In contrast, no normal sensation was noted in UAPF flap and PIPF. Diminished light touch was achieved only in 1 flap each in the grafts with UAPF flap (1/8, 12.5%) and PIPF (1/8, 12.5%). For intergroup differences for s2PD, m2DP, and SWM, the Wilcoxon signed-rank test demonstrated significant differences in sensory recovery for each parameter ($p<0.05$). The fingers with AVF grafts showed optimal sensory recovery, followed by those with SPBRA flaps. Eight finger pulps (2 from each group) reconstructed by using sensate flaps showed s2PD of 5 mm (5–8 mm), normal sensation (filament level, 2.36–2.83) for 4 fingers, and diminished light touch (filament level, 3.22–3.61) for 4 fingers (Table 4).

At 9–18 months postoperatively, the patients self-evaluated cosmetic recovery: for the recipient site, the AVF grafts reported the highest satisfaction (9/11, 81.8%), while for the donor sites, the SPBRA flaps were rated the highest (8/10, 80.0%, Table 2). No defatting operations were required in the fingers grafted with AVFs; however, the number of flaps that needed secondary defatting when fingers were grafted with the SPBRA flap, UAPF flap, and PIPF was 4, 5, and 5, respectively (Table 2, Figures 1, 2, 3).

Discussion

In our study, we found that AVF could be used for broader therapeutic indications than the other 3 flaps. First, composite AVF with a vascularized tendon was an optimal choice for one-stage reconstruction of dorsal composite finger injuries as compared with multi-stage reconstruction or grafting of non-vascularized tendons [22,23]. Recent studies have indicated that a vascularized tendon can be integrated into AVFs and SPBRA flaps for finger reconstruction of skin and tendon defects [24,25]. In theory, a vascularized palmaris longus in the SPBRA flap is possible; however, its clinical application remains a problem due to the long distance (average, 2.2–3.0 cm) between the originating point of the SPBRA and the palmaris longus [24]. For a flap with a vascularized palmaris longus tendon, the length of the SPBRA flap must be greater than 3 cm. This limits the clinical application of this flap [14]. In contrast, AVF can be designed in a position centered on the palmaris longus tendon. It is easy to carry the vascularized tendon. In our study, AVFs were used in 4 fingers with extensor tendon defects, with satisfactory outcomes.

Second, AVFs could conveniently cover the wound surface, and it was possible to repair arterial defects via the flow-through technique. According to previous studies, AVFs and SPBRA flaps can be used as flow-through type flaps to reconstruct arterial defects along with skin defects, without sacrificing the main vessels. Iwuagwu et al reported that the SPBRA flap can be used as a flow-through flap to reconstruct digital arteries [25]. However, in our study, we found that the length of the SPBRA was not adequate and could not be adjusted for the vascular defects at the recipient sites. Additionally, the distal diameter of the SPBRA was not comparable to that of the recipient vessel when the injured artery was located in Verdan's injury zone III, IV, or V [26], which could hamper anastomosis. In contrast, the design and harvesting of AVFs was comparatively easier after taking the area of the wound, the length of the vascular defect, and the diameter of the proximal/distal artery into consideration. In our study, 4 fingers underwent flow-through type of AVFs to reconstruct the digit's blood supply, with satisfactory outcomes.

In our study, fingers receiving AVF grafts were more prone to developing blisters and venous congestion as compared with those receiving grafts with SPBRA flaps, PIPFs, and UAPF flaps. This is primarily because in AVFs, the primary blood supply enters and exits the flap through the venous system. In the AVF-treated fingers, blister formation occurred on 6 fingers, with significant bullae in the fingers (5/5) grafted with a flap in an antegrade perfusion fashion as compared with the finger (1/6) grafted with a flap in a retrograde perfusion fashion. These results were consistent with a previous study by Woo et al [27,28], who suggested that retrograde perfusion would enhance flap perfusion by enhancing blood flow in the periphery of AVFs, resulting in satisfactory flap survival. If the blood flows through the flap in the original anatomic direction, no resistance is posed by the venous valves. Consequently, most of the blood flows through the central vein in the flap only, which may lead to insufficient perfusion in the peripheral areas of the flap, eventually leading to blister formation or partial necrosis.

In our series, only 8 fingers received sensate flap reconstruction for finger pulp reconstruction. This is because of the following reasons: (i) In theory, all the 4 types of flaps used in this study could carry sensory nerves; however, the nerves contained in the flaps were rather small, being terminal branches of cutaneous nerves. Therefore, the identification and carrying over of the sensory nerves in the flaps during surgery was challenging. (ii) The sensation in the finger pulp is more important than that in other parts of the finger. When reconstruct finger defect apart from finger pulp by sensate free flap, one digital nerve is often sacrificed to perform an end-to-end nerve anastomosis. This can affect the sensation in the finger pulp [7,11]. Meanwhile, although the end-to-side method of nerve anastomosis can preserve the digital nerve, the achieved sensation in the flap is not always satisfactory [29,30]. (iii) According to a previous study, the fingers that received nonsensate flaps showed acceptable s2PD, even with no nerve coaptation. In addition, adequate protective sensation was obtained in the fingers [30,31]. Satisfactory sensory recovery can be obtained using non-innervated flaps for covering finger defects, especially in younger patients, with sensory recovery mainly depending on the following aspects. First, the ingrowth of the nerve ending from the peripheral and the wound bed could provide good sensory recovery when the flap is thin and narrow. Second, the finger is a highly innervated area and contains numerous nerve endings for regeneration. Third, relatively young patients show improved regeneration and recovery [31].

In the present study, among the for 4 types of nonsensate flaps, the fingers receiving grafts with AVFs showed superior sensory recovery as compared with the other types. Yan et al. reported that sensate AVFs resulted in s2PD of 6–13 mm [23]. Woo et al. [32] demonstrated that in 8 cases (8/20) that underwent reconstruction of palmar soft tissue defects using sensate venous flaps, the average s2PD was 10 mm. Additionally, in patients undergoing reconstruction of the dorsum of the hand, an average s2PD of 13 mm or protective sensation was attained [31]. In this study, the averaged s2PD for fingers with AVF grafts was 7 mm, and normal sensation was achieved in 5 of 11 fingers postoperatively. These results demonstrate that AVFs are effective for sensory recovery through nerve regeneration surrounding the recipient site. Yokoyama et al. reported that sensory improvement can be obtained by finger palmar surface reconstruction without grafting of the subcutaneous nerve. He suggested the presence of the reinnervation effect in venous flaps without neurorrhaphy, when reconstructing fingertip defects [33]. Most importantly, venous flaps are thinner than conventional arterial flaps because they consist only of skin, the venous plexus, and subcutaneous fat, which may theoretically facilitate good sensory recovery through nerve regeneration surrounding the recipient site [34].

Interestingly, satisfactory sensory recovery was also obtained in the SPBRA flap group. Sensory recovery is better when the number of sensory nerves contained in the flap is greater [35,36]. We speculated that this result was associated with the abundant number of sensory nerves contained in these flaps, i.e., the palmar cutaneous branch of the median nerve, the branches of the superficial radial nerve, and/or the lateral antebrachial cutaneous nerve can be included in SPBRA flaps [24]. In contrast, the sensory recovery in the fingers receiving grafts of UAPF flaps and PIPFs was poor, mainly due to the few sensory nerves contained in those flaps. Based on these results, we propose that AVFs and SPBRA flaps integrated with sensory nerves should be used for the reconstruction of skin defects on the palmar side of the fingers and fingertips.

The shortest mean surgical duration was noted in cases receiving AVFs, including 4 fingers with an extensor tendon defect and 4 fingers with a bilateral arteria digitalis defect. The AVF design is convenient, and its use obviates the need to identify the vessel by preoperative color Doppler. The elevation of AVFs can be performed quicker than the other type of flaps, as elaborate dissection and careful skin perforator protection is not needed. For the other three types of flaps, it requires a considerable amount of time to identify the perforator and dissect it intraoperatively. This may be the main reason why operations involving the other three types of flaps take considerably longer.

Regarding the cosmetic appearance of the donor/recipient sites, optimal appearance was noted in the AVFs, mainly due to the following reasons: The AVFs were thinner than the SPBRA flaps, PIPFs, and UAPF flaps, which contained skin, subcutaneous tissues, deep fascia, and additional tissues to protect the vascular pedicle, in contrast to only skin and subcutaneous tissue in the AVFs. Further, 5 of the 10 SPBRA flap grafts were graded as good (5/10) for cosmetic appearance of the fingers, which was superior to that for grafting with UAPF flaps and PIPFs, possibly because subcutaneous fat distribution in the wrist and radial sides was thinner than that in the ulnar side of the wrist and the dorsal part of the forearm. Further, the SPBRA flap was designed to be parallel to the wrist's transverse striations, and only a transverse scar remained after the donor sites were sutured. These factors contributed to the optimal degree of satisfaction with regard to the cosmetic appearance of the donor sites for the SPBRA flaps.

The disadvantage of the 4 free flaps described here includes the technical demands of microsurgery, which are not an obstacle for most hand surgeons. However, compared to the use of traditional pedicled flaps, the long operation duration is a drawback of free flap transfer. Vascular anastomosis is main reason for the longer surgical duration, particularly in cases with complications such as vasospasm. Moreover, venous congestion due to a low amount of venous return is the most common reason for the failure of free flap transfer. In the present study, we attempted to anastomose 2 veins instead of 1 vein to avoid venous congestion. This may be a reason for the longer operative time. However, improvement in the microsurgery skill of the surgeon may reduce the operative time. Nevertheless, the risks caused by longer operative time and donor site dehiscence should be considered; however, these were not observed in our series.

In conclusion, the forearm of the ipsilateral extremity is an acceptable donor site for AVFs, SPBRA flaps, UAPF flaps, and PIPFs for the reconstruction of small- and moderate-sized soft tissue skin defects in the fingers. These flaps are suitable for covering finger defects because they are thin, pliable, and hairless, with low donor site morbidity. The optimal cosmetic appearance was observed for recipient sites in patients with AVF grafts. The vascularized palmaris longus tendon could be incorporated into the flap for reconstructing tendon defects and restoring digital circulation via a flow-through flap. AVFs were most useful among the 4 types of flaps studied here because of the simpler technique, wider range of indications, and better sensory recovery and cosmetic appearance. Among SPBRA flaps, UAPF flaps, and PIPFs, optimal sensory recovery was obtained with SPBRA flap grafts together with satisfactory cosmetic appearance and minimal donor site injury.

Author Contributions

Conceived and designed the experiments: LYJ CXC. Performed the experiments: LYJ JHS ZHX ZXP DXH. Analyzed the data: LCL. Wrote the paper: LYJ. Assessment of the overall outcomes of the patients: JX. Final approval of the manuscript: CXC.

References

1. Foucher G, Boulas HJ, Braga Da Silva J (1991). The use of flaps in the treatment of fingertip injuries. World J Surg. 15(4): 458–462.
2. Foucher G, Delaere O, Citron N, Molderez A (1999). Long-term outcome of neurovascular palmar advancement flaps for distal thumb injuries. Br J Plast Surg. 52(1): 64–68.
3. Kappel DA, Burech JG (1985). The cross-finger flap. An established reconstructive procedure. Hand Clin. 1(4): 677–683.
4. Li YF, Cui SS (2005). Innervated reverse island flap based on the end dorsal branch of the digital artery: surgical technique. J Hand Surg Am. 30(6): 1305–1309.
5. Moschella F, Cordova A (2006). Reverse homodigital dorsal radial flap of the thumb. Plast Reconstr Surg. 117(3): 920–926.
6. Toia F, Marchese M, Boniforti B, Tos P, Delcroix L (2013). The little finger ulnar palmar digital artery perforator flap: anatomical basis. Surg Radiol Anat. 35(8): 737–740.
7. Gu JX, Pan JB, Liu HJ, Zhang NC, Tian H, et al (2014). Aesthetic and sensory reconstruction of finger pulp defects using free toe flaps. Aesthetic Plast Surg. 38(1): 156–163.
8. Gillies H, Millard DR (1957). The principles and Art of Plastic surgery. London: Butterworth.
9. Huang SH, Wu SH, Lai CH, Chang CH, Wangchen H, et al (2010). Free medial plantar artery perforator flap for finger pulp reconstruction: report of a series of 10 cases. Microsurgery. 30(2): 118–124.
10. Lin CH, Lin YT, Sassu P, Wei FC (2007). Functional assessment of the reconstructed fingertips after free toe pulp transfer. Plast Reconstr Surg. 120(5): 1315–1321.
11. Hsieh JH, Wu YC, Chen HC, Chen YB (2009). Posterior auricular artery sensate flap for finger pulp reconstruction. J Trauma. 67(2): E48–E50.
12. Lee HB, Tark KC, Rah DK, Shin KS (1998). Pulp reconstruction of fingers with very small sensate medial plantar free flap. Plast Reconstr Surg. 101(4): 999–1005.
13. Yoshimura M, Shimada T, Imura S, Shimamura K, Yamauchi S (1987). The venous skin graft method for repairing skin defects of the fingers. Plast Reconstr Surg. 79(2): 243–250.
14. Yang JW, Kim JS, Lee DC, Ki SH, Roh SY, et al (2010). The radial artery superficial palmar branch flap: a modified free thenar flap with constant innervation. J Reconstr Microsurg. 26(8): 529–538.
15. Ishiko T, Nakaima N, Suzuki S (2009). Free posterior interosseous artery perforator flap for finger reconstruction. J Plast Reconstr Aesthet Surg. 62(7): e211–215.
16. Inada Y, Tamai S, Kawanishi K, et al (2004). Free dorsoulnar perforator flap transfers for the reconstruction of severely injured digits. Plast Reconstr Surg. 114(2): 411–420.
17. Ozaksar K, Toros T, Sügün TS, Bal E, Ademoğlu Y, et al (2010). Reconstruction of finger pulp defects using homodigital dorsal middle phalangeal neurovascular advancement flap. J Hand Surg Eur Vol. 35(2): 125–129.
18. Chi Z, Gao W, Yan H, Li Z, Chen X, et al (2012). Reconstruction of totally degloved fingers with a spiraled parallelogram medial arm free flap. J Hand Surg Am. 37(5): 1042–1050.
19. Hamdi M, Coessens BC (1996). Distally planned lateral arm flap. Microsurgery. 17(7): 375–379.
20. Chen HC, Tang YB, Noordhoff MS (1991). Four types of venous flaps for wound coverage: a clinical appraisal. J Trauma. 31(9): 1286–1293.
21. Kim SW, Jung SN, Sohn WI, Kwon H, Moon SH (2013). Ulnar artery perforator free flap for finger resurfacing. Ann Plast Surg. 71(1): 72–75.
22. Chen CL, Chiu HY, Lee JW, Yang JT (1994). Arterialized tendocutaneous venous flap for dorsal finger reconstruction. Microsurgery. 15(12): 886–890.
23. Yan H, Fan C, Zhang F, Gao W, Li Z, et al (2013). Reconstruction of large dorsal digital defects with arterialized venous flaps: our experience and comprehensive review of literature. Ann Plast Surg. 70(6): 666–671.
24. Omokawa S, Ryu J, Tang JB, Han J (1997). Vascular and neural anatomy of the thenar area of the hand: its surgical applications. Plast Reconstr Surg. 99(1): 116–121.
25. Iwuagwu FC, Orkar SK, Siddiqui A (2013). Free superficial palmar branch of the radial artery flap for the reconstruction of defects of the volar surface of the digits, including the pulp. Plast Reconstr Surg. 131(2): 308e–309e.
26. Verdan C (1975). Primary and Secondary Repair of Flexor and Extensor Tendon Injuries. In: J. E. Flynn (Ed.), Hand Surgery, Baltimore: Williams & Wilkins.
27. Woo SH, Jeong JH, Seul JH (1996). Resurfacing relatively large skin defects of the hand using arterialized venous flaps. J Hand Surg Br. 21(2): 222–229.
28. Woo SH, Seul JH (2001). Pre-expanded arterialised venous free flaps for burn contracture of the cervicofacial region. Br J Plast Surg. 54(5): 390–395.
29. Brunelli GA, Brunelli F, Brunelli GR (1995). Microsurgical reconstruction of sensory skin. Ann Acad Med Singapore. 24(4 Suppl): 108–112.
30. Kleinert HE, McAlister CG, MacDonald CJ, Kutz JE (1974). A critical evaluation of cross finger flaps. J Trauma. 14(9): 756–763.
31. Kushima H, Iwasawa M, Maruyama Y (2002). Recovery of sensitivity in the hand after reconstruction with arterialised venous flaps. Scand J Plast Reconstr Surg Hand Surg. 36(6): 362–367.
32. Woo SH, Kim KC, Lee GJ, Ha SH, Kim KH, et al (2007). A retrospective analysis of 154 arterialized venous flaps for hand reconstruction: an 11-year experience. Plast Reconstr Surg. 119(6): 1823–1838.
33. Yokoyama T, Hosaka Y, Kusano T, Morita M, Takagi S (2006). Finger palmar surface reconstruction using medial plantar venous flap: possibility of sensory restoration without neurorrhaphy. Ann Plast Surg. 57(5): 552–556.
34. Yan H, Gao W, Zhang F, Li Z, Chen X, et al (2012). A comparative study of finger pulp reconstruction using arterialised venous sensate flap and insensate flap from forearm. J Plast Reconstr Aesthet Surg. 65(9): 1220–1226.
35. Waris T, Rechardt L, Kyösola K (1983). Reinnervation of human skin grafts: a histochemical study. Plast Reconstr Surg. 72(4): 439–447.
36. Lai CH, Lai CS, Huang SH, Lin SD, Chang KP (2010). Free medial plantar artery perforator flaps for the resurfacing of thumb defects. Ann Plast Surg. 65(6): 535–540.

9

Multipaddled Anterolateral Thigh Chimeric Flap for Reconstruction of Complex Defects in Head and Neck

Canhua Jiang[a], **Feng Guo**[a], **Ning Li***, **Wen Liu**, **Tong Su**, **Xinqun Chen**, **Lian Zheng**, **Xinchun Jian**

Department of Oral and Maxillofacial Surgery, Xiangya Hospital, Central South University, Changsha, Hunan, China

Abstract

The anterolateral thigh flap has been the workhouse flap for coverage of soft-tissue defects in head and neck for decades. However, the reconstruction of multiple and complex soft-tissue defects in head and neck with multipaddled anterolateral thigh chimeric flaps is still a challenge for reconstructive surgeries. Here, a clinical series of 12 cases is reported in which multipaddled anterolateral thigh chimeric flaps were used for complex soft-tissue defects with several separately anatomic locations in head and neck. Of the 12 cases, 7 patients presented with trismus were diagnosed as advanced buccal cancer with oral submucous fibrosis, 2 tongue cancer cases were found accompanied with multiple oral mucosa lesions or buccal cancer, and 3 were hypopharyngeal cancer with anterior neck skin invaded. All soft-tissue defects were reconstructed by multipaddled anterolateral thigh chimeric flaps, including 9 tripaddled anterolateral thigh flaps and 3 bipaddled flaps. The mean length of skin paddle was 19.2 (range: 14–23) cm and the mean width was 4.9 (range: 2.5–7) cm. All flaps survived and all donor sites were closed primarily. After a mean follow-up time of 9.1 months, there were no problems with the donor or recipient sites. This study supports that the multipaddled anterolateral thigh chimeric flap is a reliable and good alternative for complex and multiple soft-tissue defects of the head and neck.

Editor: Fabio Santanelli, di Pompeo d'Illasi Sapienza, University of Rome, School of Medicine and Psychology, Italy

Funding: The National Natural Sciences Foundation of China (Grant No. 81000445) and the State Key Specialist Construction Projects of China provided funding. The funders had no role in study design, data collection and analysis, decision to publish, or preparation of the manuscript.

Competing Interests: The authors have declared that no competing interests exist.

* Email: liningbeta@hotmail.com

[a] These authors contributed equally to this work.

Introduction

Though relatively uncommonly, complex soft-tissue defects of head and neck which involve multiple and nonadjacent anatomic sites can arise after radically surgery of advanced-staged malignancies or multiple lesions of the upper aerodigestive tract. Meanwhile, immediate flap reconstruction is the gold standard for surgical treatment for the defects after tumor ablation. However, functional and aesthetic reconstruction of complex and multiple defects in head and neck is still a major surgical challenge, because the reconstruction of multiple and nonadjacent defects demand a flexible and feasible flap with multiplanar configuration and multiple paddles [1]. There are several reconstructive choices open to the clinician, including local cutaneous flaps, pedicled fasciocutaneous flaps and microsurgical free flaps. It is usually not applicable for local and pedicled flaps to reconstruct such complex defects because of their limited soft-tissue amount and less versatile design, while using two or more individual flaps for multiple defects might be an opinion, but not the best. An ideal reconstructive procedure for multiple and complex three-dimensional defects should be performed in a single stage operation, which not only can reduce operative time but also prevent likelihood of postoperative complications.

For multiple and complex soft-tissue defects, reconstruction with three-dimensional microvascular flaps is often the preferred alternative. The free anterolateral thigh (ALT) flap, as first described by Song et al [2] in 1984, is a versatile and reliable reconstructive option. This flap has already been a workhorse flap for head and neck reconstruction in recent decades [3,4]. The advantages of ALT flap include consistent and reliable anatomy, long vascular pedicle, the feasibility to create multiple skin paddles by recruiting additional perforators, the flexibility to reconstruct composite defects by recruiting different tissue types, and low donor site morbidity. Based on multiple cutaneous perforators originated from the descending branch of the lateral circumflex femoral artery (LCFA), free ALT flap can be harvested with multiple skin paddles for multiple and complicated soft-tissue defects, which can eliminate the need for two or more separately flaps and vascular anastomosis [5–7]. In this study, we present our experience with free multipaddled ALT chimeric flap for functional and aesthetical reconstruction of complex head and neck soft-tissue defects involving multiple nonadjacent anatomic sites in a single operation.

Patients and Methods

Between May 2009 and August 2012, a total of 12 consecutive patients with head and neck cancer indicated for radical resection and complex soft-tissue reconstruction with multipaddled ALT chimeric flaps were enrolled. Of the 12 cases, 11 were men and

Table 1. Statistical description of case series.

No.	Age/Sex	Aetiology	TNM stage	Reconstructed area	Flap size (W × L cm)	Donor-site scar (W/L cm)	Follow-up (month)
1	46/M	Right BC with OSF	T3N1M0	Right through-and-through cheek	P: 4×6	0.7/25	8
					M: 6×9		
				Left buccal mucosa	D: 3×5		
2	34/M	Left BC with OSF	T4N2aM0	Left through-and-through cheek	P: 5×7	0.5/23	10
					M: 6×8		
				Right buccal mucosa	D: 2.5×4		
3	43/M	Left TC and BC with multiple leukoplakia	T3N0M0 (TC)	Right tongue mucosa	P: 3×5	1.0/26	12
			T2N0M0 (BC)	Left partial tongue	M: 5×7		
				Left buccal mucosa	D: 6×8		
4	56/M	Recurrent HC with neck skin invasion	T4N0M0	Pharyngoesophagus	P: 7×12	0.6/24	6
				Anterior neck skin	D: 7×8		
5	58/M	Recurrent Left BC with right buccal OSF scar	T3N0M0	Left through-and-through cheek	P: 7×8		
					M: 7×10		
				Right buccal mucosa	D: 3×5		
6	62/M	Left TC with OSF	T3N1M0	Left buccal mucosa	P: 3×6	0.8/22	18
				Left half tongue	M: 5×8		
				Right buccal mucosa	D: 3×5		
7	54/M	Right BC with OSF	T3N1M0	Right through-and-through cheek	P: 5×6	0.5/21	8
					M: 7×8		
				Left buccal mucosa	D: 4×4		
8	51/M	HC with neck skin invasion	T4N1M0	Pharyngoesophagus	P: 6×10	0.8/19	7
				Anterior neck skin	D: 5×7		
9	43/M	Left BC with OSF	T3N2aM0	Left through-and-through cheek	P: 4×7	1.2/22	10
					M: 6×8		
				Right buccal mucosa	D: 3×5		
10	54/M	HC with neck skin invasion	T4N1M0	Pharyngoesophagus	P: 6×9		
				Anterior Neck skin	D: 4×5		
11	33/F	Left BC with OSF	T3N1M0	Left through-and-through cheek	P: 5×7	0.9/20	14
					M: 6×9		
				Right buccal mucosa	D: 3×4		
12	34/M	Right BC with OSF	T3N0M0	Right through-and-through cheek	P: 3×6	0.6/22	8
					M: 7×9		
				Left buccal mucosa	D: 4×5		

Abbreviations: BC, buccal cancer; TC, tongue cancer; HC, hypopharyngeal cancer; OSF, oral submucous fibrosis; P, proximal paddle; M, middle paddle; D, distal paddle; W, width; L, length.

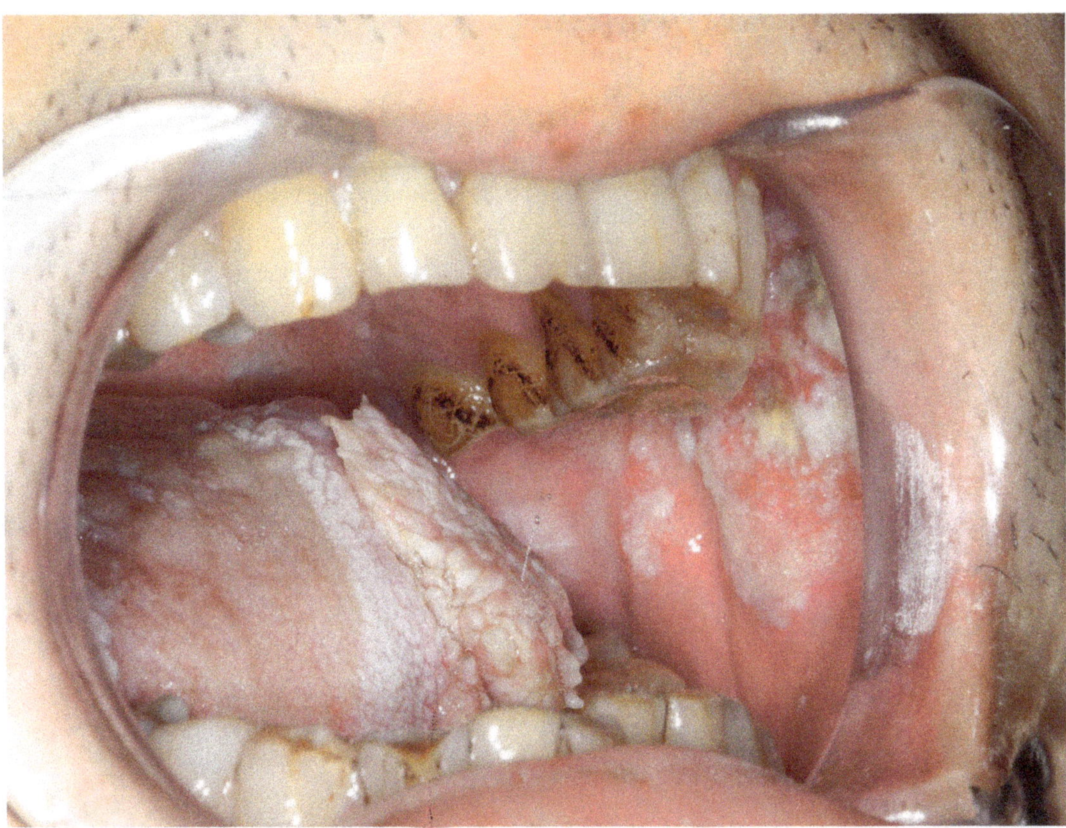

Figure 1. Preoperative view of two primary tumors. Note that the left tongue cancer (T3N0M0) and left buccal cancer (T2N0M0) were not directly adjacent.

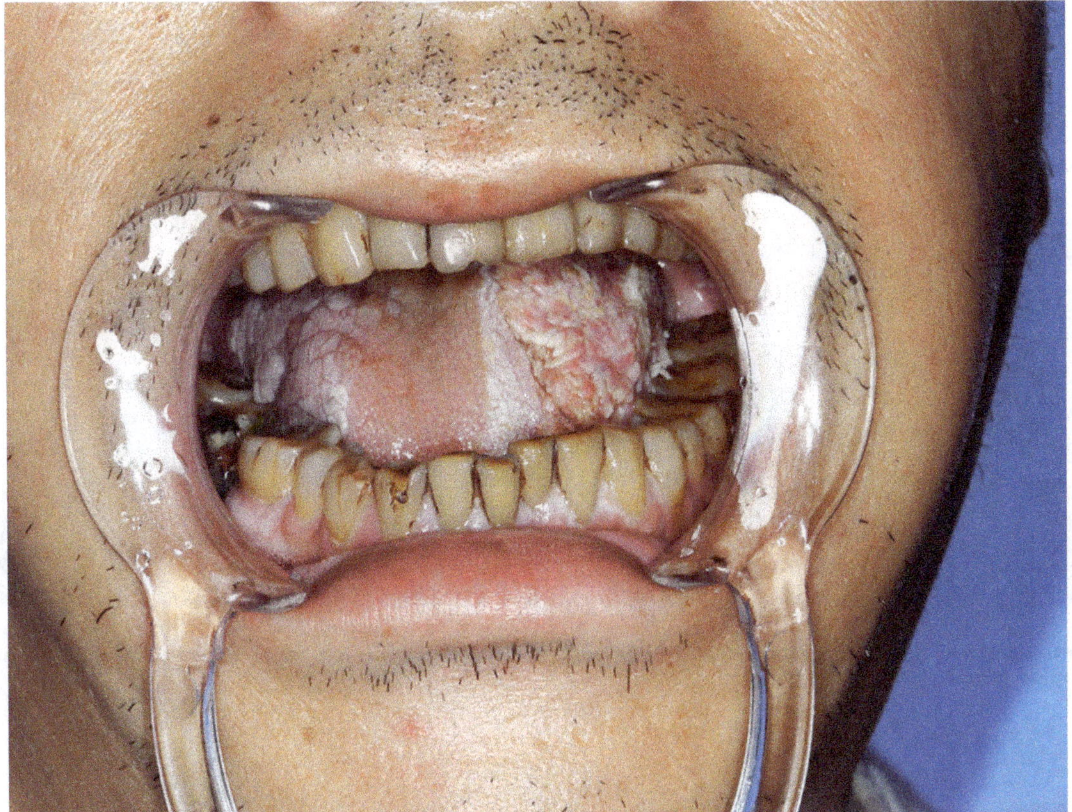

Figure 2. Preoperative view of left tongue cancer and right tongue mucosa leukoplakia. The extensive mucosa leukoplakia (3×4 cm^2) of right tongue was indicated to be resected.

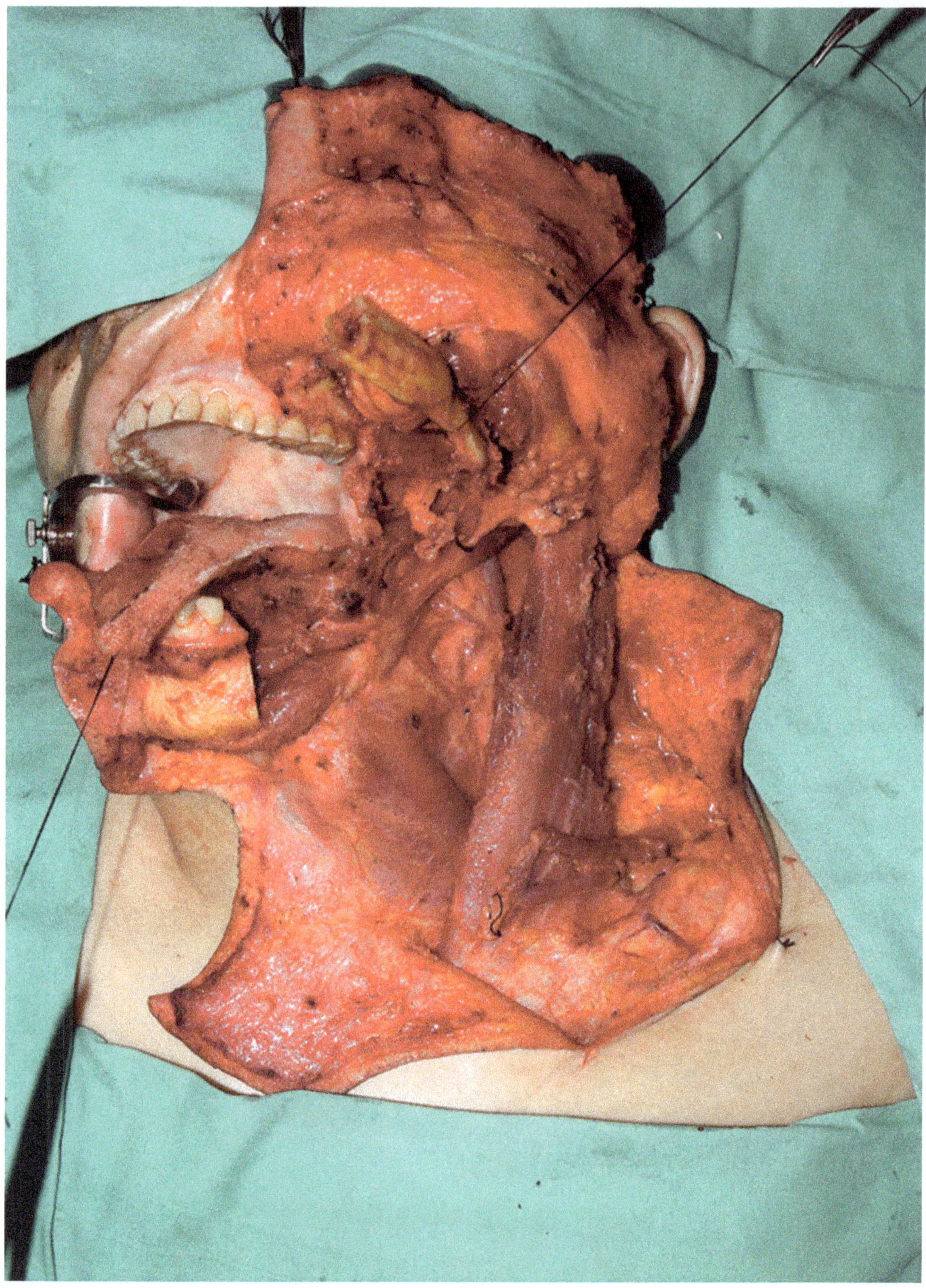

Figure 3. Intraoperative view of three individual defects involved left half tongue, left buccal mucosa, and right tongue mucosa after the radical cancer ablation.

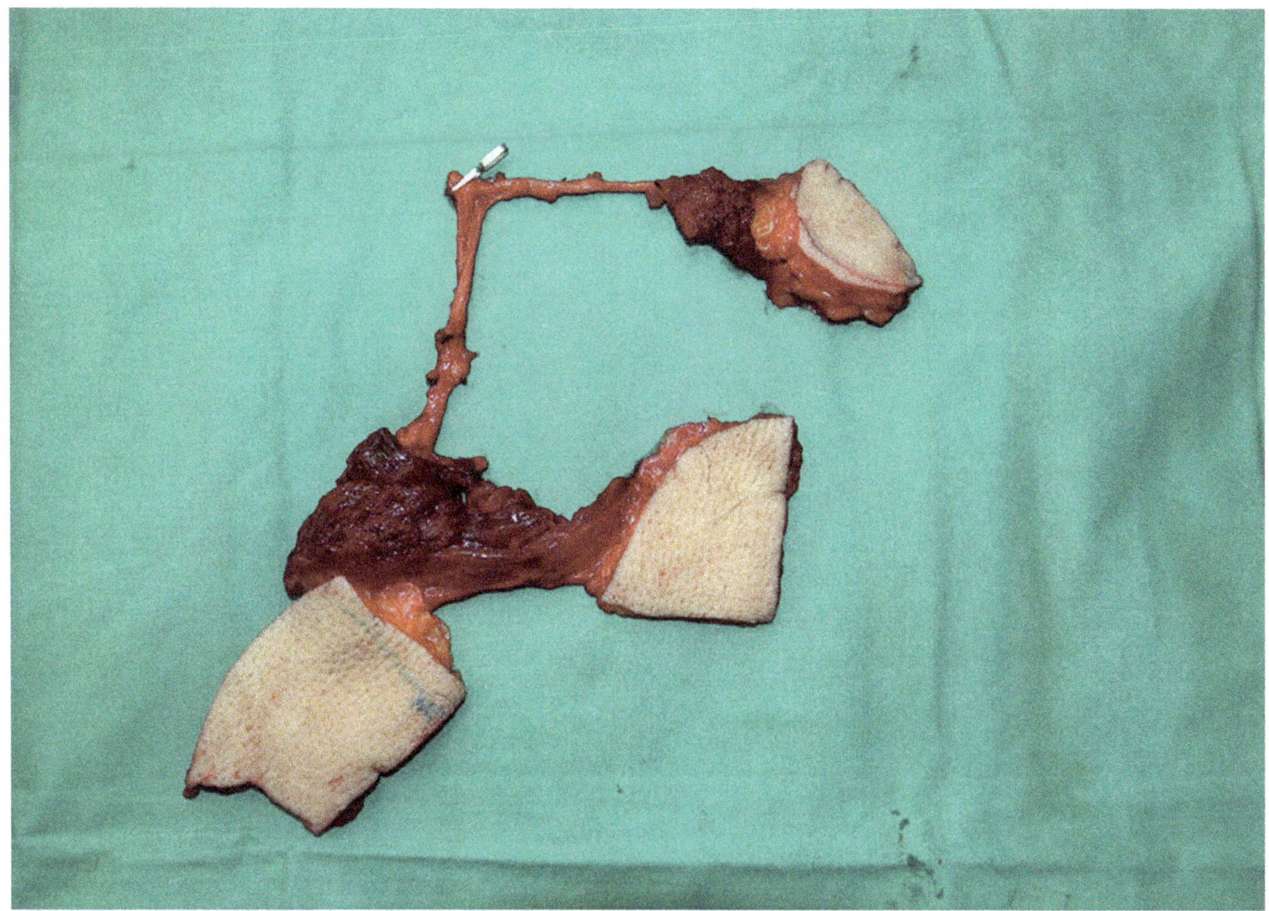

Figure 4. Intraoperative view after elevation of the tripaddled free ALT musculocutaneous flap.

only 1 was woman, with a mean age of 47.3 years (range, 33 to 62 years). None presented with distant metastases at the time of surgery. Tumor size was T4 in 4 patients (33.3%) and T3 in 8 cases (66.7%). The baseline data about 12 cases are shown in Table 1.

After radical ablation of cancer and other relative lesions, the resulting soft-tissue defects were classified into three types according to the locations of soft-tissue defects: type I, patient with advanced buccal mucosa cancer in one site and oral submucous fibrosis (OSF) of contralateral buccal mucosa (n = 7, Case 1, 2, 5, 7, 9, 12, 13); type II, patient with oral cancer and multiple oral mucosa lesions (leukoplakia or OSF) (n = 2, Case 3, 6); type III, patient with primary or recurrent hypopharyngeal cancer which has also invaded anterior neck skin (n = 3, Case 4, 8, 11).

The study followed the ethical guidelines of the Ministry of Health, China. Protocols applied in this study and the publish of patients' details have been approved by the Hospital Ethical Committee of the Xiangya Hospital. The individuals in this manuscript have given written informed consent to publish these case details.

Reconstructive Procedures

All patients were examined preoperatively by using a portable Super Dopplex D900 non-directional hand-held Doppler probe (Huntleigh Diagnostics, Glamorgan, UK) to predict the vessel perforators originated from the branches of the lateral circumflex femoral artery on the left or right anterolateral thigh. Enough separately and suitable perforators should be detected on at least one thigh. Patients without enough perforators on both thighs were excluded. All defects were soft tissue. The relevant surgical technique has previously been described [8,9]. Briefly, a line was drawn between the anterior–superior iliac spine and the midpoint of the lateral border of the patella on the donor thigh in supine position. The locations of main cutaneous perforators were detected using ultrasound Doppler preoperatively. Skin paddles were designed around the detected perforators. The pedicle of the multipaddled ALT flap was supplied by the descending branch or transverse branch of the lateral circumflex femoral vessels. A medial incision was made above the rectus femoris muscle and continued underneath the deep fascia of vastus lateralis to identify the located cutaneous perforators with intramuscular dissection. Perforators were then dissected in a retrograde fashion until arriving at the descending branch of the lateral circumflex femoral artery. For some cases, a small segment of vastus lateralis muscle around perforator was included as additional volume to augment the dead space and decrease tissue retraction after postoperative radiotherapy. And partial deep fascial cuff and soft-tissue around the perforator was left to prevent the vessel spasm and facilitate the fixation of perforator. The integrity of lateral cutaneous nerve was preserved carefully to decrease the risk of postoperative lateral thigh paresthesia. All skin paddles of multipaddled ALT flap was checked for viability and then transferred to the defect with vessel anastomosis. We usually select two recipient veins for anastomosis,

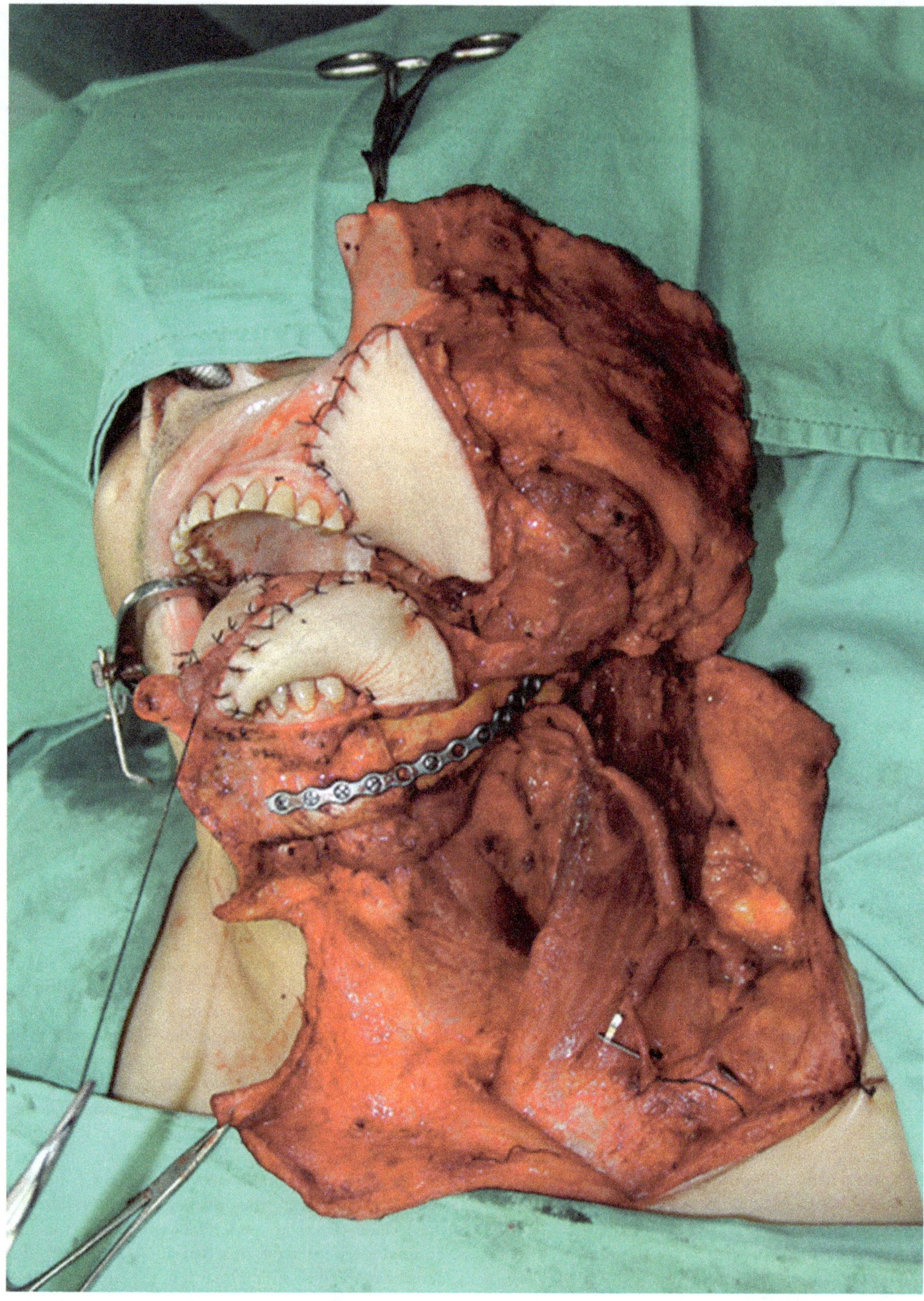

Figure 5. Intraoperative view of three separately skin paddles covering left buccal, left tongue, as well as right tongue mucosa defect respectively. Vascular anastomosis was made between the artery of the flap and the left superior thyroid artery and between the veins of the flap and the external jugular vein as well as a branch of internal jugular vein.

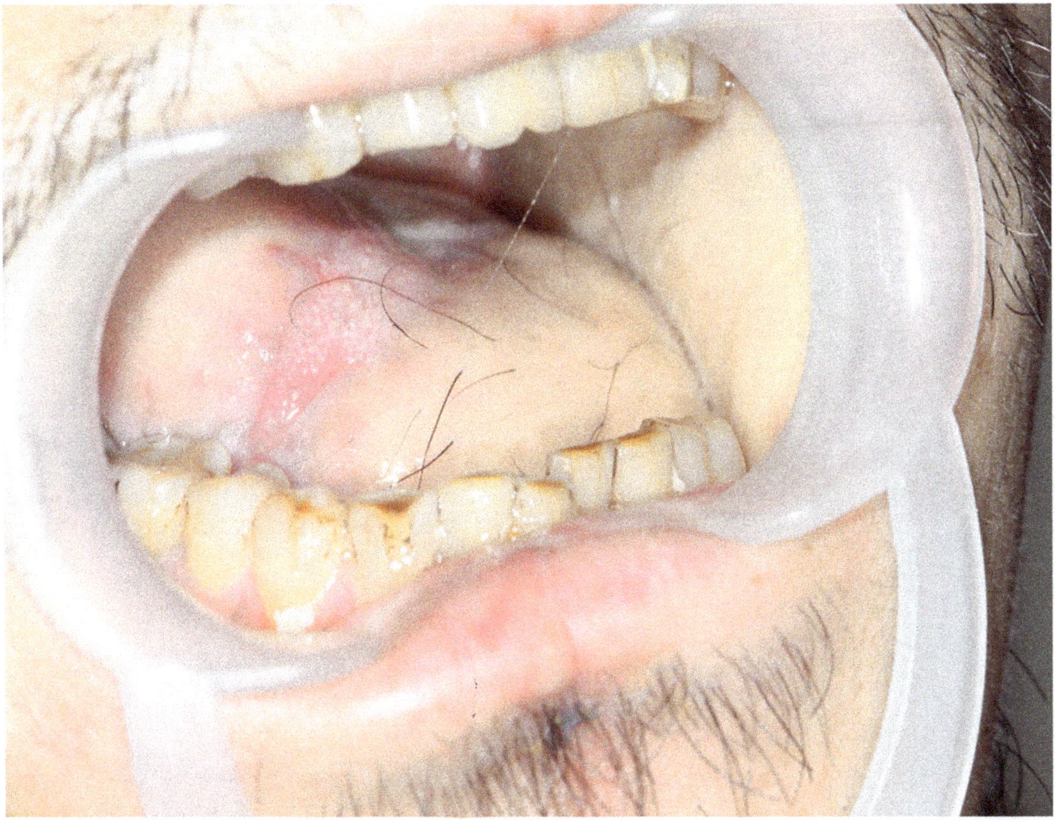

Figure 6. Appearance 2 months after operation with complete flap survival.

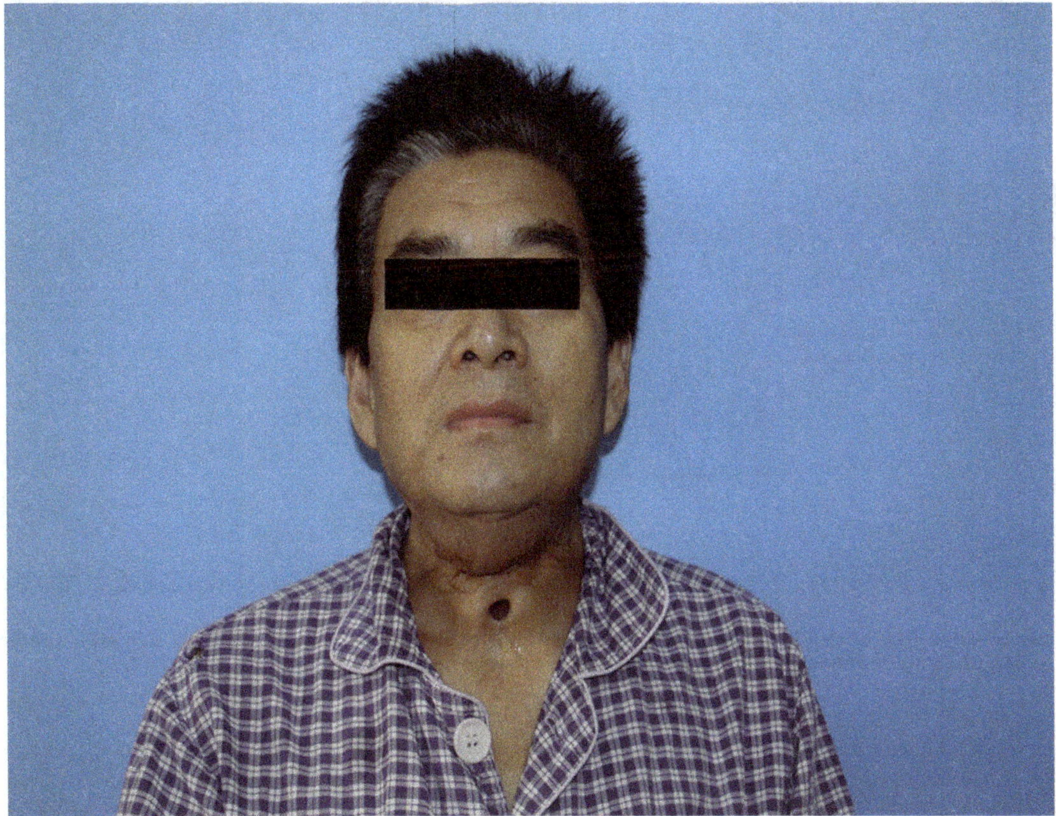

Figure 7. Preoperative view of a recurrent hypopharyngeal cancer invaded the anterior neck skin.

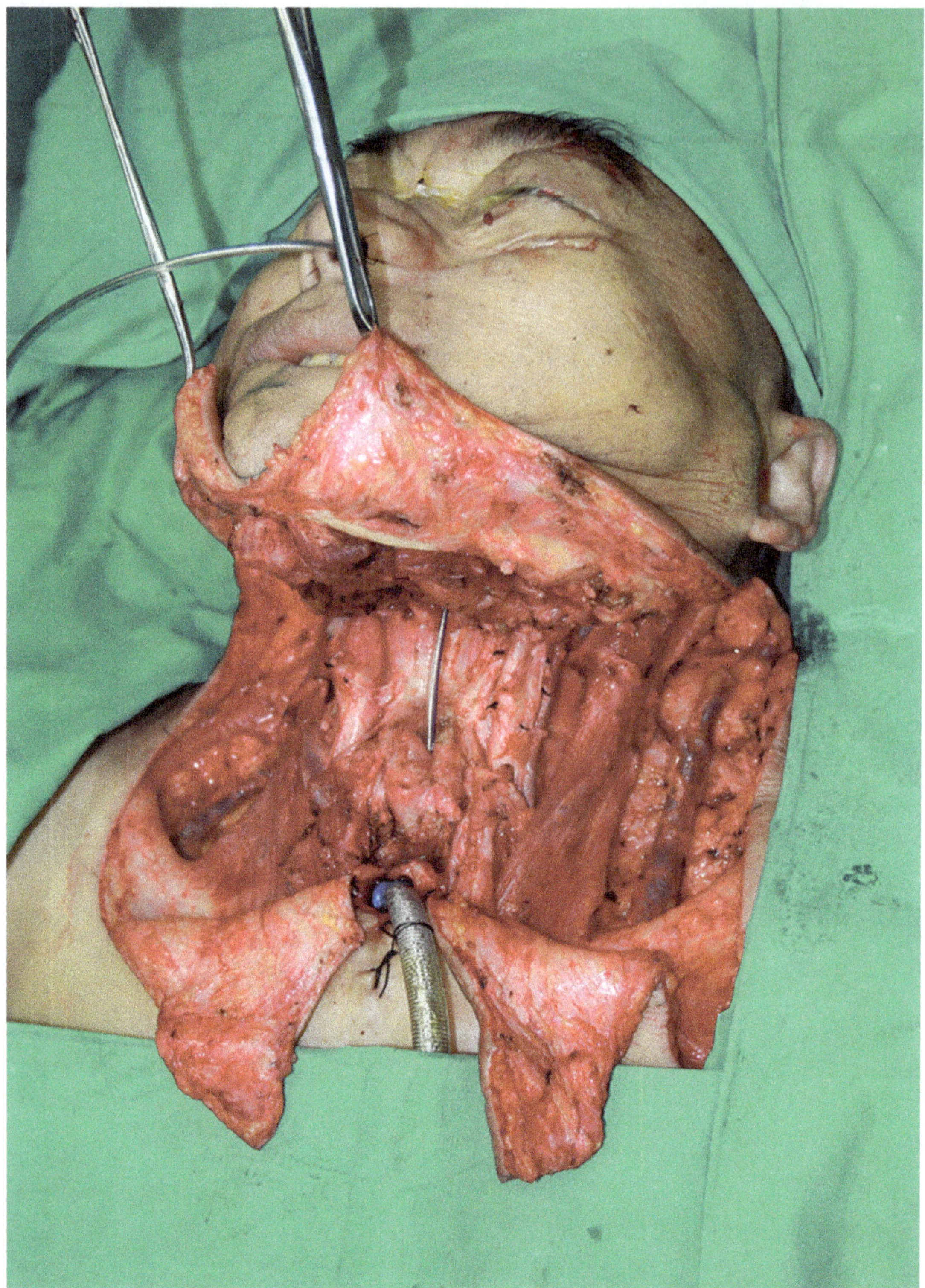

Figure 8. Intraoperative view of the resulting defects involved a part of esophagus and anterior neck skin after a radical salvage surgery including pharyngoesophagus, anterior neck skin and bilateral neck dissection.

which can secure the venous return of the flap. Hemostasis and drainage should maintained adequately to prevent hematoma formation and the flap should be monitored carefully by clinical examination for color and capillary refill during the early postoperative period. For excluded cases due to insufficient perforators, contralateral or bilateral ALT flaps could be supplementary to reconstruct all defects.

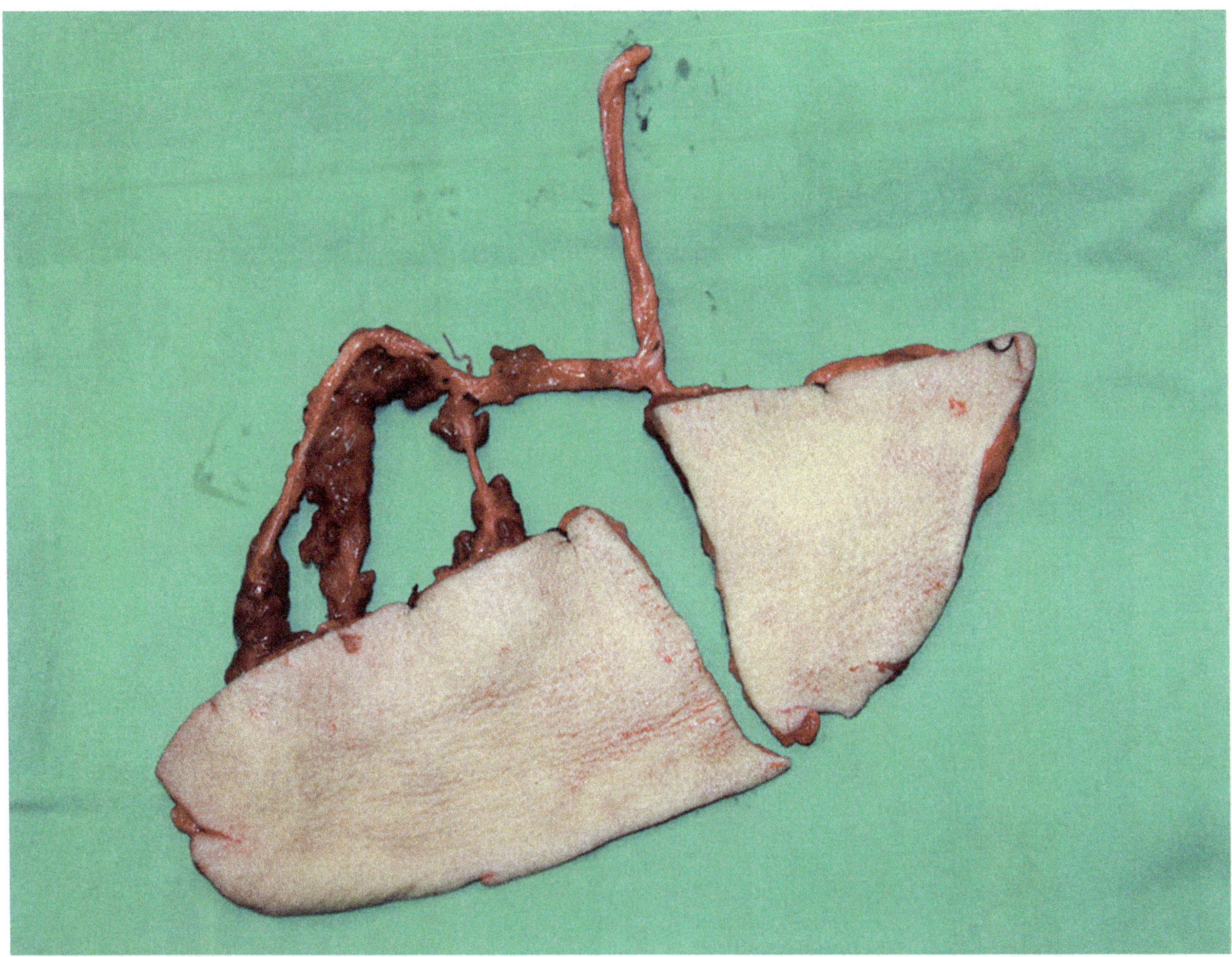

Figure 9. Intraoperative view after harvest of bipaddled free ALT fasciocutaneous flap.

In our present study, for type I patients, after radical ablation, the bilateral complex defects involved full-thickness cheek on one side and contralateral buccal mucosa. Tripaddled ALT musculocutaneous flap was raised, and the proximal and middle paddles were chimeric and restored for the full-thickness cheek defects, while the distal paddle for the contralateral mucosa defect.

For type II patients, after surgical resection of tongue cancer and oral multiple lesions, resulting soft-tissue defects included unilateral or bilateral tongue and buccal mucosa. Tripaddled ALT musculocutaneous flap was used to reconstruction the 3-dimensional defects. The proximal and distal flaps were used to repair the bilateral mucosa defects respectively, and the middle one for tongue defect.

For type III patients, the invaded pharyngoesophagus and anterior neck skin were radical resected. Bipaddled ALT fasciocutaneous or musculocutaneous flap was raised. The larger skin flap was whole or near circumferential to reconstruct the pharyngoesophagus, while the remaining for the skin defect.

Results

Initially, 13 cases were selected for this study. One was excluded due to no enough perforators intraoperatively, although Doppler showed enough perforator signals preoperatively in the operated thigh. For the remaining 12 cases, multipaddled ALT fasciocutaneous or musculocutaneous chimeric flaps were harvested to reconstruction complex 3-dimensional defects in head and neck. The mean length of skin paddle was 19.2 (range: 14–23) cm and the mean width was 4.9 (range: 2.5–7) cm. All flaps survived and all donor sites were closed primarily. After a mean follow-up time of 9.1 (5–18) months, there were no problems with the donor or recipient sites. All patients underwent postoperative radiotherapy.

Case report

Case 1. A 43-year-old man (case number 3 in Table 1) presented with left tongue cancer (T3N0M0), left buccal cancer (T2N0M0) and extensive mucosa leukoplakia on right tongue (Fig. 1 and 2) underwent a radical ablation of all oral lesions and left functional neck dissection. The resulting defects involved left half tongue, left buccal mucosa ranging from the gingival buccal sulcus of maxilla to left hyomandibular furrow of mandible, and right tongue mucosa (Fig. 3). One-staged reconstruction by tripaddled free ALT musculocutaneous flap was performed on the left thigh (Fig. 4). Partial vastus lateralis was included around the musculocutaneous perforator for augmentation of dead space. The distal skin paddle (6×8 cm^2) was used to cover the left buccal defect, the middle one (5×7 cm^2) for left half-tongue defect, and the proximal paddle (3×5 cm^2) for right tongue defect (Fig. 5). The donor-site defect was closed primarily. Three skin paddles

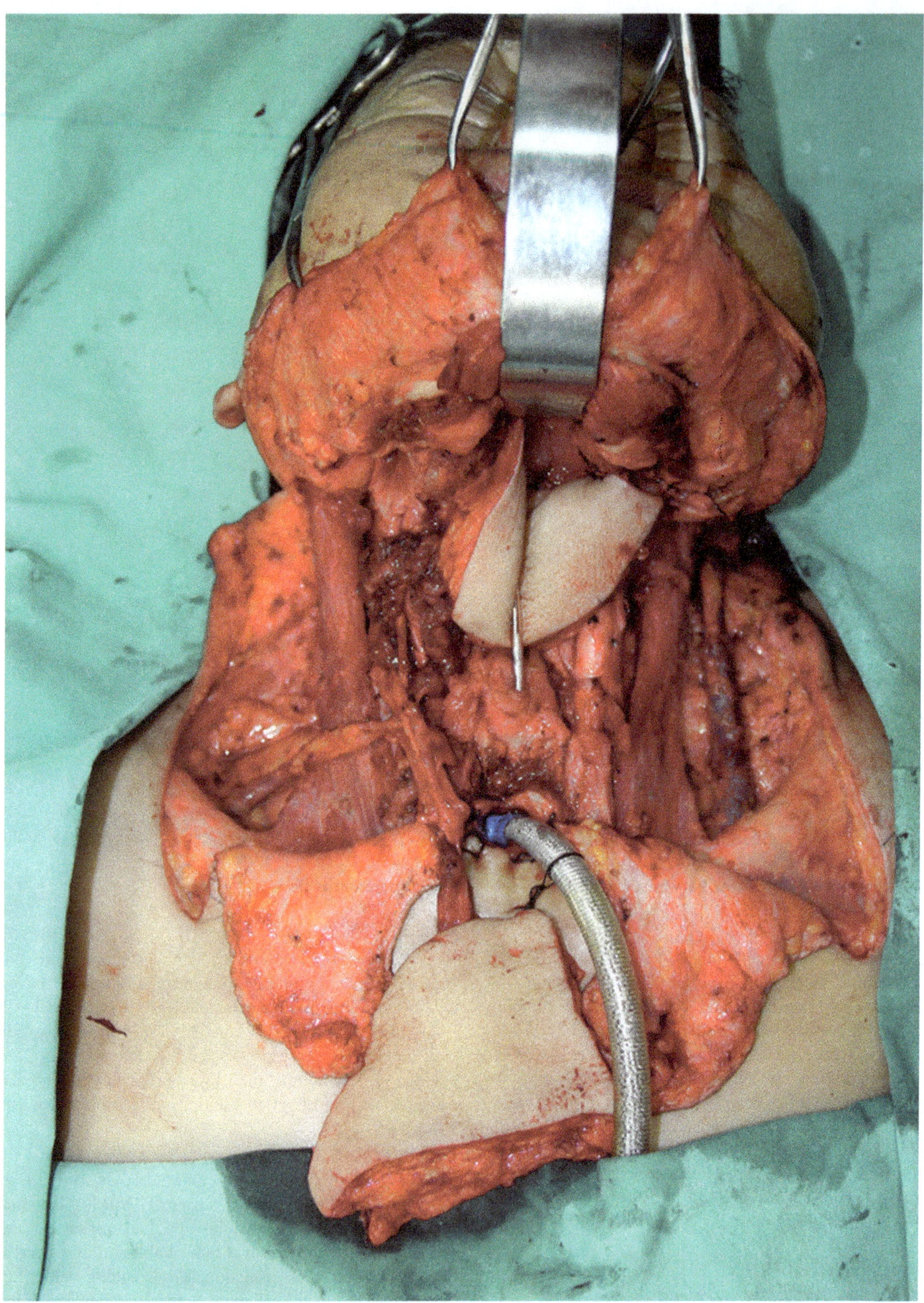

Figure 10. Intraoperative view of two separately skin paddles reconstructing neoesophagus and anterior neck skin respectively. The distal paddle with two separately perforators was tubularized by itself to form a neoesophagus.

were all survival, and no recurrence occurred during 12-month follow-up (Fig. 6).

Case 2. A 56-year-old male patient (case number 4 in Table 1) presented with a local recurrent hypopharyngeal cancer that invaded the esophagus and anterior neck skin (Fig. 7). A salvage resection involving the cancer, esophagus, anterior neck skin and bilateral neck dissection was performed. The resulting defects involved a part of circumferential esophagus and anterior

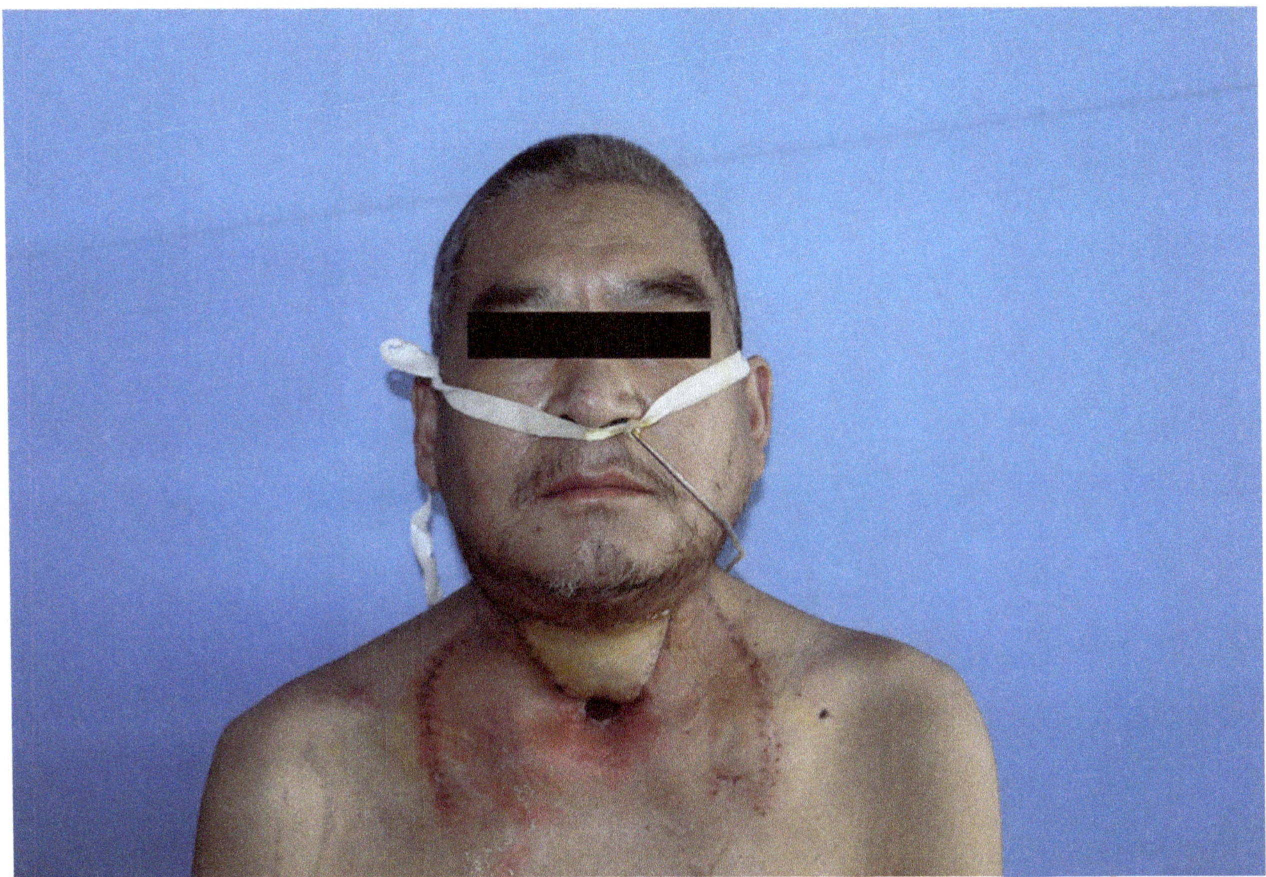

Figure 11. Appearance 14 days after operation with complete flap survival.

neck skin (Fig. 8). A bipaddled ALT fasciocutaneous flap was harvested (Fig. 9). The distal paddle (7×12 cm^2) was tubularized by itself to form a neoesophagus, while the proximal paddle (7×8 cm^2) for the defect of anterior neck skin, which also could monitor the inner free flap (Fig. 10). The flap survived completely without any complications (Fig. 11). Patient had good functional outcome without fistula or stricture formation. However, this was the only one patient who complained of fatigue while ascending and descending stairs for 2 months after operation, and felt obvious recovery at 4 months after operation.

Case 3. A 54-year-old male patient (case number 7 in Table 1) was presented with the right buccal tumor and progressive trismus of about 6-month duration which was caused by severe OSF (Fig. 12). The patient underwent a radical surgery for right buccal cancer, a transversal release of left OSF tissue, and right functional neck dissection. After ablation, the bilateral buccal defects were noted, including a left buccal mucosa defect (3×4 cm^2), and a right through-and-through cheek defects which involved the intraoral defect (6×8 cm^2) and the outer skin defect (4×6 cm^2) (Fig. 13). A free ALT musculocutaneous flap with three independent skin paddles was harvested (Fig. 14). The distal paddle was used to resurface the left mucosa defect, and two remaining paddles were chimeric to reconstruct the right full-thickness cheek defects. The donor site was closed primarily. All skin paddles of the ALT flap were survival, and the postoperative month opening of the patient was improved obviously (Fig. 15).

Discussion

There are several tissue organs with different locations and configuration in head and neck, and reconstruction of multiple and complex soft-tissue defects after radical surgery in this region demands a flap with three-dimensional requirement of both volume and surface. Two or more free flap transfers for complex defects in a single operation are frequently encountered, nevertheless there are several disadvantages of limited availability of recipient vessels, having to do two or more sets of microvascular anastomosis and a possible longer operating time.

Free ALT flap has become an important option for reconstruction of multiple anatomical locations in head and neck, which is often attributed to its multiple advantages: a long pedicle with good caliber, a large and pliable skin territory with the ability to design more than one skin paddle depending on the perforator anatomy, and the ability of two teams to work at the same time [10]. The most important advantage of ALT flap for multiple and complex defects is the fact that this flap can be harvested to include skin only or both skin and muscle, or as a chimeric flap with separately perfused skin paddles for multiple anatomical locations Longo et al [11–13] perfomed unipaddled or bipaddled free ALT perforator flaps for complex but adjacent defect locations in head and neck. However, there is few literature concerned on the reconstruction of more complex soft-tissue defects involving two or more nonadjacent anatomic sites. For such complex defects, ALT flap should be designed as multiple separately skin paddles to cover multiple defects in different anatomical regions simultaneously.

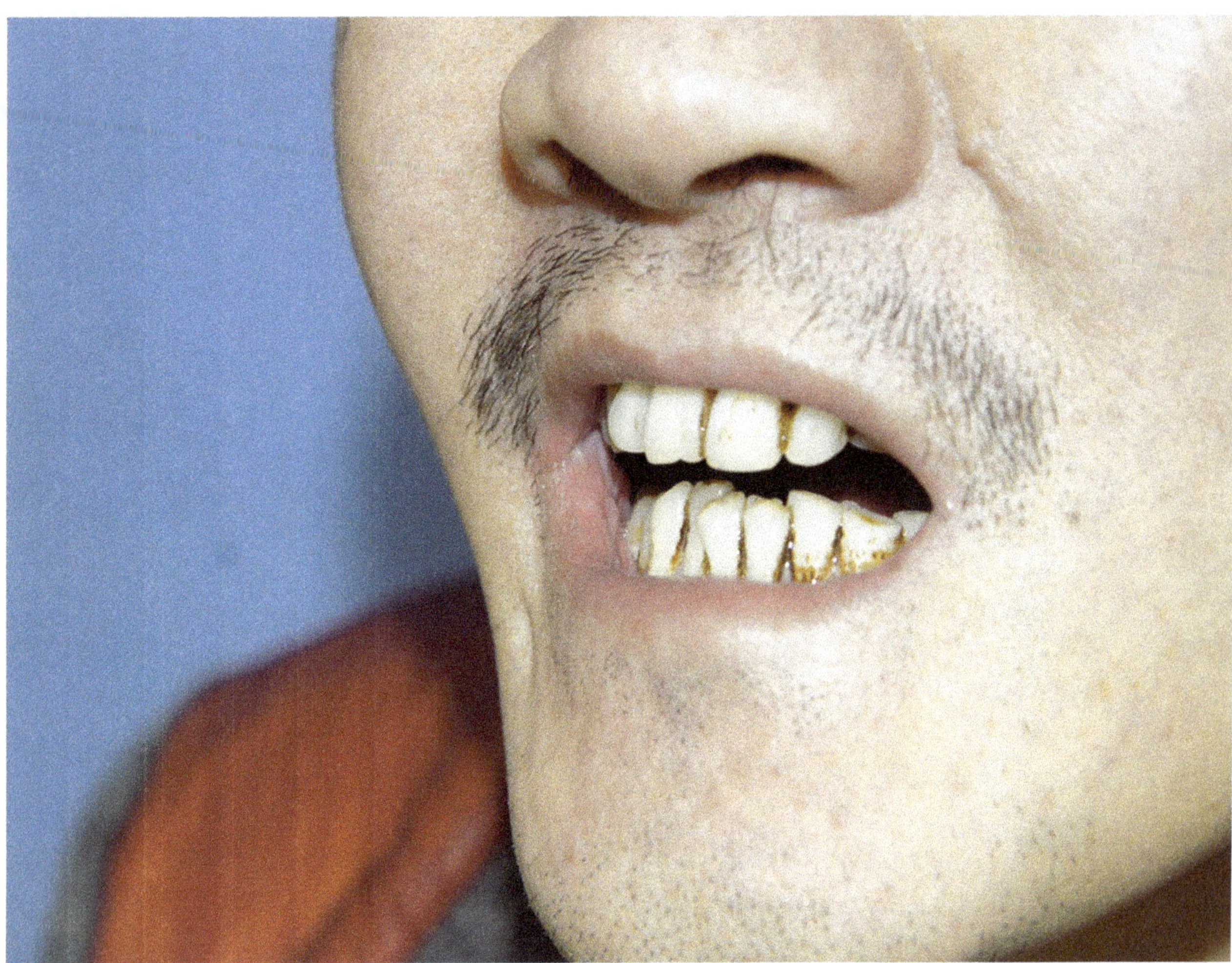

Figure 12. Preoperative view of trismus due to right buccal cancer and left OSF. The preoperative month opening was severely limited.

In our present series, all three types of complex soft-tissue defects are unsuitable to be reconstructed by an unipaddled free ALT flap with a single perforator, because there were at least two nonadjacent defect locations in one patient. Especially for type I patients presented with advanced buccal cancer and contralateral OSF, a radical ablation of buccal cancer was primary and imperative, however it was also necessary to release contralateral OSF buccal mucosa and correct the trismus [14]. OSF is a chronic oral mucosal disease primarily affecting oral cavity and always leads to the restriction of mouth opening, eventually impairing the ability to eat, speak and dental care [15]. For these OSF cases, a free multipaddled ALT flap should be designed to recover bilateral buccal defects, including a full-thickness cheek defects in one side and contralateral buccal defect. However, for cases with type III defect, a single free ALT flap with a single perforator might be a supplementary option for cases with no enough Intraoperative perforator by de-epithelializing the skin between the two paddles like the method introduced by Tan et al [16], Nevertheless, overmuch folding and looping of one flap can always increase the flap necrosis, while the design of individually perfused paddles with separately perforators can reduce the risk.

For the harvest of multipaddled free ALT flap, at least two separately and safe perforators based on descending branch of lateral circumflex femoral artery (dbLCFA) should be found intraoperatively on one thigh. However, one of principal uncertainties of free ALT flap is the variation of the perforator's anatomy and the occasional absence of satisfactory perforators. Kimata et al. [17] and Wei et al. [18] considered that 2 to 3 cutaneous perforators can be found to run through the medial edge of vastus lateralis. From our experience and the work of others, at least 1 suitable cutaneous perforator could be always found [19]. The first perforator with the largest diameter can be always found to exit within a 5-cm-diameter circle centered at the midpoint of the line between the anterior superior iliac crest and the superolateral border of the patella. Although 5–6% cases with absent cutaneous perforators were also described in some earlier studies, the small size of those presented perforators was considered as the likely reason for being overlooked [20,21]. Although preoperative Doppler examination is commonly used to map out ALT cutaneous perforators, operator dependence and false positive are its main disadvantages. Shaw et al. [22] speculated that false positives represented either pure muscular perforators, or signals from the main descending branch because of their proximity to the tip of the probe when the intervening layer of fat is minimal. Chiu et al. considered that preoperative multi-detector computed tomographic angiography (CTA) could be performed to map perforator and evaluate the dominant vascularity in the suitable thigh before transferring chimeric ALT

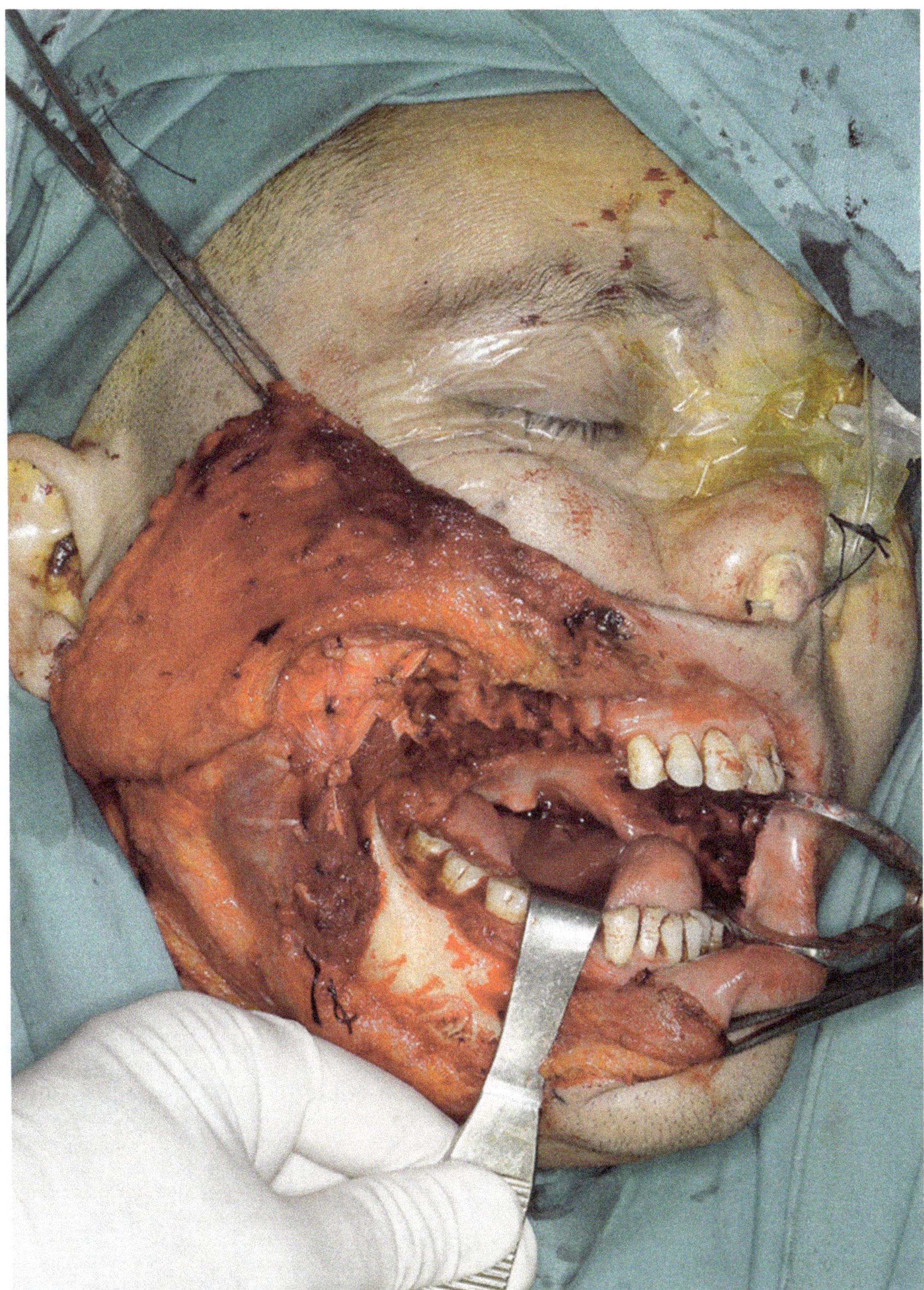

Figure 13. Intraoperative view of right full-thickness cheek defects and left buccal mucosa defect after the radical cancer surgery.

flaps [23]. However, it was hard for CTA to show the direct location of cutaneous perforators just like Doppler for surgeons. While in our enrolled cases, we can find at least 2 or 3 reliable cutaneous perforators intraoperatively on one thigh with the help of preoperative Doppler examination. So although there are many methods to locate the perforators, in our experience a handheld Doppler probe has adequate sensitivity for perforator location. Meanwhile, we agree with the free-style flap harvest concept, which means any cutaneous perforators located by a handheld Doppler probe can potentially be harvested by retrograde

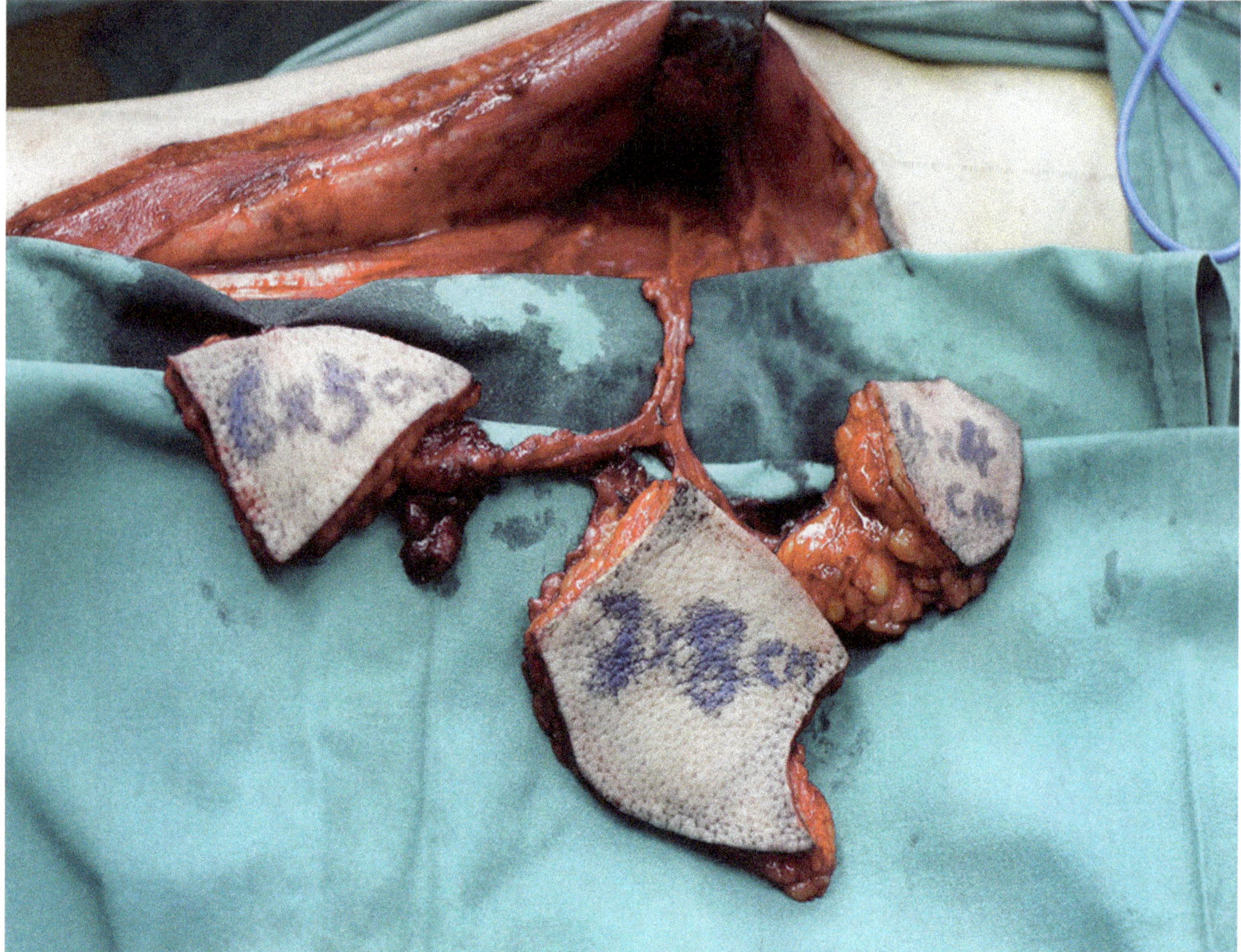

Figure 14. Intraoperative view after harvest of a tripaddled free ALT musculocutaneous flap.

dissection as a free flap, regardless of regional anatomy. However, in our present study, for the only abandoned patient, who was an old female patient, it was a very rare case that we only found a single reliable cutaneous perforators on each thigh intraoperatively, although preoperative Doppler showed at least 2 perforators in one thigh The too small size of the presented perforators and moderate dystrophy of the case might be the main reasons. The more microsurgical experience and careful manipulation should be needed. However, for the rare patient in our present study, two unipaddled ALT flaps from both thighs had to be harvested to recover multiple defects in her head and neck.

In our present study, a small segment of vastus lateralis muscle around perforator was included in the majority of cases as additional volume to augment the dead space raised after radical cancer ablation and prevent tissue retraction of postoperative radiotherapy [19]. Meanwhile, we usually leave partial soft-tissue or a small deep fascial cuff around the perforator to prevent the vessel spasm, especially perforators and limit the risk of damage to the vessel. So the free ALT flaps in our cases were the musculocutaneous or fasciocutaneous flaps, not the perforator flap as classically described [24]. Free ALT musculocutaneous flap does not affect quadriceps muscular function, because only the vastus lateralis is dissected and still three bellies of the quadriceps can provide good functional synergy [25]. Meanwhile, careful preservation of the lateral cutaneous nerve and femoral motor nerve branches can decreases the risk of complications, such as lateral thigh paresthesia, musculoskeletal dysfunction, and compartment syndrome [26]. However, Anatomical variations include the nerve passing through the pedicle of the ALT flap, or passing between perforators, seen in 28% of a 36-human cadaveric thigh dissection study [27]. The close course of the vascular pedicle with the femoral motor nerve branch innervating the vastus lateralis could lead to nerve damage during flap elevation, resulting in knee extension weakness [28]. In our present study, only one patient (Case 2) complained of fatigue while ascending and descending stairs for 2 months after operation. This might be attributed to the intraoperative temporary damage of the femoral motor nerve branches in the vastus lateralis. Early physical therapy plays an important role in minimizing the weakness of the vastus lateralis [29]. However, in comparison with salvage reconstruction of the advanced cancer, this could be considered negligible.

Moreover, the selection of recipient vessel is also very important to avoid flap failure [30]. Although the vessels of the ALT flap match closely to the recipient vessels in head and neck, radical surgery of cancer in head and neck could usually cause the recipient vascular impairment or resection. There are two veins of different sizes accompanying the artery of the ALT flap, while many authors believed that only one accompanying vein

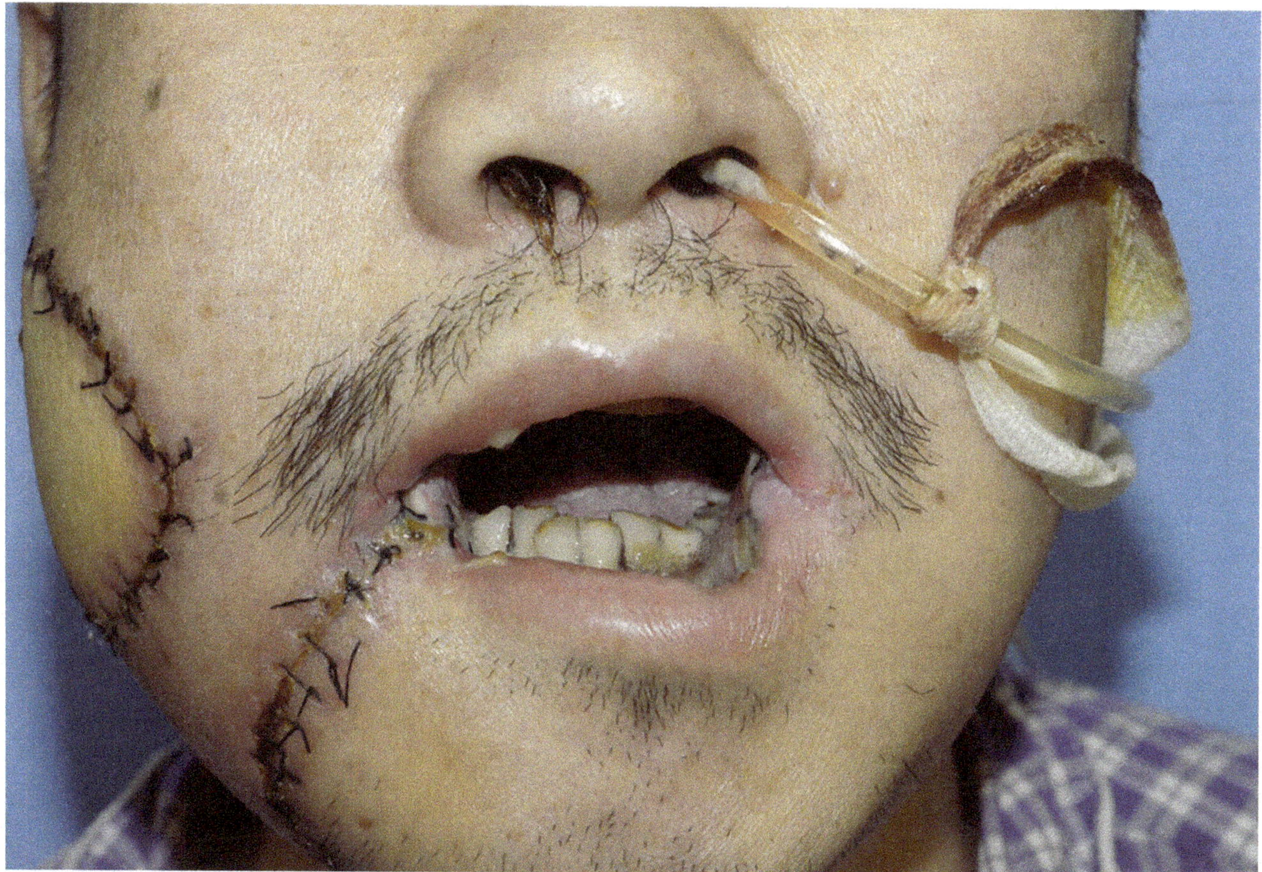

Figure 15. Early postoperative view of two proximal chimeric paddles restoring right full-thickness cheek defects and the distal paddle restoring left buccal defect. The postoperative month opening was obviously improved.

anastomosis was enough for venous return [31]. Kimata et al [32] prefers to check the quality of venous back-flow and choose an appropriate vein for anastomosis after the anastomosis of the artery has been completed, because the flow strength of venous return sometimes differs between the two veins, unrelated to venous size. Rubino C [33] reported that flow rate measured postoperatively on flap arteries is significantly correlated with flap weight. In order to avoid congestion of the multiple ALT flap and postoperative complications, we usually chose a branch of internal jugular vein and the external jugular vein as the two recipient veins for anastomosis. It can secure the venous return of the flap and no flap congestion occurred in our series.

Conclusion

In our experience, we believe that the multipaddled ALT chimeric flap is a reliable option for the reconstruction of complex soft-tissue defects with multiple different spatial orientations in head and neck, because it can provide several independent skin paddles for multiple separately defects simultaneously with minimal donor site morbidity.

Author Contributions

Conceived and designed the experiments: CJ FG NL TS XC XJ. Analyzed the data: NL WL LZ. Contributed to the writing of the manuscript: NL.

References

1. Longo B, Nicolotti M, Ferri G, Belli E, Santanelli F (2013) Sagittal split osteotomy of the fibula for modelling the new mandibular angle. J Craniofac Surg 24:71–74.
2. Song YG, Chen GZ, Song YL (1984) The free thigh flap: a new free flap concept based on the septocutaneous artery. Br J Plast Surg 37:149–159.
3. Koshima I, Hosoda S, Inagawa K, Urushibara K, Moriguchi T (1998) Free combined anterolateral thigh flap and vascularized fibula for wide, through-and-through oromandibular defects. J Reconstr Microsurg 14:529–534.
4. Koshima I (2000) Free anterolateral thigh flap for reconstruction of head and neck defects following cancer ablation. Plast Reconstr Surg 105:2358–2360.
5. Park CW, Miles BA (2011) The expanding role of the anterolateral thigh free flap in head and neck reconstruction. Curr Opin Otolaryngol Head Neck Surg 19:263–268.
6. Huang WC, Chen HC, Jain V, Kilda M, Lin YD, et al. (2002) Reconstruction of through-and-through cheek defects involving the oral commissure, using chimeric flaps from the thigh lateral femoral circumflex system. Plast Reconstr Surg 109:433–441.
7. Lai CL, Ou KW, Chiu WK, Chen SG, Chen TM, et al. (2012) Reconstruction of the complete loss of upper and lower lips with a chimeric anterolateral thigh flap: a case report. Microsurgery 32:60–63.
8. Wong CH, Wei FC (2009) Microsurgical free flap in head and neck reconstruction. Head Neck 32: 1236–1245.
9. Jiang C, Guo F, Li N, Huang P, Jian X, et al. (2013) Tripaddled anterolateral thigh flap for simultaneous reconstruction of bilateral buccal defects after buccal camcer ablation and severe oral submucous fibrosis release: A case report. Microsurgery 33:667–671.
10. Koshima I, Fukuda H, Yamamoto H, Moriguchi T, Soeda S, et al. (1993) Free anterolateral thigh flaps for reconstruction of head and neck defects. Plast Reconstr Surg 92:421–430.
11. Longo B, Pagnoni M, Ferri G, Morello R, Santanelli F (2013) The mushroom-shaped anterolateral thigh perforator flap for subtotal tongue reconstruction. Plast Reconstr Surg 132:656–665.

12. Longo B, Ferri G, Fiorillo A, Rubino C, Santanelli F (2013) Bilobed perforator free flaps for combined hemitongue and floor-of-the-mouth defects. J Plast Reconstr Aesthet Surg 66:1464–1469.
13. Longo B, Paolini G, Belli E, Costantino B, Pagnoni M, et al. (2013) Wide excision and anterolateral thigh perforator flap reconstruction for dermatofibrosarcoma protuberans of the face. J Craniofac Surg 24:597–599.
14. Jiang C, Guo F, Li N, Huang P, Jian Y, et al. (2013) Tripaddled anterolateral thigh flap for simultaneous reconstruction of bilateral buccal defects after buccal camcer ablation and severe oral submucous fibrosis release: A case report. Microsurgery 33:667–671.
15. Pindborg JJ, Sirsat SM (1966) Oral submucous fibrosis. Oral Surg Oral Med Oral Pathol 22:764–779.
16. Tan NC, Yeh MC, Shih HS, Nebres RP, Yang JC, et al. (2011) Single free anterolateral thigh flap for simultaneous reconstruction of composite hypopharyngeal and external neck skin defect after head and neck cancer ablation. Microsurgery 31:524–528.
17. Kimata Y, Uchiyama K, Ebihara S, Sakuraba M, Iida H, et al. (2000) Anterolateral thigh flap donor-site complications and morbidity. Plast Reconstr Surg 106:584–589.
18. Wei FC, Jain V, Celik N, Chen HC, Chuang DC, et al. (2002) Have we found an ideal soft-tissue flap? An experience with 672 anterolateral thigh flaps. Plast Reconstr Surg 109: 2219–2226.
19. Wei FC, Celik N, Chen HC, Cheng MH, Huang WC (2002) Combined anterolateral thigh flap and vascularized fibula osteoseptocutaneous flap in reconstruction of extensive composite mandibular defects. Plast Reconstr Surg 109:45–52.
20. Yu P (2004) Characteristics of the anterolateral thigh flap in a Western population and its application in head and neck reconstruction. Head Neck 26:759–769.
21. Rozen WM, Ashton MW, Pan WR, Kiil BJ, McClure VK, et al. (2009) Anatomical variations in the harvest of anterolateral thigh flap perforators: a cadaveric and clinical study. Microsurgery 29: 16–23.
22. Shaw RJ, Batstone MD, Blackburn TK, Brown JS (2010) Preoperative Doppler assessment of perforator anatomy in the anterolateral thigh flap. Br J Oral Maxillofac Surg 48:419–422.
23. Chiu WK, Lin WC, Chen SY, Tzeng WD, Liu SC, et al. (2011) Computed tomography angiography imaging for the chimeric anterolateral thigh flap in reconstruction of full thickness buccal defect. ANZ J Surg 81:142–147.
24. Van Landuyt KH, Monstrey SJ, Hamdi M, Matton GE, Allen RJ, et al. (2003) The "Gent" consensus on perforator flap terminology: preliminary definitions. Blondeel PN. Plast Reconstr Surg 112:1378–1383.
25. Hanasono MM, Skoracki RJ, Yu P (2010) A prospective study of donor site morbidity after anterolateral thigh fasciocutaneous and myocutaneous free flap harvest in 220 patients. Plast Reconstr Surg 125:209–214.
26. Collins J1, Ayeni O, Thoma A (2012) A systematic review of anterolateral thigh flap donor site morbidity. Can J Plast Surg 20:17–23.
27. Rozen WM, le Roux CM, Ashton MW, Grinsell D (2009) The unfavorable anatomy of vastus lateralis motor nerves: A cause of donor-site morbidity after anterolateral thigh flap harvest. Plast Reconstr Surg 123:1505–1509.
28. de Vicente JC, de Villalaín L, Torre A, Peña I (2008) Microvascular free tissue transfer for tongue reconstruction after hemiglossectomy: A functional assessment of radial forearm versus anterolateral thigh flap. J Oral Maxillofac Surg 66:2270–2275.
29. Zhang Q, Qiao Q, Yang X, Wang H, Robb GL, et al. (2010) Clinical application of the anterolateral thigh flap for soft tissue reconstruction. J Reconstr Microsurg 26:87–94.
30. Baumeister S, Follmar KE, Zenn MR, Erdmann D, Levin LS (2008) Strategy for reoperative free flaps after failure of a first flap. Plast Reconstr Surg 122:962–971.
31. Demirtas Y, Neimetzade T, Kelahmetoglu O, Guneren E (2010) Free anterolateral thigh flap for reconstruction of car tire injuries of children's feet. Foot Ankle Int 31:47–52.
32. Kimata Y, Uchiyama K, Ebihara S, Nakatsuka T, Harii K (1998) Anatomic variations and technical problems of the anterolateral thigh flap: a report of 74 cases. Plast Reconstr Surg 102:1517–1523.
33. Rubino C, Ramakrishnan V, Figus A, Bulla A, Coscia V, et al. (2009) Flap size/flow rate relationship in perforator flaps and its importance in DIEAP flap drainage. J Plast Reconstr Aesthet Surg. 62(12):1666–70.

10

Tanshinon IIA Injection Accelerates Tissue Expansion by Reducing the Formation of the Fibrous Capsule

Qingxiong Yu[1⁹], Lingling Sheng[1⁹], Mei Yang[2], Ming Zhu[1], Xiaolu Huang[1], Qingfeng Li[1]*

1 Department of Plastic and Reconstructive Surgery, Shanghai Ninth People's Hospital, Shanghai Jiao Tong University, School of Medicine, Shanghai, P.R. China, **2** Division of Plastic Surgery, Southern Illinois University School of Medicine, Springfield, Illinois, United States of America

Abstract

The tissue expansion technique has been applied to obtain new skin tissue to repair large defects in clinical practice. The implantation of tissue expander could initiate a host response to foreign body (FBR), which leads to fibrotic encapsulation around the expander and prolongs the period of tissue expansion. Tanshinon IIA (Tan IIA) has been shown to have anti-inflammation and immunoregulation effect. The rat tissue expansion model was used in this study to observe whether Tan IIA injection systematically could inhibit the FBR to reduce fibrous capsule formation and accelerate the process of tissue expansion. Forty-eight rats were randomly divided into the Tan IIA group and control group with 24 rats in each group. The expansion was conducted twice a week to maintain a capsule pressure of 60 mmHg. The expansion volume and expanded area were measured. The expanded tissue in the two groups was harvested, and histological staining was performed; proinflammatory cytokines such as tumor necrosis factor-α (TNF-α), interleukin-6 (IL-6) and interleukin-1β (IL-1β) and transforming growth factor-β (TGF-β) were examined. The expansion volume and the expanded area in the Tan IIA group were greater than that of the control group. The thickness of the fibrous capsule in the Tan IIA group was reduced with no influence on the normal skin regeneration. Decreased infiltration of macrophages, lower level of TNF-α, IL-6, IL-1β and TGF-β, less proliferating myofibroblasts and enhanced neovascularization were observed in the Tan IIA group. Our findings indicated that the Tan IIA injection reduced the formation of the fibrous capsule and accelerated the process of tissue expansion by inhibiting the FBR.

Editor: Cheryl A. Stoddart, University of California, San Francisco, United States of America

Funding: This study was supported by the National Key Project of Scientific and Technical Supporting Programs funded by the Ministry of Science & Technology of China (no. 2012BAI11B03) and Shanghai Jiaotong University School of Medicine Doctoral Innovation Foundation (BXJ201230). The funders had no role in study design, data collection and analysis, decision to publish, or preparation of the manuscript.

Competing Interests: The authors have declared that no competing interests exist.

* Email: dr.liqingfeng@yahoo.com

⁹ These authors contributed equally to this work.

Introduction

The tissue expansion technique has been in use for many years in plastic surgery. It's a process of implanting a silicon sac subcutaneously and regularly injecting saline into the sac, in this process, new skin forms under the mechanical stretch, providing a supply of tissue similar in color, structure and adnexal distribution to the adjacent skin for a perfect repair [1]. Tissue expansion is a very useful technique and has a wide range of clinical applications, especially for repairing of large skin defect.

Tissue expansion is a safe and reliable method for reconstruction; however, it is also a time-consuming procedure. In clinical practice, 4–6 months are usually needed to achieve adequate expansion. Such long time expansion not only causes distress in patients, but also increases the incidence of complications such as infection, and the rupture or exposure of the tissue expander.

According to previous studies of tissue expansion, there are two important histological changes occurring during expansion. The first one is tissue regeneration, which is correlated with cell proliferation and neovascularization of expanded tissue. The other change is the formation of fibrous capsule. In our previous studies, we have been trying to promote tissue expansion by enhancing skin regeneration. Stem cells, such as bone marrow derived stem cells (BM-MSCs) [2], adipose tissue derived stem cells (ADSCs) [3], and stromal vascular fraction (SVF) [1] have been found effective in accelerating tissue expansion and promoting skin growth. In this study, we aimed to reduce fibrous capsule formation during tissue expansion, which may potentially increase the efficiency of tissue expansion technique and the efficacy of stem cell therapy during tissue expansion.

The fibrous capsule forms, because the tissue expander, as a foreign body, initiates a foreign body response (FBR) after implanted in vivo, which is characterized by macrophage infiltration and fibrotic encapsulation around the expander to "seal off" the expander [4]. The Jun N-terminal kinase (JNK) and NF-κB inflammatory pathways and proinflammatory cytokines such as tumor necrosis factor-α (TNF-α), interleukin-6 (IL-6) and interleukin-1β (IL-1β) are involved in the FBR, according to our previous experiment [5].

During tissue expansion, inelastic capsule augments the mechanical resistance to the expander, which significantly prolongs the expansion time [6]. The capsule also causes the contracture of expanded flap, which reduces available expanded skin for repair surgery, impairs reconstruction, and usually leads to extra surgeries or even re-expansion. Many efforts have been made to explore a wide range of substances, topical or systemic delivered, to reduce the formation of fibrous capsule to shorten the tissue expansion process [7,8]. However, these agents are limited in clinical application because of their toxic effects.

Tanshinone (Danshen) is an herbal medicine derived from the dried root of *Salvia miltiorrhiza Bunge*, which has a wide clinical use in China and other countries for hundreds of years [9,10], Tanshinon IIA (Tan IIA), the main component of Tanshinone, has drawn extensive attention because of its therapeutic efficacy in cardiovascular diseases, metabolic diseases and cancers. As a multi-target drug, its molecular targets include transcription factors, ion channels, apoptosis regulating proteins, growth factors and inflammatory mediators [11]. The Tan IIA we used in this study is a finished pharmaceutical product purchased from Shanghai No. 1 Biochemical & Pharmaceutical Co. Ltd. (Shanghai, P.R. China), The English name of this product is Sulfotanshinone Sodium Injection, it is a sulfonated form of Tan IIA. The formula of this compound is C19H17NaO6S (Fig. 1A). The Tan IIA acquires enhanced water solubility in a sulfonated form and the drug efficacy is improved. This chemical drug meets a criterion of Chinese sanitation industry standard WS-10001-(HD-1014)-2002. The effective component accounted for more than 98% of the chemical and the impurity content is below 1%.The aim of this study was to evaluate the effectiveness of systemically delivered Tan IIA on the process of tissue expansion and the formation of the fibrous capsule during tissue expansion.

Materials and Methods

1. Ethics Statement

The Animal Care and Use Committee of Shanghai Jiaotong Medical University approved all of the experiments in accordance with the Declaration of the National Institutes of Health Guide for Care and Use of Laboratory Animals (Publication No. 85-23, revised 1996). All of the surgeries were performed under sodium pentobarbital anesthesia, and all efforts were made to minimize suffering.

2. Animal preparation

Sprague-Dawley male adult rats, weighing 220–250 g each, were obtained from the Animal Center (Shanghai Experimental Animal Center, China). The rats were kept in a temperature-controlled habitat under a 12 h light/dark cycle and fed a standard laboratory diet and watered libitum.

3. Cell culture and Tan IIA treatment

Three-day-old SD rats were sacrificed with 3% sodium pentobarbital to harvest the skin fibroblasts according to the method reported previously [12]. The cells of passage 3–4 were seeded at 1×10^3 cells per well in 96-well plates with 100 µl culture medium. After being treated with Tan IIA (Shanghai No. 1 Biochemical & Pharmaceutical Co. Ltd, Shanghai, China) of different concentrations, 10 µl of Cell Counting Kit-8 (CCK-8) solution (Dojindo, Kumamoto, Japan) was added to each well, and the plates were incubated at 37°C for 3 h. The supernatants were aspirated and transferred into a new 96-well plate, and the optical density at 450 nm was read on a Microplate Reader (Bio-Rad, Hercules, CA, USA). The effect of Tan IIA on the viability of the adherent monolayer fibroblasts was presented as the % of cytoviability using the following formula: % cytoviability = A450 of treated cells/A450 of control cells ×100%. Three independent experiments were performed.

The cell apoptosis was measured with Annexin V-FITC and PI (BD Bioscience, San Jose, CA, USA) using a detection kit. The cells were harvested, washed once with cold PBS, and resuspended in 500 µl of binding buffer with a number of 1×10^5 cells, followed by staining with Annexin V-FITC and PI solution in the dark for 15 min at room temperature. The cells were centrifuged at 1000 rpm for 5 min, and the pellets were resuspended in 500 µl of binding buffer. After filtration, the percentage of cell apoptosis was determined using flow cytometry (BD FACSCalibar, San Jose, CA, USA).

4. Tissue expanding model and Tan IIA injection

Forty-eight SD rats were anaesthetized with 3% sodium pentobarbital at 0.13 ml/100 g and shaved. The 10 ml tissue expanders were implanted in the back of the rats as previously described, and 10 ml of physiological saline was injected through the tissue expander pot immediately after the implantation [7]. The expansion was conducted twice a week with an internal pressure maintained 60 mmHg, monitored by a simple self-made apparatus composed of a sphygmomanometer and a three-way pipe [1]. After a preliminary study, we chose 10 mg/kg/day as an appropriate dose for Tan IIA injection; The rats in the Tan II A group received daily intraperitoneal injection of Tan IIA for 28 days, and the rats in the control group received physiological saline injection.

5. Expansion volume and expanded area

The expansion ended after 4 weeks, and the water volume in the expander pockets of each group was added to perform the statistical analysis. The expanded skin was scanned using a Konica Minolta Vivid 910 fw 3D laser scanner (Konica Minolta, Tokyo, Japan) and the images were imported into Mimics CAD/CAM software (Konica Minolta, Tokyo, Japan) to create three-dimensional images of the expanded tissue to measure area of the expanded skin.

6. Histological staining

Expanded tissue specimens were collected at day 7, 14 and 28 (n = 6 for each group) postoperatively, and fixed with 4% paraformaldehyde for 24 h, and embedded in paraffin. Histological staining was performed on 4 µm section. The hematoxylin-eosin (H&E) staining was performed to observe the thickness of the whole skin layers and the fibrous capsule. Immunohistochemistry staining with vimentin (Santa Cruz, CA, USA) for fibroblasts, with CD68 (Abcam, Cambridge, UK) for macrophages, with α-smooth muscle actin (α-SMA; Santa Cruz, CA, USA) for myofibroblasts, with CD31 (Abcam) for capillaries and proliferating-cell nuclear antigen (PCNA; Abcam) for proliferating cells was performed. The steps were identical to those same as described in a previous report [3].

7. Protein level of cytokines

For the detection of growth factors, 0.5 g of tissue on the above area of tissue expander from each group was collected (n = 6 for each group). The tissues were homogenized in 500 µl of tissue protein extraction reagent (CWBIO, Beijing, China) and 5 µl of PMSF (Sigma-Aldrich). After centrifuging at 10000 rpm for 10 min, the supernatant was collected for the assay of TNF-α, IL-1β, IL-6 and TGF-β using a Protein Quantibody Array kit according to the manufacturer's instructions (R&D Systems, Minneapolis, USA). The signals were visualized by using a laser scanner equipped with a Cy3 wavelength. The data were extracted with microarray analysis software programs (GenePix, ScanArray Express, ArrayVision, or MicroVigene).

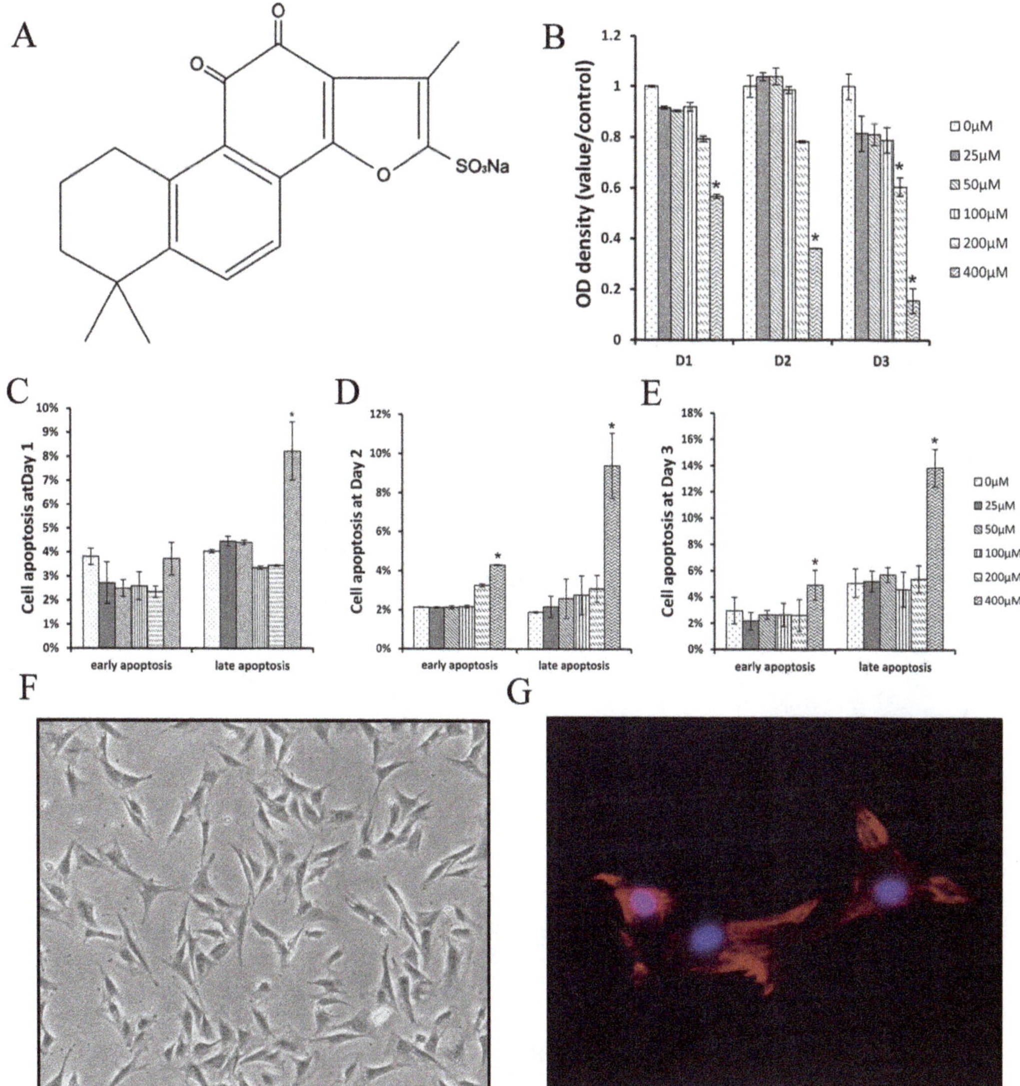

Figure 1. The molecular structure of Tan IIA used in the study (A). The effect of Tan IIA on the viability (B) and apoptosis (C–E) of dermal fibroblasts *in vitro* from days 1 to 3. Dermal fibroblasts demonstrate a spindle shape under optical microscope (F, 40×) and are positive stained with vimentin (G, 200×). There was no remarkable change as the concentration of Tan IIA varied when compared with 0 μM, except with 400 μM, showing that a low Tan IIA concentration could not influence the fibroblasts. Mean ± SD; $^*P<0.05$.

8. Statistical analysis

All of the quantitative variables were analyzed with the SPSS 13.0 program (SPSS, Inc., Chicago, IL, USA). All of the values were expressed as mean ± SD. The analysis of variance followed by Student's test was used to determine the significant differences between the two groups. Values of $P<0.05$ were considered statistically significant.

Results

1. Effect of Tan IIA on the viability and apoptosis of fibroblasts

The effect of Tan IIA on the growth of the fibroblasts was examined with CCK-8 and Annexin V/PI. After exposure to Tan IIA at concentrations of 0, 25, 50, 100, 200, 400 μM, the viability and apoptosis of the fibroblasts showed no evident change when compared with that without Tan IIA treatment, except at the concentration of 400 μM. In this high concentration, the viability of fibroblasts was inhibited and the percentage of apoptosis was increased. All of these results suggested that a low concentration of Tan IIA should not influence the growth of fibroblasts (Fig. 1 B–E).

2. Tan IIA accelerated tissue expansion

The inflation volume was measured to evaluate the effect of Tan IIA on tissue expansion. Four weeks later, the Tan IIA group had a higher inflation volume (55.88±5.56 ml) when compared with the control group (37.00±0.82 ml) (n = 6, $P<0.01$). The difference between the two groups appeared at the second week (39.83±1.57 ml in the Tan IIA group and 31.63±1.25 ml in the control group (n = 6, $P<0.05$)). Consistent with the expansion volume, the expanded area began to show a difference at day 14 and became evidently at day 28. There was no significant difference at day 7 (n = 6, $P>0.05$) (Fig. 2).

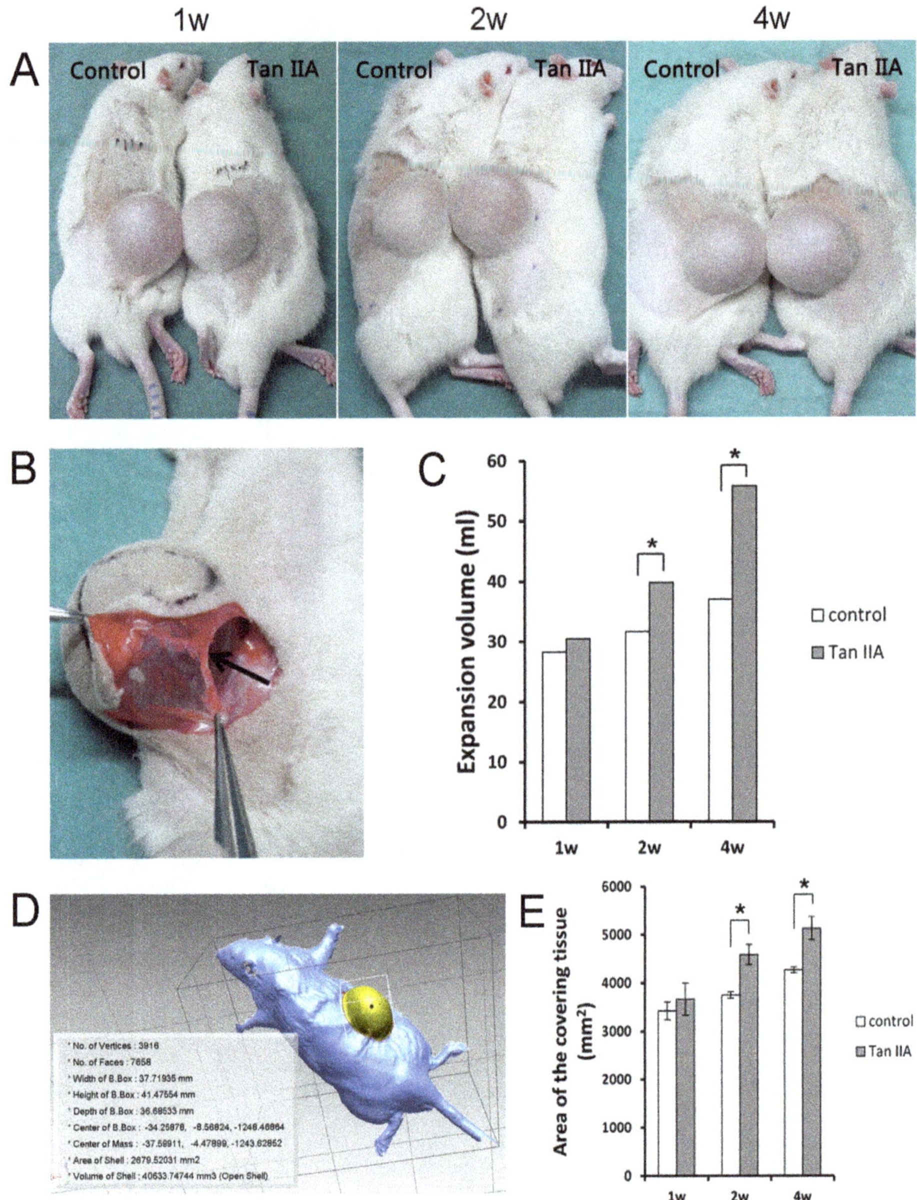

Figure 2. After the Tan IIA injection, the expansion volume was much greater than that of the control group at day 14 and 28 (A and C). The arrow in B showed the fibrous capsule formed around the tissue expander. The expanded area was measured using the Konica Minolta Vivid 910 fw 3D laser scanner (D), and there were significant differences between the two groups at day 14 and 28 (E). Mean ± SD; **P*<0.05.

3. The thickness of the expanded skin and the fibrous capsule

The thickness of the entire skin layer was measured, including the epidermis, dermis and subcutaneous tissue. At day 28, the skin thickness in the Tan IIA group (1111.9±21.96 μm) showed no significant difference (n = 6, $P>0.05$) compared with the control group (1083.2±16.53 μm). The thickness of the fibrous capsule in the control group was much thicker than that in the Tan IIA group at all of the time points (n = 6, $P<0.05$) The fibrous capsule measured in this study was the internal layer in contact with the implant, which was irregular and filled with collagen. The layer of parallel fibers combined with the capillaries as well as the layer of panniculus carnosus was not included (Fig. 3).

4. The proliferating cells in the expanded tissue

The PCNA-positive cells were distributed in all of the layers in the expanded tissue, especially in the basal layer and at the tissue-material interface. There was no difference in the positive cells in the basal layer between the Tan IIA group and the control group at all of the time points ($P>0.05$), showing that Tan IIA did not influence skin growth. The density of the PCNA-positive cells at the tissue-material interface in the Tan IIA group was much less than that in the control group, which might contribute to the reduced formation of the fibrous capsule (Fig. 3).

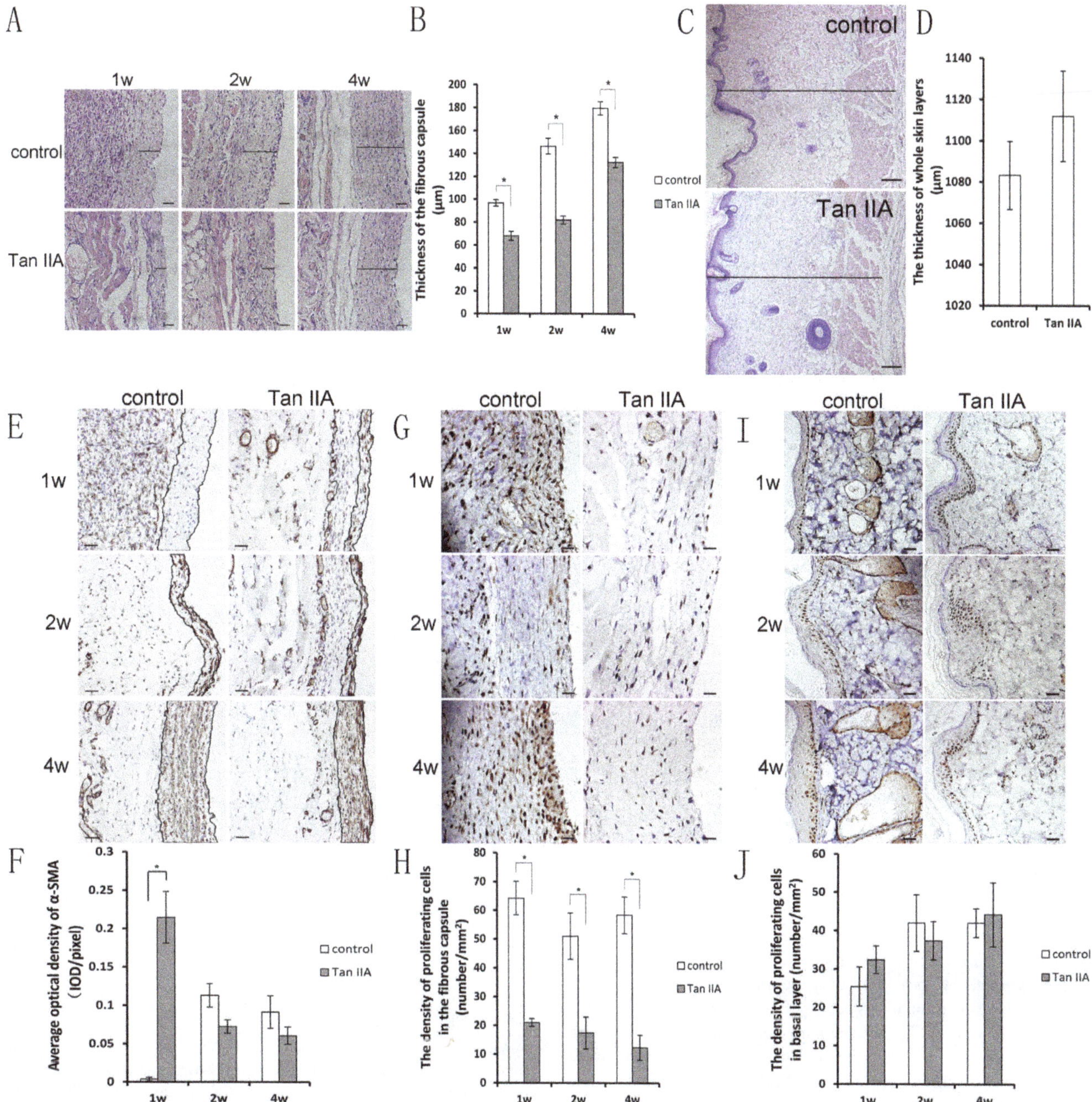

Figure 3. The thickness of the fibrous capsule in the Tan IIA group was much less than that in the control group at all of the time points (A and B), and the thickness of the whole skin layers, except the fibrous capsule, showed no difference (C and D). There were fewer α-SMA positive myofibroblasts in the fibrous capsule in the Tan IIA group (E and F), and their proliferation was much lower (G and H). The proliferating cells in the basal layer in the two groups showed no difference (I and J). The area within the black lines in E was calculated for the α-SMA density. The scale bars in E, G and I were ×200. Mean ± SD; $^{*}P<0.05$; Bar in C, 40 μm; Bar in E, G, and I, 200 μm.

5. Tan IIA injection enhanced the neovascularization of the expanded skin

Anti-CD31 immunohistochemical staining was used to determine the degree of neovascularization of the membrana carnosa, which provide the blood supply for the fibrous capsule. No difference of capillary density was found between the two groups at day 7 (n = 10, $P>0.05$). However, the capillary density in Tan IIA group was clearly increased after 14 days ($45\pm4.7/mm^2$ at day 14 and $26\pm2.50/mm^2$ at day 28), compared with the control group ($17\pm2.78/mm^2$ at day 14 and $14\pm1.24/mm^2$ at day 28) (n = 10, $P<0.05$), signifying that systematically injection of Tan IIA could effectively enhance the viability of the capillary vessel (Fig. 4).

6. Tan IIA inhibited the infiltration of macrophages and secretion of inflammatory cytokines

The macrophages showed a persistent infiltration, and were primarily located at the tissue-material interface in both the Tan IIA and control groups. However, less macrophages were observed

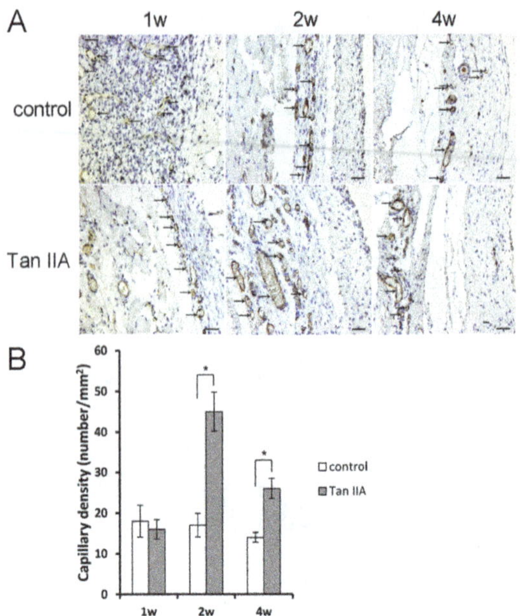

Figure 4. The capillary density in the membrana carnosa, which provides the blood supply for the fibrous capsule, was much higher in the Tan IIA group than in the control group at days 14 and 28, indicating that the Tan IIA injection could promote neovascularization. Mean ± SD; *$P<0.05$; Bar, 200 μm.

in the tissue from the Tan IIA group compared with the control, especially at day 7 (Fig. 1). Inflammatory cytokines, IL-6, TNF-α, IL-1β and TGF-β showed higher expression in the expanded tissue at all of the time points in the control group, however, in the Tan IIA group, these four cytokines presented a lower expression (Fig. 5).

Discussion

Repairing a defect resulting from wound or surgical resection is challenging, and the best tissue for such coverage is the one similar to the original. A local flap may be the best solution to this problem. However for a large defect, local flap cannot provide sufficient coverage. The use of tissue expanders presents a promising alternative. The advantages of tissue expansion were summarized by Schmidt et al. as follows: the best tissue match with defect areas, the lack of a wound at the donor site and the maintenance of the vascular supply [13]. However, tissue expansion is a time consuming procedure. During months of expansion, it is suffering and inconvenient for the patient and the probability of all kinds of unexpected events, such as infection and rupture, also increases. Finding a simple and effective measure to speed up the expansion process has very important clinical implication.

Capsule formation is a chronic-proliferative inflammation process [14,15], and is determined by the physico-chemical properties of the implants as well as the various biological components, to which the implant is exposed after implantation [16]. Periprosthetic fibrosis is a reaction to a foreign body and begins at the moment of implantation of the prosthesis and lasts until its stabilization. Myofibroblasts are the main cells in the fibrous capsule. In the FBR process, dermal fibroblasts are activated and migrate to the fibrous capsule layer. Vimentin positive fibroblasts in the capsule tissue decrease over time, and some of them transdifferentiate into myofibroblasts under TGF-β regulation [17]. The activated myofibroblasts proliferate and synthesize collagen, resulting in material encapsulation [18,19]. Our results showed that lower concentration of Tan IIA had no influence on the viability and apoptosis of fibroblasts, however, α-SMA positive myoblasts in the fibrous capsule was much less after Tan IIA application. It seems that Tan IIA could inhibit the trasndifferentiating of fibroblasts into myofibroblasts. This may relate to the inhibition of TGF-β expression. The reduced density of the proliferating myofibroblasts in the fibrous capsule led to less collagen deposition and fibrous capsule formation. The result was consistent with the study reported by Laitung et al [20], who found that less number of myofibroblasts in the tissue around tissue expanding devices led to lower capsular formation and contracture.

The cell proliferation in the stratum basele, which plays an important role in skin growth, was not influenced by the Tan IIA treatment. Similarly in the *in vitro* study, Tan IIA treatment with a low dosage did not inhibit the fibroblast proliferation and did not promote fibroblast apoptosis. The thickness of the whole skin layers was not influenced, and there was no difference between the two groups at the end of tissue expansion. These results indicated that the capsule formation in the Tan IIA group was inhibited but that the skin growth was not influenced. The greater inflation volume with the larger expansion area in the Tan IIA group was positively correlated with decreased capsule thickness. In our earlier experiment, 20 mg/kg of Tan IIA was injected every day, and at approximately 14 days, the expanded skin of some rats underwent necrosis. The result was consistent with our in *vitro* study, which showed that high concentration (400 μM) may inhibit the fibroblast proliferation and promote fibroblast apoptosis. So in this study we chose 10 mg/kg/day as a safe and effective drug dose.

The expanded tissue had a high vascularity that was considered superior to surgical delayed flaps [21]. High neovascularization of a tissue flap before transplantation is critical to its postoperative survival. The histologic examination showed that Tan IIA treatment could enhance angiogenesis, which was evidenced by the increased number of blood vessels, providing the newly formed tissue with sufficient nutriments and oxygen to improve the viability of the expanded skin. In this study, thickness of the fibrous capsule decreased, however, the capillary density was not decreased.

Fibrous capsule formation is a complicated multifactorial process. The severity of capsule contracture has a positive linear correlation with the degree of local inflammatory reactions [22]. When the tissue expanders are implanted, the injury and ischemia caused by the surgical procedure initiate an acute inflammatory cascade. In the long term expansion period, the acute inflammatory transfer into a chronic pattern because the tissue expander as a non-removable injurious stimuli. In this process a protein layer adsorbs to the biomaterial surface, and macrophages, the main cells participating into FBR, adhere to the surface via interaction of adhesion receptors with the adsorbed proteins [23]. Our results showed that Tan IIA markedly reduced the infiltration of CD68-positive macrophages and the expression of inflammatory cytokines in the local tissue. This chronic inflammatory inhibiting effect explained less fibrous capsule formation in the Tan IIA group. Tan IIA inhibits the chronic inflammatory which shows little relation with infection defense but a pathological state of the body to non-removable injurious stimuli. Chronic inflammation can always lead to tissue destruction and fibrosis, including the fibrous capsule formed after material implantation. So Tan IIA could inhibit fibrous capsule formation without infection defense

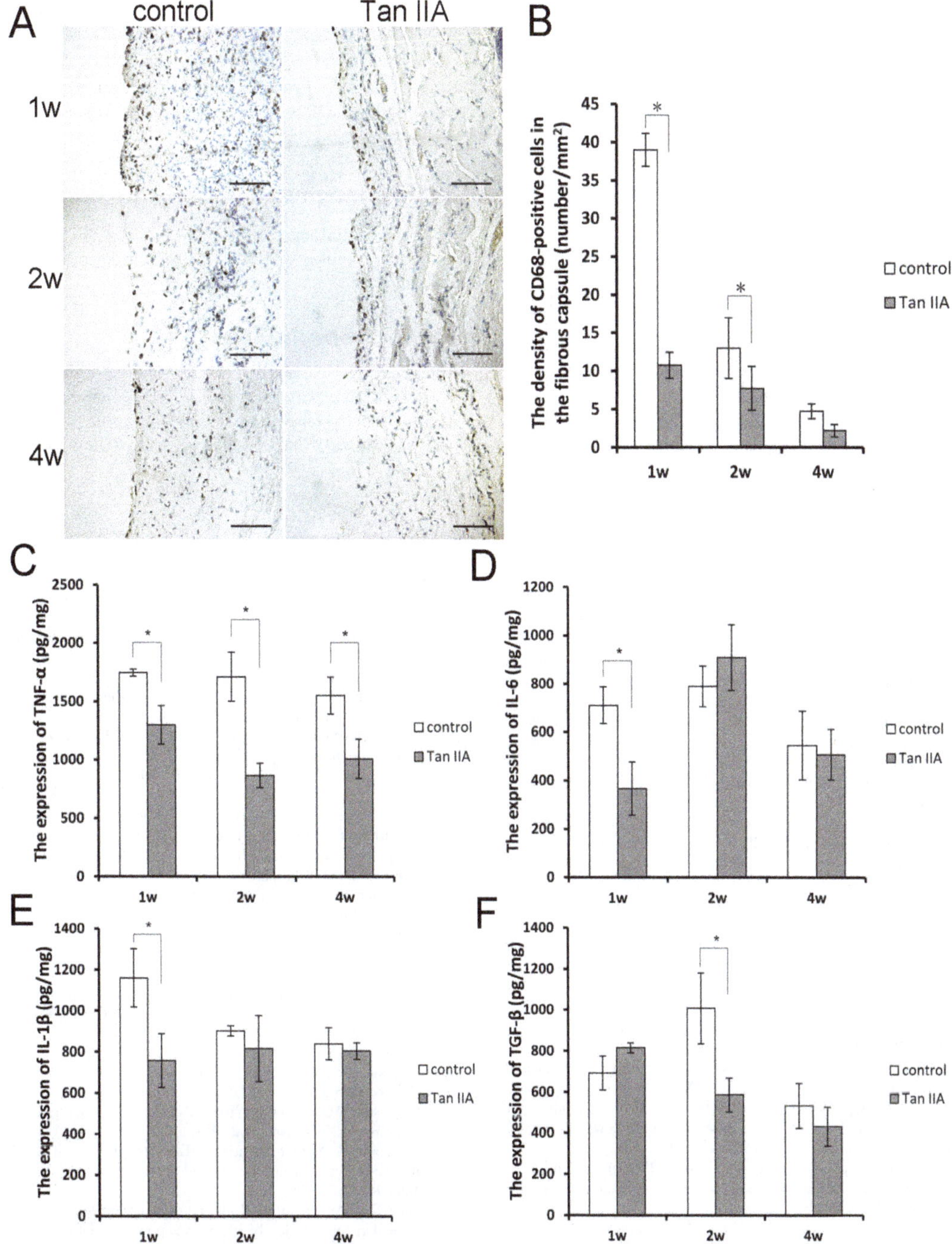

Figure 5. There was less infiltration of the CD68-positive macrophages at the tissue-material interface in the Tan IIA group when compared with the control group, particularly at day 7 (A and B). The inflammatory cytokines, IL-6, TNF-α, IL-1β and TGF-β showed higher expression in the expanded tissue at all of the time points in the control group, and after the Tan IIA treatment, these three cytokines presented lower expression (C–F). Mean ± SD; *$P<0.05$; Bar, 200 μm.

function impairment. Since the use of Tan IIA has a long history and the long-term practice proved it to be a safe and effective traditional Chinese medicine (TCM) preparations, we think it is safe to use Tan IIA to reduce the formation of fibrous capsule around the expander. And in our experiment all rats receiving Tan IIA injection had no sign of infection.

Macrophages produce growth factors and fibrocyte-stimulating cytokines, such as IL-6, TNF-α, IL-1β and TGF-β [13]. In our study, the expression of these cytokines decreased in the Tan IIA group. The TNF-α secreted by macrophages could recruit more macrophages to the target tissue, and there is positive feedback between them. In our previous study, we demonstrated that the NF-κB and JNK pathways were the major pathways activated in the tissue expansion model [5]. NF-κB is one of the central players in the cascade, and it is initiated and plays a crucial role in regulating inflammatory signal transduction and cytokine production. Research showed that Tan IIA could suppress the TNF-α expression after cellular oxygen-glucose deprivation/recovery

(OGD/R) in a dose-dependent manner and this suppression was mimicked by BAY 11-7082, a commercial NF-κB inhibitor [24]. Another study demonstrated that Tan IIA could reduce the levels of IL-6, TNF-α and IL-1β by markedly inhibiting the activation of NF-κB and the mitogen-activated protein kinases (MAPKs) pathways in a spinal cord injury model [25]. All these results indicated that Tan IIA could inhibit NF-κB pathway and down regulate the expression of kinds of inflammatory cytokines. IL-1 and TGF-β have been showed to have an important regulatory effect on fibroblast proliferation and collagen synthesis [26–28]. High levels of TGF-β and IL-1 could potentially result in significant fibrosis surrounding silicone implants *in vivo*. The TGF-β1 inhibitor peptide was significantly effective in achieving a reduction in periprosthetic fibrosis after silicone implants placements [29]. This explains the fibrous capsule formation inhibiting effect of Tan IIA in our experiment.

Our results suggested that pharmacological control of capsular formation and neovascularization in the course of tissue expansion was feasible by means of systemic application of Tan IIA. With Tan IIA, the expansion can proceed in a safer, more rapid and efficacious manner, relieving patients' discomfort and lowering the total cost of the procedure. Extensive study is still needed to test the long-term safety of Tan IIA and to evaluate its mechanisms of action.

Acknowledgments

We thank Yimin Liang, Rui Jin, Yan Zheng and Jinjun Chen for kindly technical assistance and Shuai Shao for help with animal raise and experiment.

Author Contributions

Conceived and designed the experiments: Q-XY L-LS MY Q-FL. Performed the experiments: Q-XY L-LS. Analyzed the data: Q-XY X-LH. Contributed reagents/materials/analysis tools: MZ X-LH. Wrote the paper: Q-XY L-LS MY. Final approval of manuscript: Q-FL.

References

1. Sheng L, Yang M, Du Z, Yang Y, Li Q (2012) Transplantation of stromal vascular fraction as an alternative for accelerating tissue expansion. J Plast Reconstr Aesthet Surg 66: 551–557.
2. Yang M, Li Q, Sheng L, Li H, Weng R, et al. (2011) Bone marrow-derived mesenchymal stem cells transplantation accelerates tissue expansion by promoting skin regeneration during expansion. Ann Surg 253: 202–209.
3. Sheng L, Yang M, Liang Y, Li Q (2013) Adipose tissue-derived stem cells (ADSCs) transplantation promotes regeneration of expanded skin using a tissue expansion model. Wound Repair Regen 21: 746–754.
4. Higgins DM, Basaraba RJ, Hohnbaum AC, Lee EJ, Grainger DW (2009) Gonzalez-Juarrero M: Localized immunosuppressive environment in the foreign body response to implanted biomaterials. Am J Pathol 175: 161–170.
5. Sheng L, Yu Q, Xie F, Li Q (2014) Foreign body response induced by tissue expander implantation. Mol Med Rep 9: 872–876.
6. Raposio E, Santi PL (1999) Topical application of DMSO as an adjunct to tissue expansion for breast reconstruction. Br J Plast Surg 52: 194–197.
7. Tang Y, Luan J, Zhang X (2004) Accelerating tissue expansion by application of topical papaverine cream. Plast Reconstr Surg 114: 1166–1169.
8. Lee P, Squier CA, Bardach J (1985) Enhancement of tissue expansion by anticontractile agents. Plast Reconstr Surg 76: 604–610.
9. Fu J, Huang H, Liu J, Pi R, Chen J, et al. (2007) Tanshinone IIA protects cardiac myocytes against oxidative stress-triggered damage and apoptosis. Eur J Pharmacol 568: 213–221.
10. Li J, Xu M, Fan Q, Xie X, Zhang Y, et al. (2011) Tanshinone IIA ameliorates seawater exposure-induced lung injury by inhibiting aquaporins (AQP) 1 and AQP5 expression in lung. Respir Physiol Neurobiol 176: 39–49.
11. Xu S, Liu P (2013) Tanshinone II-A: new perspectives for old remedies. Expert Opin Ther Pat 23: 149–153.
12. Yin S, Cen L, Wang C, Zhao G, Sun J, et al. (2010) Chondrogenic transdifferentiation of human dermal fibroblasts stimulated with cartilage-derived morphogenetic protein 1. Tissue Eng Part A 16: 1633–1643.
13. Schmidt SC, Logan SE, Hayden JM, Ahn ST, Mustoe TA (1991) Continuous versus conventional tissue expansion: experimental verification of a new technique. Plast Reconstr Surg 87: 10–15.
14. Siggelkow W, Faridi A, Spiritus K, Klinge U, Rath W, et al. (2003) Histological analysis of silicone breast implant capsules and correlation with capsular contracture. Biomaterials 24: 1101–1109.
15. Prantl L, Schreml S, Fichtner-Feigl S, Poppl N, Eisenmann-Klein M, et al. (2007) Clinical and morphological conditions in capsular contracture formed around silicone breast implants. Plast Reconstr Surg 120: 275–284.
16. Joseph J, Mohanty M, Mohanan PV (2010) Role of immune cells and inflammatory cytokines in regulation of fibrosis around silicone expander implants. J Mater Sci Mater Med 21: 1665–1676.
17. Li AG, Quinn MJ, Siddiqui Y, Wood MD, Federiuk IF, et al. (2007) Elevation of transforming growth factor beta (TGFbeta) and its downstream mediators in subcutaneous foreign body capsule tissue. J Biomed Mater Res A 82: 498–508.
18. Ratner BD (2002) Reducing capsular thickness and enhancing angiogenesis around implant drug release systems. J Control Release 78: 211–218.
19. Ratner BD, Bryant SJ (2004) Biomaterials: where we have been and where we are going. Annu Rev Biomed Eng 6: 41–75.
20. Laitung JK, McClure J, Shuttleworth CA (1987) The fibrous capsules around static and dynamic implants: their biochemical, histological, and ultrastructural characteristics. Ann Plast Surg 19: 208–216.
21. Bozkurt A, Groger A, O'Dey D, Vogeler F, Piatkowski A, et al. (2008) Retrospective analysis of tissue expansion in reconstructive burn surgery: evaluation of complication rates. Burns 34: 1113–1118.
22. Poeppl N, Schreml S, Lichtenegger F, Lenich A, Eisenmann-Klein M, et al. (2007) Does the surface structure of implants have an impact on the formation of a capsular contracture? Aesthetic Plast Surg 31: 133–139.
23. Franz S, Rammelt S, Scharnweber D, Simon JC (2011) Immune responses to implants - a review of the implications for the design of immunomodulatory biomaterials. Biomaterials 32: 6692–6709.
24. Wu WY, Wang WY, Ma YL, Yan H, Wang XB, et al. (2013) Sodium tanshinone IIA silate inhibits oxygen-glucose deprivation/recovery-induced cardiomyocyte apoptosis via suppression of the NF-kappaB/TNF-alpha pathway. Br J Pharmacol 169: 1058–1071.
25. Yin X, Yin Y, Cao FL, Chen YF, Peng Y, et al. (2012) Tanshinone IIA attenuates the inflammatory response and apoptosis after traumatic injury of the spinal cord in adult rats. PLoS One 7: e38381.
26. Heppleston AG, Styles JA (1967) Activity of a macrophage factor in collagen formation by silica. Nature 214: 521–522.
27. Tavazzani F, Xing S, Waddell JE, Smith D, Boynton EL (2005) In vitro interaction between silicone gel and human monocyte-macrophages. J Biomed Mater Res A 72: 161–167.
28. Miller KM, Anderson JM (1988) Human monocyte/macrophage activation and interleukin 1 generation by biomedical polymers. J Biomed Mater Res 22: 713–731.
29. Ruiz-de-Erenchun R, Dotor de las Herrerias J, Hontanilla B (2005) Use of the transforming growth factor-beta1 inhibitor peptide in periprosthetic capsular fibrosis: experimental model with tetraglycerol dipalmitate. Plast Reconstr Surg 116: 1370–1378.

11

Flapless versus Conventional Flapped Dental Implant Surgery

Bruno Ramos Chrcanovic[1]*, Tomas Albrektsson[1,2], Ann Wennerberg[1]

1 Department of Prosthodontics, Faculty of Odontology, Malmö University, Malmö, Sweden,, **2** Department of Biomaterials, Göteborg University, Göteborg, Sweden

Abstract

The aim of this study was to test the null hypothesis of no difference in the implant failure rates, postoperative infection, and marginal bone loss for patients being rehabilitated by dental implants being inserted by a flapless surgical procedure versus the open flap technique, against the alternative hypothesis of a difference. An electronic search without time or language restrictions was undertaken in March 2014. Eligibility criteria included clinical human studies, either randomized or not. The search strategy resulted in 23 publications. The I^2 statistic was used to express the percentage of the total variation across studies due to heterogeneity. The inverse variance method was used for random-effects model or fixed-effects model, when indicated. The estimates of relative effect were expressed in risk ratio (RR) and mean difference (MD) in millimeters. Sixteen studies were judged to be at high risk of bias, whereas two studies were considered of moderate risk of bias, and five studies of low risk of bias. The funnel plots indicated absence of publication bias for the three outcomes analyzed. The test for overall effect showed that the difference between the procedures (flapless vs. open flap surgery) significantly affect the implant failure rates ($P=0.03$), with a RR of 1.75 (95% CI 1.07–2.86). However, a sensitivity analysis revealed differences when studies of high and low risk of bias were pooled separately. Thus, the results must be interpreted carefully. No apparent significant effects of flapless technique on the occurrence of postoperative infection (P = 0.96; RR 0.96, 95% CI 0.23–4.03) or on the marginal bone loss ($P=0.16$; MD −0.07 mm, 95% CI −0.16–0.03) were observed.

Editor: Michael Glogauer, University of Toronto, Canada

Funding: This work was supported by CNPq, Conselho Nacional de Desenvolvimento Científico e Tecnológico - Brazil. The supportive institution had no role in study design, data collection and analysis, decision to publish, or preparation of the manuscript.

Competing Interests: The authors have declared that no competing interests exist.

* Email: bruno.chrcanovic@mah.se

Introduction

When placing dental implants, a flap is traditionally elevated to better visualize the implant recipient site, providing that some anatomical landmarks are clearly identified and protected. When a limited amount of bone is available, a flap elevation can help implant placement to reduce the risk of bone fenestrations or perforations [1]. More recently, the concept of flapless implant surgery has been introduced for the patients with sufficient keratinized gingival tissue and bone volume in the implant recipient site. In a flapless procedure, a dental implant is installed through the mucosal tissues without reflecting a flap. The alleged reasons to choose the flapless technique are to minimize the possibility of postoperative peri-implant tissue loss and to overcome the challenge of soft tissue management during or after surgery [2]. Other alleged advantages of the flapless implant surgery include less traumatic surgery, decreased operative time, rapid postsurgical healing, fewer postoperative complications and increased patient comfort [3,4]. A disadvantage of this technique is that the true topography of the underlying available bone cannot be observed because the mucogingival tissues are not raised, which may increase the risk for unwanted perforations which in its turn could lead to esthetical problems or implant losses [5]. Moreover, there is the potential for thermal damage secondary to reduced access for external irrigation during osteotomy preparation [4].

Researchers have been trying to evaluate whether the insertion of implants by the flapless technique may influence the survival of dental implants. However, some studies may lack statistical power, given the small number of patients per group in the clinical trials comparing the techniques. Thus, we conducted a meta-analysis of previously published clinical studies to investigate whether there are any positive effects of flapless implant insertion surgery on implant failure rates, postoperative infection, and marginal bone loss in comparison with the more traditional open flap technique. The present study presents a more detailed and profound analysis of the influence of these two techniques on the implant failure rates, previously assessed in a published systematic review [6].

Materials and Methods

This study followed the PRISMA Statement guidelines [7]. A review protocol does not exist.

Objective

The purpose of the present review was to test the null hypothesis of no difference in the implant failure rates, postoperative infection, and marginal bone loss for patients being rehabilitated by dental implants being inserted by a flapless surgical procedure versus the open flap technique, against the alternative hypothesis of a difference.

Search strategies

An electronic search without time or language restrictions was undertaken in March 2014 in the following databases: PubMed, Web of Science, and the Cochrane Oral Health Group Trials Register. The following terms were used in the search strategy on PubMed:

{Subject AND Adjective}

{*Subject*: (dental implant OR dental implant failure OR dental implant survival OR dental implant success [text words])

AND

Adjective: (flapless OR flapped OR open flap [text words])}

Refining the results with the option "Dentistry Oral Surgery Medicine" selected within the filter "Research Areas", the following terms were used in the search strategy on Web of Science:

{Subject AND Adjective}

{*Subject*: (dental implant failure OR dental implant survival OR dental implant success [title])

AND

Adjective: (flapless surgery OR flapped surgery OR open flap surgery [title])}

The following terms were used in the search strategy on the Cochrane Oral Health Group Trials Register:

(dental implant OR dental implant failure OR dental implant survival OR dental implant success AND (flapless surgery OR flapped surgery OR open flap surgery))

A manual search of dental implants-related journals, including *British Journal of Oral and Maxillofacial Surgery, Clinical Implant Dentistry and Related Research, Clinical Oral Implants Research, European Journal of Oral Implantology, Implant Dentistry, International Journal of Oral and Maxillofacial Implants, International Journal of Oral and Maxillofacial Surgery, International Journal of Periodontics and Restorative Dentistry, International Journal of Prosthodontics, Journal of Clinical Periodontology, Journal of Dental Research, Journal of Oral Implantology, Journal of Craniofacial Surgery, Journal of Cranio-Maxillofacial Surgery, and Journal of Maxillofacial and Oral Surgery, Journal of Oral and Maxillofacial Surgery, Journal of Periodontology*, and *Oral Surgery Oral Medicine Oral Pathology Oral Radiology and Endodontology*, was also performed.

The reference list of the identified studies and the relevant reviews on the subject were also scanned for possible additional studies. Moreover, online databases providing information about clinical trials in progress were checked (clinicaltrials.gov; www.centerwatch.com/clinicaltrials; www.clinicalconnection.com).

Inclusion and Exclusion Criteria

Eligibility criteria included clinical human studies, either randomized or not, comparing implant failure rates in any group of patients receiving titanium dental implants by a flapless surgical procedure versus the open flap technique. For this review, implant failure represents the complete loss of the implant. Exclusion criteria were case reports, technical reports, animal studies, *In Vitro* studies, and reviews papers.

Study selection

The titles and abstracts of all reports identified through the electronic searches were read independently by the three authors. For studies appearing to meet the inclusion criteria, or for which there were insufficient data in the title and abstract to make a clear decision, the full report was obtained. Disagreements were resolved by discussion between the authors.

Quality assessment

The quality assessment was performed by using the recommended approach for assessing risk of bias in studies included in Cochrane reviews [8]. The classification of the risk of bias potential for each study was based on the four following criteria: sequence generation (random selection in the population), allocation concealment (steps must be taken to secure strict implementation of the schedule of random assignments by preventing foreknowledge of the forthcoming allocations), incomplete outcome data (clear explanation of withdrawals and exclusions), and blinding (measures to blind study participants and personnel from knowledge of which intervention a participant received). The incomplete outcome data will also be considered addressed when there are no withdrawals and/or exclusions. A study that met all the criteria mentioned above was classified as having a low risk of bias, a study that did not meet one of these criteria was classified as having a moderate risk of bias. When two or more criteria were not met, the study was considered to have a high risk of bias.

Data extraction and meta-analysis

From the studies included in the final analysis, the following data was extracted (when available): year of publication, study design (randomized controlled trial – RCT, controlled clinical trial – CCT, retrospective study), unicenter or multicenter study, number of patients, patients' age, follow-up, days of antibiotic prophylaxis, mouth rinse with chlorhexidine, implant healing period, failed and placed implants, postoperative infection, marginal bone loss, implant surface modification, use of grafting procedures, use of a surgical guide, and presence of smokers among the patients. Contact with authors for possible missing data was performed.

Implant failure and postoperative infection were the dichotomous outcomes measures evaluated. Weighted mean differences were used to construct forest plots of marginal bone loss, a continuous outcome. The statistical unit for 'implant failure' and 'marginal bone loss' was the implant, and for 'postoperative infection' was the patient. Whenever outcomes of interest were not clearly stated, the data were not used for analysis. The I^2 statistic was used to express the percentage of the total variation across studies due to heterogeneity, with 25% corresponding to low heterogeneity, 50% to moderate and 75% to high. The inverse variance method was used for random-effects or fixed-effects model. Where statistically significant ($P<.10$) heterogeneity is detected, a random-effects model was used to assess the significance of treatment effects. Where no statistically significant heterogeneity is found, analysis was performed using a fixed-effects model [9]. In the inverse variance method the weight given to each study is chosen to be the inverse of the variance of the effect estimate (i.e. one over the square of its standard error) [8]. Thus larger studies, which have smaller standard errors, are given more weight than smaller studies, which have larger standard errors. This choice of weight minimizes the imprecision (uncertainty) of the pooled effect estimate. The basic data required for the analysis are an estimate of the intervention effect and its standard error from each study [8].

The estimates of relative effect for dichotomous outcomes were expressed in risk ratio (RR) and in mean difference (MD) in millimeters for continuous outcomes, both with a 95% confidence interval (CI). Only if there were studies with similar comparisons reporting the same outcome measures was meta-analysis to be attempted. In the case where no events (or all events) are observed in both groups the study provides no information about relative probability of the event and is automatically omitted from the

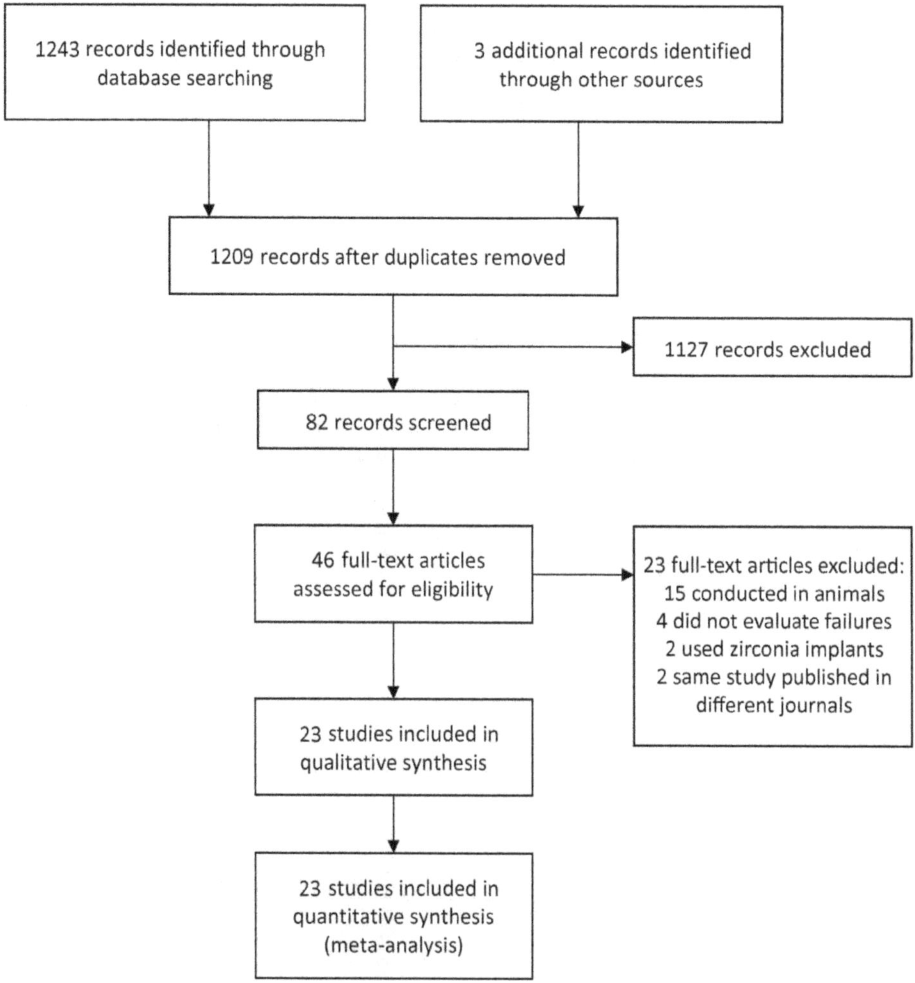

Figure 1. Study screening process – flow diagram.

meta-analysis. In this (these) case(s), the term 'not estimable' is shown under the RR column of the forest plot table. The software used here automatically checks for problematic zero counts, and adds a fixed value of 0.5 to all cells of study results tables where the problems occur.

A funnel plot (plot of effect size versus standard error) will be drawn. Asymmetry of the funnel plot may indicate publication bias and other biases related to sample size, although the asymmetry may also represent a true relationship between trial size and effect size.

The data were analyzed using the statistical software Review Manager (version 5.2.8, The Nordic Cochrane Centre, The Cochrane Collaboration, Copenhagen, Denmark, 2014).

Results

Literature search

The study selection process is summarized in Figure 1. The search strategy resulted in 1246 papers. The three reviewers independently screened the abstracts for those articles related to the focus question. The initial screening of titles and abstracts resulted in 82 full-text papers; 37 were cited in more than one research of terms. The full-text reports of the remaining 43 articles led to the exclusion of 23 because they did not meet the inclusion criteria; 15 studies were conducted in animals, 2 studies used zirconia implants, 4 studies compared the techniques but did not evaluate implant failures, and 2 articles were the same study published in different journals. Additional hand searching of the reference lists of selected studies yielded two additional papers. Thus, a total of 23 publications were included in the review.

Description of the Studies

Detailed data of the 23 included studies are listed in Table 1. Ten RCTs [1,4,10–17], seven CCTs [3,18–23] and six retrospective studies [5,24–28] were included in the meta-analysis. Only three studies [1,25,27] were multicenter. In five studies [4,12–14,17] both patients and operators/outcome assessors were blinded to the tested intervention. Six studies [3,11,12,16,17,21] had a follow-up up to 6 months, and six studies [15,18–20,22,23] with a follow-up up to 1 year.

All studies but one [26] with available data of patients' age included only adult patients. Three split-mouth design studies were performed [13,14,16]. Eight studies [1,10,13,18,21,25–27] made use of surgical guides when inserting implants through the flapless surgical technique, five studies [12,15,17,22,24] used the surgical guides in both groups, whereas in ten studies [3–5,11,14,16,19,20,23,28] the implants were inserted without any kind of surgical guide.

Table 1. Detailed data of the included studies.

Authors	Published	Patients (n) (number per group)	Patients' Age Range (Average) (years)	Follow-up visits (or range)	Failed/Placed Implants (n)	Implant failure rate (%)	*P* value (for failure rate)	Antibiotics/ mouth rinse (days)	Healing period/loading	Implant surface modification (brand)	Grafting	Observations
Kinsel and Liss [24]	2007	43 (NM)	35–80 (58)	2–10 years	13/196 (G1) 3/148 (G2)	6.6 (G1) 2.0 (G2)	0.07	NM	Immediate	TPS (SLA, Straumann, Basel, Switzerland; n = 131), sandblasted and acid-etched (SLA, Straumann, Basel, Switzerland; n = 213)	Grafting in 2 patients, with implants placed 5–6 months later	12 smokers, surgical guide (G1 and G2)
Nkenke et al. [18]	2007	10 (5, G1, 5, G2)	NM (65±10)	1 and 7 days, 12 months	0/30 (G1) 0/30 (G2)	0 (G1) 0 (G2)	NM	NM	6 months	NM	NP	Only in maxilla, use of CT-guided surgical stents (G1)
Ozan et al. [1]	2007	12 (5, G1; 7, G2)	NM (46±9)	6–14 months (mean 9±3)	0/14 (G1) 1/45 (G2)	0 (G1) 2.2 (G2)	NM	NM	3 months (maxilla) 2 months (mandible)	Sandblasted and acid-etched (SwissPlus, Zimmer Dental, Carlsbad, USA)	NP	Use of CT-guided surgical stents (G1), healing abutments screwed immediately
Villa and Rangert [19]	2007	33 (15, G1; 18, G2)	NM	10 days, 1, 3, 6 and 12 months	1/29 (G1) 1/47 (G2)	3.4 (G1) 2.1 (G2)	NM	6/14–21	Immediate and early loading	Oxidized (Brånemark Mk III and Mk IV and NobelSpeedy, TiUnite, Nobel Biocare, Göteborg, Sweden)	NP	Implants placed in infected extraction sockets, no use of a surgical guide
Cannizzaro et al. [10]	2008	40 (20, G1; 20, G2)	18–62 (40.1, G1) 19–64 (37.4, G2)	3 years	0/52 (G1) 0/56 (G2)	0 (G1) 0 (G2)	NM	3/13	Immediate loading (G1), 4 months (maxilla) and 3 months (mandible) (G2)	Sandblasted and acid-etched (SwissPlus, Zimmer Dental, Carlsbad, USA)	NP	Use of surgical templates based on diagnostic tooth arrangement (G1), 17 smokers (8, G1; 9, G2)
Covani et al. [11]	2008	20 (10, G1; 10, G2)	30–67 (NM)	6 months	1/10 (G1) 0/10 (G2)	10 (G1) 0 (G2)	NM	4/21	6 months	Titanium plasma-sprayed coated (Premium, Sweden & Martina, Padova, Italy)	All implants: grafting with a mixture of collagen gel/ corticocancellous porcine bone	Submerged implants, no use of a surgical guide, heavy smokers (> 10 cigarettes/day) were excluded

Table 1. Cont.

Authors	Published	Patients (n) (number per group)	Patients' Age Range (Average) (years)	Follow-up visits (or range)	Failed/Placed Implants (n)	Implant failure rate (%)	*P* value (for failure rate)	Antibiotics/ mouth rinse (days)	Healing period/loading	Implant surface modification (brand)	Grafting	Observations
Maló and Nobre [20]	2008	41 (20, G1; 21, G2)	19–79 (45.5)	6 months 1 year	1/32 (G1) 0/40 (G2)	3.1 (G1) 0 (G2)	NM	6/60 (rinse with hyaluronic acid)	Immediate loading	Oxidized (NobelSpeedy, TiUnite, Nobel Biocare, Göteborg, Sweden)	NP	No use of a surgical guide
Sennerby et al. [25]	2008	43 (NM)	NM (50)	1–18 months (mean 10.2)	6/76 (G1) 0/41 (G2)	7.9 (G1) 0 (G2)	NM	NM	Immediate/early (n = 95), from 6 weeks to 6 months (n = 22)	Anodically oxidized (NobelDirect, Nobel Biocare, Göteborg, Sweden)	Minor bone grafting in 8 implants	Use of a slide-over guide sleeve to evaluate and determine the position of the implant (G1) Healed sites (n = 99) Extraction sockets (n = 18)
Danza et al. [26]	2009	93 (8, G1; 85, G2)	16–89 (48)	Mean of 14 months	0/66 (G1) 9/225 (G2)	0 (G1) 4.0 (G2)	0.3311	5/NP	Immediate or after 3 months	? (3D Alpha-Biomedical s.r.l., Pescara, Italy)	NP	Use of CT-guided surgical template (G1), heavy smokers (>20 cigarettes/day) were excluded
Arisan et al. [3]	2010	52 (15, G1; 37, G2)	28–63 (48.4)	4 months	3/99 (G1) 5/242 (G2)	3.0 (G1) 2.1 (G2)	0.946	5/before surgery	2–4 months	Sandblasted and acid-etched (SPI-Element, Thommen Medical, Waldenburg, Switzerland, n = 180), sandblasted and acid-etched (XiVe, Dentsply-Friadent, Mannheim, Germany, n = 161)	NP	Use of a stereolitho-graphic surgical guide (G1) In G2: the surgical guide was used in 16 patients (101 implants), whereas in 21 patients it was not used (141 implants), heavy smokers (> 10 cigarettes/day) were excluded
Berdougo et al. [27]	2010	169 (99, G1; 76 G2)[a]	20–84 (53.1±14.5)	1–4 years	10/271 (G1) 4/281 (G2)	3.7 (G1) 1.4 (G2)	0.1	NM	NM	NM	NP	Use of an image-guided template (G1), 22 patients were smokers
Lindeboom and van Wijk [12]	2010	16 (8, G1; 8, G2)	NM (54.6±2.9, G1) NM (58.7±7.2, G2)	1 week 1 month 6 months [b]	3/48 (G1) 0/48 (G2)[b]	4.2 (G1) 0 (G2)	NM	5/7	The implants were not loaded	Oxidized (NobelReplace, Nobel Biocare, Göteborg, Sweden)	NP	Use of CT-guided surgical template (G1 and G2) No smokers
Rousseau [28]	2010	219 (121, G1; 98, G2)	23–84 (54.3±12.6)	4 weeks, 2–3 months, 2 years	3/174 (G1) 3/203 (G2)	1.7 (G1) 1.5 (G2)	0.46	NM	2–3 months	Sandblasted and acid-etched (SLA, Straumann, Basel, Switzerland)	NP	No use of a surgical guide

Table 1. Cont.

Authors	Published	Patients (n) (number per group)	Patients' Age Range (Average) (years)	Follow-up visits (or range)	Failed/Placed Implants (n)	Implant failure rate (%)	*P* value (for failure rate)	Antibiotics/ mouth rinse (days)	Healing period/loading	Implant surface modification (brand)	Grafting	Observations
Van de Velde et al. [13]	2010	14 (split-mouth design)	39–75 (55.7)	1 week, 6 weeks, 3, 6, 12 and 18 months	1/36 (G1) 0/34 (G2)	2.8 (G1) 0 (G2)	NM	NP/before surgery	Immediate loading (G1), 6 weeks (G2)	Sandblasted and acid-etched (SLA, Straumann, Basel, Switzerland)	Bone grafts/sinus lifts: performed with a minimum of 6 months before implant installation	Use of a stereolitho-graphic surgical guide (G1), heavy smokers (>10 cigarettes/day) were excluded
Cannizzaro et al. [14]	2011	40 (split-mouth design)	22–65 (44.5)	3 days, 10 days, 6 weeks, 8 weeks Every 3 months for 1 year	2/76 (G1) 2/67 (G2)	2.6 (G1) 3.0 (G2)	1.0	Preoperative/ 12	Immediate loading	Sandblasted and acid-etched (SwissPlus, Zimmer Dental, Carlsbad, USA)	NP	Nonsubmerged implants, 49 extraction sockets implants (25, G1; 24, G2), no use of a surgical guide, 20 patients were smokers
De Bruyn et al. [5]	2011	49 (NM)	20–79 (53)	1 and 3 years	0/28 (G1) 0/25 (G2)	0 (G1) 0 (G2)	NM	7/unknown number of days	3–6 months	Porous anodized surface (TiUnite, Nobel Biocare, Göteborg, Sweden)	NP	No use of a surgical guide, 10 patients were smokers
Froum et al. [15]	2011	52 (60)[c] (27, G1; 25, G2)	NM	6 months, 1 year	0/27 (G1) 0/25 (G2)	0 (G1) 0 (G2)	NM	7/NM	8–12 weeks	Anodically oxidized (NobelDirect, Nobel Biocare, Göteborg, Sweden)	NP	Use of a surgical guide (G1 and G2)
Al-Juboori et al. [16]	2012	9 (split-mouth design)	27–62 (50)	6 and 12 weeks	0/11 (G1) 0/11 (G2)	0 (G1) 0 (G2)	NM	Before surgery/ before surgery	The implants were not loaded	Sandblasted and acid-etched (SLA, Straumann, Basel, Switzerland)	NP	No use of a surgical guide
Katsoulis et al. [21]	2012	40 (17, G1; 23, G2)	47–78 (61±9)	1 week 3 months	0/85 (G1) 0/110 (G2)	0 (G1) 0 (G2)	NM	5/unknown number of days	The implants were not loaded	Oxidized (NobelReplace Select Tapered, Nobel Biocare, Göteborg, Sweden)	NP	Use of a stereolitho-graphic surgical guide (G1), 3 patients were light smokers
Marcelis et al. [22]	2012	29 (NM)	NM (48.7±16.4)	1 year of functional loading	0/16 (G1) 1/18 (G2) [d]	0 (G1) 5.6 (G2)	NM	NM	Immediate (n = 9) 2–3 months (n = 24) ≥ 6 months (n = 1)	Sandblasted + fluoride (Osseospeed, AstraTech, Mölndal, Sweden)	NP	Use of a surgical guide (G1 and G2), 3 patients were smokers
Sunitha and Sapthagiri [4]	2013	40 (20, G1; 20, G2)	25–62 (39±4)	1 week, 3 and 6 months, 1 and 2 years	0/20 (G1) 0/20 (G2)	0 (G1) 0 (G2)	NM	5/NP	NM	NM	NP	No use of a surgical guide No smokers

Table 1. Cont.

Authors	Published	Patients (n) (number per group)	Patients' Age Range (Average) (years)	Follow-up visits (or range)	Failed/Placed Implants (n)	Implant failure rate (%)	*P* value (for failure rate)	Antibiotics/ mouth rinse (days)	Healing period/loading	Implant surface modification (brand)	Grafting	Observations
Tsoukaki et al. [17]	2013	20 (10, G1; 10, G2)	30–62 (47)	1, 2, 6, and 12 weeks	0/15 (G1) 0/15 (G2)	0 (G1) 0 (G2))	NM	4/15	The implants were not loaded	Sandblasted + fluoride (Osseospeed, Astra Tech Dental, Mölndal, Sweden)	NP	Nonsubmerged implants, use of surgical guides (G1 and G2), heavy smokers (>10 cigarettes/ day) were excluded
Meizi et al. [23]	2014	155 (NM)	NM (47.5)	3–9 months	7/237 (G1) 3/107 (G2)	2.95 (G1) 2.80 (G2)	NM	5/NM	Immediate (155, G1; 29, G2) 3–6 months (160)	Sandblasted and acid-etched (Saturn, Cortex Dental, Shlomi, Israel)	NM	No use of a surgical guide, 7% of the patients were diabetics, and 8% were smokers, 215 implants in fresh extraction sockets

NM – not mentioned; G1 – group flapless surgery; G2 – group conventional flapped surgery; NP – not performed

[a]The total of patients does not equal 169 because of cases treated with both protocols or in two phases of treatment in different years.

[b]Unpublished information concerning the number of failed implants in each group was obtained by personal communication with one of the authors. In this case 3 implants were lost in the flapless group at the 6-month follow-up

[c]There were 60 patients at the beginning of the study, but only 52 completed the study with 1 year of follow-up

[d]Unpublished information concerning the number of failed implants in each group was obtained by personal communication with one of the authors.

Table 2. Results of quality assessment.

Authors	Published	Sequence generation (randomized?)	Allocation concealment	Incomplete outcome data addressed	Blinding	Estimated potential risk of bias
Kinsel and Liss [24]	2007	No	Inadequate	No	No	High
Nkenke et al. [18]	2007	No	Inadequate	No	No	High
Ozan et al. [1]	2007	Yes	Unclear	Yes	Unclear	High
Villa and Rangert [19]	2007	No	Inadequate	Yes	No	High
Cannizzaro et al. [10]	2008	Yes	Adequate	Yes	No	Moderate
Covani et al. [11]	2008	Yes	Unclear	Yes	No	High
Maló and Nobre [20]	2008	No	Inadequate	Yes	No	High
Sennerby et al. [25]	2008	No	Inadequate	Yes	No	High
Danza et al. [26]	2009	No	Inadequate	No	No	High
Arisan et al. [3]	2010	No	Inadequate	Yes	No	High
Berdougo et al. [27]	2010	No	Inadequate	No	No	High
Lindeboom and van Wijk [12]	2010	Yes	Adequate*	Yes*	Yes*	Low
Rousseau [28]	2010	No	Inadequate	No	No	High
Van de Velde et al. [13]	2010	Yes	Adequate	Yes	Yes	Low
Cannizzaro et al. [14]	2011	Yes	Adequate	Yes	Yes	Low
De Bruyn et al. [5]	2011	No	Inadequate	Yes	No	High
Froum et al. [15]	2011	Yes	Adequate	Yes	Unclear	Moderate
Al-Juboori et al. [16]	2012	Yes	Inadequate	Yes*	No	High
Katsoulis et al. [21]	2012	No	Inadequate	No	No	High
Marcelis et al. [22]	2012	No	Inadequate	Yes	No	High
Sunitha and Sapthagiri [4]	2013	Yes	Adequate	Yes	Yes	Low
Tsoukaki et al. [17]	2013	Yes	Adequate	Yes	Yes	Low
Meizi et al. [23]	2014	No	Inadequate	No	No	High

* Unpublished information was obtained by personal communication with one of the authors.

Not every article provided information about the number of failed implants or to which group the failed implants belonged to. Unpublished information concerning the number of failed implants in each group was obtained by personal communication with one of the authors in two studies [12,22]. From the 23 studies, a total of 1648 implants were placed through the flapless technique, with 51 failures (3.09%), and 1848 implants were placed through an open flap surgery, with 32 failures (1.73%). Nine studies [1,11–13,19,20,22,23,25] did not inform whether there was a statistically significant difference or not between the techniques concerning implant failure, whereas the other six studies [3,14,24,26–28] did not find statistically significant difference. There were no implant failures in eight studies [4,5,10,15–18,21].

Thirteen articles [1,3–5,11,13,15,22–27] did not report the incidence of postoperative infection. From the ten studies [10,12,14,16–21,28] that provided this information, it was observed 3 occurrences of infection in 265 patients receiving implants through the flapless technique (1.1%), and 3 episodes of postoperative infection in 252 patients receiving implants through the open flap surgery (1.2%).

Quality Assessment

Each trial was assessed for risk of bias, and the scores are summarized in Table 2. Sixteen studies were judged to be at high risk of bias [1,3,5,11,16,18–28], whereas two studies were considered of moderate risk of bias [10,15], and five studies of low risk of bias [4,12–14,17].

Meta-analysis

In this study, a fixed-effects model was used to evaluate the implant failure, since statistically significant heterogeneity was not found ($P = 0.86$; $I^2 = 0\%$). The fixed-effects model was also used when the postoperative infection outcomes were evaluated, because statistically significant heterogeneity was also not found ($P = 0.58$; $I^2 = 0\%$).

The test for overall effect showed that the difference between the procedures (flapless vs. flapped) statistically affected the implant failure rates ($P = 0.03$; Figure 2). A RR of 1.75 (95% CI 1.07–2.86) for the use of flapless surgery implies that failures when implants are inserted by the flapless surgery are 1.75 times likely to happen than failures when implants are inserted by the open flap technique. Thus, the relative risk reduction (RRR) is −75%. In other words, being the RRR negative, the insertion of implants by the flapless surgery increases the risk of implant failure by 75%. Since the RR could differ depending on the risk of bias of the studies, a sensitivity analysis was performed. The RR was examined for the groups of studies of low and high risk of bias. The reasons to not include studies of moderate risk of bias was that there were only two studies [10,15], and no events were observed in both. When all low risk of bias studies were pooled, a RR of 1.84 resulted (95% CI 0.44–7.77; $P = 0.49$; $I^2 = 0\%$), whereas

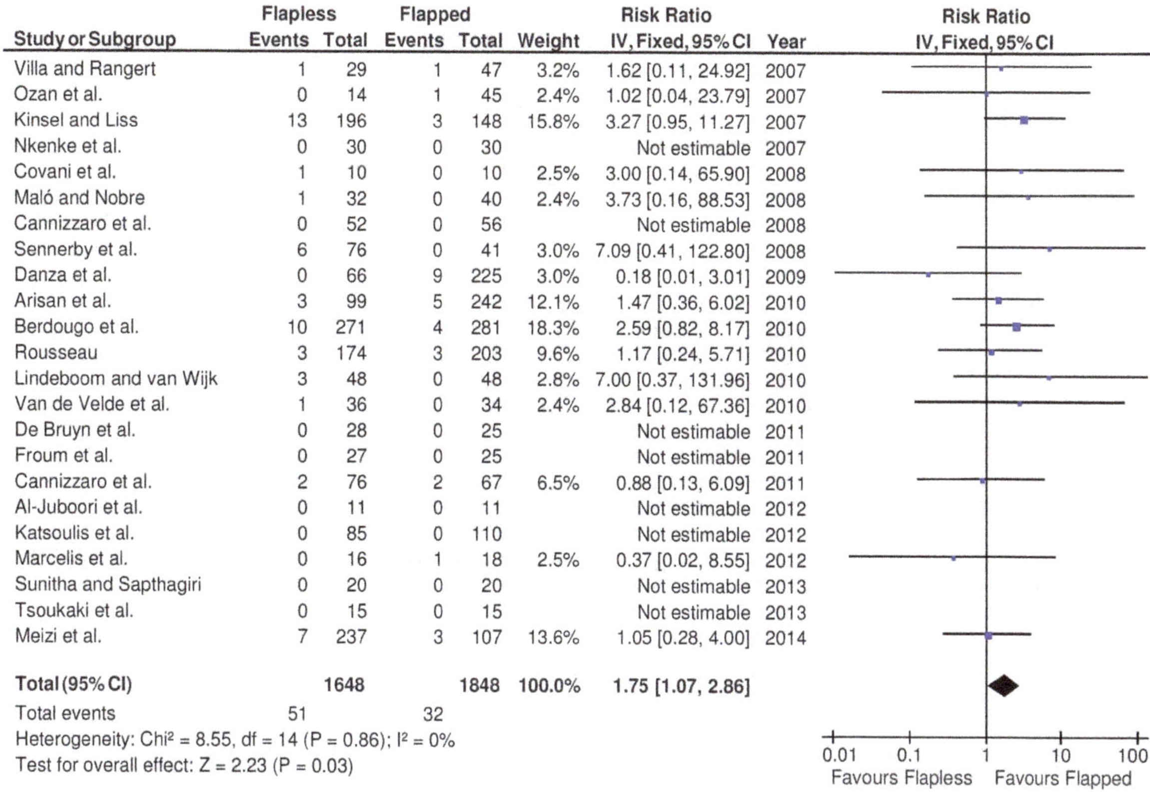

Study or Subgroup	Flapless Events	Flapless Total	Flapped Events	Flapped Total	Weight	Risk Ratio IV, Fixed, 95% CI	Year
Villa and Rangert	1	29	1	47	3.2%	1.62 [0.11, 24.92]	2007
Ozan et al.	0	14	1	45	2.4%	1.02 [0.04, 23.79]	2007
Kinsel and Liss	13	196	3	148	15.8%	3.27 [0.95, 11.27]	2007
Nkenke et al.	0	30	0	30		Not estimable	2007
Covani et al.	1	10	0	10	2.5%	3.00 [0.14, 65.90]	2008
Maló and Nobre	1	32	0	40	2.4%	3.73 [0.16, 88.53]	2008
Cannizzaro et al.	0	52	0	56		Not estimable	2008
Sennerby et al.	6	76	0	41	3.0%	7.09 [0.41, 122.80]	2008
Danza et al.	0	66	9	225	3.0%	0.18 [0.01, 3.01]	2009
Arisan et al.	3	99	5	242	12.1%	1.47 [0.36, 6.02]	2010
Berdougo et al.	10	271	4	281	18.3%	2.59 [0.82, 8.17]	2010
Rousseau	3	174	3	203	9.6%	1.17 [0.24, 5.71]	2010
Lindeboom and van Wijk	3	48	0	48	2.8%	7.00 [0.37, 131.96]	2010
Van de Velde et al.	1	36	0	34	2.4%	2.84 [0.12, 67.36]	2010
De Bruyn et al.	0	28	0	25		Not estimable	2011
Froum et al.	0	27	0	25		Not estimable	2011
Cannizzaro et al.	2	76	2	67	6.5%	0.88 [0.13, 6.09]	2011
Al-Juboori et al.	0	11	0	11		Not estimable	2012
Katsoulis et al.	0	85	0	110		Not estimable	2012
Marcelis et al.	0	16	1	18	2.5%	0.37 [0.02, 8.55]	2012
Sunitha and Sapthagiri	0	20	0	20		Not estimable	2013
Tsoukaki et al.	0	15	0	15		Not estimable	2013
Meizi et al.	7	237	3	107	13.6%	1.05 [0.28, 4.00]	2014
Total (95% CI)		**1648**		**1848**	**100.0%**	**1.75 [1.07, 2.86]**	
Total events	51		32				

Heterogeneity: Chi² = 8.55, df = 14 (P = 0.86); I² = 0%
Test for overall effect: Z = 2.23 (P = 0.03)

Figure 2. Forest plot of comparison of flapless versus open flap surgery for the event 'implant failure'.

when all high risk of bias studies were pooled, a RR of 1.73 was observed (95% CI 1.03–2.93; $P=0.04$; $I^2=0\%$).

On the other side, the meta-analysis showed that there are no apparent significant effects of flapless surgery on the occurrence of postoperative infection in patients receiving implants (RR 0.96, 95% CI 0.23–4.03; $P=0.960$; Figure 3).

Fifteen studies (1360 implants) provided information about the marginal bone loss with standard deviation, necessary for the calculation of comparisons in continuous outcomes (Figure 4). A random-effects model was used to evaluate the marginal bone loss, since statistically significant heterogeneity was found ($P=0.0002$; $I^2=66\%$). There was no statistically significant difference ($P=0.16$) between the different techniques concerning the marginal bone loss.

Publication bias

The funnel plots did not show asymmetry when the studies reporting either the outcome 'implant failure' (Figure 5), 'postoperative infection' (Figure 6), or 'marginal bone loss' (Figure 7) are analyzed, indicating absence of publication bias.

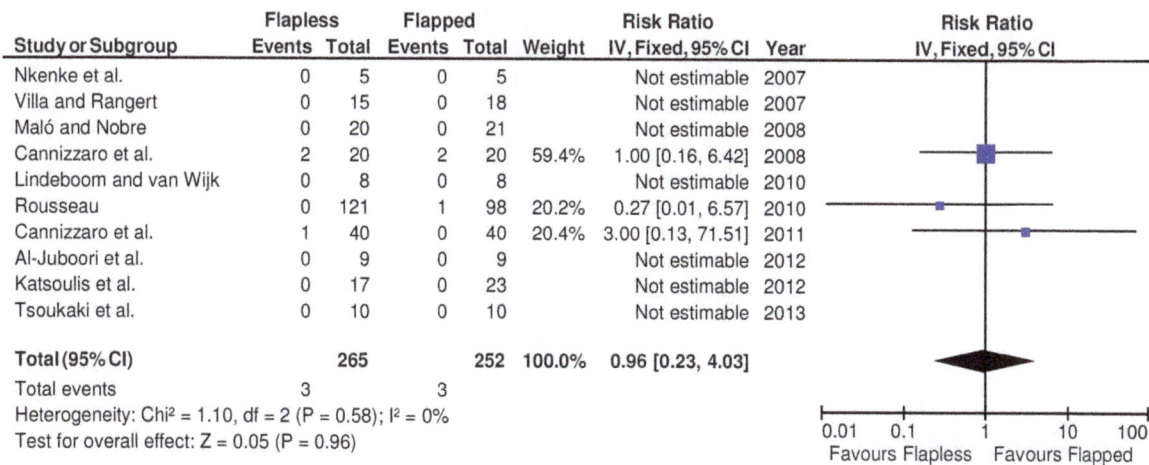

Study or Subgroup	Flapless Events	Flapless Total	Flapped Events	Flapped Total	Weight	Risk Ratio IV, Fixed, 95% CI	Year
Nkenke et al.	0	5	0	5		Not estimable	2007
Villa and Rangert	0	15	0	18		Not estimable	2007
Maló and Nobre	0	20	0	21		Not estimable	2008
Cannizzaro et al.	2	20	2	20	59.4%	1.00 [0.16, 6.42]	2008
Lindeboom and van Wijk	0	8	0	8		Not estimable	2010
Rousseau	0	121	1	98	20.2%	0.27 [0.01, 6.57]	2010
Cannizzaro et al.	1	40	0	40	20.4%	3.00 [0.13, 71.51]	2011
Al-Juboori et al.	0	9	0	9		Not estimable	2012
Katsoulis et al.	0	17	0	23		Not estimable	2012
Tsoukaki et al.	0	10	0	10		Not estimable	2013
Total (95% CI)		**265**		**252**	**100.0%**	**0.96 [0.23, 4.03]**	
Total events	3		3				

Heterogeneity: Chi² = 1.10, df = 2 (P = 0.58); I² = 0%
Test for overall effect: Z = 0.05 (P = 0.96)

Risk Ratio
IV, Fixed, 95% CI
0.01 0.1 1 10 100
Favours Flapless Favours Flapped

Figure 3. Forest plot of comparison of flapless versus open flap surgery for the event 'postoperative infection'.

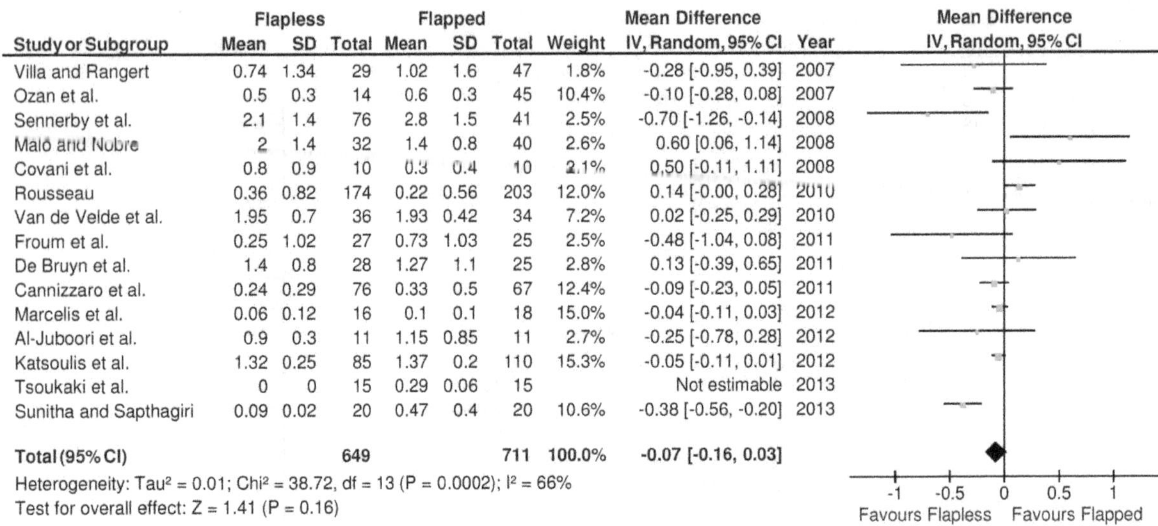

Study or Subgroup	Flapless Mean	Flapless SD	Flapless Total	Flapped Mean	Flapped SD	Flapped Total	Weight	Mean Difference IV, Random, 95% CI	Year
Villa and Rangert	0.74	1.34	29	1.02	1.6	47	1.8%	-0.28 [-0.95, 0.39]	2007
Ozan et al.	0.5	0.3	14	0.6	0.3	45	10.4%	-0.10 [-0.28, 0.08]	2007
Sennerby et al.	2.1	1.4	76	2.8	1.5	41	2.5%	-0.70 [-1.26, -0.14]	2008
Maló and Nobre	2	1.4	32	1.4	0.8	40	2.6%	0.60 [0.06, 1.14]	2008
Covani et al.	0.8	0.9	10	0.3	0.4	10	2.1%	0.50 [-0.11, 1.11]	2008
Rousseau	0.36	0.82	174	0.22	0.56	203	12.0%	0.14 [-0.00, 0.28]	2010
Van de Velde et al.	1.95	0.7	36	1.93	0.42	34	7.2%	0.02 [-0.25, 0.29]	2010
Froum et al.	0.25	1.02	27	0.73	1.03	25	2.5%	-0.48 [-1.04, 0.08]	2011
De Bruyn et al.	1.4	0.8	28	1.27	1.1	25	2.8%	0.13 [-0.39, 0.65]	2011
Cannizzaro et al.	0.24	0.29	76	0.33	0.5	67	12.4%	-0.09 [-0.23, 0.05]	2011
Marcelis et al.	0.06	0.12	16	0.1	0.1	18	15.0%	-0.04 [-0.11, 0.03]	2012
Al-Juboori et al.	0.9	0.3	11	1.15	0.85	11	2.7%	-0.25 [-0.78, 0.28]	2012
Katsoulis et al.	1.32	0.25	85	1.37	0.2	110	15.3%	-0.05 [-0.11, 0.01]	2012
Tsoukaki et al.	0	0	15	0.29	0.06	15		Not estimable	2013
Sunitha and Sapthagiri	0.09	0.02	20	0.47	0.4	20	10.6%	-0.38 [-0.56, -0.20]	2013
Total (95% CI)			**649**			**711**	**100.0%**	**-0.07 [-0.16, 0.03]**	

Heterogeneity: Tau² = 0.01; Chi² = 38.72, df = 13 (P = 0.0002); I² = 66%
Test for overall effect: Z = 1.41 (P = 0.16)

Figure 4. Forest plot of comparison of immediate nonfunctional versus immediate functional loading for the event 'marginal bone loss' (values in millimeters).

Discussion

Potential biases are likely to be greater for non-randomized studies compared with RCTs, so results should always be interpreted with caution when they are included in reviews and meta-analyses [8]. However, narrowing the inclusion criteria increases homogeneity but also excludes the results of more trials and thus risks the exclusion of significant data [29]. This was the reason to include non-randomized studies in the present meta-analysis. The issue is important because meta-analyses are frequently conducted on a limited number of RCTs. In meta-analyses such as these, adding more information from observational studies may aid in clinical reasoning and establish a more solid foundation for causal inferences [29].

The relevant question is whether the lack of a difference between the flapless and the open flap implant procedures in some studies concerning implant failure rates is a real finding or is due to the lack of statistical power, given the small number of patients per

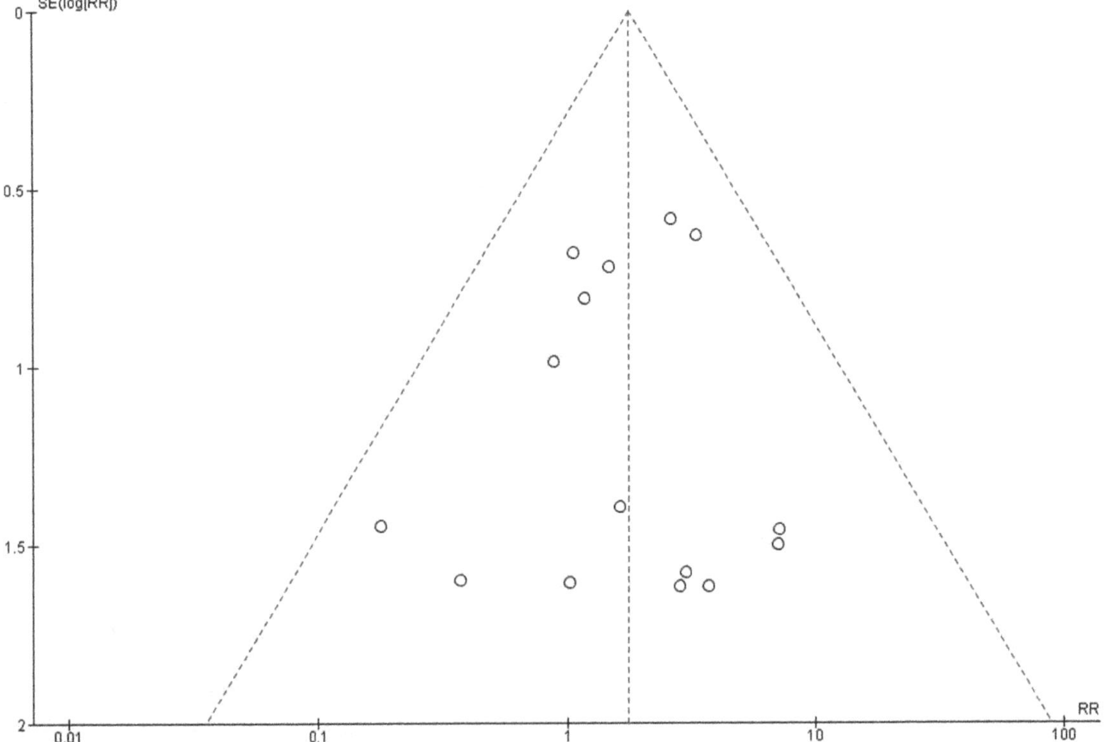

Figure 5. Funnel plot for the studies reporting the outcome event 'implant failure'.

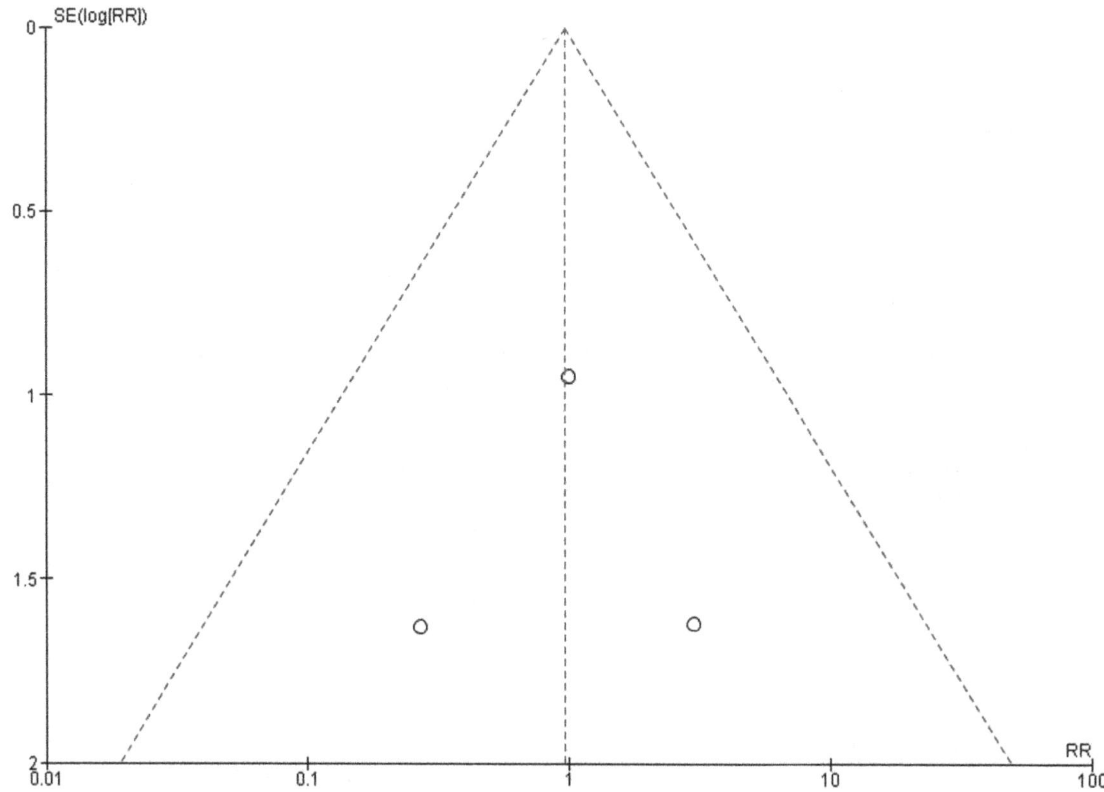

Figure 6. Funnel plot for the studies reporting the outcome event 'postoperative infection'.

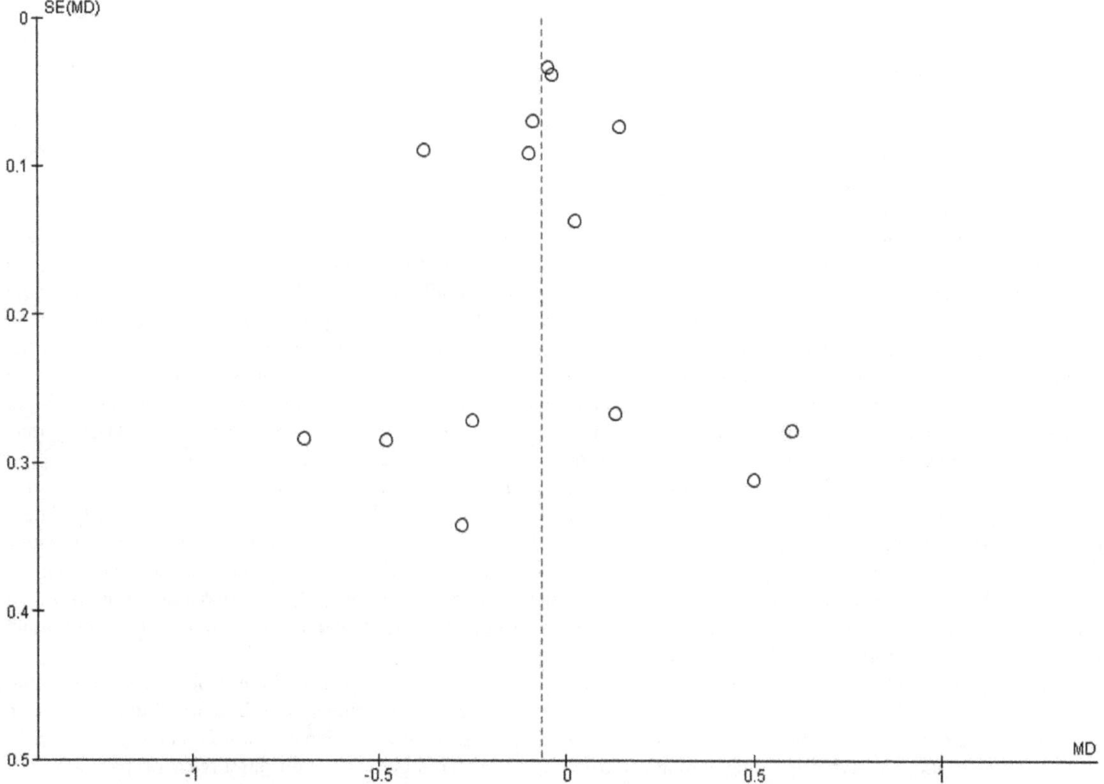

Figure 7. Funnel plot for the studies reporting the outcome event 'marginal bone loss'.

group in many studies [1,4,5,11,13,15,16–20,22,24]. However, there was a statistically and clinically significant difference ($P = 0.03$) favoring the open flap surgery was found after the meta-analyses, stressing the importance of meta-analyses to increase sample size of individual trials to reach more precise estimates of the effects of interventions. However, when studies of low and high risk of bias were pooled separately, there was a difference in the results and in the statistical significance of the RR. Thus, the results must be interpreted carefully.

One drawback found in six studies [3,11,12,16,17,21] is the fact that the patients were followed for a short period (1–6 months). Thus, only early failures could be assessed. A longer follow-up period can lead to an increase in the failure rate, especially if it extended beyond functional loading, because other prosthetic factors can influence implant failure from that point onward [30]. The success of a dental implant should be defined after a minimal period of 12 months of implant loading. Early, intermediate, and long-term success has been suggested to span 1 to 3 years, 3 to 7 years, and more than 7 years respectively [31]. Moreover, the results found in the studies differed from each other, and this difference could be due to factors such as differences in the patients included in the study or the clinicians placing and restoring the implants.

The immediate loading only in the flapless group in some studies [10,13] is a confounding factor, as well as the presence of smokers among the patients in several trials [5,10,14,21–24,27], the use of grafts [11,24,25], the use or not use of surgical guides, different prosthetic configurations, and the insertion of implants from different brands and surface treatments. Titanium with different surface modifications shows a wide range of chemical, physical properties, and surface topographies or morphologies, depending on how they are prepared and handled [32–34], and it is not clear whether, in general, one surface modification is better than another [35]. Also, there is the fact that some studies inserted some [14,23,25] or all implants in fresh extraction sockets [19]. One of these studies [19] placed all implants in infected extraction sockets. Moreover, in four studies [5,19,20,28] flapless surgery was only considered in favorable clinical conditions. Flapless surgery was considered a treatment option based on clinical examination and largely depending on the anatomical condition of the bone after clinical and radiographic inspection. Therefore, the allocation to the surgical approach was biased (selection bias), what could have masked substantial intergroup disparity.

Currently, some software systems using computed tomography scans have been proposed to aid in planning surgery and to produce surgical drilling guides to transfer the planned position to the surgical field. These guides are manufactured in such a way that they match the location, trajectory, and depth of the planned implant with a high degree of precision. As the dental practitioner places the implants, the guides stabilize the drilling by restricting the degrees of freedom of the drill trajectory and depth [36]. It was stated that by using computer-assisted surgery predictability, precision and safety in flapless dental implantology are ensured [12].

However, the precision of the whole procedure depends largely on the ability to position accurately the drill guide, and to maintain that stable position during the whole procedure [36]. In the case of the placement of implants in completely edentulous jaws, there must be a way to assure the stability of the drill guide, and this is done by fixing the surgical guide onto the bone by osteosynthesis screws. Asymmetric distribution of the screws or uneven tightening of the screws could bring the drilling template out of balance. Furthermore, a certain error is induced as the diameter of the steel tubes is slightly larger than the drill diameter [36]. Finally, the largest error is probably due to the fact that the final step in the procedure is carried out manually, depending on the surgical guide used. In these cases, implant placement cannot be done through the surgical drill guide because of present mechanical limitations. The drill guide, therefore, has to be removed before the implant is actually inserted, leaving the possibility of additional deviation [36]. Because of these reasons, the surgical drill guide may provide a false security in decreasing the risk of bone fenestrations or perforations. This may be one of the reasons why it was observed, in the present review, a higher percentage of implant failures with the flapless technique when compared with the open flap surgery.

Still concerning the precision of the implant insertion, it is worth commenting about the technique used by the study of Sennerby et al. [25]. They made use of a slide-over guide sleeve to evaluate and determine the position of the implant. This system is based on the surgeons' imprecise opinion of what is the exact direction of the implants to be placed and it is subjected to flaws, which may have led to an increasing incidence of implant bone plate fenestrations or perforations, and consequently higher implant failure in this group (7.9% versus no failure in the open flap surgery). Correct bur angulation is critical in the procedure [36]. With the CT-guide surgery, it is possible to verify in advance the presence of concavities of the vestibular and lingual/palatal bone plates surrounding the planned implant surgical site, thus planning the correct bur angulation and decreasing the chance of implant bone fenestrations or perforations.

Moreover, one *in vitro* study [37] analyzed deviations in position and inclination of implants placed with flapless surgery compared with the ideally planned position and examined whether the outcome was affected by the experience level. The authors observed that the three-dimensional location of implants installed with flapless approach differed significantly from the ideal, although neighboring teeth were present and maximal radiographical information was available, and the outcome was not influenced by the level of experience with implant surgery. It was suggested that these deviations would in a clinical situation lead to complications such as loss of implant stability, aesthetical and phonetical consequences. The authors recommended the performance of more precise measurements of soft tissue *in situ* or additional use of guiding systems.

Since flapless implant placement generally is a "blind" surgical technique, care must be taken when placing implants. Angulation of the implants affected by drilling is critical so as to avoid perforation of the cortical plates, both lingual and buccal, especially on the lingual in the mandibular molar area and the anterior maxilla [38]. Therefore, the surgeon must weigh the benefits of the flapless technique in front of the increasing risk of implant bone fenestrations or perforations, which allegedly may impair implant success or increase the implant failure rates [39]. Violation of the dental implant beyond the alveolar housing may result in infection and ultimate loss of the implant [40]. There should be no problem if the patient has been appropriately selected and an appropriate width of bone is available for implant placement [38]. Some authors [38] suggested a minimum of 7 mm of bone width and substantial training to use the appropriate technique.

Another hypothetical drawback of the flapless procedure is that it could interfere with osseointegration because of implant surface contamination and the deposition of epithelial and connective cells from the oral mucosa in the bone during surgical preparation [27].

On the other hand, a flapless procedure could have a positive effect on the early bone remodeling process, because during the surgical procedure, the bone remains covered by the periosteum.

However, the strongly tightened surgical template used in to insert implants in totally edentulous jaws may hinder access of saline water and proper cooling during the drilling procedure, which could negatively influence the implant surrounding the bone and the remodeling process during healing [21].

Concerning the marginal bone loss, one may expect that the open flap surgery may cause higher marginal bone loss due to decreased supraperiosteal blood supply because of the raising the tissue flap during the surgical procedure. Studies have demonstrated that flap reflection often results in bone resorption around natural teeth [41]. However, it was showed in five studies that the flapless technique generated more marginal bone loss around the implants [5,11,13,20,28]. The authors of some of the articles here reviewed provided some reasonable explanations for this. De Bruyn et al. [5] suggested that this was probably caused in their study due to overdoing of the countersinking procedure. More extensive widening of the crestal bone was necessary to remove enough bone as to allow proper placement of the healing abutment. By countersinking wider and deeper, the coronal portion of the implant is not always in intimate contact with the bone. In the flapped sites, the countersinking procedure was more controlled according to the guidelines of the manufacturer because visual inspection *in situ* was possible. Rousseau [28] discussed that this is due to implants being installed blindly, and thus implants are installed more deeply with the flapless technique than with the open flap technique. Therefore, a portion of the transmucosal (supracrestal) part of the implant is slightly below the crestal bone level. Because the coronal part of the implant is smooth titanium, rearrangement of bone around the neck of the implant is normal. When an open flap technique is used, the implant is installed under visual control directly at the right crestal bone position. This results in less bone rearrangement around the implant neck [28]. The results found in the study of Van de Velde et al. [13] may be related to the fact that the implants inserted through the flapless technique were immediately loaded, whereas the implants inserted through open flap surgery were loaded only after 6 weeks.

The results of the present study have to be interpreted with caution because of its limitations. First of all, all confounding factors may have affected the long-term outcomes and not just the use of flapless or open flap surgery, and the impact of these variables on the implant survival rate, postoperative infection and marginal bone loss is difficult to estimate if these factors are not identified separately between the two different procedures in order to perform a meta-regression analysis. The lack of control of the confounding factors limited the potential to draw robust conclusions. Second, some of the included studies had a retrospective design, and the nature of a retrospective study inherently results in flaws. These problems were manifested by the gaps in information and incomplete records. Furthermore, all data rely on the accuracy of the original examination and documentation. Items may have been excluded in the initial examination or not recorded in the medical chart [42,43].

The authors of the present study believe that, for a more definite conclusion, future double-blinded RCTs with larger patient samples are required to determine the real effect of flapless implant surgery on patient outcome variables.

Conclusion

The difference between the procedures (flapless vs. flapped) statistically affected the implant failure rates. However, the results must be interpreted carefully, as a sensitivity analysis revealed differences when the groups of studies of high and low risk of bias were pooled separately. No statistically significant effects of open flap surgery or flapless surgery on the occurrence of postoperative infection and on the marginal bone loss were observed.

Acknowledgments

The authors would like to thank Dr. Mohammed Jasim Al-Juboori, Dr. Georgios Romanos, and Dr. Miguel de Araújo Nobre, for having sent us their articles, and Dr. Jerome A. Lindeboom, Dr. Ignace Naert, and Dr. Wim Teughels, who provided us some missing information about their studies.

Author Contributions

Contributed to the writing of the manuscript: BRC. Conception and design of the work and acquisition of data: BRC TA AW. Meta-analysis: BRC. Interpretation of data: BRC TA AW. Revised the article critically for important intellectual content: BRC TA AW. Final approval of the version to be published: BRC TA AW.

References

1. Ozan O, Turkyilmaz I, Yilmaz B (2007) A preliminary report of patients treated with early loaded implants using computerized tomography-guided surgical stents: flapless versus conventional flapped surgery. J Oral Rehabil 34: 835–840.
2. Rocci A, Martignoni M, Gottlow J (2003) Immediate loading in the maxilla using flapless surgery, implants placed in predetermined positions, and prefabricated provisional restorations: a retrospective 3-year clinical study. Clin Implant Dent Relat Res 5(Suppl.): 29–36.
3. Arisan V, Karabuda CZ, Ozdemir T (2010) Implant surgery using bone- and mucosa-supported stereolithographic guides in totally edentulous jaws: surgical and post-operative outcomes of computer-aided vs. standard techniques. Clin Oral Implants Res 21: 980–988.
4. Sunitha RV, Sapthagiri E (2013) Flapless implant surgery: a 2-year follow-up study of 40 implants. Oral Surg Oral Med Oral Pathol Oral Radiol 116: e237–e243.
5. De Bruyn H, Atashkadeh M, Cosyn J, van de Velde T (2011) Clinical outcome and bone preservation of single TiUnit implants installed with flapless or flap surgery. Clin Implant Dent Relat Res 13: 175–183.
6. Chrcanovic BR, Albrektsson T, Wennerberg A (2014) Reasons for failures of oral implants. J Oral Rehabil 41: 443–476.
7. Moher D, Liberati A, Tetzlaff J, Altman DG; PRISMA Group (2009) Preferred reporting items for systematic reviews and meta-analyses: the PRISMA statement. Ann Intern Med 151: 264–269, W64.
8. Higgins JPT, Green S (2011) Cochrane Handbook for Systematic Reviews of Interventions Version 5.1.0. [updated March 2011]. The Cochrane Collaboration. Available: http://www.cochrane-handbook.org. Accessed 2014 Mar 3.
9. Egger M, Smith GD (2003) Principles of and procedures for systematic reviews. In: Egger M, Smith GD, Altman DG (eds). Systematic Reviews in Health Care: Meta-analysis in Context. London: BMJ books. 23–42.
10. Cannizzaro G, Leone M, Consolo U, Ferri V, Esposito M (2008) Immediate functional loading of implants placed with flapless surgery versus conventional implants in partially edentulous patients: a 3-year randomized controlled clinical trial. Int J Oral Maxillofac Implants 23: 867–875.
11. Covani U, Cornelini R, Barone A (2008) Buccal bone augmentation around immediate implants with and without flap elevation: a modified approach. Int J Oral Maxillofac Implants 23: 841–846.
12. Lindeboom JA, van Wijk AJ (2010) A comparison of two implant techniques on patient-based outcome measures: a report of flapless vs. conventional flapped implant placement. Clin Oral Implants Res 21: 366–370.
13. Van de Velde T, Sennerby L, De Bruyn H (2010) The clinical and radiographic outcome of implants placed in the posterior maxilla with a guided flapless approach and immediately restored with a provisional rehabilitation: a randomized clinical trial. Clin Oral Implants Res 21: 1223–1233.
14. Cannizzaro G, Felice P, Leone M, Checchi V, Esposito M (2011) Flapless versus open flap implant surgery in partially edentulous patients subjected to immediate loading: 1-year results from a split-mouth randomised controlled trial. Eur J Oral Implantol 4: 177–188.

15. Froum SJ, Cho SC, Elian N, Romanos G, Jalbout Z, et al. (2011) Survival rate of one-piece dental implants placed with a flapless or flap protocol – a randomized, controlled study: 12-month results. Int J Periodontics Restorative Dent 31: 591–601.
16. Al-Juboori MJ, Bin Abdulrahaman S, Jassan A (2012) Comparison of flapless and conventional flap and the effect on crestal bone resorption during a 12-week healing period. Dent Implantol Update 23: 9–16.
17. Tsoukaki M, Kalpidis CD, Sakellari D, Tsalikis L, Mikrogeorgis G, et al. (2013) Clinical, radiographic, microbiological, and immunological outcomes of flapped vs. flapless dental implants: a prospective randomized controlled clinical trial. Clin Oral Implants Res 24: 969–976.
18. Nkenke E, Eitner S, Radespiel-Tröger M, Vairaktaris E, Neukam FW, et al. (2007) Patient-centred outcomes comparing transmucosal implant placement with an open approach in the maxilla: a prospective, nonrandomized pilot study. Clin Oral Implants Res 18: 197–203.
19. Villa R, Rangert B (2007) Immediate and early function of implants placed in extraction sockets of maxillary infected teeth: A pilot study. J Prosthet Dent 97: S96–S108.
20. Maló P, Nobre MD (2008) Flap vs. flapless surgical techniques at immediate implant function in predominantly soft bone for rehabilitation of partial edentulism: a prospective cohort study with follow-up of 1 year. Eur J Oral Implantol 1: 293–304.
21. Katsoulis J, Avrampou M, Spycher C, Stipic M, Enkling N, et al. (2012) Comparison of implant stability by means of resonance frequency analysis for flapless and conventionally inserted implants. Clin Implant Dent Relat Res 14: 915–923.
22. Marcelis K, Vercruyssen M, Naert I, Teughels W, Quirynen M (2012) Model-based guided implant insertion for solitary tooth replacement: a pilot study. Clin Oral Implants Res 23: 999–1003.
23. Meizi E, Meir M, Laster Z (2014) New-design dental implants: a 1-year prospective clinical study of 344 consecutively placed implants comparing immediate loading versus delayed loading and flapless versus full-thickness flap. Int J Oral Maxillofac Implants 29: e14–e21.
24. Kinsel RP, Liss M (2007) Retrospective analysis of 56 edentulous dental arches restored with 344 single-stage implants using an immediate loading fixed provisional protocol: statistical predictors of implant failure. Int J Oral Maxillofac Implants 22: 823–830.
25. Sennerby L, Rocci A, Becker W, Jonsson L, Johansson LA, et al. (2008) Short-term clinical results of Nobel Direct implants: a retrospective multicentre analysis. Clin Oral Implant Res 19: 219–226.
26. Danza M, Zollin I, Carinci F (2009) Comparison between implants inserted with and without computer planning and custom model coordination. J Craniofac Surg 20: 1086–1092.
27. Berdougo M, Fortin T, Blanchet E, Isidori M, Bosson JL (2010) Flapless implant surgery using an image-guided system. A 1- to 4-year retrospective multicenter comparative clinical study. Clin Implant Dent Relat Res 12: 142–152.
28. Rousseau P (2010) Flapless and traditional dental implant surgery: an open, retrospective comparative study. J Oral Maxillofac Surg 68: 2299–2306.
29. Shrier I, Boivin JF, Steele RJ, Platt RW, Furlan A, et al. (2007) Should meta-analyses of interventions include observational studies in addition to randomized controlled trials? A critical examination of underlying principles. Am J Epidemiol 166: 1203–1209.
30. Sharaf B, Jandali-Rifai M, Susarla SM, Dodson TB (2011) Do perioperative antibiotics decrease implant failure? J Oral Maxillofac Surg 69: 2345–2350.
31. ten Bruggenkate CM, van der Kwast WA, Oosterbeek HS (1990) Success criteria in oral implantology: A review of the literature. Int J Oral Implantol 7: 45–51.
32. Chrcanovic BR, Pedrosa AR, Martins MD (2012) Chemical and topographic analysis of treated surfaces of five different commercial dental titanium implants. Mater Res 15: 372–382.
33. Chrcanovic BR, Leão NLC, Martins MD (2013) Influence of different acid etchings on the superficial characteristics of Ti sandblasted with Al2O3. Mater Res 16: 1006–1014.
34. Chrcanovic BR, Martins MD (2014) Study of the influence of acid etching treatments on the superficial characteristics of Ti. Mater Res 17: 373–380.
35. Wennerberg A, Albrektsson T (2010) On implant surfaces: a review of current knowledge and opinions. Int J Oral Maxillofac Implants 25: 63–74.
36. Chrcanovic BR, Oliveira DR, Custódio AL (2010) Accuracy evaluation of computed tomography-derived stereolithographic surgical guides in zygomatic implant placement in human cadavers. J Oral Implantol 36: 345–355.
37. Van de Velde T, Glor F, De Bruyn H (2008) A model study on flapless implant placement by clinicians with a different experience level in implant surgery. Clin Oral Implants Res 19: 66–72.
38. Campelo LD, Camara JR (2002) Flapless implant surgery: a 10-year clinical retrospective analysis. Int J Oral Maxillofac Implants 17: 271–276.
39. Chiapasco M, Zaniboni M (2009) Clinical outcomes of GBR procedures to correct peri-implant dehiscences and fenestrations: a systematic review. Clin Oral Implants Res 20 Suppl 4: 113–23.
40. Annibali S, Ripari M, La Monaca G, Tonoli F, Cristalli MP (2009) Local accidents in dental implant surgery: Prevention and treatment. Int J Periodontics Restorative Dent 29: 325–331.
41. Wood DL, Hoag PM, Donnenfeld OW, Rosenfeld LD (1972) Alveolar crest reduction following full and partial thickness flaps. J Periodontol 42: 141–144.
42. Chrcanovic BR, Abreu MH, Freire-Maia B, Souza LN (2010) Facial fractures in children and adolescents: a retrospective study of 3 years in a hospital in Belo Horizonte, Brazil. Dent Traumatol 26: 262–270.
43. Chrcanovic BR, Abreu MH, Freire-Maia B, Souza LN (2012) 1,454 mandibular fractures: a 3-year study in a hospital in Belo Horizonte, Brazil. J Cranio-Maxillofac Surg 40: 116–123.

12

Preparation and Characterization of Electrospun PLCL/Poloxamer Nanofibers and Dextran/Gelatin Hydrogels for Skin Tissue Engineering

Jian-feng Pan[1◔], Ning-hua Liu[1◔], Hui Sun[1*], Feng Xu[2]

1 Department of Orthopaedics, Shanghai Jiao Tong University Affiliated Sixth People's Hospital, Shanghai, China, 2 Department of Orthopaedics, Kunshan Traditional Chinese Medical Hospital, Suzhou, Jiangsu, China

Abstract

In this study, two different biomaterials were fabricated and their potential use as a bilayer scaffold for skin tissue engineering applications was assessed. The upper layer biomaterial was a Poly(ε-caprolactone-co-lactide)/Poloxamer (PLCL/Poloxamer) nanofiber membrane fabricated using electrospinning technology. The PLCL/Poloxamer nanofibers (PLCL/Poloxamer, 9/1) exhibited strong mechanical properties (stress/strain values of 9.37 ± 0.38 MPa/187.43 ± 10.66%) and good biocompatibility to support adipose-derived stem cells proliferation. The lower layer biomaterial was a hydrogel composed of 10% dextran and 20% gelatin without the addition of a chemical crosslinking agent. The 5/5 dextran/gelatin hydrogel displayed high swelling property, good compressive strength, capacity to present more than 3 weeks and was able to support cells proliferation. A bilayer scaffold was fabricated using these two materials by underlaying the nanofibers and casting hydrogel to mimic the structure and biological function of native skin tissue. The upper layer membrane provided mechanical support in the scaffold and the lower layer hydrogel provided adequate space to allow cells to proliferate and generate extracellular matrix. The biocompatibility of bilayer scaffold was preliminarily investigated to assess the potential cytotoxicity. The results show that cell viability had not been affected when cocultured with bilayer scaffold. As a consequence, the bilayer scaffold composed of PLCL/Poloxamer nanofibers and dextran/gelatin hydrogels is biocompatible and possesses its potentially high application prospect in the field of skin tissue engineering.

Editor: Xiaohua Liu, Texas A&M University Baylor College of Dentistry, United States of America

Funding: The authors have no funding or support to report.

Competing Interests: The authors have declared that no competing interests exist.

* Email: sunshine20002000@126.com

◔ These authors contributed equally to this work.

Introduction

Adult skin consists of two tissue layers: a keratinized stratified epidermis and an underlying thick layer of collagen-rich dermal connective tissue providing support and nourishment. Because the skin serves as a protective barrier against the outside world, any break in it must be rapidly and efficiently mended [1]. Full thickness grafts, consisting of the epidermis and the full thickness of the dermis, are commonly used in plastic and reconstructive surgery [2]. However, the donor site following the harvest of a full thickness graft has no epidermal elements from which new skin can regenerate. So the grafts must be taken from sites of the body where the donor defects can be primarily closed. This limits the harvest of full thickness grafts clinically. Tissue-engineered skin replacements such as cultured autologous and allogenic keratinocytes grafts, autologous or allogenic composites, acellular biological matrices, and cellular matrices including biological substances such as fibrin sealant and various types of collagen and hyaluronic acid (HA) have opened new options to treat such massive skin loss [3].

Electrospinning is an effective technique to produce polymer nanofibers. It involves using a strong electrical field to rapidly stretch a polymer solution into fine filaments. The solvent evaporation from the filaments leads to the formation of dry or semi-dry fibres, which deposit randomly on the collector forming a nonwoven mat in most cases. In previous studies, synthetic biodegradable polymers, such as poly (lactic acid) (PLA) [4], poly (glycolic acid) (PGA) [5], poly (lactide-co-glycolide) (PLGA) [6], poly (e-caprolactone) (PCL) [7], poly (glycolide-co-caprolactone) (PGCL) [8] and poly (L-lactide-co-e-caprolactone) (PLCL) [9–10] were developed for vessel or skin tissue engineering. Among them, PLCL is well known as an elastic biodegradable material; therefore, it was applied as tissue engineering scaffolds to mimic the natural stratified epidermis. However, the hydration and degradation of PLCL contributes to an acidic microenvironment, which is not in favor of the skin regeneration. Poloxamers are non-ionic surfactants and have wide-ranging applications in various biomedical fields including drug delivery and medical imaging [11–12]. With use of PLCL/poloxamer blended nanofibers the formation of acidic microenvironment associated with PLCL degradation was prevented as poloxamer neutralizes the production of lactic acid during PLCL degradation in the body.

Underlying the epidermis is thick layer of collagen-rich dermis. It provides physical strength and flexibility to the skin, as well as being the matrix that supports the extensive vasculature, lymphatic system and nerve bundles. The dermis is relatively acellular, being composed predominantly of an extracellular matrix (ECM) of interwoven collagen fibrils. Gelatin, a collagen-hydrolyzed protein with unique gelation behavior under room temperature has been widely researched in food and pharmaceutical industries [13–15]. Based on previous studies, by altering the carboxyl groups to amino groups through the reaction with ethane diamine, gelatin could stay liquid state at room temperature [16–17]. While dextran was oxidized by sodium periodate to obtain aldehyde groups, the dextran could react with gelatin to form a hydrogel filling in the dermis defect area. Therefore, we fabricated a bilayer scaffold composed of a PLCL/Poloxamer nanofiber upper layer and a dextran/gelatin hydrogel sublayer to mimic the physical structure of the normal skin more accurately.

In this study, the physical properties, mechanical strength and biocompatibility of two separate biomaterials were investigated. For electrospun PLCL/poloxamer nanofibers, morphological characterization was determined through SEM and hydrophilicity was assessed with water contact angle method by a drop shape analysis system. Then the mechanical performance was examined to determine whether the samples can withstand the applied stress. For dextran/gelatin hydrogels, biodegradation was investigated by immersing the samples in PBS for 21 days to determine weight loss over time. The water absorption property of hydrogels was determined by swelling tests after 24 hours of incubation in phosphate buffered saline (PBS). Cell proliferation and viability tests were done to evaluate the biocompatibility of the scaffolds in vitro. The results of the tests performed determined which conditions were optimal to construct the bilayer scaffold that will be used for skin tissue engineering applications.

Materials and Methods

Materials

PLCL was purchased from DaiGang biomaterial Co., Ltd. (ShanDong, China). Poloxamer, dextran, N-(3-Dimethylamino-propyl)-N′-ethylcarbodiimide hydrochloride crystalline (EDC), gelatin, sodium periodate, Tetrahydrofuran (THF), ethylenedia-mine(ED) and N, N-dimethylformamide (DMF) were purchased from Sigma-Aldrich (St Louis, MO, USA). Fetal bovine serum (FBS), phosphate buffered saline (PBS), Dulbecco's modified Eagle's medium (DMEM), Live/Dead Viability Assay Kit, collagenase II, penicillin-streptomycin solution, trypsin-EDTA and other culture media and reagents were purchased from Gibco Life Technologies Corporation (Carlsbad, CA, USA). CCK-8 was purchased from Dojindo Corporation (Kumamoto, Japan). Tissue culture flasks were obtained from BD Biosciences Corporation (San Jose, CA, USA). Mouse pre-osteoblast cells (MC3T3-E1) were obtained from the institute of Biochemistry and Cell biology (Chinese Academy of Sciences, China).

Preparation of scaffolds

1. Electrospun PLCL/Poloxamer membranes. The mixed solvent of THF and DMF (v/v = 1/1) was used to prepare the electrospinning solutions at a polymer concentration of 8 wt%. In order to investigate the hydrophilicity enhancement of Poloxamer on PLCL fibers, two different compositions of PLCL and Poloxamer mixtures (9/1, 3/1, w/w) were prepared. The electrospinning solution was ejected at a speed of 1.0 mL/h under a fixed electrical potential of 16 kV with a distance of 20 cm between tip of the needle and the collector. All electrospun fibers were deposited on a rotating collector consists of aluminum foil to form a thin fibrous membrane. The fibrous mats were placed in vacuum drying at room temperature to completely remove any solvent residue.

2. Dextran/gelatin hydrogels. Dextran was oxidized by reacting with sodium periodate as reported. Briefly, dextran solution was prepared by dissolving 10 g of dextran in 100 ml of distilled water. 6.34 g of $NaIO_4$ (dissolved in 100 ml of distilled water) was added dropwise to the dextran solution. The solution was stirred at room temperature for 6 hours and shielded from light. Then 2 ml of ethylene glycol was added to terminate the oxidation reaction. The resulting solution was dialyzed exhaustively for 3 days against water and lyophilized to obtain the final dextran.

The carboxyl groups in gelatin were converted into amino groups by reaction with ED in the presence of EDC. Gelatin was dissolved in 100 ml of phosphate buffered solution (PBS) to a final concentration of 5 wt% at room temperature and 16 ml of ethylenediamine was added. Immediately after that, the pH of solution was adjusted to 5.0 by adding hydrochloric acid (HCl). After that 2.3 g of EDC was added into the gelatin solution. The molar ratio of the carboxyl groups on gelatin chains, EDC and ED was 1:2:40. The reaction mixture was stirred at room temperature overnight, and then dialyzed against distilled water for 48 hours to remove the excess ED and EDC. The dialyzed solution was freeze-dried at −80°C to obtain a modified gelatin.

Dextran was dissolved in PBS to achieve a concentration of 10% (wt/vol%) and gelatin was diluted to achieve a 20% (wt/vol%) solution. While the two solutions were mixed together, the hydrogels were formed rapidly through a Schiff-base reaction between aldehyde groups and amino groups. The mixture solution was injected into round molds and then incubated at 37°C for gel forming.

3. Bilayer scaffold. Following the characterization of the electrospun PLCL/Poloxamer nanofibers and dextran/gelatin hydrogels, the 9/1 PLCL/Poloxamer nanofiber membrane and 5/5 dextran/gelatin hydrogel were shown to display favorable physical properties and cell-material interactions [18–19]. A bilayer scaffold was fabricated using these two materials by underlaying and casting method. 9/1 PLCL/Poloxamer nanofiber membrane was fabricated and was laid in a 6-well tissue culture plate. Then 5 ml of dextran/gelatin solution at the ratio of 5/5 was poured on the surface of 9/1 PLCL/Poloxamer membrane to form hydrogel and get bilayer scaffolds.

Characterization of electrospun PLCL/Poloxamer membranes

1. Fiber size analysis. To evaluate the morphology and fiber diameters of electrospun fibers, materials were gold-coated and observed using scanning electron microscope (SEM, JSM-5600LV, JEOL, Japan) at an accelerating voltage of 20 kV. For each sample (n = 3), five random spots were captured to generate micrographs, and at least 20 different fibers were randomLy selected for further measurement using ImageJ software, version 1.46r.

2. Pore Size Measurements. A CFP-1100-AI capillary flow porometer (PMI Porous Materials Int. USA) was used in this study to measure the pore size. Galwick with a defined surface tension of 21 dynes cm^{-1} (PMI Porous Materials Int. USA) was used as the wetting agent for porometry measurements. Electrospun fibrous scaffolds were cut into 3×3 cm^2 squares and then soaked into the wetting agent. The soaked scaffolds were placed in adapting pan and sealed with O-rings for porometry measurement.

3. Tensile test. To ensure the mechanical properties of fibrous mats falls in the physiological range of human skin, mats were placed in phosphate buffered saline (PBS, Gibco, Invitrogen,

USA) for 30 min and subsequently conducted following standard mechanical test. The fabric materials (200 μm in thickness) were punched into rectangular strips (70 mm×7 mm, n = 5) and characterized by a tensile test (Instron 5567, Canton, MA). The stress-strain curves of these materials were constructed from the load-deformation curves recorded at a stretching speed of 0.5 mm/s. Ultimately the tensile strength, Young's modulus and elongation at break were obtained from plotted stress–strain curves. Tensile property values reported here represent an average of the results for tests run on at least five samples.

4. Measurement of water contact angle. To determine the influence of poloxamer on the hydrophilicity of PLCL, water contact angle test was measured using a commercial drop shape analysis system (Data Physics SCA20, Germany). The fabric materials were cut into pieces approximately 1×1 cm (n = 6) and air-dried at room temperature for 48 h, then 3 μL deionized droplets were gently deposited on each sample through a micro syringe, images were captured at 2 s after the water droplet was dripped on the surface of materials, and the contact angle was measured by the inbuilt software in the machine.

Characterization of dextran/gelatin hydrogels

1. Swelling analysis. To study the swelling kinetics of the modified hydrogels, the dextran/gelatin hydrogels at different ratios (3/7, 4/6, 5/5, 6/4, 7/3) were frozen at −80°C and lyophilized in a vacuum oven. The dry hydrogels were weighed (W_d) and then immersed in PBS at 37°C. After 24 h of incubation, the samples were removed from the PBS and the water on the surface was quickly wiped out with a filter paper so that the swollen weight could be measured (W_s) accurately. The swelling ratio (SR) was then calculated according to the following equation: $SR = W_s/W_d$.

2. In vitro degradation. To determine the weight loss due to hydrolytic degradation, hydrogels were divided into four groups (day 3, day 7, day 14, day 21) for time-control degradation study. The samples (n = 3) were prepared from blending 10 wt% dextran and 20 wt% gelatin aqueous solutions in different ratios (3/7, 4/6, 5/5, 6/4, 7/3) and pre-swollen in PBS overnight. Subsequently, the weight of the sample was record as W_0 and the hydrogels were completely submerged in PBS at 37°C. At different time intervals, the samples were removed from the solution, blotted dry and then weighed to determine the weight of the remaining mass (W_1). The PBS was replaced every 3 days and the experiments were performed in triplicate. The weight loss (%) was calculated as the following formula: weight loss = $(W_0-W_1)/W_0 \times 100\%$.

3. Compression test. The hydrogels were also characterized by compression stress-strain measurements using a Dejie DXLL-20000 materials testing instrument at 25°C. Based on the early screening studies, samples were incubated in PBS at 37°C for 24 h before test in order to reach completely swelling equilibrium. After measuring diameter and thickness of the specimens, they were put on the lower plate and compressed by the upper plate at a strain rate of 1 mm/min. The initial compressive modulus was determined by the average slope in a range of 0–10% strain from the stress-strain curves. The fracture stress, determined from the peak of the stress-strain curve, was also reported. All compression testing groups had a sample quantity of n = 3.

Biological assess of electrospun PLCL/Poloxamer membranes and dextran/gelatin hydrogels

1. Cell isolation and culture. Animal procedures related to adipose tissue isolation were approved by the Shanghai JiaoTong University Ethical Committee. After the 10% chloral hydrate (350 mg/kg) anesthesia of rats, abdominal adipose tissue (approximately 5 g) was obtained from bilateral inguinal region of SD rats and washed with PBS for 15 min. Tissue was minced by sharp dissection into 1 mm^3 pieces, and directly exposed to PBS containing 0.1% collagenase type I (Sigma–Aldrich, St. Louis, MO) for enzymatic digestion. After 60 min incubation at 37°C with mild agitation (40 rpm), an equal volume of Dulbecco's modified Eagle's medium (DMEM, Gibco) containing 10% FBS was added to stop enzymatic digestion. Then the mixed solution was filtered through a 70 μm nylon mesh and the filter liquor was transferred into a 15 mL centrifuge tube, finally the cellular pellet was isolated via centrifugation 1500 rpm for 10 min at room temperature. Cells were dispensed into tissue culture flasks (Corning Glass Works, Corning, NY) containing 5 mL complete medium. ADSCs were incubated in a 5% CO_2 incubator at 37°C, and medium was changed every 3 days.

2. Cell viability assay of electrospun PLCL/Poloxamer membranes. Cell viability was determined using a CCK-8 Assay Kit. Electrospun matrices were cut into 12 mm diameter circles and sterilized by immersion in 70% ethanol for 1 h, subsequently they were washed with PBS (supplemented with 500 U/mL penicillin and 500 U/mL streptomycin) and DMEM three times separately. ADSCs were suspended in complete medium and seeded with a density of 5×10^3 cells per each sample, and they were also seeded on tissue culture plate (TCP) as a control group. Then the 24-well tissue culture plate was incubated under a humidified atmosphere of 5% CO_2 at 37°C. The culture medium was exchanged every day. After 1, 3 and 7 days culture, 400 μl CCK-8 mixed solution (400 μl medium containing 40 μl CCK-8 reaction solution) was added to each well and incubated for 2 hours at 37°C. Then the medium with CCK-8 was transferred to 96-well tissue culture plate and the absorbance was read at 450 nm. All experiments were carried out in triplicate.

3. Cell viability assay of dextran/gelatin hydrogels. For this assay, each 300 μl mixed solution was injected into 24-well tissue culture plate and formed hydrogel at 37°C. Cell suspension with cell density of 1×10^6 cells/mL was injected on the surface of hydrogel. The cell-seeding hydrogels were incubated at 37°C in a humidified atmosphere of 5% CO_2. The culture medium was exchanged every day. After 1, 3 and 7 days culture, 400 μl CCK-8 mixed solution (400 μl medium containing 40 μl CCK-8 reaction solution) was added to each well and incubated for 2 hours at 37°C. Then the medium with CCK-8 was transferred to 96-well tissue culture plate and the absorbance was read at 450 nm. All experiments were carried out in triplicate.

4. Cytotoxicity assay of bilayer scaffold. The cytotoxicity assay of bilayer scaffold was quantified using the CCK-8 assay for 1, 3, 7 and 14 days through a Transwell system (Costar 3422). Briefly, the adipose-derived stem cells suspension with cell density of 1×10^6 cells/mL was injected in 24-well culture plates. The bilayer scaffold was placed within the upper chambers and the upper chambers were inserted in 24-well culture plates. ADSCs seeded in 24-well culture plate without upper chamber served as control group. The complete medium was added and culture plates were incubated at 37°C in a humidified atmosphere of 5% CO_2. The culture medium was exchanged every three days. After 1, 3, 7 and 14 days culture, the culture medium was removed and 400 μl medium containing 40 μl CCK-8 reaction solution was added to each well and incubated for 4 hours at 37°C and 5% CO_2. Then the medium with CCK-8 was transferred to 96-well tissue culture plate and the absorbance was read at 450 nm using a multidetection microplate reader (MK3, Thermo, USA). All experiments were carried out in triplicate.

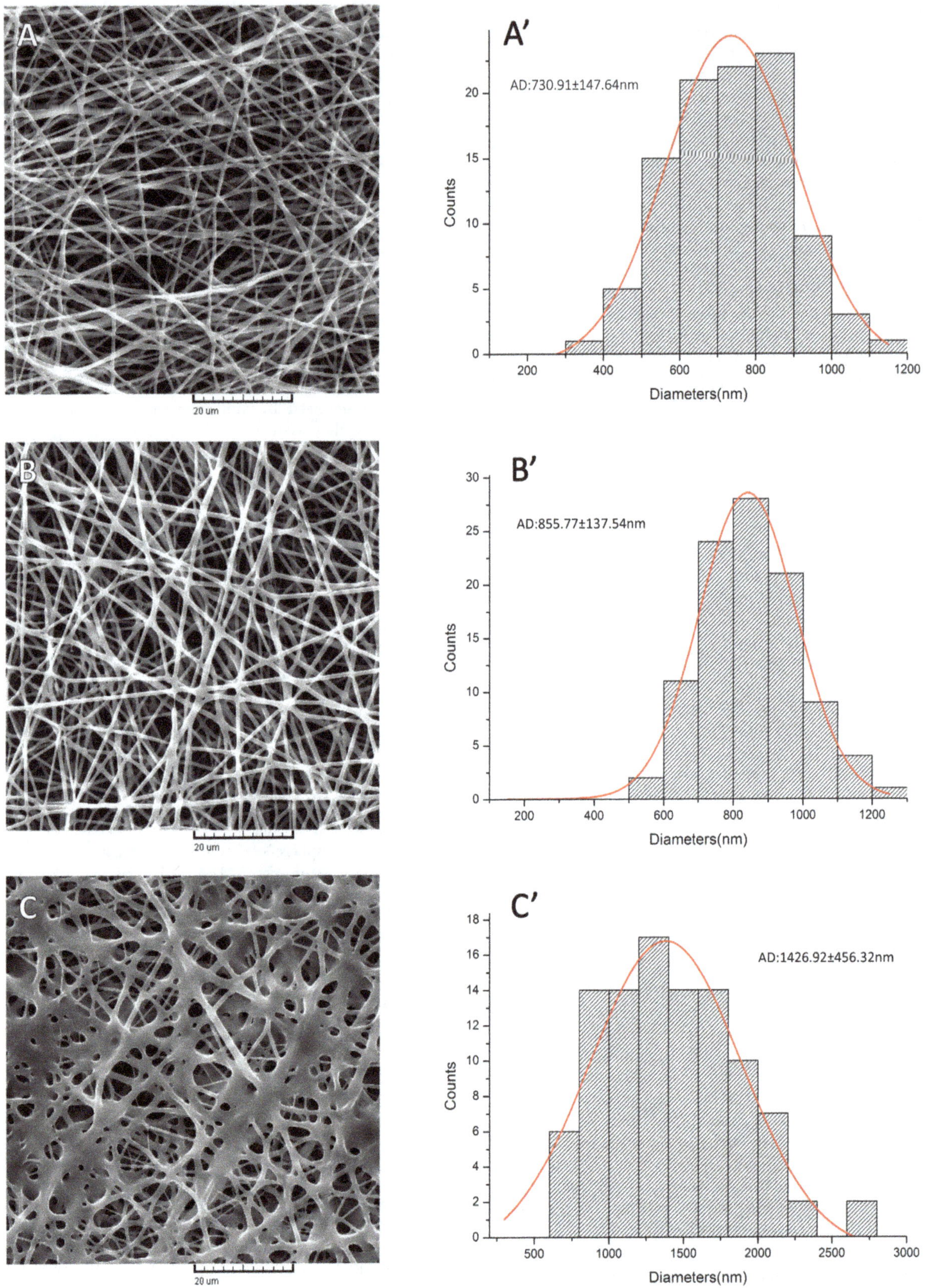

Figure 1. SEM images of electrospun PLCL/Poloxamer nanofibers with different weight ratio of PLCL to Poloxamer: (A) 1/0; (B) 9/1; (C) 3/1.

Statistical Analysis

Values are expressed as mean ± SD. One-way analysis of variance (ANOVA) was used to discern the statistical difference between groups. Repeated-measures analysis of variance (rMANOVA) and Least-significant difference (LSD) were utilized to compare the between-subjects effects of time and group. For all analyses, a two-tailed P value of less than 0.05 indicated statistical significance. Statistical analysis was conducted using SPSS 16.0 for Windows (SPSS, Chicago, USA).

Results

Electrospun PLCL/Poloxamer membranes

1. Morphology of PLCL and PLCL/Poloxamer nanofibers. The SEM morphologies of PLCL and PLCL/Poloxamer nanofibers were shown in Figure 1. Smooth surface and interconnected porous structures of PLCL and PLCL/Poloxamer nanofibers have been obtained. From the micrographs, it is clear that the ratio of PLCL/Poloxamer significantly affected the fiber diameter distributions. The average diameter of PLCL nanofibers from 8 wt% solution is 730.91±147.64 nm, while PLCL/Poloxamer nanofibers of 9/1 and 3/1 have the average diameters of 855.77±137.54 nm and 1426.92±456.32 nm respectively. Fiber average diameters gradually increased with increasing Poloxamer content. At the same time, an enhanced non-uniformity and non-homogeneity of fibers was also noted as the Poloxamer increased.

2. Pore Diameter Analyses. Microscale and nanoscale porous structure of electrospun nanofibrous scaffolds play critical roles for cellular growth and tissue regeneration because the highly porous network of interconnected pores provides nutrients and gas exchange for cell proliferation. SEM showed that the nanofibers had a solid surface with interconnected voids, so that a porous structure was present. Pore diameters of PLCL and PLCL/Poloxamer nanofibers were shown and summarized in Table 1. When blended ratios ranged from 1/0 to 9/1 mean pore diameter increased with increasing the content of Poloxamer. According to a published report [20], as expected the fiber diameter increased, the average pore size of the scaffolds increased. With increasing the content of Poloxamer, the fiber diameter increased so that the pore diameter increased. However, mean pore diameter of 3/1 PLCL/Poloxamer nanofibers was smaller than that of 9/1 PLCL/Poloxamer nanofibers. This may be caused the fact that a large amount of fibers accumulated disorderly and bonded together in 3/1 PLCL/Poloxamer nanofibers showed in Figure 1. Therefore, the pore structure of scaffolds might be jammed with increasing bonded fibers. As expected that cells infiltrated the scaffolds with lager pore diameters and the nanofibrous scaffold with small pore diameter exhibited reduced cellular infiltration. So the 9/1 PLCL/Poloxamer nanofibers might mimic the native ECM and promote cell more spreading in skin tissue engineering.

3. Water contact angle assay. The surface hydrophilic property plays an important role in cell adhesion, spreading, and proliferation on the biomaterials surfaces. To investigate the influence of different blending ratios on the surface hydrophilic property of electrospun PLCL and PLCL/Poloxamer nanofibers, the water contact angle measurement was done and shown in Figure 2. The pure PLCL nanofibers showed a contact angle of about 127.56°±13.74°, indicating that the surface was hydrophobic. In contrast, the electrospun PLCL/Poloxamer nanofibers exhibited more hydrophilic properties, which have an apparent decrease in contact angle. As the Poloxamer content increased, the contact angle of blended nanofibers decreased to approximately 0°. Therefore, the surface wettability of hybrid nanofibers can be obtained by introducing Poloxamer in the blended PLCL/Poloxamer nanofibers.

4. Mechanical properties. Mechanical properties of PLCL/Poloxamer nanofibers are critical for their successful application in skin tissue engineering. For example, a major cause of graft failure in skin substitutes is ischemic and nutrient-deprived, which is often caused by the compliance mismatch between the graft and the host skin tissue [21–22]. Therefore, the appropriate mechanical compatibility between PLCL/Poloxamer nanofibers and host skin tissues is a requirement for functioning soft tissue substitutes. Tensile tests were performed on all scaffolds to determine whether the tensile strength properties were favorable for use as a skin graft. Figure 3 shows the typical tensile stress–strain curve of electrospun PLCL and PLCL/Poloxamer nanofibers. The ultimate tensile strength, tensile modulus and elongation at break were summarized in Table 2. The tensile strength and modulus of nanofiber substrates lie well within the range of those of human skin. It is desirable that the tensile properties are similar to those of human skin, providing it with good resilience and compliance to movement as a skin graft. On the other hand, the nanofibrous scaffolds have a larger ultimate strain compared with human skin. This reinforces its potential as a skin graft, since it could still cover the wound when immobilized at a wound site under a high tensile strength. It can also be observed that the PLCL/Poloxamer nanofibers showed higher tensile strength and ultimate strain than PLCL nanofibers. Moreover, the average tensile strength of PLCL/Poloxamer nanofibers (9/1) was 9.37±0.38 MPa with an ultimate strain of 187.43±10.66% when compared with 7.23±0.16 MPa and 158.54±6.67% for PLCL nanofibers, 7.85±0.65 MPa and 215.23±16.41% for PLCL/Poloxamer nanofibers(3/1). It indicates that the introduction of hydrophilic Poloxamer can improve the electrospinnability, thus forming nanofibers with solid surface and interconnected structures which can be benefit for the enhancement of mechanical properties. Thus, it is possible to create hybrid scaffolds with desirable mechanical property for engineering of various soft tissues by selecting the optimum blend ratios of two components. The blended PLCL/Poloxamer nanofibers with PLCL/Poloxamer ratio of 9/1 were selected for further studies as they exhibited better comprehensive properties including hydrophilicity, pore diameter and mechanical strength than other ones.

Table 1. Pore diameter of PLCL and PLCL/Poloxamer nanofibers with various blend ratios.

PLCL/Poloxamer ratio	Specimen thickness (mm)	Mean pore diameter ± SD (μm)	Largest pore diameter (μm)	Smallest pore diameter (μm)
1/0	0.07	1.73±0.44	2.85	0.96
9/1	0.05	2.05±0.39	3.03	1.01
3/1	0.10	1.57±0.65	2.60	0.92

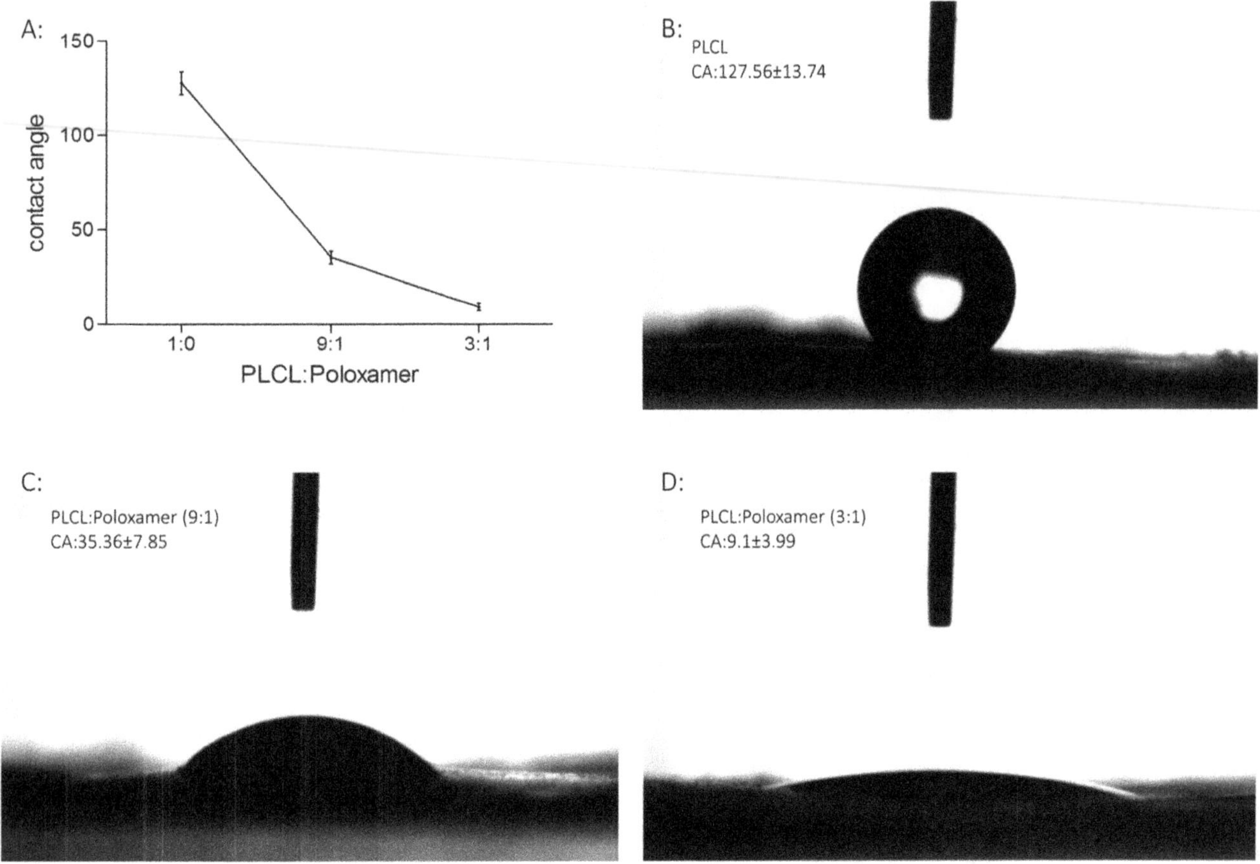

Figure 2. Digital pictures of water contact angles of electrospun PLCL/Poloxamer nanofibers with different weight ratio of PLCL to Poloxamer: (B) 1/0; (C) 9/1; (D) 3/1.

Dextran/gelatin hydrogels

1. Morphology. As shown in Figure 4A, dextran and gelatin solutions were mixed and the gel can be formed in a short time. The dextran/gelatin hydrogel was transparent and yellowish in color. In this study, all hydrogel samples were flash-frozen at −80°C in liquid nitrogen and lyophilized. After that, the corresponding cross-section of the dry samples was observed and the freeze-dried hydrogel was yellowish and porous (Figure 4B). Figure 4C and 4D showed the SEM micrographs of freeze-dried hydrogels. All hydrogels showed good interconnected porous structures with an average pore sizes ranging from approximately 50–200 μm. The interconnected porous structure is necessary for scaffolds to promote nutrient and gas diffusion, allow cellular ingrowth and retain high water. Therefore, the hydrogels might be suitable as carriers for cell delivery in skin tissue engineering.

2. Swelling analysis. The swelling behavior is an important property of tissue engineering scaffold because it relates to the diffusion of signaling molecules and nutrients. Figure 5 indicates the swelling results of freeze-dried dextran/gelatin hydrogels in PBS. The dry hydrogels could absorb large quantity of water from 19.47 to 43.45 times of their original dry weight, suggesting that they could be good scaffolds to retain tissue fluid and nutrients in vivo. Figure 5 also revealed the relationship between the swelling ratio of the dextran/gelatin hydrogels and the dextran content in the hydrogels. Generally, the swelling ratio of a hydrogel is related to physic-chemical factors, such as the crosslinking density, gel composition, network structure, etc.

The swelling ratio decreased rapidly from 43.45 to 19.47 with the increase of dextran's content from 30 to 50%, which can be ascribed to the increase of crosslinking degree. Thereafter, with an elevation of dextran's content from 50 to 70%, the crosslinking density in the hydrogels declined and the swelling ratio increased slightly from 19.47 to 25.94. In this regard, the variation of the swelling ratio corresponds well with the information of the gelation time depicted in Figure 3. It is also worthwhile to notice that group 5/5 exhibited apparently different swelling property compared with groups of 3/7 and 4/6. We ascribe this obvious decline on swelling ratio to the decrease content of gelatin, which have a strong ability to absorb water. From the clinical aspect, over load swelling ratio of the scaffolds may cause pressure to the surrounding tissues. In contrast, under load swelling ratio of the scaffolds would result in insufficient nutrients exchanged from surrounding circumstances. Meanwhile, the scaffolds with inadequate swelling ratio may escape from the implant point easily. Therefore, the dextran/gelatin hydrogel with an adjustable swelling property can meet those requirements by changing the ratio of components.

3. In vitro degradation. The degradation of five composite hydrogels was monitored as by incubating in PBS at 37°C, as shown in Figure 6. Apparently, the ratio of dextran and gelatin has great impact on the weight loss of samples. Concretely, the 3/7 dextran/gelatin hydrogel exhibited the fastest degradation rate and totally degraded after 7 days. By contrast, 4/6 and 5/5 groups showed a more controllable degradation rate due to higher crosslinking density. Since gelatin can be easily solubilized in

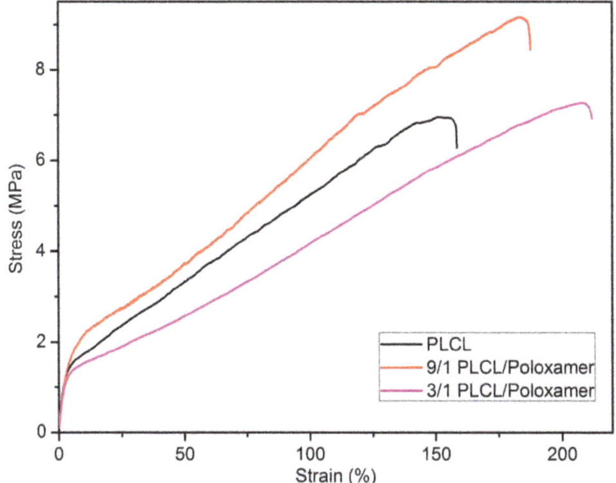

Figure 3. Stress-strain curves for electrospun PLCL/Poloxamer nanofibers with different weight ratio of PLCL to Poloxamer.

aqueous environment, groups of 6/4 and 7/3 with an incline of gelatin have the strongest resistance to degradation that they could still hold more than 50% of the initial weight after three weeks. Generally, it takes at least 14 days for the stem cells seeded in hydrogels to generate extracellular matrices for epidermal formation. So the results indicate that the degradation rate of the dextran/gelatin hydrogels could be modulated by altering the dextran content of hydrogel to match epidermal tissue formation.

4. Mechanical properties. The effects of the difference ratio of dextran and gelatin on the mechanical properties were also evaluated. All mechanical tests were carried out at 37°C with fully hydrated hydrogel samples which were free from any physical imperfection. Figure 7 shows force-displacement curve for all the compositions. Compressive force corresponding to the same displacement value showed an increasing trend with an increase in dextran amount (from 3/7 to 5/5). The effect may be explained on the basis of formation of denser and condensed networks, which are rigid and thus require more stress to compress. Also, a representative compression curve is shown in Figure 8. As seen in the figure, all of the five groups show linear elastic behavior at low stress, non-linear switching strain at intermediate stress and linear elastic behavior at high stress. The modulus increases as the strain increases. This causes the stress at 50%–60% strain to be significantly larger than the stress at 10%–50% strain. The 6/4, 7/3, 5/5 dextran/gelatin have demonstrated the higher initial modulus than 4/6 and 3/7 hydrogel, which can be ascribed to the prefect crosslinking density and limited swelling property. The 3/7 and 4/6 dextran/gelatin hydrogels showed the worse mechanical property due to their great swollen condition. It can also be observed that the fracture strain of hydrogels increased slightly with the increase of gelatin content. The 3/7 dextran/gelatin hydrogel underwent higher deformation before failure than others although it failed at a lower stress. In general, all hydrogels deformed much less than 70%. This can be explained on the basis of the large pore size and high water content of the hydrogel. The imbibed water molecules migrate from the regions under load towards the unloaded regions thus resulting in deformation of the hydrogels as observed. For present purposes, the skin can be approximated as a bilayer, consisting of the epidermis (modulus, 140 to 600 kPa; thickness, 0.05 to 1.5 mm) and the dermis (modulus, 2 to 80 kPa; thickness, 0.3 to 3 mm) [23–24]. For the trends analyzed, the dextran/gelatin was suitable as the dermis substitute since the compressive modulus is close to the clinical range of modulus that will be expected for a material placed under the epidermis.

Biocompatibility of the samples

1. Cell viability assay of electrospun PLCL/Poloxamer membranes. Adipose derived stem cells were used to determine the ability of the PLCL/Poloxamer membranes to support cell viability and proliferation. ADSCs were seeded onto various electrospun scaffolds and cultured. At different time points (1, 3, 7 and 10 days) the viability of ADSCs was determined by CCK-8 test and the values of absorbance at 450 nm were showed in Figure 9. The statistical analysis revealed that ADSCs had an increased metabolic activity on the electrospun PLCL/Poloxamer membranes with the increase of culture time, indicating the PLCL/Poloxamer membranes were able to support cell proliferation. And after 1, 3, 7 and 10 days in vitro culture, There was no significant difference in cell viability between the 9/1 group and the 3/1 group, while cell viability in PLCL/Poloxamer groups are significantly greater than PLCL group. The result may be explained on the basis of high hydrophilicity of PLCL/Poloxamer nanofibers, which facilitates the diffusion of tissue fluid and nutrients to support cell viability and proliferation. With the introduction of poloxamer, greater hydrophilic properties resulted in smaller contact angle as observed through water contact angle assay. The surface wettability is an important factor governing oxygen and nutrient permeability since the tissue fluid diffuses easily throughout the surface of membranes with high hydrophilicity.

2. Cell viability assay of dextran/gelatin hydrogels. Mouse pre-osteoblast cells were used to demonstrate the ability of the dextran/gelatin hydrogels to support cell proliferation since the dextran/gelatin hydrogels mimic natural extracellular matrix (ECM) of the dermis, which supports the extensive vasculature. The CCK-8 Assay was implemented to quantitatively assess cell viability of cells cultured on the hydrogels after 1, 3 and 7 days. As shown in Figure 10, there was a significant effect of gelatin

Table 2. Mechanical properties of PLCL and PLCL/Poloxamer nanofibers at various blend ratios compared with human skin.

	PLCL/Poloxamer			
Property	**1/0**	**9/1**	**3/1**	**Human skin**
Tensile strength (MPa)	7.23±0.16	9.37±0.38	7.85±0.65	5–30
Tensile modulus (MPa)	47.65±2.24	47.49±5.44	46.86±2.54	15–150
Elongation at break (%)	158.54±6.67	187.43±10.66	215.23±16.41	35–115

Values represent the average ± standard deviation.

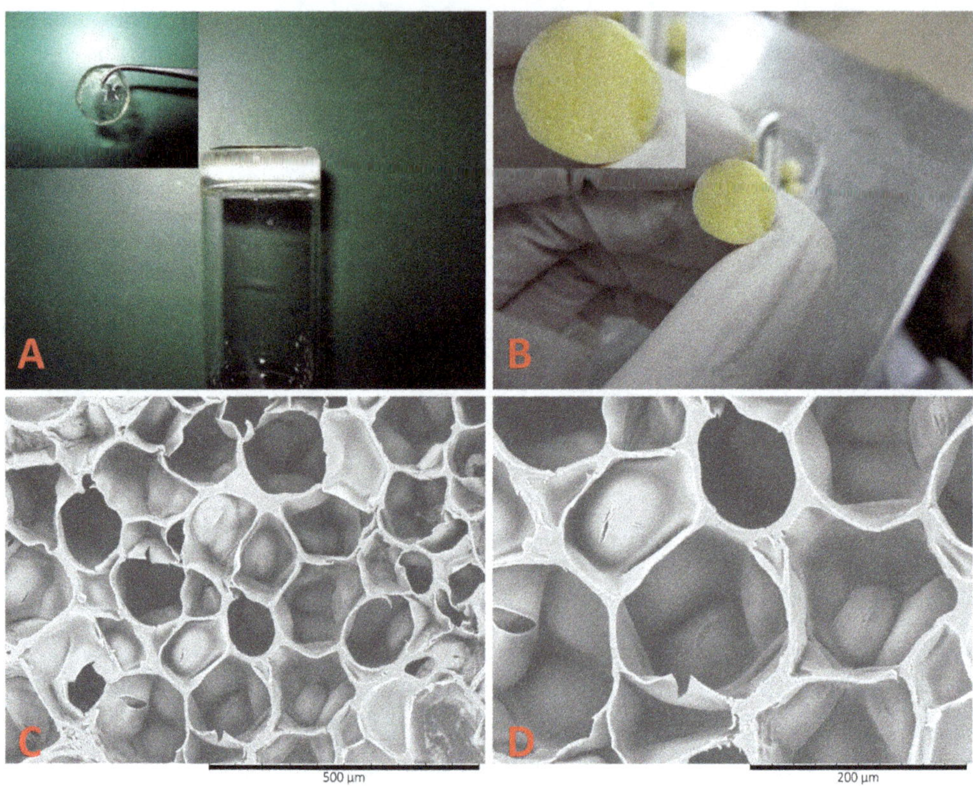

Figure 4. Morphology of the dextran/gelatin hydrogels. A: Gross view of the dextran/gelatin hydrogel; B: Gross view of lyophilized dextran/gelatin hydrogel; C: SEM micrograph of lyophilized dextran/gelatin hydrogel. Scale bar represents 500 µm. D: SEM micrograph of lyophilized dextran/gelatin hydrogel. Scale bar represents 200 µm.

concentration ($p<0.05$) and culture time ($p<0.05$) on cell viability. The statistical analysis revealed that cells had an increased metabolic activity on the hydrogels with the increase of incorporated gelatin. After 3 days culture, cells cultured on the hydrogels were stained with Live/Dead staining solution. In the fluorescence microscope it is showed that the hydrogel became a little adverse to cell responses such as the attachment, spreading and proliferation of cells with the ratio of dextran/gelatin change from 3/7 to 7/3. One possible explanation is that the side effect caused by the aldehyde groups in oxidized dextran hampered the adhesion of cells on matrix surface. After 7 days in vitro culture, cells on the surface of hydrogels remained viable and proliferative compared with the day 1 and 3 group, indicating the good cytocompatibility of hydrogels. These results implied that dextran/gelatin hydrogels might be good scaffold materials which have excellent biocompatibility.

3. Cytotoxicity assay of bilayer scaffold. In addition to examining the two biomaterials that will comprise the bilayer scaffold, cytotoxicity assay data was also obtained on the constructed bilayer scaffold to determine if the bilayer composition affected the final result. Figure 11 shows the cell viability cocultured with bilayer scaffold compared to TCP. There was no statistically significant difference between the bilayer scaffold group and control group ($p>0.05$), indicating that the bilayer

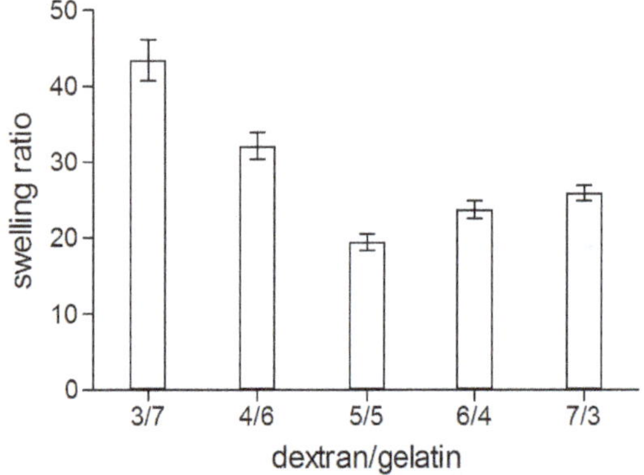

Figure 5. The swelling ratio of dextran/gelatin hydrogels with different volume ratio.

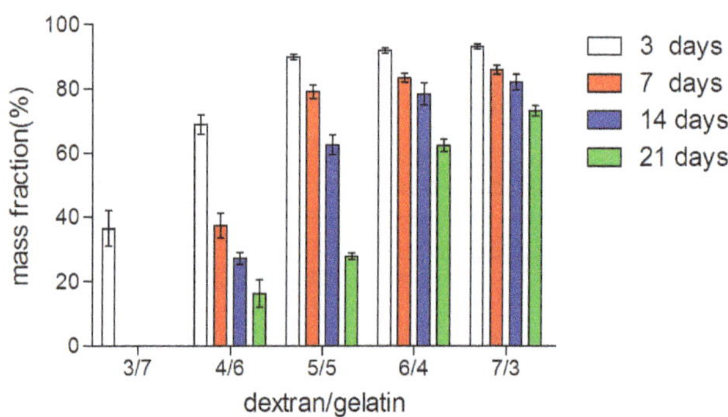

Figure 6. The degradation of dextran/gelatin hydrogels with different volume ratio.

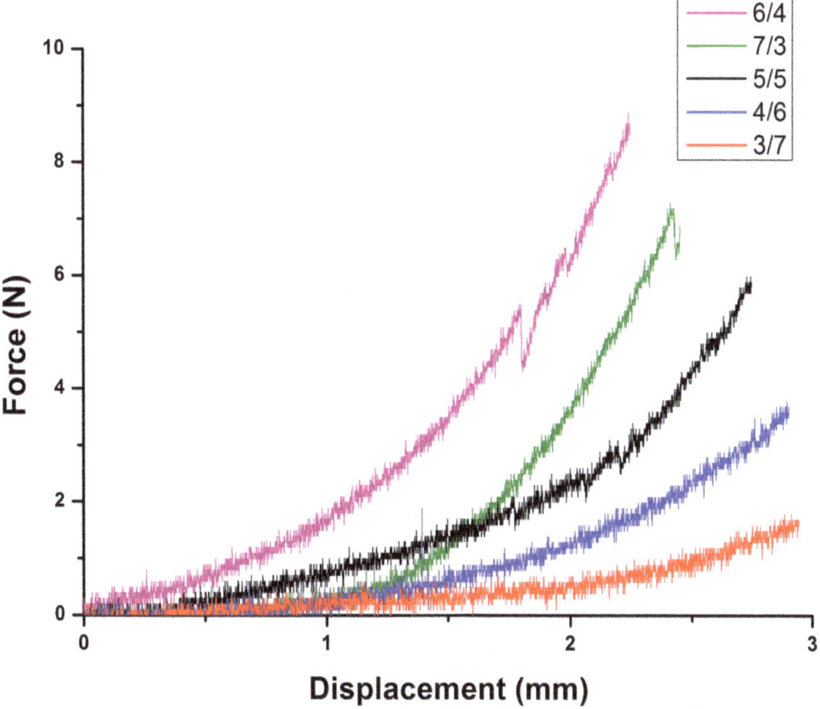

Figure 7. Force-displacement curves for all the compositions of dextran/gelatin hydrogels.

scaffold has no toxicity on cell viability. The statistical analysis revealed that cells had an increased metabolic activity with the increase of culture time. After 14 days culture, cells cocultured with or without bilayer scaffold were also stained with Live/Dead staining solution. In the fluorescence microscope the live and dead cells exhibit green-fluorescent and red-fluorescent. There was no visual difference between control group and bilayer scaffold group. The cells in two groups reached complete confluence and had an organized arrangement. All of them exhibited green-fluorescent morphology. Cells cocultured with bilayer scaffold remained

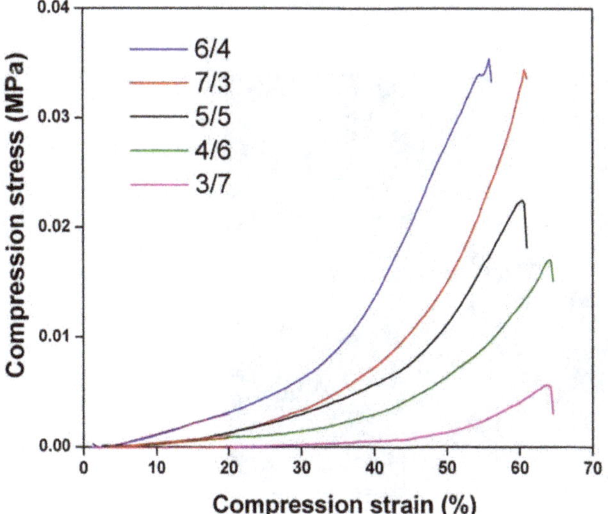

Figure 8. Stress-strain curves for all the compositions of dextran/gelatin hydrogels.

viable and proliferative. These results implied that the degradation products derived from bilayer scaffold did not inhibit key metabolic pathways of cells.

Discussion

In this study, we analysed the characteristics of electrospun PLCL/poloxamer nanofibers and dextran/gelatin hydrogels with the goal of fabricating a bilayer scaffold for skin tissue engineering applications. Electrospun nanofibers have received more and more attention to be used as tissue engineering scaffolds since they have the nanofibrous porous structure, which can mimic the native Extracellular Matrix (ECM) [25–28]. Utilizing electrospinning technology, PLCL and poloxamer can be processed into nanofiber membranes. PLCL is a synthetic biodegradable copolymer which is approved by FDA for both wound closure and orthopedic applications [29–30]. However, the hydrophobic property has restricted its applications. Poloxamer, which was also approved by FDA for human use, consists of hydrophilic poly(ethylene oxide) (PEO) and hydrophobic poly(propylene oxide) (PPO) blocks arranged in tri-block structure: PEO-PPO-PEO. Due to its amphiphilic character poloxamer displays surfactant properties including ability to interact with the surfaces of hydrophobic membranes [31]. In this study, poloxamer was used as a hydrophilic additive to PLCL membranes. The water contact angle of PLCL/poloxamer membranes decreased with the increase of incorporated poloxamer, indicating the addition of poloxamer improved the hydrophilicity. This may be provided by pore surface exposure of the hydrophilic PEO chains in poloxamer molecules entrapped within the PLCL/poloxamer membranes.

PLCL and poloxamer was blended together to be electrospun into nanofibers. The mechanical properties and biocompatibility of the obtained nanofibers were investigated. Pure PLCL nanofibers had the breaking strength of 7.23 MPa and elongation

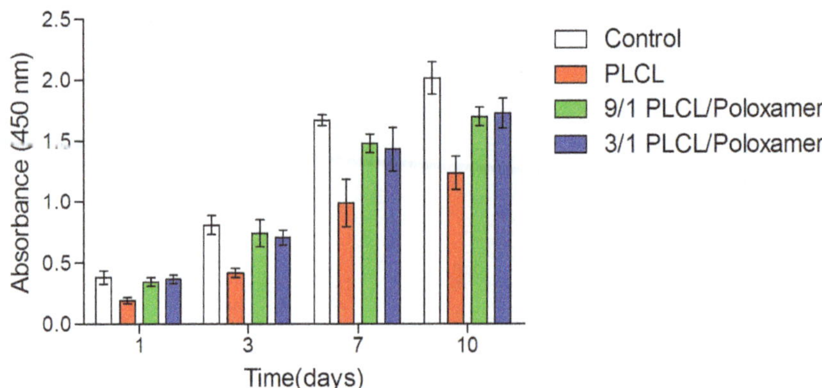

Figure 9. The proliferation of adipose-derived stem cells cultured on electrospun PLCL and PLCL/Poloxamer nanofibers in the CCK-8 assay: the absorbance of these medium with CCK-8 was read at 450 nm.

at break of 158%. When a small amount poloxamer was added in (content of 10%), the PLCL/Poloxamer nanofibers reached the higher tensile strength of 9.37 MPa, and it still keep the elasticity with the elongation at break of 187%. But with the further increasing of poloxamer content the mechanical properties of PLCL/poloxamer nanofibers decreased. Tensile strength and modulus of PLCL/poloxamer nanofiber membranes lie within the range of values suitable for human skin [32], providing these scaffolds with good resilience and compliance to movement as a skin graft.

Cell viability studies with adipose-derived stem cells demonstrated that PLCL/poloxamer nanofibers significantly promoted cell proliferation in comparison with PLCL nanofibers, especially when the weight ratio of PLCL to poloxamer was 9:1. PLCL/poloxamer nanofibers showed better mechanical properties and biocompatibility than PLCL. One possible explanation is that the

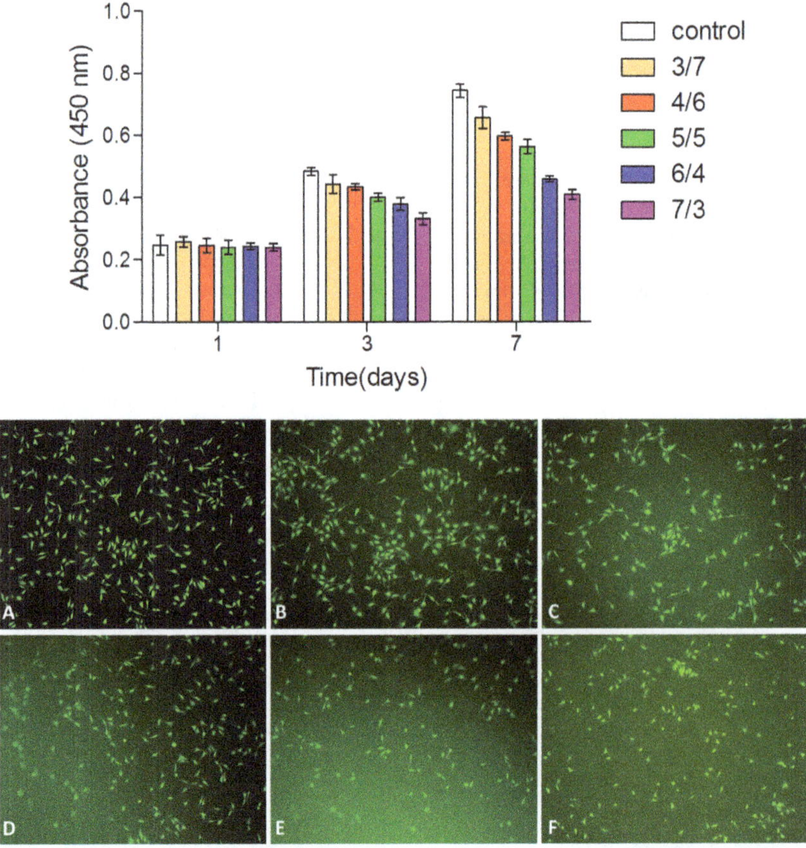

Figure 10. The proliferation of cells cultured on dextran/gelatin hydrogels in the CCK-8 assay: the absorbance of these medium with CCK-8 was read at 450 nm. Cells cultured on the hydrogels were stained with Live/Dead staining solution (A: tissue culture plate; B: 3/7; C: 4/6; D: 5/5; E: 6/4; F: 7/3).

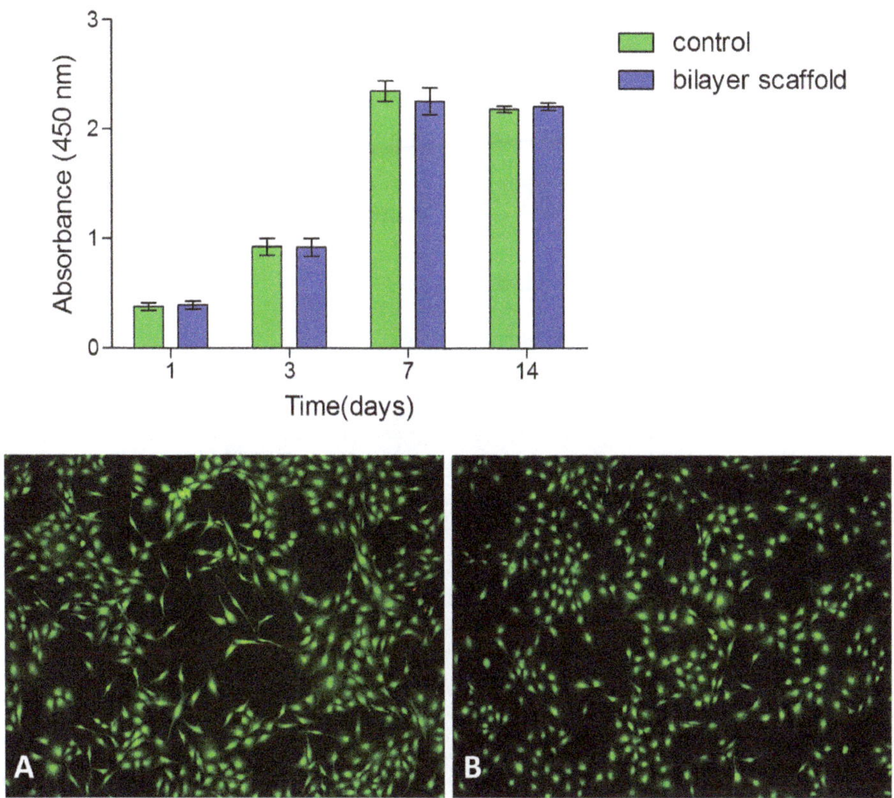

Figure 11. The proliferation of cells co-cultured with the bilayer scaffold in the CCK-8 assay. Cells were stained with Live/Dead staining solution (A: tissue culture plate; B: bilayer scaffold).

introduction of hydrophilic Poloxamer improves the electrospinnability thus forming hydrophilic nanofibers with interconnected and solider structure which facilitates the diffusion of tissue fluid and nutrients to support cell viability and proliferation. So that, the best way to get tissue engineering scaffolds with both excellent mechanical properties and biocompatibility is to combine two distinct materials together to form the blend nanofibers via electrospinning technology.

Native skin is composed of two layers with distinct qualities. One of the most used, commercially available skin substitute is Integra [33], which is a bilayer scaffold composed of a silicone upper layer and a collagen-glycosaminoglycan porous sublayer. Thus, the bilayer scaffold composed of PLCL/poloxamer nanofiber upper layer and dextran/gelatin hydrogel sublayer should more accurately mimic the physical structure of the normal skin. The two separate layers have distinct functions which help the bilayer scaffold adapt to the complex environment of wound healing. The upper, PLCL/poloxamer nanofiber layer serves as a protective barrier against the outside world and integrates with the host skin tissue. The tensile strength and hydrophilic property provides good resilience and compliance to movement as a skin graft. The lower, dextran/gelatin hydrogel layer provide a highly swollen three-dimensional environment similar to soft tissues and fills in the hypodermis defect area. The swollen and biodegradable property allows for the ingrowth of surrounding native stem cells while maintaining significant amounts of tissue fluid on the wound bed and promoting diffusion of nutrients and cellular waste through the elastic networks.

Hydrogels are prepared by swelling cross-linked structures in water or biological fluids. Methods of preparing the hydrogel networks include chemical cross-linking(Schiff-based reaction, click reaction), environmentally or physiologically responsive cross-linking(self-assembly, thermosensitivity, pH-sensitivity) and photopolymerization [34–36]. Injectable hydrogels have gained widespread applications as three-dimensional tissue engineering scaffolds due to their advantages of taking the shape of a cavity and providing a good fit or interface between the hydrogel and host tissue. Moreover, various therapeutic molecules and even cells can be incorporated by simply mixing with the precursor solution prior to injection [37–38]. Dextran/gelatin hydrogel was fabricated through Schiff-based reaction between aldehyde groups and amino groups without the addition of a chemical crosslinking agent. Dextran and gelatin offer the advantage of being very similar to macromolecular substances of extracellular matrix and complete degradation by enzymes in vivo. The proliferation phase of the wound healing process is said to be about 3 weeks [39]. Therefore, a scaffold intended for temporary skin replacement should not completely disintegrate before this time to be able to perform its template function. Except dextran/gelatin hydrogel with the ratio of 3/7, other hydrogels meet this criterion and can support the proliferation of cells to repair the wound in skin tissue engineering. In respect of biocompatibility, with the ratio of dextran/gelatin change from 3/7 to 7/3, the matrix became adverse to cell viability and proliferation. So the bilayer scaffold consisting of 9/1 PLCL/poloxamer nanofiber upper layer and 5/5 dextran/gelatin hydrogel sublayer should be suitable to mimic the physical structure of the normal skin. And the results demonstrated that the bilayer scaffold has shown favorable in vitro biocompatibility as an acellular scaffold aimed to aid wound healing.

Conclusions

In the present study, we prepared two different biomaterials and investigated the characteristics to fabricate a bilayer scaffold for skin tissue engineering applications. A bilayer design was conceived for an artificial skin substitute where distinct qualities of the two layers can be combined to enhance wound healing. The electrospun PLCL/Poloxamer nanofibers (9/1) displayed the optimal mechanical strength and biocompatible properties. The dextran/gelatin hydrogel (5/5) is a fast in situ forming scaffold that can support cell viability while possessing critical physical properties (mechanical strength and degradation) required for a skin tissue scaffold. The proposed combination of these two biomaterials can open more possibilities for wound treatment and rehabilitation as one system may not be sufficient to answer the complex environment in wound treatment and skin regeneration. This work provides a strategy for the design and fabrication of nanofiber-hydrogel bilayer scaffolds mimicking the structure of the normal skin for wound repair.

Author Contributions

Conceived and designed the experiments: JFP NHL HS. Performed the experiments: NHL JFP. Analyzed the data: JFP NHL HS FX. Contributed reagents/materials/analysis tools: HS. Wrote the paper: JFP NHL.

References

1. Martin P (1997) Wound healing–aiming for perfect skin regeneration. Science 276: 75–81.
2. Adams DC, Ramsey ML (2005) Grafts in dermatologic surgery: review and update on full-and split-thickness skin grafts, free cartilage grafts, and composite grafts. Dermatol Surg 31: 1055–1067.
3. Priya SG, Jungvid H, Kumar A (2008) Skin tissue engineering for tissue repair and regeneration. Tissue Eng Part B Rev 14: 105–118.
4. Ignatova M, Manolova N, Markova N, Rashkov I (2009) Electrospun non-woven nanofibrous hybrid mats based on chitosan and PLA for wound-dressing applications. Macromol Biosci 9: 102–111.
5. Hajiali H, Shahgasempour S, Naimi-Jamal MR, Peirovi H (2011) Electrospun PGA/gelatin nanofibrous scaffolds and their potential application in vascular tissue engineering. Int J Nanomedicine 6: 2133–2141.
6. Liu SJ, Kau YC, Chou CY, Chen JK, Wu RC, et al. (2010) Electrospun PLGA/collagen nanofibrous membrane as early-stage wound dressing. J Memb Sci 355: 53–59.
7. Chong EJ, Phan TT, Lim IJ, Zhang YZ, Bay BH, et al. (2007) Evaluation of electrospun PCL/gelatin nanofibrous scaffold for wound healing and layered dermal reconstitution. Acta Biomater 3: 321–330.
8. Lee SH, Kim BS, Kim SH, Choi SW, Jeong SI, et al. (2003) Elastic biodegradable poly(glycolide-co-caprolactone) scaffold for tissue engineering. J Biomed Mater Res A 66: 29–37.
9. Jeong SI, Kim SH, Kim YH, Jung Y, Kwon JH, et al. (2004) Manufacture of elastic biodegradable PLCL scaffolds for mechano-active vascular tissue engineering. J Biomater Sci Polym Ed 15: 645–660.
10. Kim SH, Kwon JH, Chung MS, Chung E, Jung Y, et al. (2006) Fabrication of a new tubular fibrous PLCL scaffold for vascular tissue engineering. J Biomater Sci Polym Ed 17: 1359–1374.
11. Jeong B, Bae YH, Lee DS, Kim SW (1997) Biodegradable block copolymers as injectable drug-delivery systems. Nature 388: 860–862.
12. Spitzenberger TJ, Heilman D, Diekmann C, Batrakova EV, Kabanov AV, et al. (2006) Novel delivery system enhances efficacy of antiretroviral therapy in animal model for HIV-1 encephalitis. J Cereb Blood Flow Metab 27: 1033–1042.
13. Gómez-Guillén MC, Giménez B, López-Caballero ME, Montero MP (2011) Functional and bioactive properties of collagen and gelatin from alternative sources: A review. Food Hydrocoll 25: 1813–1827.
14. Fu Y, Xu K, Zheng X, Giacomin AJ, Mix AW, et al. (2012) 3D cell entrapment in crosslinked thiolated gelatin-poly (ethylene glycol) diacrylate hydrogels. Biomaterials 33: 48–58.
15. Watanabe R, Hayashi R, Kimura Y, Tanaka Y, Kageyama T, et al. (2011) A novel gelatin hydrogel carrier sheet for corneal endothelial transplantation. Tissue Eng Part A 17: 2213–2219.
16. Mo X, Iwata H, Ikada Y (2010) A tissue adhesives evaluated in vitro and in vivo analysis. J Biomed Mater Res A 94: 326–332.
17. Mo X, Iwata H, Matsuda S, Ikada Y (2000) Soft tissue adhesive composed of modified gelatin and polysaccharides. J Biomater Sci Polym Ed 11: 341–351.
18. Seliktar D (2012) Designing cell-compatible hydrogels for biomedical applications. Science 336: 1124–1128.
19. Li WJ, Laurencin CT, Caterson EJ, Tuan RS, Ko FK (2002) Electrospun nanofibrous structure: a novel scaffold for tissue engineering. J Biomed Mater Res 60: 613–621.
20. Li D, Frey MW, Joo YL (2006) Characterization of nanofibrous membranes with capillary flow porometry. J Memb Sci 286: 104–114.
21. Supp DM, Boyce ST (2005) Engineered skin substitutes: practices and potentials. Clin Dermatol 23: 403–412.
22. Boyce ST, Warden GD (2002) Principles and practices for treatment of cutaneous wounds with cultured skin substitutes. Am J Surg 183: 445–456.
23. Kuwazuru O, Saothong J, Yoshikawa N (2008) Mechanical approach to aging and wrinkling of human facial skin based on the multistage buckling theory. Med Eng Phys 30: 516–522.
24. Pailler-Mattei C, Bec S, Zahouani H (2008) In vivo measurements of the elastic mechanical properties of human skin by indentation tests. Med Eng Phys 30: 599–606.
25. Hassanzadeh P, Kharaziha M, Nikkhah M, Shin SR, Jin J, et al. (2013). Chitin nanofiber micropatterned flexible substrates for tissue engineering. J Mater Chem B Mater Biol Med 1: 4217–4224.
26. Sun X, Cheng L, Zhao J, Jin R, Sun B, et al. (2014). bFGF-grafted electrospun fibrous scaffolds via poly (dopamine) for skin wound healing. J Mater Chem B Mater Biol Med 2: 3636–3645.
27. Rieger KA, Birch NP, Schiffman JD (2013). Designing electrospun nanofiber mats to promote wound healing–a review. J Mater Chem B Mater Biol Med 1: 4531–4541.
28. Kim Y, Kim G (2013). Collagen/alginate scaffolds comprising core (PCL)-shell (collagen/alginate) struts for hard tissue regeneration: fabrication, characterisation, and cellular activities. J Mater Chem B Mater Biol Med 1: 3185–3194.
29. Jung Y, Kim SH, You HJ, Kim SH, Kim YH, et al. (2008) Application of an elastic biodegradable poly (L-lactide-co-ε-caprolactone) scaffold for cartilage tissue regeneration. J Biomater Sci Polym Ed 19: 1073–1085.
30. Jeong SI, Lee AY, Lee YM, Shin H (2008). Electrospun gelatin/poly (L-lactide-co-ε-caprolactone) nanofibers for mechanically functional tissue-engineering scaffolds. J Biomater Sci Polym Ed 19: 339–357.
31. Batrakova EV, Kabanov AV (2008) Pluronic block copolymers: evolution of drug delivery concept from inert nanocarriers to biological response modifiers. J Control Release 130: 98–106.
32. Jin G, Prabhakaran MP, Ramakrishna S (2011) Stem cell differentiation to epidermal lineages on electrospun nanofibrous substrates for skin tissue engineering. Acta Biomater 7: 3113–3122.
33. Heimbach DM, Warden GD, Luterman A, Jordan MH, Ozobia N, et al. (2003) Multicenter postapproval clinical trial of Integra dermal regeneration template for burn treatment. J Burn Care Rehabil 24: 42–48.
34. Peppas NA, Huang Y, Torres-Lugo M, Ward JH, Zhang J (2000) Physicochemical foundations and structural design of hydrogels in medicine and biology. Annu Rev Biomed Eng 2: 9–29.
35. Lin G, Cosimbescu L, Karin NJ, Gutowska A, Tarasevich BJ (2013) Injectable and thermogelling hydrogels of PCL-g-PEG: mechanisms, rheological and enzymatic degradation properties. J Mater Chem B Mater Biol Med 1: 1249–1255.
36. Ding F, Shi X, Jiang Z, Liu L, Cai J, et al. (2013) Electrochemically stimulated drug release from dual stimuli responsive chitin hydrogel. J Mater Chem B - Mater Biol Med 1: 1729–1737.
37. Yu L, Ding J (2008) Injectable hydrogels as unique biomedical materials. Chem Soc Rev 37: 1473–1481.
38. Kretlow JD, Klouda L, Mikos AG (2007) Injectable matrices and scaffolds for drug delivery in tissue engineering. Adv Drug Deliv Rev 59: 263–273.
39. Kirsner RS, Eaglstein WH (1993) The wound healing process. Dermatol Clin 11: 629–640.

13

A Novel Model of Human Skin Pressure Ulcers in Mice

Andrés A. Maldonado[1]*, Lara Cristóbal[1], Javier Martín-López[2], Mar Mallén[3], Natalio García-Honduvilla[4], Julia Buján[4]

1 Department of Plastic and Reconstructive Surgery and Burn Unit, University Hospital of Getafe, Madrid, Spain, **2** Department of Pathology, University Hospital of Puerta de Hierro, Madrid, Spain, **3** Department of Genetics, University Hospital Central de la Defensa, Madrid, Spain, **4** Department of Medical Specialties, Faculty of Medicine, University of Alcalá, Networking Research Centre on Bioengineering, Biomaterials and Nanomedicine (CIBER-BBN), Madrid, Spain

Abstract

Introduction: Pressure ulcers are a prevalent health problem in today's society. The shortage of suitable animal models limits our understanding and our ability to develop new therapies. This study aims to report on the development of a novel and reproducible human skin pressure ulcer model in mice.

Material and Methods: Male non-obese, diabetic, severe combined immunodeficiency mice (n = 22) were engrafted with human skin. A full-thickness skin graft was placed onto 4×3 cm wounds created on the dorsal skin of the mice. Two groups with permanent grafts were studied after 60 days. The control group (n = 6) was focused on the process of engraftment. Evaluations were conducted with photographic assessment, histological analysis and fluorescence in situ hybridization (FISH) techniques. The pressure ulcer group (n = 12) was created using a compression device. A pressure of 150 mmHg for 8 h, with a total of three cycles of compression-release was exerted. Evaluations were conducted with photographic assessment and histological analysis.

Results: Skin grafts in the control group took successfully, as shown by visual assessment, FISH techniques and histological analysis. Pressure ulcers in the second group showed full-thickness skin loss with damage and necrosis of all the epidermal and dermal layers (ulcer stage III) in all cases. Complete repair occurred after 40 days.

Conclusions: An inexpensive, reproducible human skin pressure ulcer model has been developed. This novel model will facilitate the development of new clinically relevant therapeutic strategies that can be tested directly on human skin.

Editor: Amit Gefen, Tel Aviv University, Israel

Funding: This study was supported by a Grant from the Fundación MAPFRE (SA/11/AYU/444). The funders had no role in study design, data collection and analysis, decision to publish, or preparation of the manuscript.

Competing Interests: The authors have declared that no competing interests exist.

* Email: mail@andresmaldonado.es

Introduction

Pressure ulcers (PU) are a high-prevalence problem in our society. It is estimated that 1.3 million to 3 million adults have a PU, with an estimated cost of $500 to $40,000 to heal each ulcer. The incidence varies greatly by clinical setting; in the hospital, for example, the incidence is estimated to be 0.4% to 38.0% [1].

Although conservative management is conducted in clinical practice (e.g., postural changes, dressing care), there is great disparity in the approach and management of these patients [2,3]. According to the American and European Pressure Ulcer Advisory Panel guidelines, nutrition is an important aspect of a comprehensive care plan for prevention and treatment of pressure ulcers (although limited evidence-based research is available) [4]. Moreover, according to Thomas [5], prescriptions should be individually tailored to persons with pressure ulcers with regard to both macro- and micronutrients. Surgical treatment is used in only a small numbers of patients. However Larson and others advocate good results with a surgical approach (without consideration of nutritional status or osteomyelitis) [6], while other authors have reported a high recurrence rate with this method [7,8].

Approaches incorporating cellular therapy and growth factors are thought to be on the horizon. The combined clinical evidence on platelet-derived growth factor (PDGF) suggests that PDGF-BB may improve healing of pressure ulcers. However, the evidence is not sufficient to recommend this treatment for routine use [9]. According to Akita et al. [10] adipose-derived stem cells can promote human dermal fibroblast proliferation by directly contacting cells and via paracrine activation in the re-epithelialization phase of wound healing. Moreover, skin substitutes were made by employing advanced tissue-engineering approaches and have been used for clinical applications, promoting the healing of acute and chronic wounds [11]. For example, bilayered bioengineered human skin equivalent (Apligraf, Novartis) has been shown to be efficacious in a case study of patients with heel PUs (level IV evidence) [12]. Additionally, growth factors could be another alternative to stem cells. According to Yang et al. [13], the expression of VEGF and bFGF in PU tissue is decreased. This leads to a reduction in angiogenesis, which may be a crucial factor in the formation of PUs.

Regarding the etiology of PUs, external pressure is viewed as the main factor. Other patient-specific factors leading to derangement in tissue perfusion may account for an observed development of a pressure ulcer [14]. It is well known that ischemia-reperfusion injury contributes to the pathophysiology of PUs more significantly than a single, prolonged ischemic insult [15]. The animal models described in the literature employ a variety of devices to apply localized pressure on the back of mouse skin, and many of these models use external magnets; this technique is based on the repetition of ischemia-reperfusion cycles [16–19]. However, all of these models are based on mouse skin, which could be a potential limitation to studying the effect of human stem cells or growth factors in the PU environment.

From our point of view, the shortage of suitable animal models together with the ethical and practical considerations for humans limits our understanding of PUs and the development of new therapies. This study aims to report a novel and reproducible PU model of human skin graft. Cell therapy, growth factors and other techniques could be applied directly to human skin instead of mouse skin.

Material and Methods

Animals

Three-week-old, male, non-obese diabetic/severe combined immunodeficiency (NOD.CB17-Prkdscid/NCrHsd) mice (n = 22) (Harlan Laboratories S.r.l. Barcelona, Spain) were used in this study. All mice were caged under standard light and temperature conditions with free access to food and water throughout the study. All experimental procedures were made to minimize suffering and they were approved by the local committee for animal welfare and were conducted in accordance with the European Community Council Directive (86/609/EEC). The ethical Committee at University of Alcalá (Madrid, Spain) approved this research.

Human skin grafts

Mice were engrafted under general anesthesia (Ohmeda, BOC Health Care) with female human skin. All human skin came from abdominoplasty or breast reduction procedures. Ethics committee from University of Alcalá (Madrid, Spain) was approved and written informed consent from all patients was obtained. Full-thickness skin grafts (FTSGs) were placed onto a 4×3 cm wound created with scalpel on the dorsal skin of the animals. Mice skin was incised down to the muscle and removed, exposing muscular layer. FTSGs were sutured in place with 4/0 nylon. Postoperative analgesia (meloxicam and buprenorphine) was provided for 3 days and the dressing was tied on for the first 5 days. Special care was taken with sterilization and postoperative animal handling due to the immunodeficient status of the mice. A total of 4 mice died in the immediate postoperative period.

Mice were classified into two groups after 60 days with permanent human skin grafts. In the control group (n = 6), mice were sacrificed after 190 days and the FTSG was removed to study the engraftment process.

Pressure ulcers

In the PU group (n = 12), mice were placed in a compression device (Fig. 1A) following the method described by Stadler et al. [17] and modified by our group in terms of the device and the timing. A modified pressure device (7 mm×5 mm) that delivered a pressure of 150 mmHg to the human FTSG was used. The exerted pressure was measured with a dynamometer (Fig. 1B). Three cycles of compression-release (8 hours of clamping after 16 hours of no compression) were applied to the human FTSG. This group was subdivided into two groups. From the first one (n = 6), biopsies were taken at 5, 25, 45 and 130 days post-cycle. From the second subgroup (n = 6), animals were used to assess PU evolution by photographic analysis. All animals were sacrificed after 190 days.

Macroscopic analysis

At the macroscopic level, the behavior of the graft was evaluated every 15 days for 60 days in the control group. In the PU group, the PU was evaluated every 7 days for 130 days after compression cycles. The evolution of the graft was analyzed morphometrically (ImageJ for Windows XP NIH Image) using photographs from days 0 to 190. These measurements were taken by 2 independent researchers who were blinded to the treatment group. The values are expressed as the means ± standard deviation.

Microscopic evaluation

At the end of the experiments, tissue specimens were collected for different studies and placed in 10% buffered formaldehyde, Bouin and Carnoy. Then the samples were dehydrated and embedded in paraffin. Tissue sections (5 µm-thick) passing through the center plane of each wound were stained with hematoxylin-eosin and Masson's trichrome for morphological assessment. Cytogenetic analysis using fluorescence in situ hybridization (FISH) for the X and Y chromosomes (sonde XA X/Y, D-5608-100-OG, MetaSystems GmbH) was also performed.

Statistical analysis

Areas of the FTSG were compared among treatment groups by ANOVA followed by the Mann-Whitney U test. Differences with $p<0.05$ were considered statistically significant.

Results

Human skin grafts

Stable human FTSGs from the control groups took successfully, as demonstrated by photographic assessment (Fig. 2A). Macro-

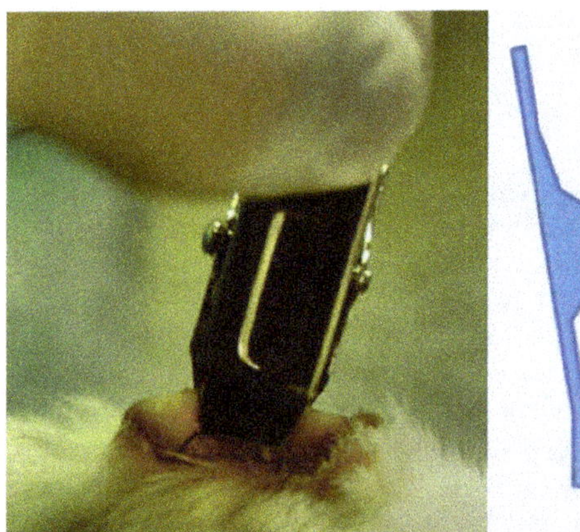

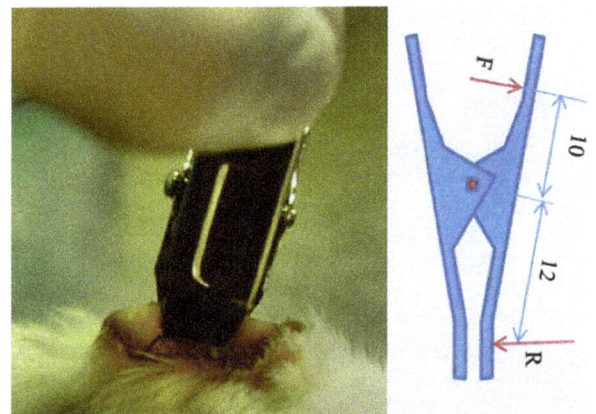

Figure 1. Compression device on the human full-thickness skin graft delivering a pressure of 150 mmHg. A, three cycles of compression (8 h of clamping after 16 h of no compression) were delivered to the human skin graft to generate the pressure ulcer. B, schematic representation of the compression device. F= force generated by the spring. R= force generated by the compression device.

scopically, the graft was soft and pliable after 60 days, resembling normal human skin (Fig. 1A–d). Human FTSGs showed uniform behavior in all studied animals. The FTSGs featured normal coloration (Fig. 2A–a) during the first few days but successively transformed into crusty skin over the first 30 days (Figs. 2A–b and 2A–c). This crust progressively disappeared and was replaced by a fully re-epithelialized area resembling normal and fine human skin after 60 days (Fig. 2A–d). Morphometrical analysis showed the effect of the contraction and retraction of the grafted skin. An important retraction of 33% of the graft was observed in the first 7 days. A progressive decrease with a retraction of 71% after 120 days was reached (Fig. 3).

In the histological analysis, a panoramic view showed (Fig. 4A) a clear delimitation between the human skin and the mouse skin. The presence of well-preserved human skin could be observed in the center of the graft which was formed by a stratified epidermis on a dermis with many papillae, resembling human skin. At higher magnification, keratinized squamous epithelium was observed on a papillae dermis with pressure corpuscles. A lymphocytic infiltrate was randomly distributed without specific accumulations. Human dermis (superficial and deep level) was well vascularized, which implies graft stability. The human skin was surrounded by a discrete and well-vascularized dermal layer from the receptor tissue (mouse). The host tissue presented the usual features of mouse skin. This animal model had a fine skin, two or three layers of keratinocytes, a papillary dermis with well-preserved hair follicles and a deep dermis with great development of adipose tissue.

The human tissue over the mouse receptors was assessed using the FISH technique (Fig. 5). Chromosomes XX from the human skin and chromosomes XY from the mouse skin were found as green-green dots (X-X) and green-red dots (X-Y). Most cells showing the Y chromosome (red dot) appeared to correspond to mouse cells infiltrating the human tissue.

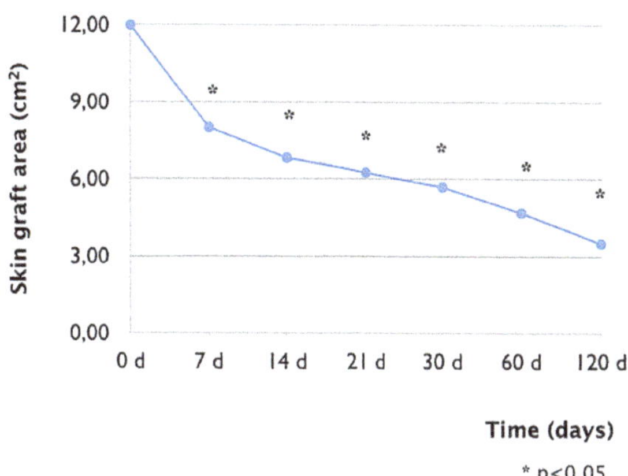

Figure 3. Area in cm^2 of the human full thickness skin graft on the back of the mice during the first 120 days after surgery. A significant reduction of the skin graft can be observed during the first week after the transplantation.

Pressure ulcers

Placing the compression device on the human skin graft for three cycles induced irreversible damage, characterizing a PU (Fig. 2B). A dermoepidermal necrotic fold covering the entire longitudinal extension under the site of the compression device was observed day 1 post-cycle (Fig. 2B–b). The ischemia produced

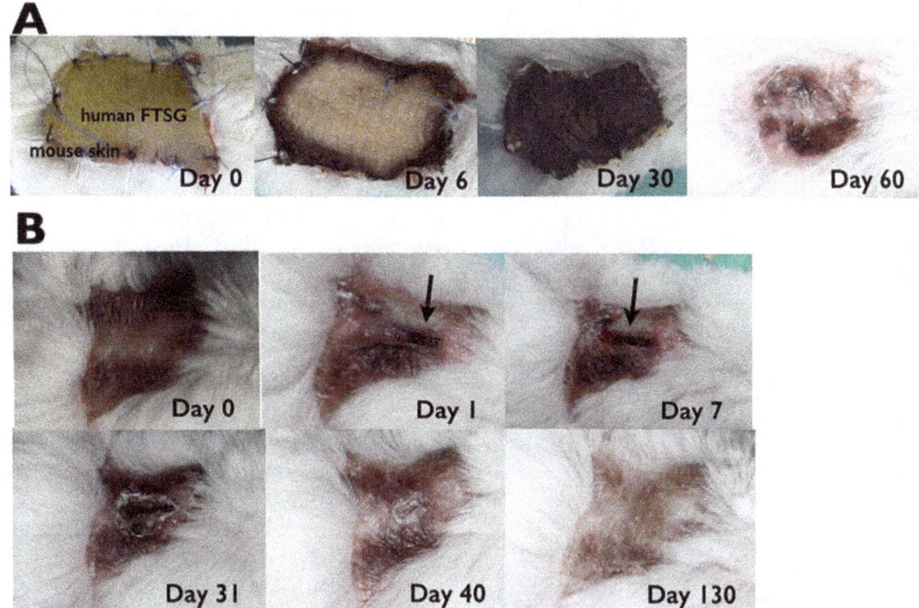

Figure 2. Photographic evolution of the human skin graft in mice. A, human full-thickness skin graft evolution from the control group. (a) Day of surgery. (b) Day 6 after surgery. (c) Day 30 after surgery. (d) Day 60 after surgery. Macroscopically, the graft was soft and pliable, resembling normal human skin. Note that the stable human full-thickness skin graft from the control groups took successfully. B, human full-thickness skin graft evolution after placing the compression device for three cycles. (a) Day before the compression device was applied. (b) Day 1 after the three compression cycles. The human skin graft remained folded with a hemorrhagic area in the center of the fold (see arrow). (c) Day 7 after compression cycles. Irreversible damage characterizing a PU can be observed. The center of the fold was occupied by a necrotic and hemorrhagic area (see arrow). (d) Day 31 after the compression cycles. Crusty remnants were observed. (e) Day 40 after compression cycles. Only a small central crusted island could be observed. (f) Day 130 after compression cycles. Complete regeneration of the graft was noticed.

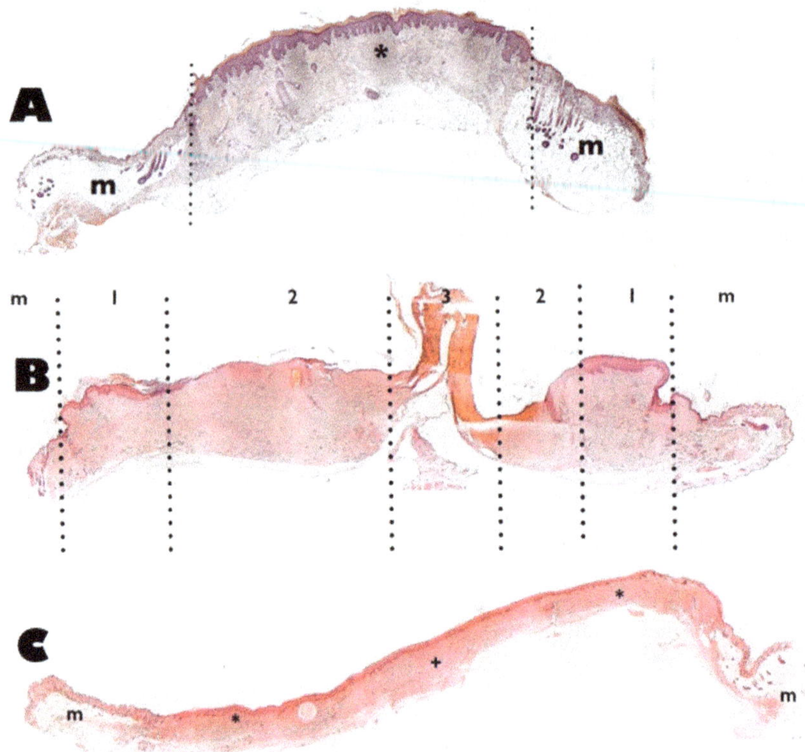

Figure 4. Histological analysis (H&E at 5x, panoramic view) of the mouse and human skin. A, human skin taken 60 days after placement of the human full-thickness skin graft. A clear delimitation between the normal human skin (*) and the mouse skin (m) can be observed. The transition between human and mouse skin has been marked with dotted lines. B, pressure ulcer over the human full-thickness skin graft. 7 days post-compression cycles. Pressure ulcer tissue can be observed as a consequence of mechanical damage. Four zones can be differentiated: m = receptor mouse skin; zone 1 = normal human skin; zone 2 = medium damage human skin; zone 3 = maximal damage human skin. C, 130 days post-compression cycles. A central area with a stratified epithelium over a non-papillary neodermis (+), a homogeneous and uniform human skin (*) and receptor mouse skin tissue (m) can be observed.

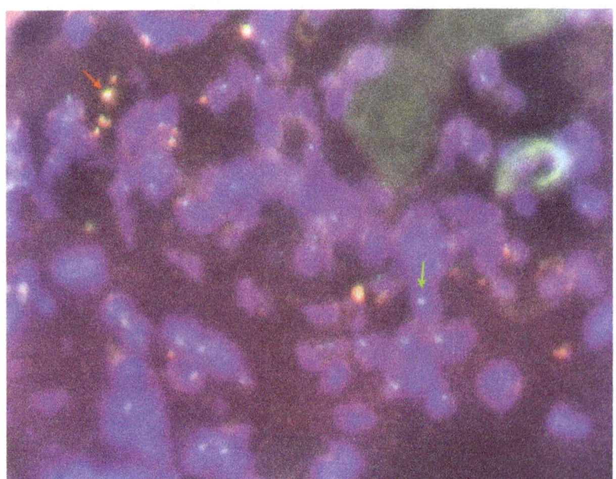

Figure 5. Fluorescence in situ hybridization (FISH) for chromosomes XX and XY. Chromosomes XX from the female human skin and chromosome XY from the male mouse skin were found as green-green dots (X-X, see green arrow) and green-red dots (X-Y, see red arrow). Most cells showing the Y chromosome (red dot) appeared to correspond to mouse cells infiltrating the human tissue.

over the next few days continued to bleed on day 7 post-cycle (Fig. 2B–c). Then, a further evolution towards a retracted and elevated lesion with crusty edges with underlying granulation tissue was observed (Fig. 2B–d). The appearance of the lesion changed completely on day 40 due to the loss of the crust and the formation of a sclerotic surface (Fig. 2B–e). Fully recovered dermoepidermal tissue then emerged. The stability of the human skin graft even after recovery of the PU was striking; the human skin had completely recovered after 130 days (Figs. 2B–a vs. 2B–f).

Histological analysis of the injured human skin was performed systematically in mice at various intervals (days 5, 25, 45 and 130 days post-cycle) after the three ischemic periods of 8 hours. Tissue ischemia was observed during the first days after the cycles of compression as a consequence of mechanical damage (Fig. 4B), reminiscent of PU tissue. The effect of the compression device induced potent tissue degeneration, necrosis in the center and full thickness skin loss involving subcutaneous tissue damage (stage III pressure ulcer). Tissue with a "U" shape was formed by dermal collagen residues. The edges of the tissue were also affected by loss of epithelialization, vascularization and cell population (Fig. 4B, zone 3). These edges were followed by skin areas showing denuded surface, epithelial desquamation and small surface areas covered with crust. The superficial dermis was composed of thick bundles of acellular collagen, while the deep dermis showed signs of cell habitability (Fig. 4B, zone 2). Compression effects were not observed in remote areas (Fig. 4B, zone l). Finally, this area was bordered by the recipient mouse tissue (Fig. 4B, zone m). The evolution of this tissue damage was studied. Total tissue recovery was observed after 130 days. Fig. 4C shows a sagittal section of the human FTSG. The repair capacity of the human skin could be assessed; zones 1 and 2 of the previous figure (Fig. 4B) were replaced by a homogeneous and uniform human skin, showing the characteristics expected for a reparative epithelium after a significant injury. The central area of Figure 4C (zone 3 in Fig. 4B) showed a stratified epithelium over a non-papillary dermis, which is characteristic of neodermis.

Discussion

Human skin grafts

In our initial experiments, human FTSG rejection was observed in all mice using semiathymic and athymic nude mice (unpublished results). Although several papers have reported human skin transplantation to the nude mice, [20–24] hypertrophic scarring of the tissue developed instead of viable normal human skin. Yang et al. [24] postulated that although nude mice are immunologically defective of T cells, there might be other immune mechanisms involved, most likely related to the strong antigenicity of the skin, remnant T cells in nude mice (extrathymic lymphocyte populations) and the enhanced role of macrophages and natural killer cells. In the same way, Lin et al. [25] published that NK cells and macrophages could be activated in the absence of T cells or xenoantibodies to directly reject xenografts. To solve this problem, male NOD.CB17-Prkdscid/NCrHsd mice were used in our model. No graft rejection was observed and a viable normal human skin was achieved after 60 days.

Other models of human skin transplantation on mice were used in order to study the rejection process. Murray et al. [26,27] transplanted 7×7 mm skin graft on a C.B-17 SCID mice. Changes that resembled skin rejection in humans were observed after 2 weeks. Waldron-Lynch et al. [28] used neonatal NOD/SCID/IL2Rc cnull mice, reconstituted with human CD34+ hematopoietic stem cells. A murine skin transplant model in humanized mice was used to test human monoclonal antibody therapy. Racki et al. [29] studied human skin transplantation on immunodeficient mice and rejection following engraftment of allogeneic peripheral blood mononuclear cells. They transplanted 1.5 cm^2 human skin graft onto NOD-scid $IL2r\gamma^{null}$ and CB17-scid bg for this purpose. Although all these models are useful for studying the immunology system and the rejection process, non of them provide enough dimensions of normal human skin as our model. Even when a fully new re-epithelialized area resembling normal and fine human skin was available after 60 days, the graft dimensions were about 5 cm^2. Although it is a 60% less than the initial dimensions (12 cm^2), this area should be enough to study the PU process or other possible skin damage.

Other models have used genetically engineered human skin on the backs of NOD/SCID mice [30–32]. Selected keratinocytes were assembled in a live fibroblast-containing fibrin dermal matrix orthotopically grafted onto mice. Although the authors presented stable human bilayer skin, we could not apply this to our model because human dermis is a more complex structure with a key role in PU generation and resolution.

Our model is based on a four-month stable human FTSG with complete dermal and epidermal layers. Studies have focused on the progress and shrinking of the graft and on the re-epithelialization after the generation of a PU. The graft has shown a high rate of shrinkage in the implant site, specially during the first 7 days. This process, which is known as primary contraction, is the immediate recoil of freshly harvested grafts as a result of the elastin in the dermis. The more dermis the graft has, the more primary the contraction that will be experienced [33]. In our model, more than half of the original size of the graft was observed after the FTSG reached a stable phase. The maximum dimensions of the back of the mice (4×3 cm) were used to achieve enough human graft after 60 days to develop the PU. The evolution of the graft was towards the initial formation of a crust related to the dermal and epidermal surface area of the graft. After 60 days, the FTSG site was denuded of a crusty layer and a new intensely keratinized and vascularized human stratified epithelium was formed.

Therefore, based on these results, we have used this experimental model to induce PUs in human skin. Skin stability was observed up to 190 days after the FTSG surgery, which demonstrates the effectiveness of our experimental model.

Pressure ulcers

PU models have been developed using mouse skin [17–19,34,35]. Our model presents a true human skin pressure ulcer model for the first time (see Table 1).

Based on the PU model presented by Stadler et al. [17], we used an original modification, replacing magnets with a mechanical compression device delivering a known, constant and controlled pressure. A modification of the magnet model was published by Wassermann et al. [18] A steel disk was implanted under the gluteus maximus muscle and pressure cycles were applied in conjunction with a magnet. This method could potentially damage the tissue underlying the implanted steel disk and, in particular, the area where the human FTSG was placed in our model. Our model differs from other models because the pressure exerted by the magnets depends on the thickness of the fold and on the position of the magnet. Moreover, we found it more reproducible to put forceps in the same position after every cycle than magnetic disks. After 3 cycles of 8 hours of clamping, irreversible tissue ischemia led to tissue necrosis, which was visible a week after the last cycle. This tissue damage was observed as an ulcer on the edges of the compression device and in the underlying deep dermal and subcutaneous tissue (stage III pressure ulcer).

Ulceration and bleeding could be observed for the rest of the first month. In all cases, recovery of the tissue continuity was evident after 40 days, which corroborated the notion that our model of ischemia had been successful in obtaining an experimental transient PU over human skin. Regenerated epidermis was characterized as a keratinized epidermis without melanocytes and with no papillary dermis, as in human skin defects. The underlying dermis demonstrated parallel bundles of mature collagen with new vascular components. Lymphocytic infiltrates were limited to the interface between the host (mouse) and the grafted (human) tissue.

This study has two main limitations. First, mice immunosuppression does not allow a normal inflammation process. However, as mentioned above, human PUs may be not only a pressure problem [14]. Systemic factors as diabetes, may produce decreased tissue perfusion, poor wound healing, slower epithelialization and immunosuppression [36]. We think that previous models [17–19,34] using completely healthy mice are distant from a clinical setting. Our immunosuppressed model would be more similar to the overall condition that many patients with PUs have: delayed wound healing, altered healing environment, etc. Moreover, from a histological point of view, our model would be more analogous to human PUs than previous models. Nevertheless, further improvements of the model remain to be performed. The second limitation involves the damaged adipose tissue under the human skin. Adipocyte cells come from the mouse, not from the human

Table 1. Characteristics of the different published pressure ulcer models.

Model	Animal	Compression device	Cycles	Tissue
Stadler et al. (2004){Stadler:2004jx}	BALB/c mouse	magnetic plates	12 h compression - 12 h release	mouse skin
Reid et al. (2004){Reid:2004ee}	C57BL/6J mouse	magnetic plates	1, 2 or 5 cycles/day of 0.5 h	mouse skin
Wassermann et al. (2009){Wassermann:2009ba}	Balb/c nu/nu nude mouse	neodymium magnet	2 h compression - 1 h release	mouse skin
Garza-Rodea et al. (2011){delaGarzaRodea:2011 kq}	NOD-LtSz-scid/scid/J mouse	magnetic disks	Only one cycle (4/8/12/14/20 h of clamping)	mouse skin
Maldonado et al.	NOD.CB17-Prkdscid/NCrHsd mouse	forceps	8 h compression - 16 h release	human skin

graft. Although that could be a limitation, we think that it should not affect the cicatrization process as the dermis and epidermis play the main role.

We believe this PU model could represent the most similar situation to human PUs at this time. Further research into any kinds of cellular (i.e. stem cells) or molecular therapies (i.e. growth factors) could be tested directly on damaged human skin after pressure without the ethical issues involved with research in humans. As we described above, the cicatrization time of this model is well-known. Improving this process on our model with new therapies, could potentially mean a direct application in the healing of human PUs.

Conclusions

To our knowledge, this is the first model where PU has been developed over human skin. In comparison with other mouse skin PU models, future therapies applied in our human skin model could be more realistically extrapolated to a human PU. We think it opens up prospects for testing different cellular or molecular therapies directly over human skin.

Acknowledgments

We thank Dr. Purificación Holguín and all the staff of the Department of Plastic Surgery and Burns, University Hospital of Getafe, Madrid, Spain; Dr. Mario Arenillas (Fundación para la Investigación Biomédica of Getafe, Spain) and Dr. José Carrasco (Department of Materials, School of Mines of Madrid, Spain).

Author Contributions

Conceived and designed the experiments: AAM LC NGH JB. Performed the experiments: AAM LC JML MM. Analyzed the data: AAM LC. Contributed reagents/materials/analysis tools: AAM LC. Wrote the paper: AAM LC JB.

References

1. Lyder CH (2003) Pressure ulcer prevention and management. JAMA 289: 223–226.
2. Levine SM, Stadler I, Sinno S, Zhang R-Y, Oskoui P, et al. (2013) Current thoughts for the prevention and treatment of pressure ulcers: using the evidence to determine fact or fiction. Ann Surg 257: 603–608.
3. Moore Z, Cowman S (2008) A systematic review of wound cleansing for pressure ulcers. J Clin Nurs 17: 1963–1972.
4. Dorner B, Posthauer ME, Thomas D, National Pressure Ulcer Advisor Panely (2009) The role of nutrition in pressure ulcer prevention and treatment: National Pressure Ulcer Advisory Panel white paper. Adv Skin Wound Care 22: 212–221.
5. Thomas DR (2014) Role of Nutrition in the Treatment and Prevention of Pressure Ulcers. Nutr Clin Pract 29: 466–472.
6. Larson DL, Hudak KA, Waring WP, Orr MR, Simonelic K (2012) Protocol management of late-stage pressure ulcers: a 5-year retrospective study of 101 consecutive patients with 179 ulcers. Plast Reconstr Surg 129: 897–904.
7. Kierney PC, Engrav LH, Isik FF, Esselman PC, Cardenas DD, et al. (1998) Results of 268 pressure sores in 158 patients managed jointly by plastic surgery and rehabilitation medicine. Plast Reconstr Surg 102: 765–772.
8. Keys KA, Daniali LN, Warner KJ, Mathes DW (2010) Multivariate predictors of failure after flap coverage of pressure ulcers. Plast Reconstr Surg 125: 1725–1734.
9. Dealey C, Clark M, Defloor T, Schoonhoven L, Vanderwee K, et al. (2009) European Pressure Ulcer Advisory Panel and National Pressure Ulcer Advisory Panel. Treatment of pressure ulcers: Quick Reference Guide. Washington DC: National Pressure Ulcer Advisory Panel.
10. Akita S, Yoshimoto H, Akino K, Ohtsuru A, Hayashida K, et al. (2012) Early experiences with stem cells in treating chronic wounds. Clin Plast Surg 39: 281–292.
11. Groeber F, Holeiter M, Hampel M, Hinderer S, Schenke-Layland K (2012) Skin Tissue Engineering—In Vivo and In Vitro Applications. Clin Plast Surg 39: 33–58.
12. Karr J (2008) Utilization of living bilayered cell therapy (Apligraf) for heel ulcers. Adv Skin Wound Care 21: 270–274.
13. Yang J-J, Wang X-L, Shi B-W, Huang F (2013) The angiogenic peptide vascular endothelial growth factor-basic fibroblast growth factor signaling is up-regulated in a rat pressure ulcer model. Anat Rec (Hoboken) 296: 1161–1168.
14. Thomas DR (2010) Does pressure cause pressure ulcers? An inquiry into the etiology of pressure ulcers. J Am Med Dir Assoc 11: 397–405.
15. Tsuji S, Ichioka S, Sekiya N, Nakatsuka T (2005) Analysis of ischemia-reperfusion injury in a microcirculatory model of pressure ulcers. Wound Repair Regen 13: 209–215.
16. Peirce SM, Skalak TC, Rodeheaver GT (2000) Ischemia-reperfusion injury in chronic pressure ulcer formation: a skin model in the rat. Wound Repair Regen 8: 68–76.
17. Stadler I, Zhang R-Y, Oskoui P, Whittaker MBS, Lanzafame RJ (2004) Development of a Simple, Noninvasive, Clinically Relevant Model of Pressure Ulcers in the Mouse. J Invest Surg 17: 221–227.
18. Wassermann E, van Griensven M, Gstaltner K, Oehlinger W, Schrei K, et al. (2009) A chronic pressure ulcer model in the nude mouse. Wound Repair Regen 17: 480–484.
19. De la Garza-Rodea de AS, Knaän-Shanzer S, van Bekkum DW (2011) Pressure Ulcers: Description of a New Model and Use of Mesenchymal Stem Cells for Repair. Dermatology 223.
20. Kischer CW, Sheridan D, Pindur J (1989) Use of nude (athymic) mice for the study of hypertrophic scars and keloids: vascular continuity between mouse and implants. Anat Rec 225: 189–196.
21. Kischer CW, Wagner HN, Pindur J, Holubec H, Jones M, et al. (1989) Increased fibronectin production by cell lines from hypertrophic scar and keloid. Connect Tissue Res 23: 279–288.
22. Shetlar MR, Shetlar CL, Kischer CW, Pindur J (1991) Implants of keloid and hypertrophic scars into the athymic nude mouse: changes in the glycosaminoglycans of the implants. Connect Tissue Res 26: 23–36.
23. Wang J, Ding J, Jiao H, Honardoust D, Momtazi M, et al. (2011) Human hypertrophic scar-like nude mouse model: Characterization of the molecular and cellular biology of the scar process. Wound Repair Regen 19: 274–285.

24. Yang DY, Li SR, Wu JL, Chen YQ, Li G, et al. (2007) Establishment of a Hypertrophic Scar Model by Transplanting Full-Thickness Human Skin Grafts onto the Backs of Nude Mice. Plast Reconstr Surg 119: 104–109.
25. Lin Y, Vandeputte M, Waer M (1997) Natural killer cell- and macrophage-mediated rejection of concordant xenografts in the absence of T and B cell responses. J Immunol 158: 5658–5667.
26. Murray AG, Petzelbauer P, Hughes CC, Costa J, Askenase P, et al. (1994) Human T-cell-mediated destruction of allogeneic dermal microvessels in a severe combined immunodeficient mouse. Proc Natl Acad Sci USA 91: 9146–9150.
27. Murray AG, Schechner JS, Epperson DE, Sultan P, McNiff JM, et al. (1998) Dermal microvascular injury in the human peripheral blood lymphocyte reconstituted-severe combined immunodeficient (HuPBL-SCID) mouse/skin allograft model is T cell mediated and inhibited by a combination of cyclosporine and rapamycin. Am J Pathol 153: 627–638.
28. Waldron-Lynch F, Deng S, Preston-Hurlburt P, Henegariu O, Herold KC (2012) Analysis of human biologics with a mouse skin transplant model in humanized mice. Am J Transplant 12: 2652–2662.
29. Racki WJ, Covassin L, Brehm M, Pino S, Ignotz R, et al. (2010) NOD-scid IL2rgamma(null) mouse model of human skin transplantation and allograft rejection. Transplantation 89: 527–536.
30. Río M, Larcher F, Serrano F, Meana A, Muñoz M, et al. (2002) A Preclinical Model for the Analysis of Genetically Modified Human Skin In Vivo. Hum Gene Ther 13: 959–968.
31. García M, Escamez MJ, Carretero M, Mirones I, Martínez-Santamaría L, et al. (2007) Modeling normal and pathological processes through skin tissue engineering. Mol Carcinog 46: 741–745.
32. Carretero M, Guerrero-Aspizua S, Del Río M (2011) Applicability of bioengineered human skin: From preclinical skin humanized mouse models to clinical regenerative therapies. Biobugs 2: 203–207.
33. Thorne C, Grabb WC, Beasley RW (2007) Techniques and principles in Plastic Surgery. Grabb and Smith's Plastic Surgery. 6th ed. Philadelphia: Lippincott Williams & Wilkins. pp. 7.
34. Reid RR, Sull AC, Mogford JE, Roy N, Mustoe TA (2004) A novel murine model of cyclical cutaneous ischemia-reperfusion injury. J Surg Res 116: 172–180.
35. Salcido R, Popescu A, Ahn C (2007) Animal models in pressure ulcer research. J Spinal Cord Med 30: 107–116.
36. Gantwerker EA, Hom DB (2012) Skin: Histology and Physiology of Wound Healing. Clin Plast Surg 39: 85–97.

14

Survival of Skin Graft between Transgenic Cloned Dogs and Non-Transgenic Cloned Dogs

Geon A Kim[1], Hyun Ju Oh[1], Min Jung Kim[1], Young Kwang Jo[1], Jin Choi[1], Jung Eun Park[1], Eun Jung Park[1], Sang Hyun Lim[2], Byung Il Yoon[3], Sung Keun Kang[2], Goo Jang[1], Byeong Chun Lee[1]*

1 Department of Theriogenology & Biotechnology, College of Veterinary Medicine, Seoul National University, Seoul, Republic of Korea, **2** Central Research Institutes, K-stem cell, Seoul, Republic of Korea, **3** Laboratory of Histology and Molecular Pathogenesis, College of Veterinary Medicine, Kangwon National University, Chuncheon, Gangwon-do, Republic of Korea

Abstract

Whereas it has been assumed that genetically modified tissues or cells derived from somatic cell nuclear transfer (SCNT) should be accepted by a host of the same species, their immune compatibility has not been extensively explored. To identify acceptance of SCNT-derived cells or tissues, skin grafts were performed between cloned dogs that were identical except for their mitochondrial DNA (mtDNA) haplotypes and foreign gene. We showed here that differences in mtDNA haplotypes and genetic modification did not elicit immune responses in these dogs: 1) skin tissues from genetically-modified cloned dogs were successfully transplanted into genetically-modified cloned dogs with different mtDNA haplotype under three successive grafts over 63 days; and 2) non-transgenic cloned tissues were accepted into transgenic cloned syngeneic recipients with different mtDNA haplotypes and vice versa under two successive grafts over 63 days. In addition, expression of the inserted gene was maintained, being functional without eliciting graft rejection. In conclusion, these results show that transplanting genetically-modified tissues into normal, syngeneic or genetically-modified recipient dogs with different mtDNA haplotypes do not elicit skin graft rejection or affect expression of the inserted gene. Therefore, therapeutically valuable tissue derived from SCNT with genetic modification might be used safely in clinical applications for patients with diseased tissues.

Editor: Pascale Chavatte-Palmer, INRA, France

Funding: This study was supported by Rural Development Administration (#PJ008975022014), Korea Institute of Planning and Evaluation for Technology (#311062-04-3SB010), NATURE CELL (#2014-0082), Research Institute for Veterinary Science, Nestle Purina PetCare, Natural Balance Korea, and the BK21 plus program. The funders had no role in study design, data collection and analysis, decision to publish, or preparation of the manuscript.

Competing Interests: The authors received funding from NATURE CELL CO., LTD, Nestle Purina PetCare, and Natural Balance Korea. There are no further patents, products in development or marketed products to declare. This does not alter our adherence to all the PLOS ONE policies on sharing data and materials.

* Email: bclee@snu.ac.kr

Introduction

Somatic cell nuclear transfer (SCNT) produces genetically identical cloned animals [1]. Moreover, canine SCNT combined with transgenic technologies can make genetically identical cloned dogs with functional genetic modifications that could be used for gene therapy [2]. For example, transgenic cloned dogs could be used in replacement of diseased (malfunctioning/worn out) organs. However, tissues derived from transgenic cloned dogs, reprogrammed from somatic cells with enucleated oocytes, had not yet investigated whether they are immunologically identical tissues or cell sources of transplantation. Especially, effects of red fluorescent protein (RFP) expression using genetically identical animal models derived from SCNT have not been described and this is a critical subject since RFP has been used as a potential marker for clinical trials of gene therapy [3–5].

In addition, SCNT uses oocytes from animals unrelated to the prospective transplant recipient, oocyte-derived mitochondrial DNA (mtDNA) derived antigen could lead to rejection problems in kidney transplant [6] or not in skin transplant [7,8]. Although tissues derived from SCNT, using the recipient's somatic cells as nuclear donors, provide identical genetics, the absence of immune rejection has not yet been confirmed in cloned dogs.

To our knowledge, no previous report has mentioned *in vivo* skin immune responses against tissue expressing foreign gene or the capable effects of mitochondrial derived minor antigen in cloned animals. Here, we firstly evaluated the anti-foreign gene or minor antigen derived immune responses in cloned dogs with the following design: (1) for investigation of mtDNA derived antigen compatibility, skin graft was performed between transgenic cloned dogs with different mtDNA haplotypes; (2) furthermore, skin graft was also performed between transgenic cloned dogs and non-transgenic cloned dogs for examination of immunogenicity of foreign gene.

Materials and Methods

1. Animals

Two genetically identical cloned female beagles (C1, C2) were generated by SCNT using a beagle fetal fibroblast cell line (BF3) described in a previously study [9]. Transgenic cloned female beagles (R1, R2, R3 and R5) were also produced by SCNT using BF3 transfected with RFP [2].

Non-related controls (Co1, Co2) were healthy age-matched normal female beagles purchased from commercial kennels (Marshall Beijing Biotech Ltd., Beijing, China). All animals used in this study were cared for in accordance with recommendations described in "The Guide for the Care and Use of Laboratory Animals" published by the Institutional Animal Care and Use Committee (IACUC) of Seoul National University (approval number; SNU-110915-2). Dog housing facilities and the procedures performed met or exceeded the standards established by the Committee for Accreditation of Laboratory Animal Care. All surgery was performed under isoflurane anesthesia, and all efforts were made to minimize suffering.

2. DNA extractions and PCR reaction

Blood was collected from two control beagles and six female cloned beagles 4 years of age for DNA extractions, blood typing and blood cross-matching. Approximately 10 ml of blood were collected from the jugular vein into tubes containing EDTA as anticoagulant and used for peripheral blood mononuclear cell isolation and DNA extraction, and 3 ml of blood in plain tubes were collected to provide serum samples for antibody levels. Blood samples were kept at 38°C to maintain cell viability.

Freshly retrieved non-coagulated blood samples were mixed with RBC lysis buffer (Invitrogen, Carlsbad, CA, USA) at room temperature for 15 min. Genomic DNA was isolated according to the manufacturer's protocol. Extracted DNA samples were stored at −30°C. DLA class I (MHC class I) and II (MHC class II) typing analysis was performed by means of PCR and sequencing. The polymorphic exon 2 and exon 3 of the DLA-88 gene was amplified using PCR primers [10]. The polymorphic exon 2 of the *DRB1, DQA* and *DQB* genes was also amplified using PCR primers [11]. For PCR, Maxime PCR PreMix kit (iNtRON Biotechnology, Inc., Gyeongi, Korea) was used. In each PCR tube, 1 μl of genomic DNA, 1 μl (10 pM/μl) of forward primer, 1 μl (10 pM/μl) of reverse primer and 17 μl of sterilized distilled water were added according to the manufacturer's instructions. These components were then mixed and centrifuged briefly. PCR was done using a PCR machine (Biometra, Goettingen, Germany). PCR amplification was carried out for 1 cycle with denaturing at 94°C for 5 min, and subsequently for 30 cycles with denaturing at 94°C for 40 sec, annealing at 63°C (*DLA-DRB1*), 55°C (*DLA-DQA1*) and 66°C (*DLA-DQB1*) for 40 sec, extension at 72°C for 40 sec, and a final extension at 72°C for 5 min. Amplified PCR product was run on the gel by gel electrophoresis (Mupid-exu, Submarine electrophoresis system, Advance, Japan) at 100 V for 20 min. A 2% agarose gel was prepared using agarose (Invitrogen) and 1X TAE buffer. The stain (RedSafe, iNtRON Biotechnology Inc.) was used at a concentration of 2.5 μl per 50 ml of gel. After running gels, images were made under ultraviolet light. PCR product was sequenced directly using the Big Dye Terminator kit (Applied Biosystems, Foster City, CA, USA). Sequencing was performed on an automated DNA sequencer model 377 or capillary model 3110 (Applied Biosystems).

3. Sequencing of Mitochondrial DNA haplotype

For mitochondrial DNA analysis, the oligonucleotide primers were synthesized over the hypervariable regions (forward, 5′-CCTAAGACTTCAAGGAAGAAGC-3′; reverse, 5′-TTGACTGAATAGCACCTTGA-3′) of the complete nucleotide sequence of canine mtDNA (GenBank accession no. U96639). Isolated genomic DNA sample were dissolved in 50 ul TE buffer and used for PCR amplifications. It were performed in a 50 μl volume containing 5 μl of 10× reaction buffer containing 1.5 mM MgCl2, 0.2 mM dNTPs, 0.2 μM each primer, 1.5 U Taq DNA polymerase (Intron, Kyunggi, Korea). Starting denaturing for 1 cycle at 95°C for 3 minutes, subsequently denaturation at 94°C for 30 seconds, annealing at 57°C for 30 seconds, extension at 72°C for

Table 1. Mitochondrial DNA sequences of non-transgenic cloned dog (C2) and four transgenic cloned dogs (R1, R2, R3 and R5).

Sample	Nucleotide positions																					
	15435	15483	15508	15526	15595	15611	15612	15620	15627	15632	15639	15643	15650	15652	15781	15800	15814	15815	15912	15955	16025	16083
Reference[1]	G	C	C	C	C	T	T	T	A	C	T	A	T	G	C	T	C	T	C	C	T	A
C2	G	C	C	T	T	T	C	T	A	C	G	G	T	A	C	T	C	T	C	T	T	A
R1	G	C	C	C	C	T	T	T	A	C	T	A	T	G	C	T	T	T	C	C	T	A
R2	G	C	C	C	C	T	T	T	A	C	A	A	T	G	C	T	T	T	C	C	C	A
R3	G	C	C	C	C	T	T	C	G	C	A	A	T	G	C	T	T	T	C	T	T	A
R5	G	T	C	C	C	T	T	T	G	C	A	A	T	G	C	T	T	T	C	C	T	A

[1] GenBank accession number :U96639 (Kim et al., 1998).

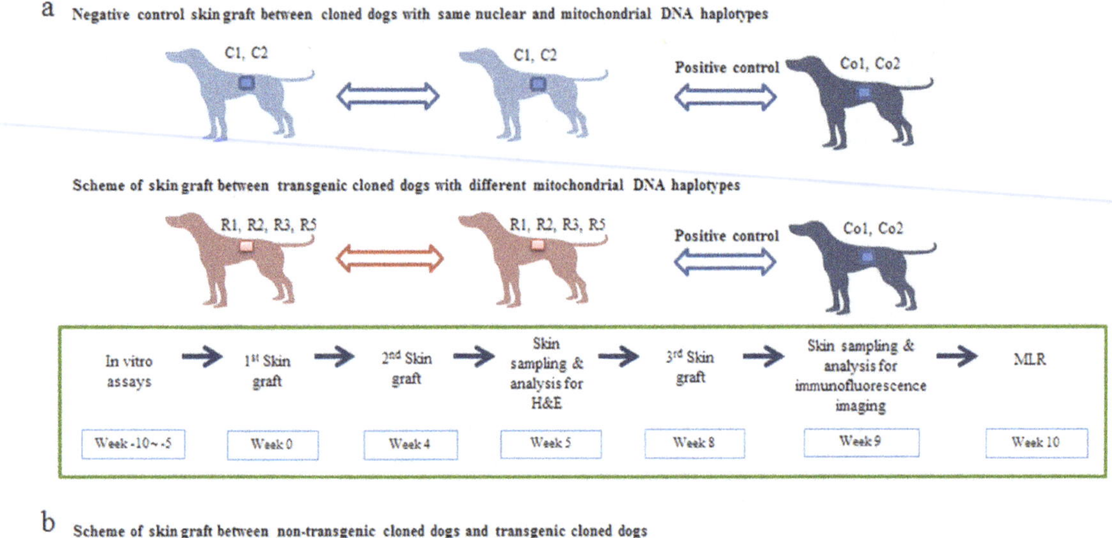

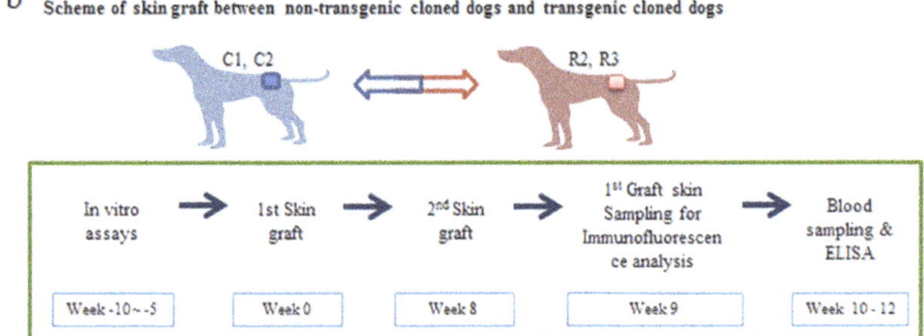

Figure 1. Experimental design and image analysis result between cloned dogs. (a) Experimental design and timeline of skin graft between cloned dogs with different mitochondrial haplotypes. As negative control, auto grafts as well as cloned dogs with same mtDNA haplotype (C1, C2) were used. Before skin graft, all *in vitro* assays were performed. For H&E staining, immunofluorescence imaging, 1st skin graft fragments were analyzed. (b) Experimental design and timeline between transgenic cloned dogs and non-transgenic cloned dogs. Before skin graft, all *in vitro* assays were performed. All dogs were tested twice for each skin graft, then skin samplings were performed. For immunofluorescence imaging, 1st skin graft fragments were analyzed. RFP expression were monitored until 63 days after skin graft.

30 seconds of 35 cycles, and a final extension at 72°C for 3 minutes were carried out. After purification of PCR products using a Gel Extraction Kit (Qiagen, Hilden, Germany), they were sequenced with an ABI3100 instrument (Applied Biosystems). Their identities with mtDNA were confirmed by BLAST search (http://blast.ncbi.nlm.nih.gov/).

4. Blood crossmatching and blood typing

Blood collection was performed from the jugular vein of all cloned dogs (R1, R2, R3, R5, C1 and C2) into an evacuated tube containing EDTA as anticoagulant. Collected samples were submitted to a commercial laboratory kit (Antech Diagnostics, Phoenix, AZ, USA). Blood type was confirmed using the tube agglutination method with antiserum; consisting of 6 types of monoclonal antibodies for canine blood typing [12].

The blood crossmatching test was done on EDTA-treated blood using the tube agglutination method. Isolated RBCs of all dogs were washed 3 times with 0.9% saline, and a 4% RBC suspension was made from the washed cells. RBC suspensions from cloned beagles (C1) were combined with equal volumes of another cloned beagle's serum (C2) and the reverse reaction was also performed. All mixtures were incubated at 37°C for 20 min, centrifuged and then assessed for hemolysis or agglutination. Agglutination was evaluated by comparing the color of supernatant in the test tube with those of the control sample. Each sample was shaken until all red blood cells in the "button" at the bottom of the tube had become suspended. Again, the degree of RBC clumping of the test sample was compared with that of the auto-mixture of RBC and plasma. When the plasma was clear, no clumping of RBCs was detected at 400× magnification, these results were considered as negative. A positive result showed agglutination resembling stacked coins. Images were obtained using a microscope, the ProgRes Capture camera system, and the ProgRes Capture 2.6 software (JENOPTIK, Jena, Germany).

5. Peripheral blood mononuclear cell isolation and mixed lymphocyte reactions

Blood was collected from two control dogs and six female cloned dogs before and 10 weeks after skin graft. EDTA-treated whole blood was transferred to 50 ml conical centrifuge tubes. An equal volume of phosphate buffered solution (PBS, Gibco, Carlsbad, CA, USA) was mixed with the sample prior to the isolation process. Peripheral blood mononuclear cells (PBMC) were isolated from EDTA-treated blood using lymphocyte separation medium on a Ficoll-paque gradient (Ficoll-Paque Plus, GE Healthcare, Pittsburgh, PA, USA). Mixed lymphocyte reactions were modified from the previous reports [13–15]. Washed cells were diluted in culture medium (RPMI1640, Gibco) supplemented with 10% FBS to 2×10^6 cells/ml. To stimulate proliferation of lymphocytes, PBMCs were preincubated with 2 ug/ml of phytohemagglutin for 24 h before mix reaction. Then 50 ul of this cell suspension was added into each well of a 96-well

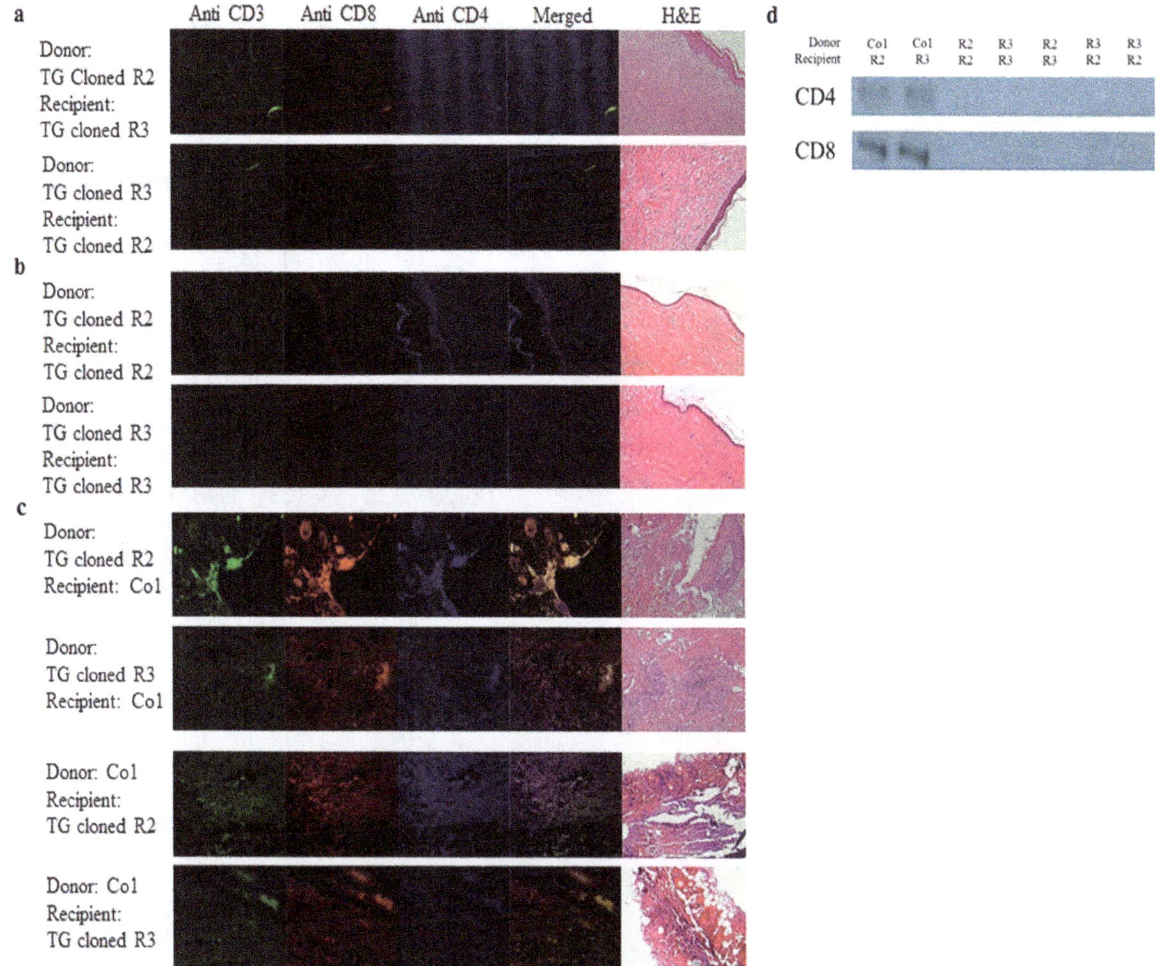

Figure 2. Absence of *in vivo* immunogenicity in skin grafts between cloned dogs with different mitochondrial DNA sequences. No evidence with infiltration of T cell was detected in the skin segments transplanted into the recipient dogs with different mitochondrial haplotypes (a). Sections from skin segments of autografts were used as negative controls (b). Sections from skin segments of cloned dogs transplanted into control dogs were used as positive controls (c). Western blot analysis confirms high protein levels of CD4 and CD8 in the positive controls, whereas CD4 and CD8 expression intensities were significantly lower in allograft of cloned dogs with different mitochondrial haplotypes (d). Upper lane indicates the donor dog and lower lane means recipient dog.

microplate except for the wells required for the blank and cultured at 37.5°C in a water-saturated atmosphere containing 5% CO_2. Each cell combination was tested in quadruplicate in a flat-bottomed micro plate containing 0.1 ml of culture medium per well. The mixture was cultured for 5 days and then pyrimidine analogue, bromodeoxyuridine labeling reagent (Cell proliferation ELISA, Roche Applied Science, Indianapolis, IN, USA) was added and re-incubated for 24 h. After removing the labeling medium, results are expressed as absorbance units at 450 nm wavelength read by a micro plate reader, Sunrise (Tecan Sunrise, Hayward, CA, USA). Time-course kinetics was studied by harvesting on day 7 of culture.

6. DNA walking

For confirmation of the transgene (RFP) location, PCR was performed with a DNA Walking SpeedUP Kit (Seegene Inc., Seoul, Korea) and products were gel purified (QIAquick PCR purification kit; QIAGEN, Valencia, CA, USA), and DNA strands were directly sequenced (Macrogen, Seoul, Korea; http://www.macrogen.com) using a custom-synthesized primer (5′-TCACAGAAGTATGCCAAGCGA-3′). The sequences, except for known sequences, including primers of each product were aligned by sequence homology analysis using the Basic Local Alignment Search Tool (BLAST) at the National Center for Biotechnology Information (NCBI) GenBank (http://blast.ncbi.nlm.nih.gov/).

7. Skin graft

For skin graft procedures, experimental dogs were anesthetized with ketamine hydrochloride (6 mg/kg) after pretreatment with xylazine (0.05 mg/kg), and were maintained with 2% isoflurane in oxygen. A flank skin segment 1.5 cm×1.5 cm was excised from each donor dog. Simultaneously, the same sized skin piece was excised from recipient dogs, and the excised skin was grafted by suturing into the graft bed of the same region of an anesthetized recipient dog. Bandages were changed every day after surgery and the grafts were observed weekly.

For examination of effects mtDNA haplotypes differences among cloned dogs, skin grafts of three times were performed

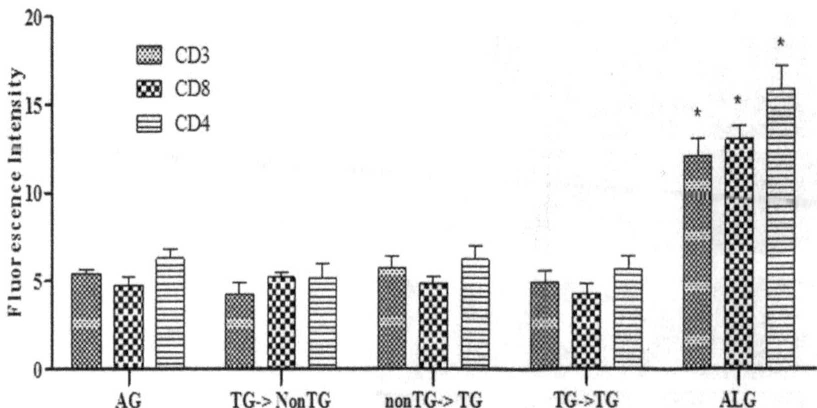

Figure 3. Expression levels of CD3, CD4 and CD8 of skin grafts between cloned dogs using fluorescence image analysis. Immunological response level of CD3, CD4 and CD8 were similar in AG (autograft), TG-> NonTG (donor: transgenic dog, recipient: non-transgenic cloned dogs), NonTG->TG (donor: non-transgenic dog, recipient: transgenic cloned dogs) and TG cloned dogs (donor: transgenic dog, recipient: transgenic cloned dogs). However, Both of ALG (allograft) between TG dogs and non-related control dogs and allograft between non-TG dogs and non-related control dogs shows significantly higher intensity of immunological response ($p<0.05$). Results are presented as mean ± SEM. Replication number is at least 8 times.

every 4 weeks between non-transgenic cloned dogs with same mtDNA haplotype and between transgenic cloned dogs with disparate mtDNA haplotypes. Accepted tissues were maintained until 9 weeks after skin graft. Biopsies of skin were performed after 63 days after first skin graft. A flank skin segment of 1st graft with size of 0.5 cm×1.5 cm including donor and recipient tissue were excised for H&E staining at 5 weeks of skin graft and remnant tissue were excised for immunofluorescence imaging and western blot at later.

8. Histological and immunofluorescence analysis

Immuno-staining of canine skin immune cells was carried out on formaldehyde-fixed sections using a rabbit monoclonal antibody to CD3 (1:100, ab94756, Abcam, Cambridge, MA, USA), visualized with an anti-rabbit polyclonal DyLight 488 (1:200, ab96895, Abcam) antibody. In these sections, CD4 and CD8 cells were counterstained with a CD4 (1:100, LS c122857, Lifespan Bioscience Inc., Seattle, WA, USA) and CD8 (1:200, ab22505, Abcam) specific antibody detected with a DyLight 405 (1:200, 3069-1, Abcam) and DyLight 649 (1:200, ab98389, Abcam) coupled secondary antibody. Skin sections were also processed for assessing expression of RFP using rabbit polyclonal RFP antibody (1:200, ab62341, Abcam) and visualized with an anti-rabbit polyclonal DyLight 488 (1:200, ab96895, Abcam) antibody. Sections were counterstained with 4′, 6′-diamidino-2-phenylindole (DAPI).

Histology was done by fixing skin fragment in 4% neutral formalin and embedding in paraffin; sections were stained with standard hematoxylin and eosin (H&E) procedures. Fluorescent and bright field images were obtained with a Leica DMI 6000B microscope using a DFC350 camera and LAS software (Leica Microsystems Pty Ltd., North Ryde, Australia) and analyzed by a computer-assisted image analysis system (Metamorph version 6.3r2; Molecular Devices Corporation, PA, USA). To maintain a constant threshold for each image and to compensate for subtle variability of the immune-fluorescent imaging, we only counted cells that were at least 70% lighter than the average level of each positive control image after background subtraction. All image analytical procedures described above were performed blind without knowledge of the experimental scheme.

9. Western blot

Skin fragments of graft was excised and homogenized in PRO-PREP protein extraction solution (iNtRON Biotechnology, Inc.) using a tissue homogenizer. After measuring protein concentration using Nanodrop 2000 (Thermo fischer scientific, Seoul, Korea), equal amounts of proteins were loaded on 10% SDS-PAGE. Proteins were electrophoresed and blotted onto polyvinylidene fluoride membranes. The membranes were blocked with 5% skim milk in TBS with 0.1% Tween-20 and incubated with primary antibodies for 2 hours at room temperature. Monoclonal CD4 and CD8 antibodies were used as markers for immune rejection. Subsequently, membranes were incubated with goat anti-mouse IgG, anti-rat IgG (Pierce, Rockford, IL, USA) with horse radish peroxidase conjugation for 1 h at room temperature. Then, WEST-one^{TM} Western blot detection system (iNtRON Biotechnology, Inc.) was added and visualized after exposing the membrane to X-ray film.

10. Statistical Analysis

The data of mixed lymphocyte reaction, image analysis of immunocytochemistry and western blot were analyzed using one-way ANOVA and a protected least significant different (LSD) test using general linear models to determine differences among experimental groups. Data were analyzed using GraphPad Prism software (GraphPad Software Inc., San Diego, CA, USA). Absorbance mean values were considered significantly different when the P-value was less than 0.05. The observations of mixed lymphocyte reaction among experimental groups were replicated at least 8 times.

Results and Discussions

It has been reported that immune rejection can occur when tissues of genetically identical SCNT cloned animals were transplanted to each other, due to the tissues having different maternally-derived antigens [6,16,17]. Antigens derived from mtDNA in accelerated skin rejection in syngeneic rodent recipients [18,19]. It has also been generally assumed that genetically-engineered tissues with insertion of a foreign gene could invoke immune-rejection by the recipient even in inbred mice [20]. Using embryonic stem cells derived from SCNT, the complete rescues of

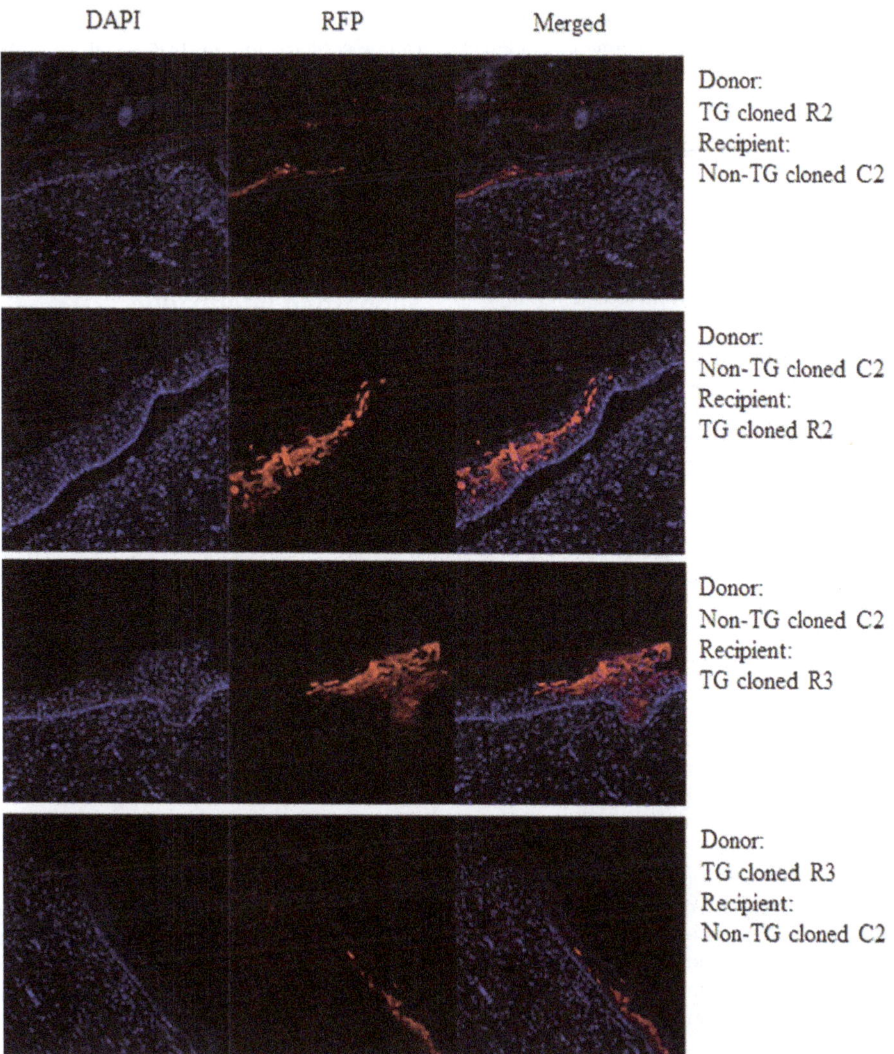

Figure 4. Maintenance of foreign gene expression between transgenic cloned beagle with foreign genes and non-transgenic cloned dogs. No expression of foreign gene in non-transgenic dog (C2) recipient was maintained in skin graft of transgenic cloned dog (R2). The limit between donor and recipient were not changed until 63 days after skin graft.

genetic defect with genetically-engineered cell therapy were not observed [21]. Engraftment of hematopoietic precursor cells differentiated from SCNT or induced pluripotent stem cells (iPSCs) was only successful in the absence of natural killer cells and immunogenicity of iPSCs was reported [21–23].

In the present study, cloned dogs produced by SCNT had different mtDNA haplotypes (Table 1), because canine SCNT used oocytes obtained from several oocyte donor dogs and the oocyte mtDNA was still present after the SCNT procedure. To examine the immunogenicity of skin tissue derived from syngeneic grafts exhibiting different mtDNA haplotypes, we initially performed *in vitro* molecular typing of dog leukocyte antigen (DLA), mixed lymphocyte reaction (MLR) and blood cross-matching using cells derived from cloned dogs with different mtDNA haplotypes (Fig. S1). Despite the different mtDNA haplotypes, they had no effects on *in vitro* immunological compatibility.

To gain insights into the therapeutic applicability of canine skin tissues with different mtDNA haplotypes, skin grafting between cloned dogs was performed to determine immunological compatibility *in vivo* (Fig. 1). Whereas allogeneic Co 1 (non-related control dogs) skin fragments were rapidly rejected in R2 (transgenic cloned dog) and R3 (transgenic cloned dog) recipients with massive infiltration of CD4+, CD8+ T cells, infiltration, edema and perivascular inflammation 7 days after 2nd skin graft, skin tissues of R2 and R3 were accepted in R3 and R2 recipients as well as autografts, without any evidence of immune rejection (Fig. 2). Likewise, skin segments from cloned dogs with different mtDNA sequences did not induce immune rejection in the recipient cloned dogs (Fig. S2). In MLR of 10 weeks after 3rd skin graft, we couldn't detect any sign of mtDNA derived minor antigen immunogenicity with no significant differences compared to those of MLR before skin graft (data not shown).

In mice, mtDNA encoded proteins could elicit rejection by innate immunity in a setting where the genomic DNA matched [24,25]. Furthermore, kidneys transplanted between cloned pigs differing in some mtDNA genes rejected those grafts [6]. Therefore, different antigenicity of grafts from different tissues could be also considered. In our experiment, despite a high level of diversity of mtDNA haplotypes heteroplasmy among domestic dogs [26], skin grafts were successfully accepted in at least 20 donor-recipient combinations. In cattle and pigs, it was shown that SCNT-derived tissues were not rejected by the immune system of the nucleus donor after SCNT in skin graft [7,27,28]. Our findings suggest that differences of canine mtDNA haplotypes could not elicit skin graft rejection among cloned dogs, as previously observed in cattle and pigs.

We also showed genetic identity between tissues of non-transgenic cloned dogs (C1, C2) derived from beagle fibroblasts (BF3) [9] and tissues of transgenic cloned dogs (R1, R2, R3 and R5) derived from BF3 transfected with RFP (Table S1.) [2]. Immunological compatibility between these dogs was completely established through *in vitro* tests such as DLA typing and MLR (Fig. S1). Skin tissues of non-transgenic cloned dogs were transplanted into transgenic cloned dogs and *vice-versa*. Skin tissues derived from cloned dogs were transplanted with no immune rejection, as determined by T cell infiltration of peri-graft skin sections after 7 days of 2nd skin graft. Despite insertion of the foreign gene RFP in transgenic cloned dogs, skin tissue from RFP transgenic cloned dogs was completely accepted in non-transgenic cloned dog recipients (Fig. 3, Fig. S3). These finding indicate that foreign gene insertion in cloned dogs did not induce a T cell-dependent skin graft rejection response in syngeneic recipients. It has been suggested that the nuclear reprogramming process in SCNT could result in surface expression of proteins and molecules unknown to the immune system of the graft recipients. In this regard, in inbred mice, enhanced GFP (eGFP) skin transplantation causes an acute reaction [29]. It was proved that eGFP also induce immune responses that interfere with its applicability in gene insertion of mouse [30]. However, our results suggest that inserted foreign gene, RFP has no immunological effects on the antigens of transgenic cloned dogs against to the non-transgenic cloned dogs. It also suggested that non-transgenic cloned dogs produced by SCNT using transfected cells have no immune regulatory effect on the host immune system and that the canine SCNT process did not result in surface expression of immunogenic molecules. Nonetheless, the possibility of immune rejection of other foreign genes, for example, pathogenically relevant transgene in clinical science remains to be confirmed.

Finally we examined whether functional expression of RFP was maintained in skin tissue grafts. During the course of this experiment, the expression level of RFP positive skin tissues were maintained for at least 63 days after surgery and RFP positive cells were detected in the epidermis, hair follicles and sebaceous glands (Fig. 4 and Table S1). It has been suggested that the co-expression of selection markers can limit or abrogate the persistence of expression of therapeutic genes [31,32]. The potential success of gene therapy or production of transgenic cloned dogs may depend on long-term transgene expression to cure or slow down the progression of disease. In addition, there were no host immune responses to the skin grafts among transgenic dogs and non-transgenic cloned dogs, and it appears that the level and duration of RFP transgene expression was not affected. This also indicates possible successful of therapeutic transplantation of tissues or cells derived from transgenic cloned dogs. In addition, the insertion site of the RFP gene into genomic DNA is not the same in all experimental dogs (Table S2). If the RFP gene insertion site can affect the immune response, it should affect the results of syngeneic skin grafting. However, no immune rejection was apparent in skin grafts with different transgene insertion sites. Our findings indicate that SCNT-derived somatic cells with or without foreign genes can be accepted in syngeneic recipients.

Our study established that tissues derived from canine SCNT can be accepted in syngeneic recipients despite different mtDNA haplotypes. We also provide evidence that skin segments containing a foreign gene are sufficiently acceptable to syngeneic recipients with or without the foreign gene. Taken together, these data indicate that SCNT using transgenic technology can support immunological compatibility between genetically engineered tissues and patients and thereby help to accelerate clinical therapeutic research and its applications.

Supporting Information

Figure S1 Immunological feature of transgenic dogs and non-transgenic dogs. (a) Molecular typing of dog leukocyte antigen, DLA-88 (MHC class I), DRB, DQA1, DQB1(MHC class II) polymorphic region in all cloned dogs (C1, C2, R1, R2, R3, and R5). (b) *In vitro* immunogenicity test using mixed lymphocyte reaction between all experimental dogs before skin graft. (c) Blood typing. (d) Analysis of blood crossmatching in all cloned dogs and control dogs.

Figure S2 Fluorescence image analysis of skin grafts between cloned dogs with different mtDNA haplotypes

Figure S3 Absence of *in vivo* immune rejection between non-transgenic dogs and transgenic dogs. (a) Positive control of skin graft, as donor skin segments were derived from non-related control dogs (Co1, Co2), they were completely rejected in the graft bed in transgenic cloned dogs (R2, R3). (b) However, skin grafts between a transgenic cloned dog, R2 and a non-transgenic cloned dog, C1 showed no apparent immune rejection. Similarly, as shown in (c) R2 - C2, (d) R3-C1, (e) R3-C2, there was no immune rejection in these grafts as well. (f) Western blot analysis of the skin graft between cloned dogs confirmed the expression of CD4 and CD8 protein only in the graft between cloned dogs and non-related control dogs.

Figure S4 Foreign gene expression between skin graft of two transgenic dogs (R2, R3). Red fluorescent protein expression in skin graft was maintained after 63 days skin graft in syngenic graft beds.

Table S1 Genetic background for microsatellite analysis of two non-transgenic cloned dogs and four transgenic cloned dogs.

Table S2 Insertion site of foreign gene, RFP in transgenic cloned dogs.

Acknowledgments

We thank Won Woo Lee for critical reading of the manuscript. We would also like to thank Dr, Barry D. Bavister for his valuable editing of the manuscript.

Author Contributions

Conceived and designed the experiments: GAK HJO MJK SKK GJ BCL. Performed the experiments: GAK YKJ JC JEP EJP SHL. Analyzed the data: GAK HJO BIY BCL. Contributed reagents/materials/analysis tools: JEP BIY BCL. Wrote the paper: GAK HJO SKK BCL.

References

1. Lee BC, Kim MK, Jang G, Oh HJ, Yuda F, et al. (2005) Dogs cloned from adult somatic cells. Nature 436: 641.
2. Hong SG, Kim MK, Jang G, Oh HJ, Park JE, et al. (2009) Generation of red fluorescent protein transgenic dogs. Genesis 47: 314–322.
3. Chang RS, Suh MS, Kim S, Shim G, Lee S, et al. (2011) Cationic drug-derived nanoparticles for multifunctional delivery of anticancer siRNA. Biomaterials 32: 9785–9795.
4. Lee CY, Li JF, Liou JS, Charng YC, Huang YW, et al. (2011) A gene delivery system for human cells mediated by both a cell-penetrating peptide and a piggyBac transposase. Biomaterials 32: 6264–6276.
5. Kinoshita Y, Kamitani H, Mamun MH, Wasita B, Kazuki Y, et al. (2010) A gene delivery system with a human artificial chromosome vector based on migration of mesenchymal stem cells towards human glioblastoma HTB14 cells. Neurol Res 32: 429–437.
6. Kwak HH, Park KM, Teotia PK, Lee GS, Lee ES, et al. (2013) Acute rejection after swine leukocyte antigen-matched kidney allo-transplantation in cloned miniature pigs with different mitochondrial DNA-encoded minor histocompatibility antigen. Transplant Proc 45: 1754–1760.
7. Martin MJ, Yin D, Adams C, Houtz J, Shen J, et al. (2003) Skin graft survival in genetically identical cloned pigs. Cloning Stem Cells 5: 117–121.
8. Theoret CL, Dore M, Mulon PY, Desrochers A, Viramontes F, et al. (2006) Short- and long-term skin graft survival in cattle clones with different mitochondrial haplotypes. Theriogenology 65: 1465–1479.
9. Hong SG, Jang G, Kim MK, Oh HJ, Park JE, et al. (2009) Dogs cloned from fetal fibroblasts by nuclear transfer. Anim Reprod Sci 115: 334–339.
10. Burnett RC, DeRose SA, Wagner JL, Storb R (1997) Molecular analysis of six dog leukocyte antigen class I sequences including three complete genes, two truncated genes and one full-length processed gene. Tissue Antigens 49: 484–495.
11. Kennedy LJ (2007) 14th International HLA and Immunogenetics Workshop: report on joint study on canine DLA diversity. Tissue Antigens 69 Suppl 1: 269–271.
12. Ogawa H, Galili U (2006) Profiling terminal N-acetyllactosamines of glycans on mammalian cells by an immuno-enzymatic assay. Glycoconj J 23: 663–674.
13. Gluckman JC (1980) [Modification of mixed lymphocyte reactivity between DLA-identical dog sibs, after in vivo sensitization]. C R Seances Acad Sci D 290: 105–108.
14. Kolb HJ, Rieder I, Grosse-Wilde H, Scholz S, Kolb H, et al. (1975) Canine marrow grafts in donor-recipient combinations with one-way nonstimulation in mixed lymphocyte culture. Transplant Proc 7: 461–464.
15. Widmer MB, Bach FH (1972) Allogeneic and xenogeneic response in mixed leukocyte cultures. J Exp Med 135: 1204–1208.
16. Do M, Jang WG, Hwang JH, Jang H, Kim EJ, et al. (2012) Inheritance of mitochondrial DNA in serially recloned pigs by somatic cell nuclear transfer (SCNT). Biochem Biophys Res Commun 424: 765–770.
17. Hiendleder S (2007) Mitochondrial DNA inheritance after SCNT. Adv Exp Med Biol 591: 103–116.
18. Chan T, Fischer Lindahl K (1985) Skin graft rejection caused by the maternally transmitted antigen Mta. Transplantation 39: 477–480.
19. Lindahl KF, Burki K (1982) Mta, a maternally inherited cell surface antigen of the mouse, is transmitted in the egg. Proc Natl Acad Sci U S A 79: 5362–5366.
20. Andersson G, Illigens BM, Johnson KW, Calderhead D, LeGuern C, et al. (2003) Nonmyeloablative conditioning is sufficient to allow engraftment of EGFP-expressing bone marrow and subsequent acceptance of EGFP-transgenic skin grafts in mice. Blood 101: 4305–4312.
21. Rideout WM 3rd, Hochedlinger K, Kyba M, Daley GQ, Jaenisch R (2002) Correction of a genetic defect by nuclear transplantation and combined cell and gene therapy. Cell 109: 17–27.
22. Hanna J, Wernig M, Markoulaki S, Sun CW, Meissner A, et al. (2007) Treatment of sickle cell anemia mouse model with iPS cells generated from autologous skin. Science 318: 1920–1923.
23. Zhao T, Zhang ZN, Rong Z, Xu Y (2011) Immunogenicity of induced pluripotent stem cells. Nature 474: 212–215.
24. Ishikawa K, Toyama-Sorimachi N, Nakada K, Morimoto M, Imanishi H, et al. (2010) The innate immune system in host mice targets cells with allogenic mitochondrial DNA. J Exp Med 207: 2297–2305.
25. Loveland B, Wang CR, Yonekawa H, Hermel E, Lindahl KF (1990) Maternally transmitted histocompatibility antigen of mice: a hydrophobic peptide of a mitochondrially encoded protein. Cell 60: 971–980.
26. Webb KM, Allard MW (2009) Mitochondrial genome DNA analysis of the domestic dog: identifying informative SNPs outside of the control region. J Forensic Sci 54: 275–288.
27. Lanza RP, Chung HY, Yoo JJ, Wettstein PJ, Blackwell C, et al. (2002) Generation of histocompatible tissues using nuclear transplantation. Nat Biotechnol 20: 689–696.
28. Oiso N, Fukai K, Kawada A, Suzuki T (2013) Piebaldism. J Dermatol 40: 330–335.
29. Lu F, Gao JH, Mizuro H, Ogawa R, Hyakusoku H (2007) [Experimental study of adipose tissue differentiation using adipose-derived stem cells harvested from GFP transgenic mice]. Zhonghua Zheng Xing Wai Ke Za Zhi 23: 412–416.
30. Stripecke R, Carmen Villacres M, Skelton D, Satake N, Halene S, et al. (1999) Immune response to green fluorescent protein: implications for gene therapy. Gene Ther 6: 1305–1312.
31. Riddell SR, Elliott M, Lewinsohn DA, Gilbert MJ, Wilson L, et al. (1996) T-cell mediated rejection of gene-modified HIV-specific cytotoxic T lymphocytes in HIV-infected patients. Nat Med 2: 216–223.
32. Bonini C, Ferrari G, Verzeletti S, Servida P, Zappone E, et al. (1997) HSV-TK gene transfer into donor lymphocytes for control of allogeneic graft-versus-leukemia. Science 276: 1719–1724.

Optimizing Radiation Dose Levels in Prospectively Electrocardiogram-Triggered Coronary Computed Tomography Angiography Using Iterative Reconstruction Techniques: A Phantom and Patient Study

Yang Hou[1], Jiahe Zheng[1], Yuke Wang[1], Mei Yu[1], Mani Vembar[2], Qiyong Guo[1]*

1 Department of Radiology, Shengjing Hospital of China Medical University, Shenyang, China, **2** CT Clinical Science Philips Healthcare, Cleveland, Ohio, United States of America

Abstract

Aim: To investigate the potential of reducing the radiation dose in prospectively electrocardiogram-triggered coronary computed tomography angiography (CCTA) while maintaining diagnostic image quality using an iterative reconstruction technique (IRT).

Methods and Materials: Prospectively-gated CCTA were first performed on a phantom using 256-slice multi-detector CT scanner at 120 kVp, with the tube output gradually reduced from 210 mAs (Group A) to 125, 105, 84, and 63 mAs (Group B–E). All scans were reconstructed using filtered back projection (FBP) algorithm and five IRT levels (L2-6), image quality (IQ) assessment was performed. Based on the IQ assessment, Group D(120 kVp, 84 mAs) reconstructed with L5 was found to provide IQ comparable to that of Group A with FBP. In the patient study, 21 patients underwent CCTA using 120 kV, 210 mAs with FBP reconstruction (Group 1) followed by 36 patients scanned with 120 kV, 84 mAs with IRT L5 (Group 2). Subjective and objective IQ and effective radiation dose were compared between two groups.

Results: In the phantom scans, there were no significant differences in image noise, contrast-to-noise ratio (CNR) and modulation transfer function (MTF) curves between Group A and the 84 mAs, 63 mAs groups (Groups D and E). Group D (120 kV, 84 mAs and L5) provided an optimum balance, producing equivalent image quality to Group A, at the lowest possible radiation dose. In the patient study, there were no significant difference in image noise, signal-to-noise ratio (SNR) and CNR between Group 1 and Group 2 ($p = 0.71$, 0.31, 0.5, respectively). The effective radiation dose in Group 2 was 1.21 ± 0.14 mSv compared to 3.20 ± 0.58 mSv (Group 1), reflecting dose savings of 62.5% ($p < 0.05$).

Conclusion: iterative reconstruction technique used in prospectively ECG-triggered 256-slice coronary CTA can provide radiation dose reductions of up to 62.5% with acceptable image quality.

Editor: Ge Wang, Virginia Tech, United States of America

Funding: This work was supported by two provincial government funds–Innovative Research Team of Liaoning Educational Committee (LT2010105) and Science and Technique Foundation of Shenyang(F12-193-9-35). The funders had no role in study design, data collection and analysis, decision to publish, or preparation of the manuscript.

Competing Interests: MV is an employee of Philips Healthcare. However, all other authors had complete unrestricted access to the study data at all stages of the study and controlled the inclusion of all data and information that might have represented a conflict of interest otherwise.

* E-mail: guoqy@vip.sina.com

Introduction

In the past decade, with the development of multi-detector spiral computed tomography (CT), coronary computed tomography angiography (coronary CTA) has increasingly become a noninvasive method of choice for the rule-out of coronary artery disease [1–5] owing to its high sensitivity. However, despite radiation dose reduction technologies implemented by the CT manufacturers, concerns persist. Therefore, coronary CT should continue to follow the principle of "ALARA" (as low as reasonably achievable).

The use of various basic techniques for coronary CTA such as decreasing tube voltage and current, shortening/optimizing scan length, electrocardiogram (ECG) tube current modulation, prospective gating and application of prospectively ECG-triggered, high-pitch scan mode have resulted in halving radiation dose every two years since 2005 [6]. However, in order to consistently achieve further radiation dose reductions, these methods have to be supplemented by newer reconstruction technologies which can

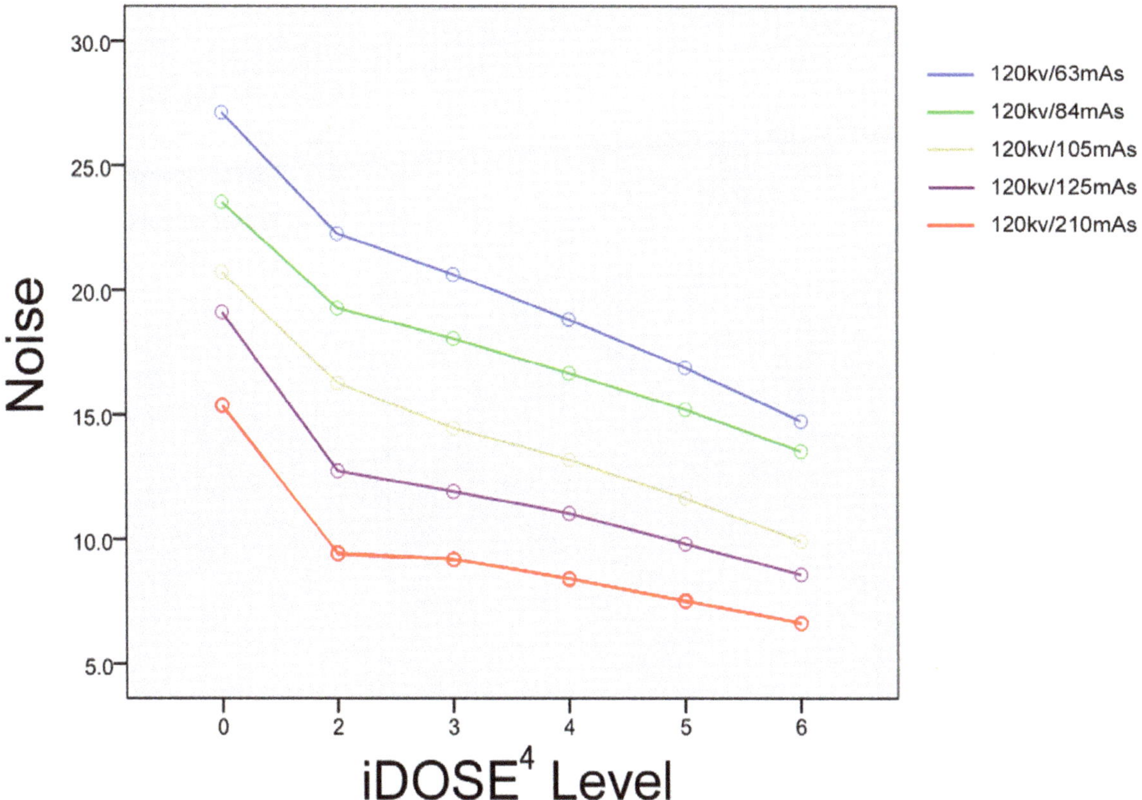

Figure 1. Noise reduction in images reconstructed with iDOSE^4 in phantom. At equal radiation doses, iDose^4 reconstruction algorithm yielded lower image noise than FBP reconstruction algorithm, and with increased iDose^4 level, image noise decreased in a linear manner.

help address the limitations (i.e., increased image noise) of the currently used filtered back projection (FBP) reconstruction algorithms. Iterative reconstruction techniques (IRT) have been recently introduced, offering an innovative solution for reducing CT radiation dose. They can markedly lower image noise, effectively increase signal-to-noise ratio (SNR) and contrast-to-noise ratio (CNR), and achieve equivalent, or in some cases, better image quality (IQ) compared to routine-dose FBP reconstruction. Recent work has shown that IRT can enable dose reductions in chest and abdominal CT in the range of 32–65% depending on the patients' body mass index (BMI) [7–15]. Likewise, the use of IRT has also been investigated in coronary CTA, demonstrating radiation dose reductions in the range of 40–76% compared to FBP while retaining the image quality [7–21].

However, these early works did not investigate the level of tube output reductions (along with the corresponding levels/strengths of IRT) that can be safely employed beyond which the image quality will be negatively impacted. For this reason, we first performed prospectively ECG-triggered 256-slice multi-detector coronary CTA in phantoms, with a constant tube voltage (120 kV) and a 'standard' tube current, followed by scans performed with gradually decreasing tube currents. Images from scans obtained with decreasing tube output were reconstructed with corresponding levels of IRT to maintain a certain noise level and compared to FBP reconstructions used for the scans performed with the standard tube output. Once a threshold of tube output reduction was identified (with the corresponding IRT level) that would provide IQ comparable to FBP from the standard scans, this was extended to a patient study, with prospectively gated axial coronary CTA performed in two demographically matched cohorts – one scanned with standard tube output and reconstructed with FBP and the other with tube reduction determined from the phantom scans and reconstructed with the appropriate level of IRT. Thus, the minimal radiation dose for 256-slice multi-detector coronary CTA using IRT without loss of clinical information could be determined.

Materials and Methods

Ethics Statement

The study protocol was approved and the study was performed under the supervision of the ethics committee of the Shengjing Hospital of China Medical University (Shenyang 110004, China) (no. 2012PS26K). Participants provided their written informed consent to participate prior to the study onset.

Phantom Study

Catphan 500 phantom (Phantom Laboratory, Cambridge, NY, USA) with CTP528 and CTP401 modules were used to evaluate objective image quality (image noise, CNR and modulation transfer function (MTF)) and subjective image quality (artifact, nodule conspicuity, detectable minimal nodule size, overall image quality).

Acquisition protocol. We used prospective ECG-gated scanning and image reconstruction on a 256-slice multi-detector CT scanner (Brilliance iCT; Philips Healthcare, Cleveland, OH, USA). The scan parameters include a detector configuration of 128×0.625 mm (detector collimation); slice thickness 0.9 mm; gantry rotation time 0.27 second; display field-of-view, 22 cm; and scan length 8 cm. An ECG signal was generated using a simulator

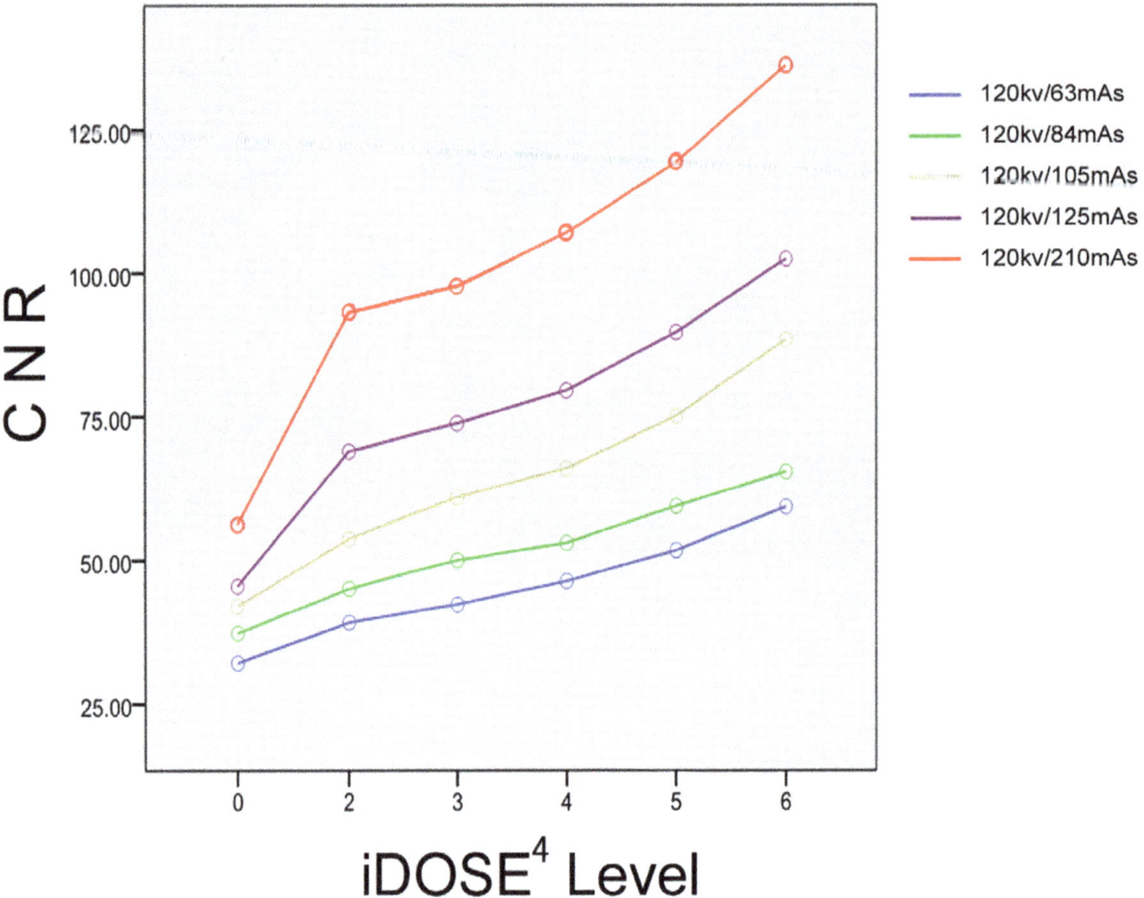

Figure 2. CNR increase in images reconstructed with iDOSE^4 in phantom. At equal radiation doses, iDose^4 reconstruction produced higher CNR than FBP reconstruction, and the CNR was increased in a linear manner with increased iDose^4 level.

set to a heart rate of 60 beats/min. Scans were performed using our institutional protocol (i.e., routine protocol), with the tube voltage set to 120 kVp and the tube current – x-ray ON time product (i.e., the tube output) of 210 mAs (i.e., Group A). The trigger time was set at 75% of the R-R interval without the buffer zone. With the tube voltage kept at 120 kVp, the tube output was gradually reduced to 125 mAs (Group B), 105 mAs (Group C), 84 mAs (Group D), and 63 mAs (Group E). The reduction rate in radiation dose for each effective tube current time product was 40%, 50%, 60%, 70%, compared to our routine dose.

CT image reconstruction and evaluation. The routine-dose and reduced-dose scan series were reconstructed using FBP and IRT (iDose^4, Philips Healthcare, Cleveland, OH, USA). The description of the IRT used in this study has been explained in prior work [17]. Five IRT levels (L2, 3, 4, 5, 6) were used in each scan series with a coronary kernel (XCC). These levels were designed to attain a certain noise reduction factor to compensate for any noise increase resulting from lowering the tube output. [16,17] Thirty scans were reconstructed to evaluate the noise and contrast to noise ratio (CNR).

Objective image quality: Measurement of image noise, CNR and MTF. For each CT images series, image noise and CNR were measured by a radiologist blinded to the scanning and reconstruction methods at the CTP401 module of the Catphan phantom; the noise was defined as the standard deviation (SD) of pixel values in background within a 10-mm diameter circular region of interest (ROI). The CT number of the Teflon objects in a 13-mm diameter area in the same slice was measured using a circular ROI cursor. CNR values were calculated as follows: (CTa-CTb)/SDb, where CTa and CTb are the CT numbers of the acrylic objects and the background ROI, and SDb is the standard deviation of the attenuation values of the background [20]. Mean noise and CNR were calculated from the noise and CNR measurements of 10 continuous images in Z direction.

The effects of different radiation doses and different IRT levels on image noise and CNR were investigated. noise and CNR curves are shown in Figures 1 and 2. The IRT images from each low-dose group with a noise value similar to images reconstructed by routine-dose FBP reconstruction algorithm were included for later analysis.

The modulation transfer function (MTF) was measured from CTP 528 module images reconstructed using FBP from routine-dose scans (120 kV, 210 mAs) and IRT from the reduced dose scans and the curves were plotted.

Evaluation of subjective image quality. The subjective image quality (IQ) scoring was performed on CTP 401 module images reconstructed using FBP on routine-dose (120 kV, 210 mAs) scans (Group A) and and IRT from reduced-dose scans (Groups B:125 mAs, C:105 mAs, D:84 mAs, E:63 mAs). The artifacts (including graininess, streaks, plastic-look), nodule conspicuity, detectable minimal nodule size, and overall IQ of images were evaluated. The above mentioned images were independently

Table 1. Image noise and CNR in each phantom group.

Item	120 KV+210 mAs/FBP (Group A)	120 KV+125 mAs/L3 (Group B)	120 KV+105 mAs/L4 (Group C)	120 KV+84 mAs/L5 (Group D)	120 KV+63 mAs/L6 (Group E)	F	P
Image noise	15.4±0.8	11.9±1.7	13.2±0.6	15.2±1.1[†]	14.8±1.4[†]	16.4	<0.001
	(14.1–16.9)	(10.6–16.2)	(12.2–14.1)	(13.5–16.7)	(13.0–17.8)		
CT value of Teflon spheres	965.8±3.7	968.2±2.0	967.8±2.8	966.1±6.4	965.3±3.4	1.1	0.4
	(962.0–973.9)	(965.2–971.7)	(963.9–973.3)	(958.1–975.0)	(957.7–970))		
CT value of background	100.9±8.4	98.7±1.3	97.7±1.4	98.0±1.8	98.7±2.0	0.9	0.4
	(97.3–124.6)	(96.0–99.9)	(95.5–100.2)	(95.1–101.6)	(96.4–102.5)		
CNR	56.2±2.8	73.9±8.4	66.0±3.0	59.5±2.3[†]	59.3±5.3[†]	20.7	<0.001
	(51.3–61.0)	(53.9–82.0)	(53.9–82.0)	(56.9–63.8)	(48.7–66.8)		

Note: [†]indicates no significant statistical difference compared to group A; CNR: contrast-to-noise ratio; L: IRT level.

scored by two experienced radiologists blinded to the reconstruction algorithm. The objective IQ of IRT reconstructions was recorded on a 4-point scale, where 1 = unacceptable with respect to diagnostic quality, 2 = suboptimal diagnostic quality and poor image quality compared to Group A, 3 = good diagnostic quality and image quality equal to Group A, and 4 = excellent diagnostic quality and superior image quality compared to Group A. With respect to minimal detectable nodule size, the acrylic spheres we used ranged from 2 to 10 mm. Data were recorded. The mean scores from these two radiologists were used as the final scores. Based on above subjective and objective indices, the IRT reconstructions with IQ equivalent to routine-dose reconstruction (Group A) were selected.

Patient Study

Population studied. Over a period of two months (March-April 2012), a total of 56 consecutive patients (34 males and 23 females) were prospectively enrolled in the study. In the first month, 21 patients underwent coronary CTA using the routine institutional protocol (120 kV, 210 mAs) (Group 1). In the second month, 36 patients underwent coronary CTA using a reduced tube-output (120 kV, 84 mAs) (Group 2). The study protocol was approved by our institution's ethics committee, and written informed consent was obtained from each subject.

Exclusion criteria: BMI<20 or>30, severe renal inadequacy (creatinine clearance rate ≤120 μmol/L); pregnant; known allergies to iodinated contrast agent; severe arrhythmia; cardiac function or thrombolysis in myocardial infarction (TIMI) flow<‴ Grade III after coronary artery stenting or coronary artery bypass grafting (CABG).

Acquisition protocol. A 256-slice MDCT scanner (Brilliance iCT; Philips Healthcare, Cleveland, OH, USA) was used. Automatic bolus tracking (Bolus Pro, Philips Healthcare) was used with a region of interest (ROI) in the ascending aorta at the level of pulmonary artery. The scans were initiated under full inspiration 6 seconds after a pre-determined signal attenuation threshold of 180 HU was attained. A volume of 60–70 mL of contrast media (Iohexol 350; GE Healthcare, Shanghai, China), followed by 20 mL saline was intravenously injected at a flow rate of 5 mL/s into the antecubital vein through the use of dual-tube high pressure syringe (Ulrich REF XD 2051) equipped with an 18-gauge catheter. The coronary CTA scan parameters were as follows: tube potential = 120 kVp; effective tube current-time product = 210, 84 mAs for routine-dose group and low-dose group, respectively; detector configuration = 128×0.625 mm; rotation time = 270 ms; field of view = 250 mm; slice thickness = 0.9 mm; increment = 0.45 mm. The scan trigger was centered around a physiologic cardiac phase of ventricular diastasis corresponding to 75% of the R-R interval, with a ±5% buffer used when the fluctuation of heart rate was >5 beats/min. Prior to CT examination, patients with heart rate >70 beats/min were administered oral ß-receptor blockers 12.5–25 mg (Metoprolol Succinate sustained-release tablets, AstraZeneca, Sweden) to decrease and stabilize the heart rate.

CT data reconstruction and image analysis. Images from the routine-dose (Group 1) acquisitions were reconstructed using FBP algorithm. The low-dose acquisitions (Group 2) were reconstructed using an IRT with the appropriate level (L5) to account for any increase in noise caused by the lowered tube output. A standard-sharp reconstruction kernel (XCC) was used in all image reconstructions. The matrix size of reconstructed images was 512×512.

Subjective evaluation of image quality. Transverse image data from each group was analyzed using an advanced cardiac

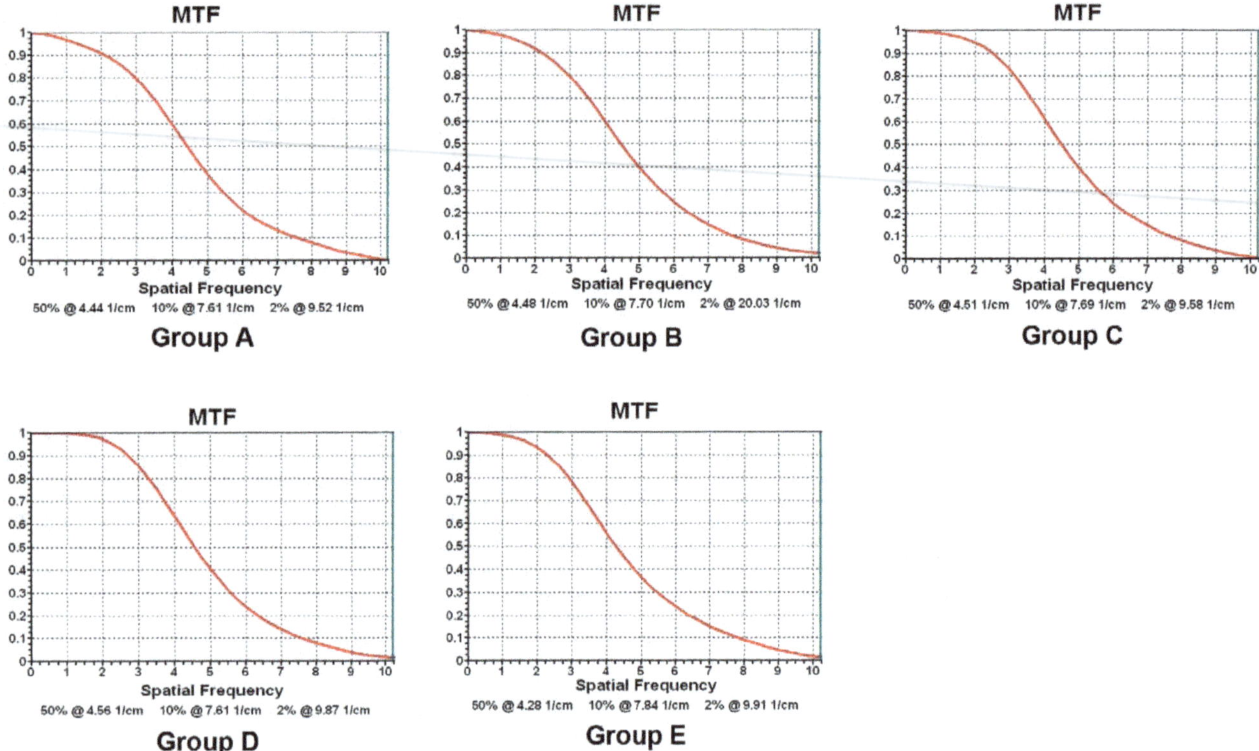

Figure 3. MTF curves of the phantom scans. No significant differences are observed between Group A and each of the low-dose iterative reconstruction groups (Groups B–E).

application (Cardiac Viewer and Comprehensive Cardiac Analysis) on a dedicated CT workstation (Extended Brilliance Workspace Version 4.01, Philips Healthcare). In addition to the transverse images, curved multi-planar reformats of the left anterior descending (LAD) artery, left circumflex (LCX) artery, and right coronary artery (RCA) were used to evaluate image quality as judged by overall image acceptability, contrast between blood vessels and the surrounding tissues, lumen edge sharpness and subjective noise in vessels with diameters $\geq$1.5 mm. These characteristics were evaluated using a 4-point grading scale: 4: excellent image quality, very good contrast, very clear and sharp lumen edge, and very low noise; 3: good image quality, good contrast, sharp lumen edge, and low noise; 2: fair image quality and contrast, blurred lumen edge, and high noise; 1: poor image quality and contrast, blurred lumen edge, and very high noise. Image quality was evaluated by two experienced (>5 years) cardiac radiologists who were blinded to scan conditions and patients' clinical data. If necessary, a third radiologist was asked to adjudicate the differences in order to obtain a consensus score.

Objective evaluation of image quality. A 2-cm^{2}ROI was identified within the aortic root at the level of the origin of the left main coronary artery. The mean CT value (HU) within the ROI was measured and its standard deviation was noted down as the image noise of the aorta. The SNR was calculated using the formula: SNR = signal$_{ao}$/noise$_{ao}$. The CT value of pericardial fat surrounding the left main coronary artery at the same level was measured, and the ROI size was designated as the maximum area without vessels. The CNR was calculated using the formula: CNR = (HU$_{ao}$ – HU$_{fat}$)/image noise$_{ao}$. [22].

Measurement of radiation dose. The CTDI$_{vol}$ and dose-length product (DLP) values during the scans were recorded. The estimated effective dose (ED) was derived as the product of the DLP and a conversion coefficient k, (ED = DLP×k), where k is the conversion coefficient for chest (k = 0.014 mSv mGy^{-1} cm^{-1}) [23].

Statistical Analysis

Statistical analysis was performed using commercially available software (SPSS 17.0, SPSS, Chicago, IL, USA). Continuous variables were expressed as mean ± standard deviation. Continuous variables and demographic data were compared by a paired Student's t-test. The kappa test was used to test inter-reader agreement in subjective evaluation of image quality. When discrepancy exists, a third radiologist was asked to give evaluation, and the consistent score was taken as the final scoring result. If the score from the three radiologists was different, the radiologists would discuss the case until an agreement was reached. The Mann-Whitney U test was used to test for differences in subjective evaluation of image quality between two groups. A level of $P<0.05$ was considered statistically significant.

Results

Phantom Study

Comparison of phantom objective indices. As expected, a reduction in the tube output resulted in corresponding increases in the image noise. The use of the IRT addressed this increase in image noise. For a given tube output, the IRT reconstruction algorithm yielded lower image noise compared to FBP, with increasing levels of IRT offering increasing noise reductions in a linear manner (Figure 1).

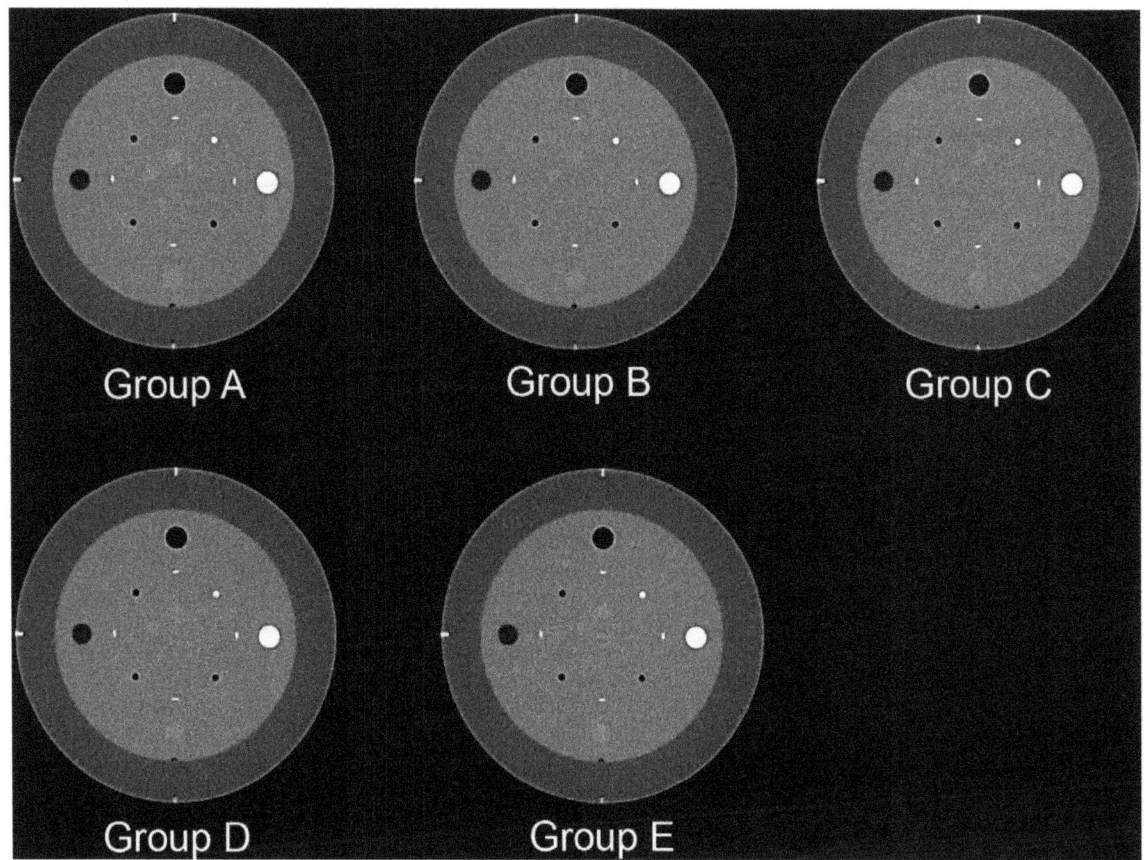

Figure 4. Phantom images acquired with routine dose(120 kv, 210 mAs) and different low dose (120 kv, 125–63 mAs) scan. A: 120 KV, 210 mAs with FBP reconstruction. B: 120 KV, 125 mAs with iDose^4 reconstruction (L3). C: 120 KV, 105 mAs with iDose^4 reconstruction (L4). D: 120 KV, 84 mAs with iDose^4 reconstruction (L5). E: 120 KV, 63 mAs with iDose^4 reconstruction (L6). The subjective image quality score was equivalent between Group D and Group A. The score of nodule conspicuity in the Group E was significantly lower than that in the Group A.

There were no significant differences in mean CT values of the background and the Teflon spheres between each low-dose group and routine-dose FBP group ($p = 0.4$). At equal radiation doses, IRT reconstruction produced higher CNR than FBP reconstruction, with the CNR increasing in a linear manner with increased IRT level (Figure 2).

IRT levels L3, L4, L5, L6 were used for 125 mAs (Group B), 105 mAs (Group C, 84 mAs (Group D), and 63 mAs (Group E) sequences respectively, to compensate for the increased image noise caused by decreased tube output to achieve the noise and CNR equivalent to or better than those of images reconstructed with FBP at 120 kV and 210 mAs.

There were no significant differences in image noise and CNR between routine-dose FBP group (Group A) and the 84 mAs, 63 mAs groups (i.e., Groups D and E respectively). The image noise and CNR in the Groups B and C were significantly superior to those of the routine-dose FBP group (Group A). The image noise and CNR in each group are shown in Table 1.

There was no significant difference in MTF curves between Group A and low-dose iterative reconstruction groups (Groups B–E), *i.e.*, there was no significant difference in spatial resolution among the groups (Figure 3).

Comparison of phantom subjective image quality. The center-slice images of CTP401 module in each dose group are

Table 2. Subjective image quality scores for phantoms in different dose groups.

Item	120 KV+210 mAs /FBP (Group A)	120 KV+125 mAs /L3 (Group B)	120 KV+105 mAs /L4 (Group C)	120 KV+84 mAs /L5 (Group D)	120 KV+63 mAs /L6 (Group E)
Artifact	3	4	3	3	3
Nodule conspicuity	3	3	3	3	2
Detectable minimal nodule size (mm)	4	4	4	4	6
Overall image quality	3	4	3.5	3	2

FBP: filtered back projection; L: IRT level.

Table 3. Comparison of general data and objective image quality of patients between Group 1 (routine-dose FBP reconstruction) and Group 2 (120 KV+84 mAs/IRT L5 reconstruction).

Item	Group 1	Group 2	t	P
Age (year)	54±18 (34-75)	52±10 (28-77)	−0.58	0.56
Sex (male/ female)	15/6	20/16	2.97†	0.09†
Body mass index	25.40±2.06	25.45±2.15	−1.28	0.2
	(22.83-28.68)	(23.16-29.10)		
Heart rate	62±6 (47-69)	59±6 (49-69)	−1.16	0.25
Heart rate viability	1.72±1.15 (0-5)	1.16±1.07 (0-5)	−1.88	0.07
Scan length	12.92±1.62	12.76±1.20	−0.44	0.66
	(10.92-16.35)	(10.96-18.78)		
CT_{aorta}	421.30±43.63	444.46±50.85	−1.75	0.09
	(354.4-558.1)	(352.7-540.1)		
CT_{fat}	−99.21±18.84	−91.97±17.92	1.44	0.16
	(−74.5-−151.3)	(−59.0-−124.3)		
Image noise	35.49±9.44	36.54±10.70	0.37	0.71
	(24.0-59.1)	(19.1-69.4)		
SNR	12.43±2.54	13.63±4.93	1.03	0.31
	(7.1-16.5)	(5.8-30.7)		
CNR	15.39±3.22	16.28±5.41	0.68	0.50
	(8.7-20.1)	(7.0-35.1)		

Note: †indicates the results of x^2. SNR: Signal-to-noise ratio, CNR: contrast-to-noise ratio.

shown in Figure 4. The subjective image quality scores in Groups B and C were better than those of Group A. The subjective image quality score was equivalent between Group D and Group A. The score of nodule conspicuity in the Group E was significantly lower than that of Group A, and the detectable minimal nodule size in Group E reached 6 mm, which was higher compared to the other groups (Table 2).

Taken together, Group D (120 kV, 84 mAs and L5 reconstruction) provided an optimum balance, producing equivalent image quality to Group A, at the lowest possible radiation dose.

Patient Study

All subjects underwent coronary CTA successfully. There were no significant differences in general data of subjects between Group 1 and Group 2 (Table 3).

There were no significant difference in image noise, SNR and CNR between Group 1 and Group 2. The subjective indices in Group 2 were slightly better than those in the Group 1 (Table 3).

The two radiologists showed very good consistency in subjective scores. The kappa value of image contrast, sharpness, objective noise and overall image quality was 0.66, 0.84, 0.84, and 0.85, respectively. In both groups, each subjective index was scored ≥3, and the IQ was good and met clinical diagnostic requirement. There were no significant differences in the index scores between the groups (Table 4, Figure 5).

The CTDI and DLP were 19.55±4.11 (Group 1) and 228.55±41.14 (Group 2), showing significant differences ($p<0.001$). The effective radiation dose in Group 2 was 1.21±0.14 mSv compared to 3.20±0.58 mSv (Group 1), reflecting dose savings of 62.5% ($p<0.05$).

Discussion

In our study, we scanned the Catphan CT phantoms using a conventional tube voltage and decreasing tube currents, measured noise and CNR of each dose group reconstructed using both FBP and IRT approaches, and identified the levels of IRT in each low dose group that provided IQ that was equivalent to the routine-dose FBP reconstruction. From the comparisons of IQ (both subjective and objective) between the routine-dose FBP group and each low- dose IRT group, the protocol of 120 kV, 84 mAs and L5 reconstruction was determined as the protocol that provided an optimal balance of IQ and radiation dose reductions. This protocol was also performed in patients with normal body habitus prospectively enrolled in a clinical study to further confirm the feasibility of this low-dose protocol.

The IRT used in this study (iDose[4]) is a fourth generation algorithm designed to reduce image artifacts and noise while maintaining the structural/anatomical information [16,17]. The use of photon statistics in the projection domain helps to iteratively reduce noise and preserve edges, and use of noise/structure models in the image domain to further reduce image noise.

The levels of IRT used in this study are designed to provide a noise reduction factor to compensate for any noise increases with the reduction in the tube output. Our phantom results showed a linear decrease in image noise with increasing levels of IRT; our experience was similar to prior work [16,17] achieving noise reduction levels of 15%–45% as the levels of the IRT was increased from L2 to L6 for a given tube output. Thus, when the tube output is reduced by 40–70%, the corresponding IRT levels can be employed to result in objective image quality which is equivalent to or better than the FBP images from the routine-dose scans (i.e., Group A). In our phantom study, the noise values in the Groups B (125 mAs) and C (105 mAs) were actually lower than that those measured in Group A, and there were no significant differences in actual noise values between Groups D & E and Group A. Lowered image noise resulted in increased CNR in Groups B and C compared to Group A; no significant differences in CNR were observed between Groups D & E (59.3±5.3 and 59.5±2.3 respectively) and Group A (56.2±2.8)($P<0.001$).

There were no significant differences in MTF value and curve shape between Group A and Groups B–E. This suggests that the IRT decreases image noise, while not negatively impacting spatial resolution. Retaining a relatively high spatial resolution is of importance for displaying coronary arteries.

The subjective evaluation scores of phantoms were similar between each low-dose iterative reconstruction group (Groups B–E) and Group A. No graininess, streak artifacts or blotchy/plastic artifacts were observed in each group. This advantage is superior to early iterative reconstruction approaches [24]. This can be attributed to the IRT used in this study which reduces noise without altering the image noise power spectrum and prevents artifacts to preserve the natural appearance of the image.

The subjective scores in Groups B and C were superior to those of Group A. Artifact, nodule conspicuity, minimal detectable nodule size and overall IQ in Group D were equivalent to those in the Group A. The nodule conspicuity and minimal detectable nodule size in the Group E were slightly lower than those in the Group A. These results may be related to the slightly decreased spatial resolution [11]. Our phantom experimental results showed that according to the "ALARA" principle, a tube voltage of 120 kVp, 84 mAs tube current x-ray on time product supple-

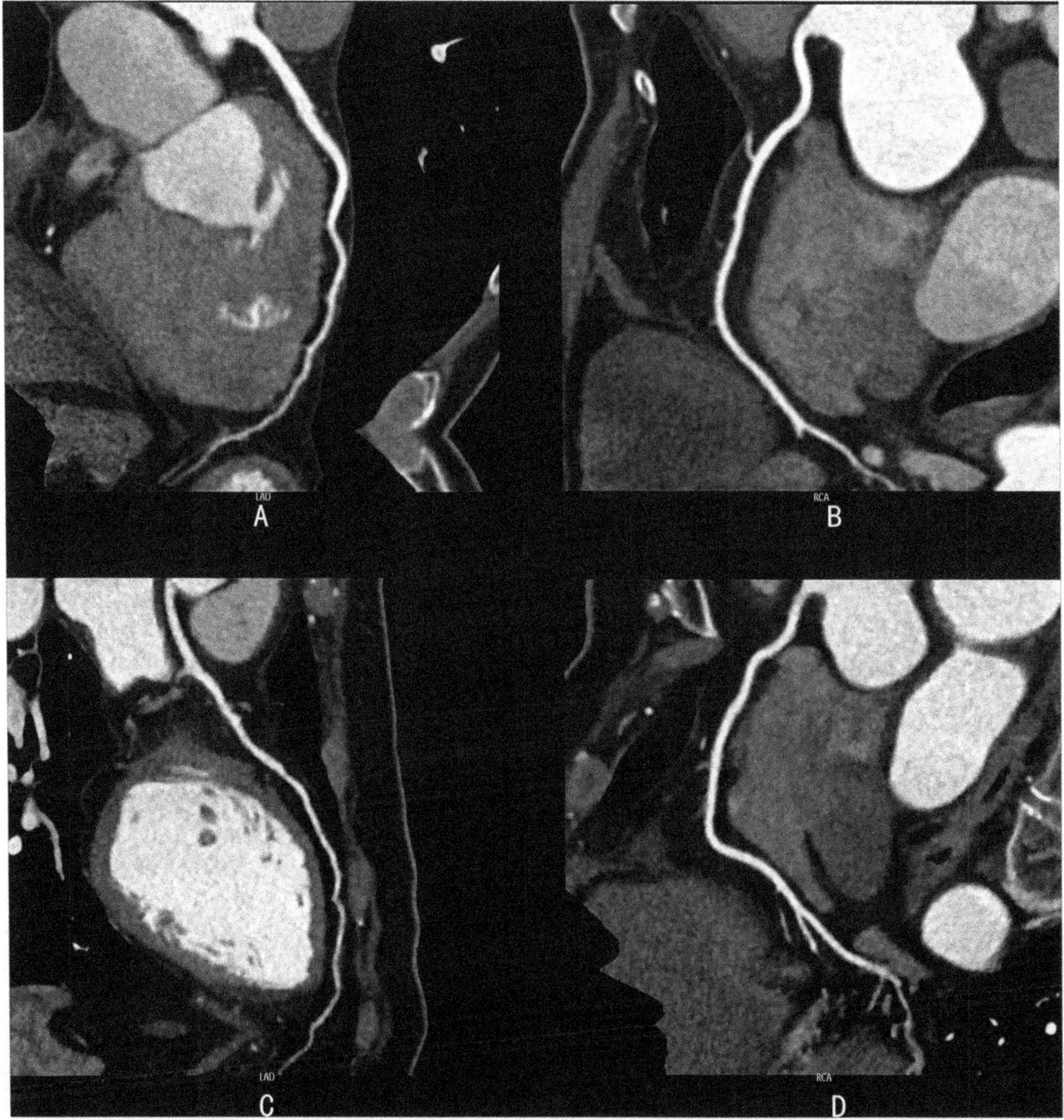

Figure 5. Representative examples of patient scans. There were no significant differences in subjective ranking for image sharpness, contrast, noise, and overall acceptability between patients belonging to Group 1 and 2. (A, B): Group 1, CPR pictures of LAD (Fig. 5A) and RCA (Fig. 5B) of a 53-year-old male with a body mass index (BMI) of 24.2 scanned at 120 kVp and 210 mAs and reconstructed with filtered back projection. Image quality (IQ) scores were 4, 4, 4, and 4 for contrast, sharpness, subjective noise, and acceptability, respectively. (C, D): Group 2, A 57-year-old male with BMI of 24.1 scanned at 120 kVp (Fig. 5C) and 84 mAs (Fig. 5D) and reconstructed with L5. IQ scores were 4, 4, 4 and 4 for contrast, sharpness, subjective noise, and acceptability, respectively.

mented by an iterative reconstruction technique of an appropriate level (L5) is the optimal combination that provides IQ comparable to the FBP reconstructions of routine-dose scans.

Recently, some studies investigating low radiation dose coronary CTA used a decreased tube voltage (80 kVp and 100 kVp) and maintained high IQ and CNR in a select group of patients with a normal body mass index [25–30]. This could be attributed to the selected energy levels being closer to the K edge of iodine, thereby increasing the contrast enhancement and thus potentially enabling a reduction of volume of contrast agent used.

However, the use of low tube voltage could also result in a larger proportion of dose absorbed by the body, potentially causing a higher degree of beam hardening effects. Since reducing the tube output (current) instead of the tube voltage only changes the effective energy and affects the x-ray penetration to a lesser extent,

Table 4. Comparison of subjective image quality between Group 1 (routine-dose FBP reconstruction) and Group 2 (120 KV+84 mAs/IRT L 5).

Item	Group 1 (score 4/3/2/1)	Group 2 (score 4/3/2/1)	U	*P*
Contrast	20/1/0/0	35/1/0/0	370.5[†]	0.69
Sharpness	20/1/0/0	31/5/0/0	343.5[†]	0.28
Objective noise	19/2/0/0	32/4/0/0	372[†]	0.85
Overall Image quality	19/2/0/0	30/6/0/0	351[†]	0.46

[†]Mann-Whitney test were used.

we used a conventional tube voltage (120 kVp) and low tube currents in this study.

The prospectively ECG-triggered coronary CTA is currently the main method to decrease the radiation dose in coronary CTA. The 256-slice multi-detector computed tomography system can achieve an axial scan range of 8 cm and allow scan of the entire heart within 3 cardiac cycles, with a rotation speed of 0.27 sec, which could relax the heart rate requirements for coronary CTA using prospective gating (i.e., increases the threshold of the upper HR limit to 75 bpm) while at the same time enabling coronary CTA imaging at well under the average background radiation levels [22,31,32].

Extending our findings from the phantom scans, we have shown that the iterative reconstruction technique used in this study (iDose4), combined with prospective ECG gating in 256-slice MDCT can significantly decrease radiation dose in patient scans without negatively impacting IQ. Results from this study showed that there were no significant differences in subjective and objective IQ between Group 2 (reduced dose patient scans) and Group 1 (routine dose). The CTDI and ED in the Group 2 were decreased by 63% and 62% respectively compared to Group 1 ($p<0.05$). The effective radiation dose in the Group 2 reached 1.21±0.14 mSv. The extent of radiation dose savings is similar to recent findings [16,19]. The dual benefits of maintaining (or even improving IQ) at low radiation dose could make the use of IRT in virtually all patient cohorts, especially in those sub-groups that are sensitive to radiation dose (younger population like infants and pediatrics) and those who require re-examination for follow-up of coronary plaque progression, percutaneous transcoronary angioplasty, coronary artery bypass grafting (CABG), etc.

The limitations of this study are as follows: (1) Our sample size was small and we did not adjust the protocol according to the BMI/body weight of the individual patients (the BMI ranged from 23 to 29 in our study). (2) We only focused on the overall image quality and did not investigate the effect of the IRT on coronary artery plaque and the diagnostic accuracy by comparing with the respective gold standards. (3) We did not evaluate the reconstruction time of the IRT compared to the conventional FBP, which may influence its wide clinical application; but the IRT used in this study had a reconstruction time of about 20 images per second making it clinically practical.

Conclusion

In conclusion, our results of phantoms and the subjects with normal body weights confirmed that the iterative reconstruction technique (iDose[4]) used in prospectively ECG-triggered 256-slice coronary CTA can greatly decrease image noise and improve image quality, while at the same time providing radiation dose reductions of up to 63%.

Author Contributions

Conceived and designed the experiments: QG YH. Performed the experiments: YH JZ YW MY. Analyzed the data: YH JZ YW MY. Contributed reagents/materials/analysis tools: JZ YW MY. Wrote the paper: YH QG MV.

References

1. Kerl JM, Schoepf UJ, Zwerner PL, Bauer RW, Abro JA, et al. (2011) Accuracy of coronary artery stenosis detection with CT versus conventional coronary angiography compared with composite findings from both tests as an enhanced reference standard. Eur Radiol 21: 1895–1903.
2. Leschka S, Stolzmann P, Desbiolles L, Baumueller S, Goetti R, et al. (2009) Diagnostic accuracy of high-pitch dual-source CT for the assessment of coronary stenoses: first experience. Eur Radiol 19: 2896–2903.
3. Janne d'Othee B, Siebert U, Cury R, Jadvar H, Dunn EJ, et al. (2008) A systematic review on diagnostic accuracy of CT-based detection of significant coronary artery disease. Eur J Radiol 65: 449–461.
4. Alkadhi H, Stolzmann P, Desbiolles L, Baumueller S, Goetti R, et al.(2010) Low-dose, 128-slice, dual-source CT coronary angiography: accuracy and radiation dose of the high-pitch and the step-and-shoot mode. Heart 96: 933–938.
5. Marwan M, Pflederer T, Schepis T, Seltmann M, Klinghammer L, et al. (2012)Accuracy of dual-source CT to identify significant coronary artery disease in patients with uncontrolled hypertension presenting with chest pain: comparison with coronary angiography. Int J Cardiovasc Imaging.
6. Raff GL. (2010) Radiation dose from coronary CT angiography: five years of progress. J Cardiovasc Comput Tomogr 4: 365–374.
7. Mitsumori LM, Shuman WP, Busey JM, Kolokythas O, Koprowicz KM (2012) Adaptive statistical iterative reconstruction versus filtered back projection in the same patient: 64 channel liver CT image quality and patient radiation dose. Eur Radiol 22: 138–143.
8. Prakash P, Kalra MK, Kambadakone AK, Pien H, Hsieh J, et al. (2012) Reducing abdominal CT radiation dose with adaptive statistical iterative reconstruction technique. Invest Radiol 45: 202–210.
9. Singh S, Kalra MK, Hsieh J, Licato PE, Do S, et al. (2010) Abdominal CT: comparison of adaptive statistical iterative and filtered back projection reconstruction techniques. Radiology 257: 373–383.
10. Kambadakone AR, Chaudhary NA, Desai GS, Nguyen DD, Kulkarni NM, et al. (2011) Low-dose MDCT and CT enterography of patients with Crohn disease: feasibility of adaptive statistical iterative reconstruction. AJR Am J Roentgenol 196: W743–752.
11. Hara AK, Paden RG, Silva AC, Kujak JL, Lawder HJ, et al. (2009) Iterative reconstruction technique for reducing body radiation dose at CT: feasibility study. AJR Am J Roentgenol 193: 764–771.
12. Singh S, Kalra MK, Gilman MD, Hsieh J, Pien HH, et al. (2011) Adaptive statistical iterative reconstruction technique for radiation dose reduction in chest CT: a pilot study. Radiology 259: 565–573.
13. Prakash P, Kalra MK, Ackman JB, Digumarthy SR, Hsieh J, et al. (2010) Diffuse lung disease: CT of the chest with adaptive statistical iterative reconstruction technique. Radiology 256: 261–269.
14. Hu XH, Ding XF, Wu RZ, Zhang MM (2011) Radiation dose of non-enhanced chest CT can be reduced 40% by using iterative reconstruction in image space. Clin Radiol 66: 1023–1029.
15. Pontana F, Duhamel A, Pagniez J, Flohr T, Faivre JB, et al (2011) Chest computed tomography using iterative reconstruction vs filtered back projection (Part 2): image quality of low-dose CT examinations in 80 patients. Eur Radiol 21: 636–643.
16. Noël PB FA, Renger B (2011) Initial performance characterization of a clinical noise-suppressing reconstruction algorithm for MDCT. Am J Roentgenol 197: 1404–1409.
17. Hou Y, Liu X, Xv S, Guo W, Guo Q (2012) Comparisons of Image Quality and Radiation Dose Between Iterative Reconstruction and Filtered Back Projection Reconstruction Algorithms in 256-MDCT Coronary Angiography. AJR Am J Roentgenol 199: 588–594.
18. Leipsic J, Labounty TM, Heilbron B, Min JK, Mancini GB, et al. (2010) Estimated radiation dose reduction using adaptive statistical iterative reconstruction in coronary CT angiography: the ERASIR study. AJR Am J Roentgenol 195: 655–660.
19. Park EA, Lee W, Kim KW, Kim KG, Thomas A, et al. (2012) Iterative reconstruction of dual-source coronary CT angiography: assessment of image quality and radiation dose. Int J Cardiovasc Imaging.

20. Wang R, Schoepf UJ, Wu R, Reddy RP, Zhang C, et al. (2012) Image quality and radiation dose of low dose coronary CT angiography in obese patients: Sinogram affirmed iterative reconstruction versus filtered back projection. Eur J Radiol.
21. Funama Y, Taguchi K, Utsunomiya D, Oda S, Yanaga Y, et al. (2011) Combination of a low-tube-voltage technique with hybrid iterative reconstruction (iDose) algorithm at coronary computed tomographic angiography. J Comput Assist Tomogr 35: 480–485.
22. Hou Y, Yue Y, Guo W, Feng G, Yu T, et al. (2012) Prospectively versus retrospectively ECG-gated 256-slice coronary CT angiography: image quality and radiation dose over expanded heart rates. Int J Cardiovasc Imaging 28: 153–162.
23. McCollough C CD, Edyvean S (2008) The measurement, reporting, and management of radiation dose in CT. Tech. Rep. 96. American Association of Physicists in Medicine, College Park.
24. Leipsic J, Labounty TM, Heilbron B, Min JK, Mancini GB, et al. (2010) Adaptive statistical iterative reconstruction: assessment of image noise and image quality in coronary CT angiography. AJR Am J Roentgenol 195: 649–654.
25. Feuchtner GM, Jodocy D, Klauser A, Haberfellner B, Aglan I, et al. (2010) Radiation dose reduction by using 100-kV tube voltage in cardiac 64-slice computed tomography: a comparative study. Eur J Radiol 75: e51–56.
26. Gutstein A DD, Cheng V, Wolak A, Gransar H, Suzuki Y, et al. (2008) Algorithm for radiation dose reduction with helical dual source coronary computed tomography angiography in clinical practice. J Cardiovasc Comput Tomogr 2: 311–322.
27. Leschka S, Stolzmann P, Schmid FT, Scheffel H, Stinn B, et al. (2008) Low kilovoltage cardiac dual-source CT: attenuation, noise, and radiation dose. Eur Radiol 18: 1809–1817.
28. Pflederer T, Rudofsky L, Ropers D, Bachmann S, Marwan M, et al. (2009) Image Quality in a Low Radiation Exposure Protocol for Retrospectively ECG-Gated Coronary CT Angiography. AJR Am J Roentgenol 192: 1045–1050.
29. Klass O, Walker M, Siebach A, Stuber T, Feuerlein S, et al. (2009) A Prospectively gated axial CT coronary angiography: comparison of image quality and effective radiation dose between 64- and 256-slice CT. Eur Radiol 20: 1124–1131.
30. Law WY, Yang CC, Chen LK, Huang TC, Lu KM, et al. (2011) Retrospective gating vs. prospective triggering for noninvasive coronary angiography: Assessment of image quality and radiation dose using a 256-slice CT scanner with 270 ms gantry rotation. Acad Radiol 18: 31–39.
31. Hosch W, Stiller W, Mueller D, Gitsioudis G, Welzel J, et al. (2012) Reduction of radiation exposure and improvement of image quality with BMI-adapted prospective cardiac computed tomography and iterative reconstruction. Eur J Radiol 81: 3568–3576.
32. Hosch W, Heye T, Schulz F, Lehrke S, Schlieter M, et al. (2011) Image quality and radiation dose in 256-slice cardiac computed tomography: Comparison of prospective versus retrospective image acquisition protocols. Eur J Radiol 80: 127–135.

16

Geometric Facial Gender Scoring: Objectivity of Perception

Syed Zulqarnain Gilani[1]*, Kathleen Rooney[2], Faisal Shafait[1], Mark Walters[3], Ajmal Mian[1]

1 School of Computer Science and Software Engineering, The University of Western Australia, Perth, Western Australia, **2** School of Anatomy, Physiology and Human Biology, The University of Western Australia, Perth, Western Australia, **3** Cranio-MaxilloFacial Unit, Princess Margaret Hospital for Children, Perth, Western Australia

Abstract

Gender score is the cognitive judgement of the degree of masculinity or femininity of a face which is considered to be a continuum. Gender scores have long been used in psychological studies to understand the complex psychosocial relationships between people. Perceptual scores for gender and attractiveness have been employed for quality assessment and planning of cosmetic facial surgery. Various neurological disorders have been linked to the facial structure in general and the facial gender perception in particular. While, subjective gender scoring by human raters has been a tool of choice for psychological studies for many years, the process is both time and resource consuming. In this study, we investigate the geometric features used by the human cognitive system in perceiving the degree of masculinity/femininity of a 3D face. We then propose a mathematical model that can mimic the human gender perception. For our experiments, we obtained 3D face scans of 64 subjects using the 3dMDface scanner. The textureless 3D face scans of the subjects were then observed in different poses and assigned a gender score by 75 raters of a similar background. Our results suggest that the human cognitive system employs a combination of Euclidean and geodesic distances between biologically significant landmarks of the face for gender scoring. We propose a mathematical model that is able to automatically assign an objective gender score to a 3D face with a correlation of up to 0.895 with the human subjective scores.

Editor: Alessandro D'Ausilio, IIT - Italian Institute of Technology, Italy

Funding: This research was partly supported by Australian Research Council Discovery Grant DP110102399 and UWA Faculty of Engineering, Computing and Mathematics Development Grant. Syed Zulqarnain Gilani is supported by International Postgraduate Research Scholarship, and Faisal Shafait was supported by Australian Research Council grant LP110201008. The funding agencies had no role in study design, data collection and analysis, decision to publish, or preparation of the manuscript.

Competing Interests: The authors have declared that no competing interests exist.

* E-mail: zulqarnain.gilani@uwa.edu.au

Introduction

Cognitive judgements of facial attractiveness, gender and the degree of masculinity/femininity are found to be universally reproducible in people of varied cultural and ethnic backgrounds [1,2]. The Human mind has the capability to assess facial masculinity/femininity and this gender attribute plays an important role in social behaviours. Psychologists and cognitive scientists have extensively analysed the role of perceived gender (masculinity/femininity) on various socio-psychological behaviours in a number of studies (see Table. 1 for a summary).

A subjective gender score is a tangible metric that human raters assign to the degree of masculinity/femininity of a face. This is because, though sex is binary, gender is understood to be a continuum. For example, Figure 1 shows synthetic images of the same individual by varying its gender from very male to very female. In the literature these scores have also been referred to as perceptual gender scores, masculinity/femininity scores or masculinity/femininity index (referred later as masculinity index for brevity).

Subjective gender scoring has been widely used by researchers in Psychology to study the relationship between sexual dimorphism and facial attractiveness [3,4], mate choice [5,8], personal character traits [9] as well as perceived and actual health [10]. Applications of subjective gender scores in medical and health care include analysis of the effects of syndromes (e.g. Autism Spectrum Disorder) on facial masculinity/femininity [11], relationship between sexual dimorphism and semen quality [12]/facial symmetry [13]. Other uses include evaluation of the outcome of facial cosmetic surgery [14,15]. A comprehensive overview of the applications of subjective gender scoring is given in Table 1. In these studies, a number of human raters are asked to judge the masculinity/femininity of the subjects.

The process of perceptual gender rating in itself is both time and resource consuming and a challenging problem is to identify the nature of predictors or features that are employed by the human mind for this task. Some researchers have also investigated objective scores for sexual dimorphism (masculinity/femininity) using morphometric analysis [16–18]. The key idea behind calculating objective masculinity index is to use facial measurements, like distances between biologically significant landmarks or ratios of these distances, for obtaining a score of facial masculinity/femininity. For each face these measures can be used individually or collectively by adding their standardised measures or their Z-scores.

Scheib et al. [16] obtained masculinity indices by summing up the standardized facial measures of the cheek-bone prominence and relative lower face length from grayscale pictures of 40 male subjects. The authors then asked 12 female participants to rate these faces for attractiveness. Interestingly, the masculinity index

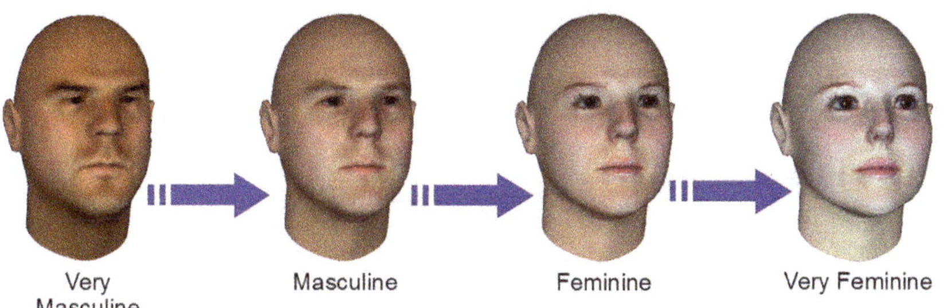

Figure 1. Facial gender is considered to be a continuum over masculinity or femininity. Figure shows morphed 3D images of the same individual with gender varying from highly masculine to highly feminine. Which geometric features do human observers employ for ascribing a score to this variation and can such scores be replicated by computer algorithms? (Note: These images have been created from a model [45,46] as we are barred from publishing images of actual subjects under ethics approval.)

correlated positively with facial attractiveness (more masculine males were more attractive) which is against the established norms [3]. In a similar study, Penton et al. [17] calculated five separate masculinity indices for each face using measures related to eye size, ratio of lower face height to total face height, cheek bone prominence, ratio of face width to lower face height and mean eyebrow height. Two dimensional pictures of 60 male and 49 female faces were used in this study. The authors did not find a correlation between these five dimorphic measurements and female-rated facial attractiveness. However, the rated attractiveness correlated positively with a composite masculinity index found by summing up the standardized Z-scores of the five individual measures. In a later study, Pound et al. [19] used the same approach to calculate a composite facial masculinity index from 2D photographs of 57 male subjects. The study aimed at analysing the correlation between circulating testosterone levels and masculinity in males. Fifty seven male subjects were first asked to predict, by seeing the photographs, the outcome of a particular wrestler in six wrestling bouts. Subjects were then shown videos of the bouts allocated to a "winning" and "loosing" condition and pre/post task testosterone levels were measured. A group of 72 participants was then asked to rate the subjects for their perceived masculinity. The authors did not find any correlation between perceived masculinity and pre/post task testosterone levels. However, post task increase in testosterone levels correlated positively with the facial masculinity index. Note that, none of these studies explored the relationship between the perceived/ rated masculinity and the objective facial masculinity index.

A more sophisticated method of obtaining the masculinity index is to first perform sex classification using discriminant analysis and then use the discriminant scores associated with each face as its masculinity index. One of the earlier attempts in that direction was made by Burton et al. [20]. The authors performed sex classification on 179 faces using a set of 16 2D and 3D Euclidean facial distances as well as their ratios and angles. The discriminant function score of each face was taken as its masculinity index and the reported sex classification accuracy using Discriminant Function Analysis (DFA) was 94%. However, the authors could

Table 1. Application of masculinity/femininity ratings in various fields of research.

Study	Reference	Subjects	Raters	Ratings
Correlation between masculinity and trustworthiness/emotions	[9]	12	40	480
Relationship between masculinity/femininity and attractiveness as well as masculinity and distinctiveness	[3] [4]	71	204	5036
Relationship between masculinity/femininity and health	[10]	310	37	11470
Relationship between masculinity/femininity and symmetry.	[13]	194	39	5599
Role of gender scores in sex classification of faces.	[47]	200	40	8000
Relationship between sexual behaviour and masculinity/femininity	[5]	362	109	40952
Womens' preference and mate choice based on masculinity of men	[48] [7]	40	20	800
Relationship between masculinity and semen quality in men	[12]	118	12	1416
Relationship between sociosexuality and gender ratings	[6]	8+50	195+17	2410
Role of masculinity in the functioning of a male endocrine system	[19]	57	72	4104
Role of masculinity and femininity in distinguishing homosexuals	[49]	95	58	5510
Effects of syndrome on masculinity/femininity	[11]	103	8	824
Comparison between masculinity (attractiveness) and intelligence as cues for health and provision of resources in mate selection	[8]	32	689	22048
Evaluating the outcome of facial cosmetic surgery in terms of perceptual attractiveness; pre and post surgery	[15] [14]	32; 20	163; 90	5216; 1800

Applications of perceptual gender ratings by employing human raters. Notice the huge number of ratings performed in case. References are provided for interested readers.

not find a positive correlation between their objective scores and the perceptual subjective scores obtained by asking 13 participants to rate the subjects' faces for masculinity/femininity. The correlation coefficient was -0.32 for male faces and -0.33 for female faces. In another study, Thornhill and Gangestad [18] used DFA based on five measures of masculinity (chin length, jaw width, lip width, eye width, and eye height) to yield 75% sex classification accuracy on 2D images of 295 subjects. Discriminant function scores were then used to measure facial masculinity. The authors then analysed the relationship between these masculinity scores and health in terms of respiratory diseases and their duration. There was a significant negative correlation for men and positive for women, between health and facial masculinity. Note that Rhodes et al. [10] did not find any such correlation between perceived masculinity and the actual health of female subjects.

A similar technique was employed by Scott et al. [21] to obtain a morphometric masculinity index. Two datasets of textured images of 20 male faces and 150 (75 male/75 female) faces were used for this purpose. Principle Component Analysis (PCA) was performed on 129 landmarks duly registered using Procrustes analysis and only 11 Principle Components (PCs) were retained. Using DFA, the authors classified facial sex with an accuracy of 96.8% in the first dataset and 98.7% in the second dataset. Discriminant function scores were used as the masculinity index. The relationship between these objective scores and perceived attractiveness was then analysed. The authors did not find any correlation between the male facial masculinity index and perceived attractiveness. However, the relationship between masculinity and attractiveness in female faces was significant and negative. Using the same approach, Stephen et al. [22] measured the masculinity index of 34 male participants using their 2D images. Interestingly, the authors found no correlation between their objective measure of sexual dimorphism and perceived attractiveness. Perhaps the absence of correlation is due to the fact that the authors have used 2D texture images in their experiments. Distances on 2D images are unable to model the facial surface accurately.

The above mentioned studies, on the one hand, highlight the importance of gender rating in evaluating various psychological and medical aspects in humans, and on the other hand, present the obvious difficulty in obtaining these scores. Our literature review shows that, so far, the methods employed for measuring objective masculinity/femininity scores fail to explain the underlying processes in perceptual gender scoring. That is why the objective scores obtained using these methods do not correlate well with subjective perceptual scores, making it difficult to use them instead of, or in combination with, perceptual scores in different studies. Note that, the main aim of these studies was to find relationship between different characteristics/attributes of the face with perceived (or objective) facial gender scores instead of looking for a direct relationship between their perceptual and objective facial masculinity/femininity. The requirement, therefore, is to understand the facial features used by humans to score the masculinity/femininity from faces and to evaluate the plausibility of reproducing these scores using objective measures. Once reliable objective measures are established, computer algorithms can be used to predict the perceived masculinity/femininity of a face with high confidence.

Understanding human perception or Human Visual System (HVS) for particular tasks has been of great interest to researchers (Note that, "Human Visual System" also refers to the anatomical structure of the visual system. However, throughout this paper we have used this term to refer to the cognitive mechanism employed by the human mind to perceptually asses and analyse visual information). Bruce et al. [23] performed Discriminant Function Analysis (DFA) for sex classification using 2D and 3D Euclidean distances extracted from 73 landmarks, the ratios of these distances and angles between them. The authors suggested that perhaps the human visual system takes into account a subset of 16 measurements to classify facial sex, since these features result in a classification accuracy of 94%. Similarly, to understand human and machine sex classification behaviour, Graf et al. [24] used 2D images as stimuli to perform perceptual as well as computational sex classification. The authors asked human subjects to visually classify the 2D images for sex. Next, they used the Principle Components of the images and several state of the art classifiers to understand human internal decision space for sex classification.

To the best of our knowledge, there is no exclusive work on understanding the broad features used by HVS to give a measure to the degree of masculinity/femininity of the face. In the absence of such an understanding, the objective scores calculated by researchers, as evident from our survey, either do not correlate significantly with the perceptual scores or go against the established findings on relationship between perceived sexual dimorphism and other facial traits. This research gap has also resulted in the lack of development of robust algorithms for objective scoring of masculinity/femininity.

There are two major cues used by humans for facial sex classification: shape and appearance. Given the 3D nature of the face, a large amount of shape information gets lost in the 2D images of the face. On the contrary, a 3D face image, although more difficult to capture, has more shape-rich information. O'Toole et al. [25] showed that 3D geometric information outperforms the texture in classifying sex of a face. Similarly, Bruce et al. [26] claimed that visually-derived semantic information like age, expression, gender etc. depend mainly on the geometric form of the perceived face. Therefore, we focus on using 3D geometric faces in this work to capture human perceptual ratings on gender. The main research questions that we want to address are the following:

- Which geometric features are used by the HVS in perceiving the degree of gender of a 3D face?
- Can a mathematical model mimic human performance and objectively rate the gender of a 3D face?

The answers to these questions will help in understanding facial sexual dimorphism and the diagnosis of related syndromes. In this study, we present 3D face models of 64 subjects in frontal, oblique and profile views to 75 raters to obtain perceptual ratings and analyse the physical features used by the raters to rate the faces. Next, we build a computational model based on the results of the perceptual study to objectively rate the gender using 3D Euclidean and geodesic features and their combinations. Using this model, we present our findings on the nature of geometric features used by the HVS in rating gender. Our results suggest that humans take into account a combination of 3D Euclidean and geodesic distances while perceiving the amount of sexual dimorphism in a face.

Materials and Methods

This study was performed at University of Western Australia (UWA) and Princess Margaret Hospital (PMH). All participants completed an informed consent form having been given written and verbal details of the tasks to be completed. The study was approved by the Princess Margaret Hospital Ethics Committee vide Approval Reference Number: 1532/EP. For developing the mathematical model for objective gender scores, the digital data was analysed anonymously. All identification features like the meta-data, texture etc. were stripped from the 3D images before hand.

Subjects

Images were obtained from participants recruited from the student body of UWA. 3D images of a total of 64 participants between the ages of 18 and 25, of varying population affinities, who had not undergone significant craniofacial surgery, and had no craniofacial abnormalities or injuries were captured for the current study. The self-reported population affinities were grouped into two categories of Europeans (Caucasian) and non-Europeans ('Other').

Fifty two percent of 64 subjects were females and 48% were males. 80% of the faces were Caucasian/European. The remaining 20% were allocated to the ethnicity category "other" which included Asians (n = 6), Blacks(n = 1), Anglo-Indian (n = 1), Eurasian (n = 2) and Indo-Chinese (n = 1). The majority (78%) of rated faces were of people between the ages of 18 and 21. Sixty eight percent of the rated subjects were born in Australia. Fourteen percent of these identified themselves as having an ethnicity other than Caucasian. The majority of the "other" group were born in Australia (46%), or in Asia (38%), the remainder having been born in Africa (n = 2). Caucasians born outside of Australia were born in Africa (n = 2), New Zealand (n = 6), and the UK (n = 6).

Raters

Raters of a similar background to the imaged subjects were recruited from within and outside the student body at The University of Western Australia. These raters were also categorised as European/Caucasian or non-European/Other.

The panel of raters (n = 75) was composed of 40 females (53%) and 35 males (47%). Sixty four of the raters were Caucasian/ European (84%). The majority, n = 48 (64%), of raters were aged between twenty one and twenty three, although the full age range extended from eighteen to twenty five. The mean age of the raters (21.9 years) was greater than that of the rated image subjects (19.9 years) ($F = 0.34, 6 + 1488 d.f., p = 0.914$). Seventy seven percent of all raters were born in Australia. Seven percent of these identified themselves as having an ethnicity other than Caucasian/European. The majority of the ethnic group Other/non-European was born in Asia (58%), or in Australia (33%), the remainder having been born in Africa (n = 1). Europeans born outside of Australia were born in Asia (n = 2), New Zealand (n = 2), and the UK (n = 4).

3D Facial Stereophotogrammetry

Three dimensional (3D) images of the faces of participants were captured using the 3dMDface 3D stereophotogrammetry system (3dMD LCC, Atlanta Georgia, USA). The 3dMDface system generates 180 degree (ear to ear) 3D images by employing the technique of triangulation. These high-resolution images are captured within 1.5 milliseconds (ms) [27]. Image capture was undertaken in an office environment under standard clinic/office lighting conditions. Subjects were positioned so that imaging of the full face from ear to ear could be achieved. Images were taken of participants with faces holding a neutral expression, and jaws in centric relation with temporomandibular joint seated and natural dental contact without clenching force.

Stimuli Preparation for Perceptual Scoring

Texture maps were stripped from the 3D images to remove features such as eyebrow shape and skin colour. Facial surface was smoothed to diminish the effects of skin texture and eyebrow coarseness. This is done in order to ensure that the raters' perceptions are based solely on facial geometry.

Processed images were prepared into individual packages of 20 randomly chosen faces for viewing on a visual display unit by each individual rater. Packages comprised equal number of males and females, drawn randomly from sex and population subgroups.

Stimuli Preparation for Objective Scoring

We annotated 23 biologically significant landmarks [28] on each image as shown in Figure 2. The motivation for using these landmarks comes from the fact that they represent the sexual dimorphism of the face [29]. These landmarks and Euclidean distances measured from them are used to measure a quantitative dimension for the morphological deviation from the normal face [28], to delineate syndromes [30] and to measure objective masculinity/femininity [21]. We have selected the facial landmarks that relate to the bony structure of the face which is effected by the ratio of testosterone to estrogen (oestrogen) during adolescence [31]. It is believed that facial masculinity is associated with levels of circulating testosterone in men [19]. Hence it is intuitive to use features extracted from these bony landmarks for facial gender scoring.

The pose of each 3D face is corrected to a canonical form based on four landmarks (Ex(L), Ex(R), N and Prn). This step is required to eliminate any error due to pose in the extraction of geodesic distances which will be discussed in detail in the Study 2 of the Experiments Section. Holes are filled and noise removed by re-sampling the 3D face on a uniform grid using the gridfit [32] algorithm. Since some portions of the face are expected to be self occluded (e.g. region around Ac) when re-sampled on a grid, we bisect the 3D face along the vertical axis at the nose tip and rotate each half by 45° before re-sampling to mitigate this problem. Besides hole filling, another advantage of bisecting and rotating the halves before re-sampling is that the resulting 3D face has a more uniform sampling in the 3D space. The processed halves are then rotated back and stitched seamlessly to form a single mesh. Figure 3 shows the different preprocessing steps.

Evaluation Criteria

The main focus of this paper is to find geometric features that are used by HVS for rating gender. Since it is well known that texture itself is very informative on sex classification [20], we used textureless 3D rendered images to avoid any bias in the results due to texture. Abdi et al. [33] show that hair is one of the major contributors in sex classification. To avoid bias resulting from this feature, ratings were obtained on 3D images with the hair concealed or cropped.

Consequent to the above considerations, raters were asked to rate each of the 64 faces for perceived masculinity/femininity and nominate the facial regions they used for this judgement. A computational model was then developed based on this study to objectively score the gender. Our evaluation criterion is the correlation between perceptual ratings and objective scores from the model. Given two random variables X and Y with n samples each, their correlation r is defined as,

$$r = \frac{\sum_{i=1}^{n} (X_i - \overline{X})(Y_i - \overline{Y})}{\sqrt{\sum_{i=1}^{n} (X_i - \overline{X})^2 \sum_{i=1}^{n} (Y_i - \overline{Y})^2}} \quad (1)$$

In each study, we depict the correlation for males and females in a plot. We also project the objective and subjective perceptual

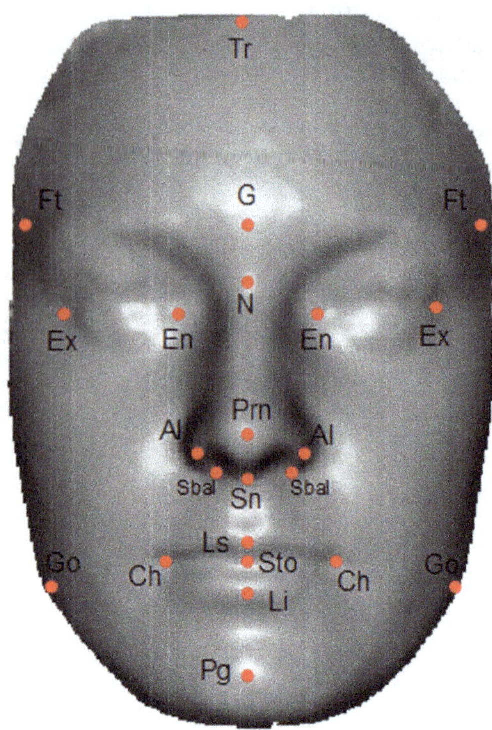

Figure 2. Landmarks used in our algorithm. 23 landmarks annotated on a shaded textureless 3D image. The image is the average face of 10 male subjects from our database.

scores on a Bland-Altman plot [34]. Bland et al. [34] proposed a technique for comparing the outcome of two methods in clinical practice. They argue that a comparison between the average of the outcomes to the difference is a better way of assessing the agreement between two different methods. The Cartesian coordinates of the Bland-Altman plot $\tau(x,y)$ are given by,

$$\tau(x_i,y_i)=\left\{\frac{O_{1i}+O_{2i}}{2},O_{1i}-O_{2i}\right\} \quad (2)$$

where $i=1,\dots,n$ are the samples of each observation O belonging to male/female class.

Perceptual Scoring

As mentioned earlier, the stimuli were prepared into individual packages of 20 randomly chosen faces for viewing on a visual display unit by each individual rater. The rater was unaware of the sex and population composition of the package. As shown in Figure 4, a series of five facial views: left profile, left oblique, straight, right oblique, right profile, were prepared for each subject and displayed on the screen. Raters were able to toggle between these images in making their ratings.

Questionnaires were presented and filled out electronically while viewing the images on a second computer screen. Raters were asked to do the following

- Fill out a personal information questionnaire detailing age, sex and population affinity.
- View each face and rate the degree of masculinity or femininity of the face on a 20 point scale.
- Nominate the facial regions that they used to make their judgement. The options available were forehead, eyes, nose, cheeks, mouth, chin, jaw and no specific features.
- Identify the sex of the individual depicted.

Objective Scoring

An overview of our gender scoring algorithm is given in Figure 5. Gender classification is an important prerequisite for obtaining objective gender scores. Using the annotated landmarks, 44 distances (22 each of the 3D Euclidean and geodesic) related to the regions indicated in Table 2 were extracted as features. Figure 6 shows some of the features used. Further details on these features are given in the Experiments Section.

We begin with feature selection which is a process of selecting the most relevant features for classification while removing the redundant ones. For this purpose we use the minimal redundancy maximal relevance (mRMR) algorithm packed in a forward-selection wrapper [35]. The algorithm first calculates the intrinsic information (relevance) within a feature and also the mutual information (redundancy) among the features to segregate different classes. Then it maximizes the relevance and minimizes the redundancy simultaneously. Let $X \in \mathbb{R}^{m\times n}$ be the feature matrix with m observations and n features, F be the target reduced feature set and c be any arbitrary class from the set of classes C, then relevance is defined by,

$$D(F,c)=\frac{1}{|F|}\sum_{x_i \in F} I(x_i;c), \quad (3)$$

and redundancy is defined by,

$$R(F)=\frac{1}{|F|^2}\sum_{x_i x_j \in F} I(x_i;x_j), \quad (4)$$

where $I(x;y)$ is the mutual information between x and y. Maximal relevance and minimal redundancy is obtained by taking the

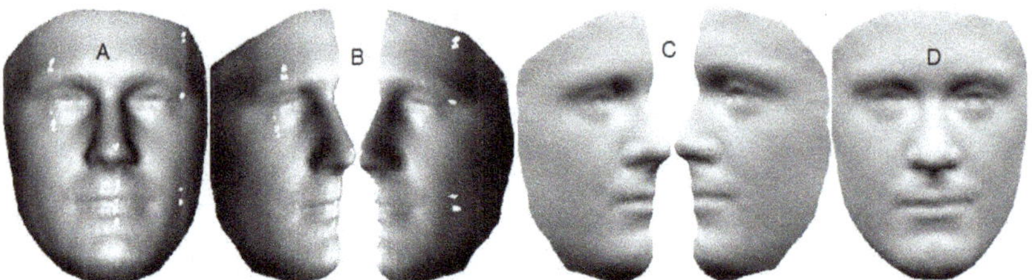

Figure 3. Different steps in preprocessing. (A) The raw input face. (B) Bisected raw face rotated by 45°. Notice the holes in the eye region. (C) Processed face. (D) Processed face stitched back seamlessly.

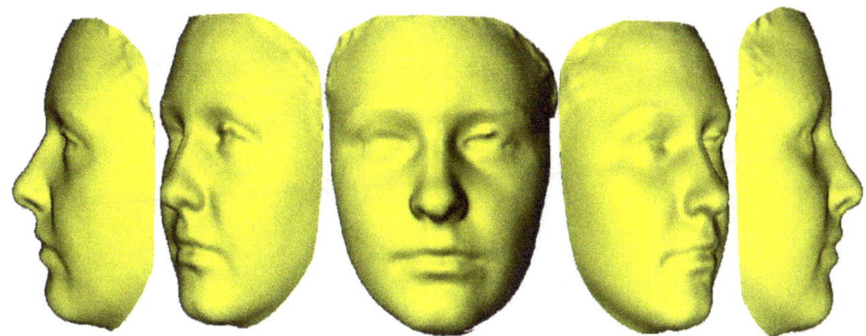

Figure 4. Facial views for perceptual rating. Series of facial views of each subject shown to raters. From left to right: left profile, left oblique, straight, right oblique, right profile.

maximum and minimum values of (3) and (4) respectively. The goal of simultaneously maximizing the relevance and minimising the redundancy is achieved by maximizing the function $\Gamma(D,R)$ where,

$$\Gamma(D,R)=D-R, \tag{5}$$

or

$$\Gamma(D,R)=\frac{D}{R}, \tag{6}$$

where equation (5) is the Mutual Information Difference and equation (6) is the Mutual Information Quotient formulation of mRMR algorithm. Since our feature set is small, we find the classification accuracy yielded by both formulations and use only the one giving the maximum accuracy on training data. The reduced number of candidate features k is selected by first obtaining n feature sets F_n using the mRMR sequential search (Eq. 5 or 6 depending on which one gives better accuracy). More specifically $F_1 \subset F_2 \subset \ldots \subset F_{n-1} \subset F_n$. Next we compare the classification accuracy for all feature subsets $F_1,,\ldots,F_k,\ldots,F_n$ $(1<k<n)$ to find a range for k where the classification accuracy is maximum. Finally, we select a compact set of features by exploiting the forward-selection wrapper [36]. The wrapper first searches for a single feature Θ_1 from the feature set F_k which gives the maximum classification accuracy. Then, from the subset $\{F_k-\Theta_1\}$ we search for another feature such that the subset $\{\Theta_1,\Theta_2\}$ gives the maximum accuracy irrespective of the previous one. This is a deviation from the original mRMR algorithm [35] which desires a feature subset that produces better or equal accuracy than the previous subset in order to minimize the number of evaluations due to the greater number of candidate features in F_k. Since our original feature set X contains fewer than 50 features and the size of candidate feature set F_k is even smaller than X, therefore, we let the wrapper evaluate all possible subsets of F_k in a forward selection scheme enabling us to find the reduced feature subset that gives the best accuracy. Consequently, we obtain a feature set $\{\Theta_1,\ldots,\Theta_p,\ldots,\Theta_k\}$ where $1<p<k$ and we select the feature subset $\{\Theta_1,\Theta_2,\ldots,\Theta_p\}$ which corresponds to the highest accuracy. Note that this is the most compact feature subset as $1<p<k<n$.

We train a Linear Discriminant Analysis (LDA) classifier using an exclusive set of training data. Let $\mathbf{X}_i \in \mathbb{R}^{m\times n_i}$ be the matrix of features of class i with n_i samples. LDA maximizes the ratio of *between-class scatter* to *within-class scatter*. Between-class scatter is defined as

$$\mathbf{S_B}=\sum_{i=1}^{c} n_i(\mu_i-\mu)(\mu_i-\mu)^\top, \tag{7}$$

and within-class scatter is defined as

$$\mathbf{S_W}=\sum_{i=1}^{c}\sum_{x_k\in Xi}(x_k-\mu_i)(x_k-\mu_i)^\top, \tag{8}$$

where μ is the mean of all classes, μ_i is the mean of class $\mathbf{X}_i$ and n_i is the number of samples in $\mathbf{X}_i$. Fisher [37] proposed to maximise the ratio between $\mathbf{S_B}$ and $\mathbf{S_W}$ relative to the projection direction by solving

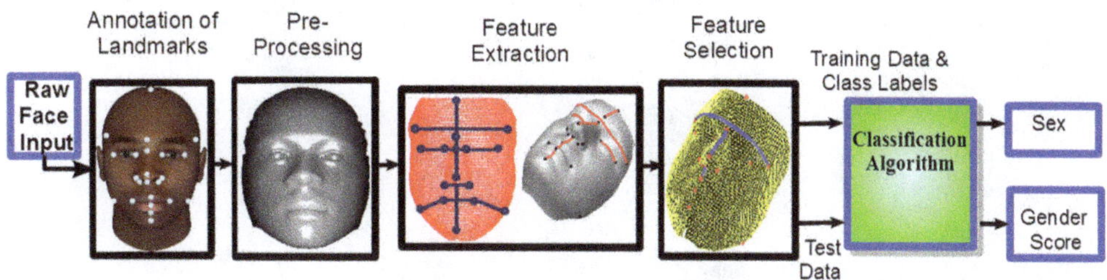

Figure 5. Block Diagram. Block diagram of the proposed gender classification and scoring algorithm. For details see the Objective Scoring Section. The synthetic images are from [45,46].

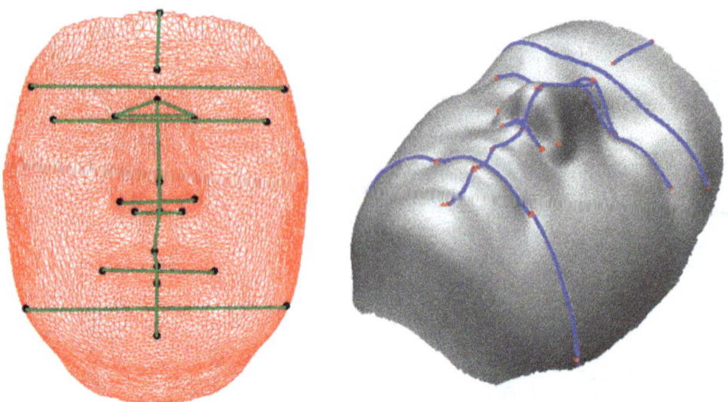

Figure 6. Features used in our algorithm. Some of the 3D Euclidean (left) and geodesic (right) distances used in gender scoring algorithm.

$$J(w) = \arg\max_{w} \frac{\mathbf{w}^\top \mathbf{S_B w}}{\mathbf{w}^\top \mathbf{S_W w}}. \quad (9)$$

By differentiating the equation with respect to **w** and equating it to zero, we get $\mathbf{S_W^{-1} S_B w} - Jw = 0$, which is a generalized eigenvalue problem and the eigenvector $\mathbf{w}^*$ of $\mathbf{S_W^{-1} S_B}$ is the desired optimal direction. Given the learnt LDA projection $\mathbf{w}^*$, a query face is classified into one of the two genders. The projection of feature vector $\mathbf{x_q}$ (of a face with unknown gender) on the LDA space is given by $x_q^* = (\mathbf{w}^*)^\top x_q$.

Gender classification is performed based on the distance between the x_q^* and the means of the projected classes μ_1^* and μ_2^* such that

$$C_q = \begin{cases} 1 & if \left\|\mu_1^* - x_q^*\right\|_2 < \left\|\mu_2^* - x_q^*\right\|_2 \\ 2 & otherwise \end{cases}, \quad (10)$$

where $\mu^* = (\mathbf{w}^*)^\top \mu$

Interestingly, the directional distance of a projected test face from the center of the projected means of the two classes gives an intuitive insight into the amount of masculinity or femininity of the face. Let $p = (\mu_1^* + \mu_2^*)/2$ be the center of the projected means. The gender score G of a test face x_i, whose gender has already been determined with Eqn. 10, is defined as

$$G = 1 - \frac{\|p - x_i^*\|_1}{2\|p - \mu^*\|_1} * \lambda \quad (11)$$

where μ^* is the projected mean of either class (1 or 2) and λ is a scaling factor for comparability with the available human perceptual ratings. In our case $\lambda = 20$. Hence we score the gender on a scale of 0 to 20 (0 being most masculine and 20 being most feminine). Figure 7 illustrates the process of scoring the gender of a query face in the LDA projected space.

Results and Analysis

Perceptual Scoring

While ratings of masculinity/femininity were clearly bimodal (Figure 8) with most males rated at the lower one third of the scale, and most females in the upper one third, a substantial proportion of images (29%) were rated in the middle one third, or perceived to be ambiguously masculine/feminine. The ratings from all the 75 raters were found to be significantly consistent ($\kappa = 0.783, p < < 0.001$) using the Fleiss Agreement Test [38].

The sex and ethnicity of the person represented in images had a significant influence on how they were rated by all groups ($F = 333.69$, $3 + 1479$ *d.f.*, $p < 0.001$). In general the perceived masculinity or femininity of the imaged subject was independent of the background of the person doing the rating. Both European male and female faces were considered to be more masculine than their non-European counterparts.

There was a strong tendency for the chin and jaw to be nominated as significant indicators in judgements of faces rated as extremely masculine (ratings 0 to 4), while the eyes, cheeks and mouth were the most frequently nominated features used in judgements of faces receiving high femininity ratings (ratings 15–20). Table 2 gives the detailed test values for each feature.

Gender was correctly identified in 86% of the instances. All sex and ethnic groups had the same ability to identify gender overall ($\chi^2 = 1.51$, 3 *d.f.*, $p = 0.680$). Raters were adept at correctly identifying sex for their own ethnic group (87.7% correct). Raters were slightly better at identifying the sex of the dominant culture when they were a minority born amongst the dominants than if they were a member of the dominant culture trying to identify the sex of one of the minorities (Europeans = 86.5% correct; non-Europeans = 83.3%). Europeans were better at classifying the sex of non-Europeans (85.5% correct) than non-Europeans were at classifying the sex of Europeans (80.5%) ($\chi^2 = 30.69$, 1 *d.f.*, $p < 0.0.001$). Gender identification errors were

Table 2. Significant facial features in perceptual gender scoring.

Feature	x^2	p	Masculinity/Femininity association
Forehead	5.28	0.071	No particular association
Eyes	23.69	<0.001	Femininity
Nose	3.08	0.214	No particular association
Cheeks	36.39	<0.001	Femininity
Mouth	23.63	<0.001	Femininity
Chin	19.38	<0.001	Masculinity
Jaw	58.29	<0.001	Masculinity
No Spec	2.97	0.227	No particular association

Chi-square and propability values for the correlation between facial features and their use in rating masculinity/femininity.

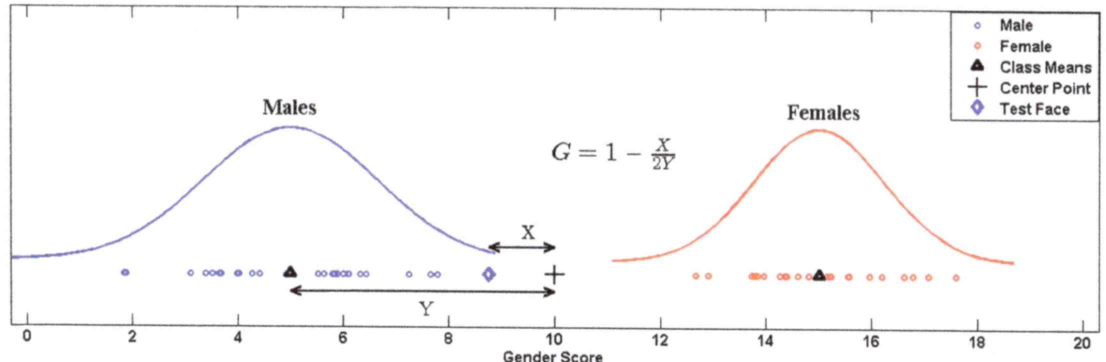

Figure 7. Gender scoring in LDA projected space. Diagram depicting the process of objectively scoring the gender in LDA space to assign a metric for masculinity/femininity of the test face.

more likely to be made amongst female faces (23% wrong) than amongst male faces (10% wrong) ($\chi^2 = 29.32$, 1 *d.f.*, $p < 0.001$). In particular, there was a strong tendency for female Europeans to be wrongly identified as males (29% wrong), while male Europeans (5% wrong) were very unlikely to be mistaken for females ($\chi^2 = 50.39$, 3 *d.f.*, $p < 0.001$). Correctly identified females were perceived to be significantly more feminine than those that were mistaken for males ($\chi^2 = 275.37$, 1+746 *d.f.*, $p < 0.001$). Correctly identified males were perceived as more masculine than those mistaken for females ($\chi^2 = 137.33$, 1+745 *d.f.*, $p < 0.001$). The ability to identify sex did not improve with the number of faces that were viewed ($\chi^2 = 26.25$, 19 *d.f.*, $p < 0.123$).

Objective Scoring

Study 1: Euclidean Measurements. Our first study constitutes obtaining objective gender scores using 3D Euclidean distances. Let $L_i = [x_i, y_i, z_i,]^\top$ be the ith landmark. The 3D Euclidean distance $D(L_i, L_j)$ between landmarks i and j is defined as,

$$D(L_i, L_j) = \|L_i - L_j\|_2 \quad (12)$$

Figure 6(Left) shows some of the 3D Euclidean distances used in this experiment.

Using 3D Euclidean distances as features, our proposed algorithm classifies 94.21% subjects correctly as males or females. The correlation between objective gender scores and the perceptual scores is 0.284 and 0.458 for males and females respectively. Figure 9(a & b, first row) show the correlation and best fit line for males and females while Figure 9(c, first row) shows the Bland-Altman plot between the objective and perceptual subjective scores.

It is evident that objective scores for masculinity and femininity do not correlate well with the perceptual subjective scores. In Figure 9(c, first row) ideally the mean of the difference of objective and subjective gender scores should have been zero. However, we can see that the mean difference line is well above zero and the width of the limits of agreement in this case is 13.86.

Clearly, 3D Euclidean distances do not seem to be the features that HVS concentrates on while scoring the facial gender. However, it is interesting to note that the forehead width (Ft-Ft), nasal bridge length (N-Prn), nasal tip protrusion (Sn-Prn), nasal width (Al-Al) and chin height (Sto-Pg) are selected as the most differentiating features by our algorithm (see Figure 10(a)). This is in line with the findings of Burton et al. [20] who performed

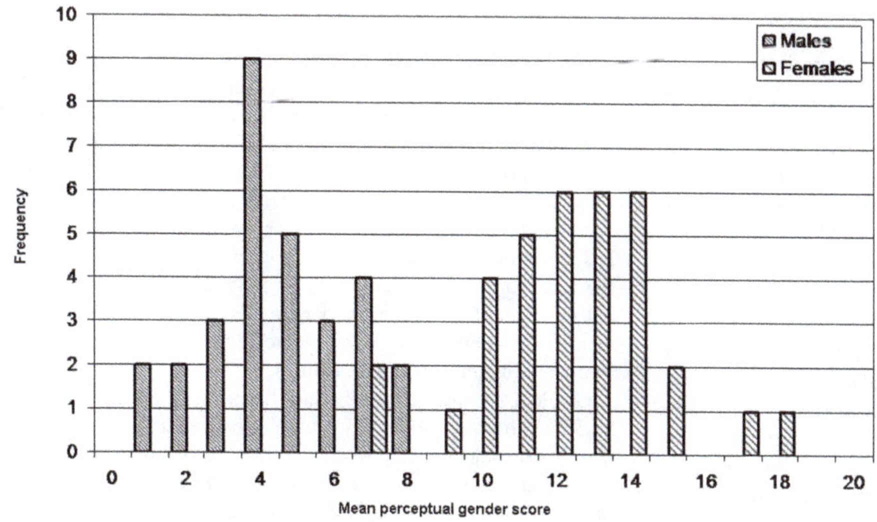

Figure 8. The perceptual subjective gender scores. A histogram of mean perceptual masculinity and femininity ratings obtained from 75 raters.

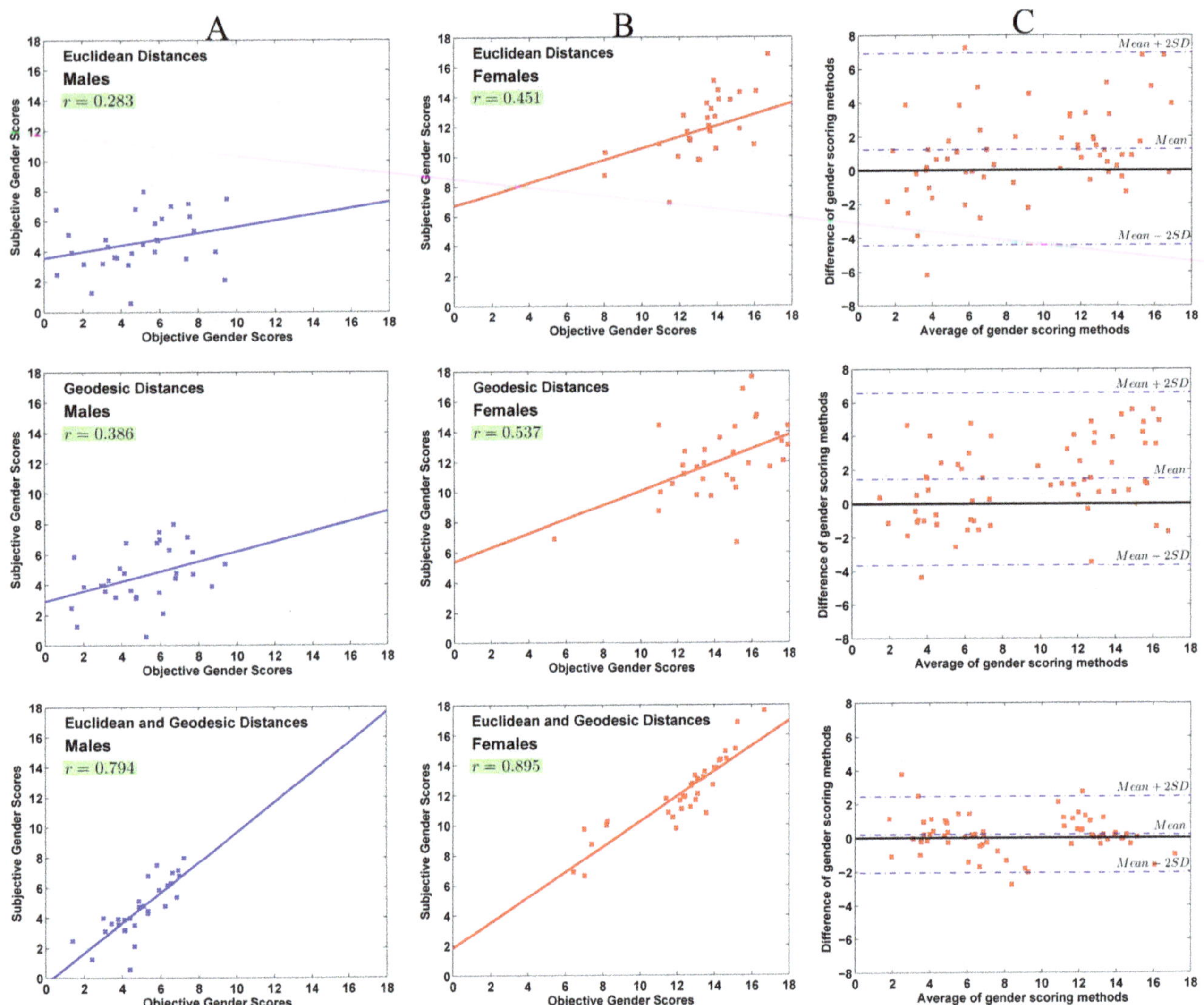

Figure 9. Results of objective gender scoring. (A) Correlation for males. (B) Correlation for females. (C) Cumulative Bland-Altman plot. Correlation and Bland-Altman plots between objective and subjective gender scores for males and females using only 3D Euclidean distances (First Row), only geodesic distances (second row) and combination of Euclidean and geodesic distances (third row).

experiments on a subset of 2D and 3D Euclidean distances. Note that the authors handpicked these features based on knowledge from existing literature, whereas our approach relies on a mathematical feature selection algorithm. This endorses the mathematical model we use for obtaining discriminant features.

Study 2: Geodesic Measurements. In the second study, we use geodesic distances to predict the facial gender scores. Some examples of the geodesics can be seen in Figure 6(Right). We define geodesic distance $m(G_{AB})$ between points A and B as the length of the curve G_{AB} generated by orthogonal projection of the Euclidean line $\overrightarrow{AB}$ on the 3D facial surface. This is precisely the reason for normalising the pose of each 3D face as variation in pose can present a different surface to the viewing angle. Less curved distances like the upper lip height (Sn-Sto) are modelled by a second order polynomial while more curved distances with multiple inflection points, like the biocular width (Ex-Ex) are modelled by higher order polynomials. Studies suggest that geodesic distances may represent 3D models in a better way as compared to 3D Euclidean distances [39]. Gupta et al. [40] argue that algorithms based on geodesic distances are likely to be robust to changes in facial expressions. In support of this argument Bronstein et al.[41] have suggested that facial expressions can be modelled as isometric deformations of the 3D surface where intrinsic properties of the surface like geodesic distances are preserved. Figure 11 depicts the variation in 3D Euclidean and geodesic distances in biocular width on two models. The left model has a protuberant nose and hence a larger geodesic distance than the right model which has a flatter nose. Euclidean distance in both the models is similar. Figure 12(a) shows some of the extracted geodesic features and Figure 12(b–c) show the process of fitting a polynomial to these features.

Geodesic distances classify facial sex with an accuracy of 98.57%. The correlation between objective gender scores and the perceptual subjective scores also increases to 0.386 and 0.537 for males and females respectively. Figure 9(a & b, second row) show the correlation and best fit line for males and females while Figure 9(c, second row) shows the Bland-Altman plot between the objective and perceptual subjective scores.

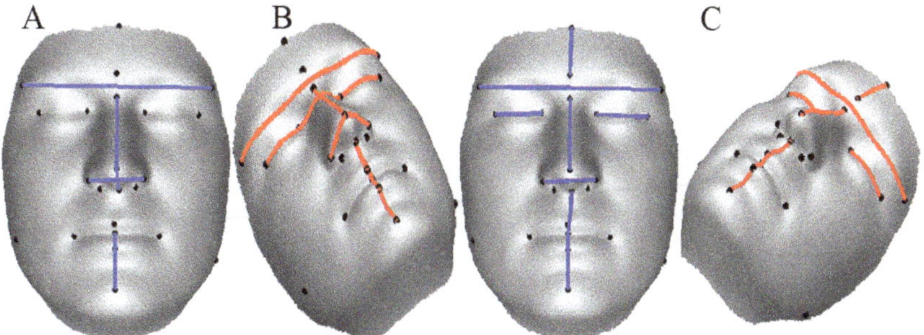

Figure 10. Most discriminating features between males and females found in the three experiments. (A) Euclidean distances only. (B) Geodesic distances only. (C) Combined Euclidean and geodesic distances.

Even though the correlation has improved, the geodesic distances alone do not seem to be the features of choice for HVS while ascribing a score to facial gender. Figure 9(c, second row) shows that the mean of the difference is still well above zero and the width of limits of agreement in this case is 13.15. Once again the forehead width (Ft-Ft), nasal bridge length (N-Prn), nasal width (Al-Prn-Al) and chin height (Sto-Pg) are amongst the most differentiating features. However, with geodesic distances, the upper lip height (Sn-Sto), eye fissure length (Ex-En) and intracanthal width (En-En) are added as the most discriminating sex classification features (see Figure 10(b)).

Study3: Combined Measurements. In the last experiment, we use a combination of 3D Euclidean and geodesic distances as our features for gender scoring. Since most of the gender discriminating features are common between the two families of distances, it seems intuitive to combine them and analyse their effect.

Equipped with a combination of 3D Euclidean and geodesic distances, our algorithm classifies facial sex with an accuracy of 99.93%. There is also a significant boost in the correlation between the objective and subjective gender scores which now is 0.794 and 0.895 for males and females respectively. The Bland-Altman plot shows the mean of the difference between the two scoring methods to be 0.21 while the width of limits of agreement is 4.95. This is a significant improvement as compared to the previous experiments. Figure 9(a & b, third row) show the correlation and best fit line for males and females while Figure 9(c, third row) shows the Bland-Altman plot between the objective and perceptual subjective scores.

The most differentiating features between the two sexes are once again common between the two families of distances. The Euclidean and geodesic distances for forehead width (Ft-Ft), nasal bridge length (N-Prn), nasal width (Al-Al), eye fissure length (Ex-En), chin height (Sto-Pg) and upper lip height (Sn-Sto) are the most discriminating features in our algorithm (see Figure 10(c)). However, this time the forehead height (Tr-G) is added to the list of discriminating features.

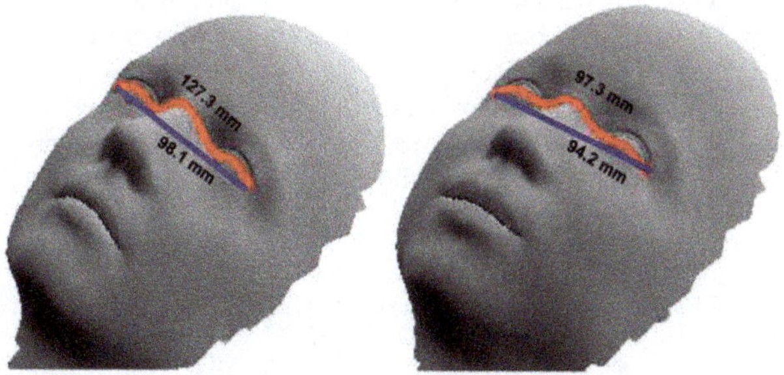

Figure 11. Robustness of geodesic distances to facial expression. Geodesic and 3D Euclidean distances of biocular width shown on two models. Left model has a protuberant nose and hence a greater geodesic distance than the right model which has a flatter nose. Euclidean distance in both the models is similar.

The above results suggest that the human visual system looks at the combination of Euclidean and geodesic distances between certain features on the face to give a gender score.

General Discussion

In the three studies involving various families of features, we have tried to find the predictors that the human visual system uses to attribute a measure to the facial gender. Beginning with 3D Euclidean distances alone, we see that there is little correlation between objective gender scores and subjective scores. This situation improves slightly when geodesic distances are used. The reason is straight forward as geodesic distances can model the facial surface curvature better than the Euclidean distances. However, the results are still below an acceptable significance threshold. Finally, when we use a combination of Euclidean and geodesic distances we see that the correlation between the two methods of scoring improves significantly and so does the agreement between them. This seems to corroborate the claim of Bruce et al. [23] that humans use a combination of predictors to perceive the sex of a face. Furthermore, as is evident from Figure 10(c), the most discriminating features from both families of distances seem to be common. This indicates that HVS might actually be taking into consideration the ratio between 3D Euclidean and geodesic distances while making a decision on the gender score of a face.

Relating the sex classification results to the gender scores in the three studies gives us a very interesting clue. In all three studies, sex classification results are very impressive. In fact, the base accuracy of 94.21% using only the 3D Euclidean distances tends to agree with the findings of Burton et al. [20] who classified facial sex with 94% accuracy using 2D and 3D Euclidean distances. However, the objective gender scores obtained with this family of distances do not significantly agree with the perceptual scores. Even when the classification results improve to 98.57% using the geodesics, the correlation between the objective and subjective gender scores remains below an acceptable significance threshold. This trend changes significantly when a combination of the two families of distances is used as predictors even though the sex classification results improve by 1.36% only. It shows that even though facial sex can be classified accurately using only the 3D Euclidean or geodesic distances, perfect and more meaningful

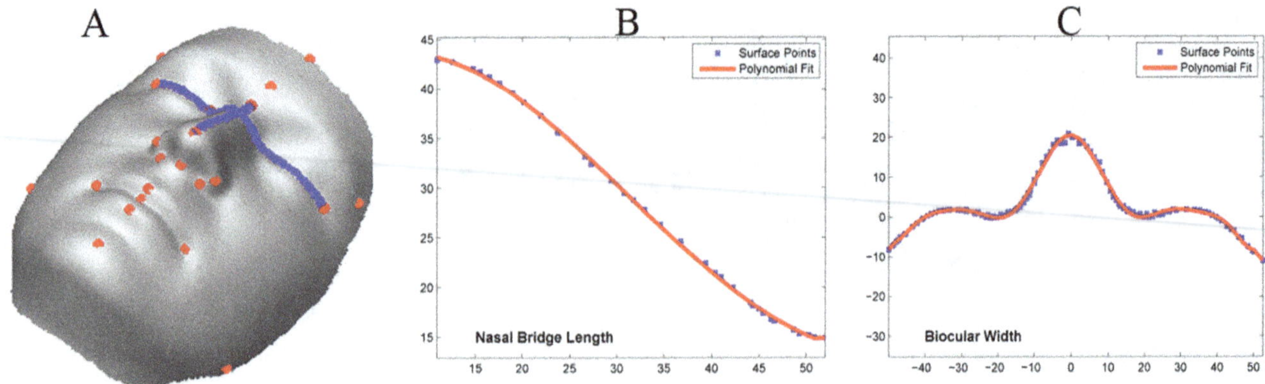

Figure 12. Modelling of geodesic curves. (A) Geodesic curves for nasal bridge length(N-Prn) and biocular width(Ex-Ex). (B–C) Fitting polynomials to these curves. Notice that N-Prn is modelled by a fourth order curve while Ex-Ex is modelled by a 14th order curve.

gender scores can only be obtained when a combination or ratio of these distances are taken as features for gender scoring.

Commenting on the method of obtaining gender scores, it is observed that a classification algorithm is a necessary prerequisite. However, the scoring result itself is invariant to the sex classification accuracy. This is evident from the gender scores obtained for females in the three experiments. There are a few female subjects who score below the boundary line of 10 giving them a more masculine gender score. This is indicative of a failure in classifying their sex but correlates very well with the perceptual subjective scores. Therefore, even though the algorithm misclassifies their sex, it still gives them a meaningful gender score which tends to agree with the subjective scores. Hence, our proposed algorithm puts the facial gender in the category of a continuum rather than binary.

From the Categorical Perception (CP) point of view, our results corroborate the findings of Armann and Bülthoff [42], that there is no evidence for naturally occurring CP for the sex of faces. Results of perceptual scoring, although bimodal, show that the gender ratings are on a continuum and do not follow a decision boundary. Consequently, a few female subjects were rated more masculine, hence crossing the decision boundary. This trend was replicated by our proposed computational model which ascribes the correct gender scores to even those subjects which fall on the other side of the decision boundary. Furthermore, the participants in Armann and Bülthoff's study [42] show a consistent bias to judge faces as male rather than female. Our findings from perceptual sex classification replicated this observation as we found a strong tendency for female Europeans to be wrongly identified as males (29% wrong), while male Europeans (5% wrong) were very unlikely to be mistaken for females ($\chi^2 = 50.39$, 3 *d.f.*, $p < 0.001$).

Our choice of features was motivated by the results from perceptual scoring. Instead of taking $\binom{L}{2}$ combinations of distances, where L is the number of landmarks, we developed our model around the facial features that our raters indicated were instrumental in giving a score. It is evident from Figure 10(c) that our algorithm also selects the features that were significant in subjective perceptual scoring. However, distances relating to the jaw (Go-Go) and mouth (Ch-Ch) were not highly discriminating. While there is no plausible reason for the mouth width (Ch-Ch) to be excluded from the list, mandible width (Go-Go) may have been excluded due to localization error of the related landmarks. Gonions (Go,L and Go,R) are a palpable landmarks indicating the extremes of the jaw and as such are very difficult to annotate consistently on 3D images.

Facial rating for attractiveness and sexual dimorphism plays an important role in planning reconstructive and cosmetic surgery. This procedure depends on a number of physiological and psychological constraints, like, age, sex, health state, structure, shape of the face and patient's needs and expectations. Patients who undergo such procedure are rated by human observers pre and post surgery to assess any improvement in perceptual attractiveness [14,15]. With the development of 3D simulation techniques to preview the aesthetical results of facial cosmetic surgery [43], our proposed algorithm can assist in predicting the attractiveness of the surgical outcome as it correlates significantly with human perceptual results. For example, secondary rhinoplasty is a nose operation carried out to correct or revise an unsatisfactory outcome from a previous rhinoplasty [44]. Lee et al. [8] have proposed a three-dimensional (3D) surgical simulation system, which can assist surgeons in planning rhinoplasty procedures. Our proposed algorithm can be used in such cases to assess the improvement in facial attractiveness of the resulting rhinoplasty through gender scoring, thus reducing the chances of further secondary procedures.

We can conclude by claiming that our proposed algorithm helps us in a better understanding of the Human Visual System. It is the first algorithm that has such a significantly high correlation with the mean perceptual scores given by 75 raters on 64 subjects. Hence, it may be possible to use these gender scores in a myriad of applications in medical and psychological fields where human raters are employed to obtain these scores.

Author Contributions

Conceived and designed the experiments: SZG KR FS AM. Performed the experiments: SZG KR. Analyzed the data: SZG KR FS MW. Contributed reagents/materials/analysis tools: MW. Wrote the paper: SZG KR AM.

References

1. Little AC, Jones BC, DeBruine LM (2011) The many faces of research on face perception. Philosophical Transactions of the Royal Society B: Biological Sciences 366: 1634–1637.
2. Leopold DA, Rhodes G (2010) A comparative view of face perception. Journal of Comparative Psychology 124: 233.

3. Rhodes G, Hickford C, Jeffery L (2000) Sex-typicality and attractiveness: Are supermale and superfemale faces super-attractive? British Journal of Psychology 91: 125–140.
4. Little AC, Hancock PJ (2002) The role of masculinity and distinctiveness in judgments of human male facial attractiveness. British Journal of Psychology 93: 451–464.
5. Rhodes G, Simmons LW, Peters M (2005) Attractiveness and sexual behavior: Does attractiveness enhance mating success? Evolution and Human Behavior 26: 186–201.
6. Boothroyd LG, Jones BC, Burt DM, DeBruine LM, Perrett DI (2008) Facial correlates of sociosexuality. Evolution and Human Behavior 29: 211–218.
7. Jones BC, Feinberg DR, Watkins CD, Fincher CL, Little AC, et al. (2013) Pathogen disgust predicts womens preferences for masculinity in mens voices, faces, and bodies. Behavioral Ecology 24: 373–379.
8. Lee AJ, Dubbs SL, Kelly AJ, von Hippel W, Brooks RC, et al. (2013) Human facial attributes, but not perceived intelligence, are used as cues of health and resource provision potential. Behavioral Ecology 24: 779–787.
9. Perrett D, Lee K, Penton-Voak I, Rowland D, Yoshikawa S, et al. (1998) Effects of sexual dimorphism on facial attractiveness. Nature 394: 884–887.
10. Rhodes G, Chan J, Zebrowitz LA, Simmons LW (2003) Does sexual dimorphism in human faces signal health? Proceedings of the Royal Society of London B: Biological Sciences 270: S93–S95.
11. Bejerot S, Eriksson JM, Bonde S, Carlström K, Humble MB, et al. (2012) The extreme male brain revisited: gender coherence in adults with autism spectrum disorder. The British Journal of Psychiatry 201: 116–123.
12. Peters M, Rhodes G, Simmons L (2008) Does attractiveness in men provide clues to semen quality? Journal of Evolutionary Biology 21: 572–579.
13. Koehler N, Simmons LW, Rhodes G, Peters M (2004) The relationship between sexual dimorphism in human faces and fluctuating asymmetry. Proceedings of the Royal Society of London B: Biological Sciences 271: S233–S236.
14. Dey JK, Ishii M, Boahene K, Byrne PJ, Ishii LE (2013) Changing perception: Facial reanimation surgery improves attractiveness and decreases negative facial perception. The Laryngoscope.
15. Chung EH, Borzabad-Farahani A, Yen SLK (2013) Clinicians and laypeople assessment of facial attractiveness in patients with cleft lip and palate treated with lefort i surgery or late maxillary protraction. International Journal of Pediatric Otorhinolaryngology.
16. Scheib JE, Gangestad SW, Thornhill R (1999) Facial attractiveness, symmetry and cues of good genes. Proceedings of the Royal Society of LondonB: Biological Sciences 266: 1913–1917.
17. Penton-Voak I, Jones B, Little A, Baker S, Tiddeman B, et al. (2001) Symmetry, sexual dimorphism in facial proportions and male facial attractiveness. Proceedings of the Royal Society of London B: Biological Sciences 268: 1617–1623.
18. Thornhill R, Gangestad SW (2006) Facial sexual dimorphism, developmental stability, and susceptibility to disease in men and women. Evolution and Human Behavior 27: 131–144.
19. Pound N, Penton-Voak IS, Surridge AK (2009) Testosterone responses to competition in men are related to facial masculinity. Proceedings of the Royal Society B: Biological Sciences 276: 153–159.
20. Burton AM, Bruce V, Dench N (1993) What's the difference between men and women? Evidence from facial measurement. Perception 22: 153–176.
21. Scott IM, Pound N, Stephen ID, Clark AP, Penton-Voak IS (2010) Does masculinity matter? the contribution of masculine face shape to male attractiveness in humans. PLoS one 5: e13585.
22. Stephen ID, Scott IM, Coetzee V, Pound N, Perrett DI, et al. (2012) Cross-cultural effects of color, but not morphological masculinity, on perceived attractiveness of men's faces. Evolution and Human Behavior 33: 260–267.
23. Bruce V, Burton AM, Hanna E, Healey P (1993) Sex discrimination: how do we tell the difference between male and female faces? Perception 22: 131–152.
24. Graf A, Wichmann FA, Bülthoff HH, Schölkopf BH (2006) Classification of faces in man and machine. Neural Computation 18: 143–165.
25. O'Toole AJ, Vetter T, Troje NF, Bülthoff HH (1997) Sex classification is better with three-dimensional head structure than with image intensity information. Perception 26: 75–84.
26. Bruce V, Young A (1986) Understanding face recognition. British journal of psychology 77: 305–327.
27. Weinberg SM, Naidoo S, Govier DP, Martin RA, Kane AA, et al. (2006) Anthropometric precision and accuracy of digital three-dimensional photogrammetry: comparing the genex and 3dmd imaging systems with one another and with direct anthropometry. Journal of Craniofacial Surgery 17: 477–483.
28. Farkas L (1994) Anthropometry of the head and face in clinical practice. Anthropometry of the Head and Face, 2nd Ed: 71–111.
29. Farkas LG, Kolar JC (1987) Anthropometrics and art in the aesthetics of women's faces. Clinics in Plastic Surgery 14: 599.
30. Aldridge K, George I, Cole K, Austin J, Takahashi T, et al. (2011) Facial phenotypes in subgroups of prepubertal boys with autism spectrum disorders are correlated with clinical phenotypes. Molecular Autism 2: 15.
31. Bardin CW, Catterall JF (1981) Testosterone: A major determinant of extragenital sexual dimorphism. Science 211: 1285–1294.
32. DErico J (2008) Surface fitting using gridfit. Technical report, MATLAB Central File Exchange.
33. Abdi H, Valentin D, Edelman B, O'Toole AJ (1995) More about the difference between men and women: evidence from linear neural network and the principal-component approach. Perception 24: 539–539.
34. Martin Bland J, Altman D (1986) Statistical methods for assessing agreement between two methods of clinical measurement. The Lancet 327: 307–310.
35. Peng H, Long F, Ding C (2005) Feature selection based on mutual information criteria of max-dependency, max-relevance, and min-redundancy. IEEE Transactions on Pattern Analysis and Machine Intelligence (PAMI) 27: 1226–1238.
36. Kohavi R, John GH (1997) Wrappers for feature subset selection. Artificial Intelligence 97: 273–324.
37. Duda R, Hart P, Stork D (2001) Pattern Classification and Scene Analysis 2nd ed.
38. Fleiss JL (1971) Measuring nominal scale agreement among many raters. Psychological Bulletin 76: 378.
39. Hamza A, Krim H (2006) Geodesic matching of triangulated surfaces. IEEE Transactions on Image Processing 15: 2249–2258.
40. Gupta S, Markey M, Bovik A (2010) Anthropometric 3D face recognition. International Journal of Computer Vision 90: 331–349.
41. Bronstein A, Bronstein M, Kimmel R (2005) Three-dimensional face recognition. International Journal of Computer Vision 64: 5–30.
42. Armann R, Bülthoff I (2012) Male and female faces are only perceived categorically when linked to familiar identities–and when in doubt, he is a male. Vision research 63: 69–80.
43. Gao J, Zhou M, Wang H, Zhang C (2001) Three dimensional surface warping for plastic surgery planning. In: IEEE International Conference on Systems, Man, and Cybernetics. IEEE, volume 3, pp. 2016–2021.
44. Bracaglia R, Fortunato R, Gentileschi S (2005) Secondary rhinoplasty. Aesthetic Plastic Surgery 29: 230–239.
45. Singular Inversions Facegen Modeller. Available: http://www.facegen.com/. Accessed 26 May 2014.
46. Blanz V, Vetter T (2003) Face recognition based on fitting a 3D morphable model. IEEE Transactions on Pattern Analysis and Machine Intelligence 25: 1063–1074.
47. Hoss RA, Ramsey JL, Griffin AM, Langlois JH (2005) The role of facial attractiveness and facial masculinity/femininity in sex classification of faces. Perception 34: 1459.
48. DeBruine LM, Jones BC, Little AC, Boothroyd LG, Perrett DI, et al. (2006) Correlated preferences for facial masculinity and ideal or actual partner's masculinity. Proceedings of the Royal Society B: Biological Sciences 273: 1355–1360.
49. Rieger G, Linsenmeier JA, Gygax L, Garcia S, Bailey JM (2010) Dissecting "gaydar": Accuracy and the role of masculinity–femininity. Archives of Sexual Behavior 39: 124–140.

17

Complications of Absorbable Fixation in Maxillofacial Surgery

Liya Yang, Meibang Xu, Xiaolei Jin, Jiajie Xu, Jianjian Lu, Chao Zhang, Tian Tian, Li Teng*

Department 2 of Cranio-maxillo-facial Surgery, Plastic Surgery Hospital, Chinese Academy of Medical Sciences and Peking Union Medical College, Beijing, P.R. China

Abstract

Background: The use of titanium during maxillofacial fixation is limited due to its palpability, mutagenic effects and interference with imaging, which lead to the requirement for subsequent removal. The use of a biologically absorbable fixation material will potentially eliminate these limitations. In this meta-analysis, we analyzed the complications of absorbable fixation in maxillofacial surgery.

Methods: We performed a systematic search of PubMed, Embase, Cochrane Central Register of Systematic Reviews and Cochrane Central Register of Controlled Trials for trials published through December 2012. Data extracted from literature were analyzed with Review manager 5.0.24.

Results: Relevant data was extracted from 20 studies (1673 participants) and revealed that patients in the absorbable group had significantly more complications than those in the titanium group (RR = 1.20; 95% CI: 1.02–1.42; P = 0.03) in all enrolled maxillofacial surgeries. For bimaxillary operation subgroup, the absorbable fixation group did not have a significant increase in complications when compared with the titanium group (RR = 1.89; 95% CI: 0.85–4.22; P = 0.12). There was no significant difference observed between the absorbable and titanium groups receiving a bilateral sagittal split ramus osteotomy (BSSRO) (RR = 1.45; 95% CI: 0.84–2.48; P = 0.18) and Le Fort I osteotomy (RR = 0.65; 95% CI: 0.34–1.23; P = 0.18). The combined results of the five trials revealed that the absorbable group had a significantly lower rate of complications compared to the titanium group (RR = 0.71; 95% CI: 0.52–0.97; P = 0.03) in fracture fixation.

Conclusion: This meta-analysis shows that absorbable fixation systems used for fixation in maxillofacial surgery do not have adequate safety profiles. Subgroup indicated the safety of absorbable fixation systems was superior during fracture fixation. The absorbable fixation systems tend to have a similar favorable safety profile as titanium fixation during Le Fort I, bimaxillary operation and BSSRO.

Editor: Samuel J. Lin, Harvard Medical School, United States of America

Funding: The authors have no support or funding to report.

Competing Interests: The authors have declared that no competing interests exist.

* E-mail: zhengxingwuke@163.com

Introduction

Essential prerequisites for bone healing of fractures and osteotomies include sufficient vascularization, immobilization of bone segments and anatomical reduction. Previously the only method of achieving this was by intraosseous wiring coupled with rigid intermaxillary (upper to lower jaw) fixation. Recent developments in biomaterials have led to the achievement of fixation using titanium. This allows patients to functionally load their masticatory system immediately following surgery [1]. However, as the need for fixation is only temporary and metallic materials cause stress shielding of the underlying bone, the removal of these plates after the bone has healed has been suggested [2]. The titanium implants are removed following bone healing in a second operation in 5–40% of the cases [3]. Moreover, titanium particles have been found in scar tissue covering these plates as well as in locoregional lymph nodes and an imperfect contact will occur between the metal plate and bone surface. Recently, it was reported that titanium miniplates is a new risk factor for the development of the bisphosphonate-related osteonecrosis of the jaw [4].

The use of the biologically inert and resorbable plates will potentially eliminate these limitations of titanium fixation, which may offer some clinical advantages for the fixation of facial bones during orthognathic surgery. Studies have demonstrated that maxillary stability can be achieved with satisfactory results when u-hydroxyapatite/poly-(L-lactic) acid (u-HA/PLLA) and poly-L-lactic acid (PLLA) plates are used, similar to titanium plates [5]. The resorbable system is a good system for rigid internal fixation in specific conditions where muscular and stress forces are not a determining factor in fragment displacement [6]. However, concerns remain about the stability of fixation, the length of time required for their degradation and especially the possibility of complications, such as foreign body reactions. Park et al. suggested that resorbable plate and screw systems (RPSSs) should be selected carefully depending on the fracture site and whether there is an accompanying infection. It is important to select the method that best fits the patient's situation [7]. The use of biodegradable plates should be recommended for minimally loaded situations [8]. In addition, the process of degradation of these devices into carbon dioxide and water may take as long as 2 years [9]. Therefore, the use of resorbable plates and screws remains unpopular for internal fixation among oral and maxillofacial surgeons. Although a number of clinical studies regarding the safety of absorbable materials in maxillofacial fixation have been recently published, there is no systemic review to analyze the exact safety of absorbable materials in maxillofacial surgery. Therefore, we performed a meta-analysis to assess the safety of absorbable materials versus metal treatments (titanium) in patients receiving maxillofacial surgery.

Materials and Methods

Data Collection

The aim of this meta-analysis was to include all publicly available data on the treatment of maxillofacial fixation with an absorbable plate and/or screws from comparative studies or randomized controlled trials (RCTs). Two authors performed systematic searches of the medical literature to identify articles from PubMed, Embase, Cochrane Central Register of Systemic Reviews and Cochrane Central Register of Controlled Trials according to a standardized protocol, to December 2012. We conducted a comprehensive literature search with the following medical subject headings: bicortical resorbable, Poly-L-Lactic Acid, PLLA, PLLA-PGA, resorbable, bio-resorbale, biodegradable and titanium, nonresorbable, and metal. For the plates and/or screws, we also performed searches for each type separately such as screw, plate, miniplate and miniscrew. The search was limited to the English language and studies conducted in humans.

Study Selection

Paired reviewers (L.-Y.Y. and M.-B.X.) independently evaluated references for eligibility using a two-stage procedure. In the first stage, all identified abstracts were evaluated for appropriateness to the study aim. All potentially relevant trials were retrieved and selected for full-text review to determine whether or not they met all eligibility criteria in the second stage. Articles that were selected by either reviewer were assessed, and the inclusion and exclusion criteria were evaluated by both reviewers in the second stage. Any disagreements were resolved by discussion. Eligibility criteria for the studies included the following: (1) Type of participants: patients who had received maxillofacial surgery, including bilateral sagittal split ramus osteotomy (BSSRO), intraoral vertical ramus osteotomy (IVRO), Le Fort I osteotomy or maxillofacial fracture fixation; (2) Intervention: fixed by plates and/or screws; (3) outcome measures: complications. After extraction, four categories (complications in bimaxillary operation, bilateral sagittal split ramus osteotomy (BSSRO), Le Fort I, and fracture fixation) were of the most interest to us; (4) Type of publication: only full papers on original patient data reporting absorbable treatment were

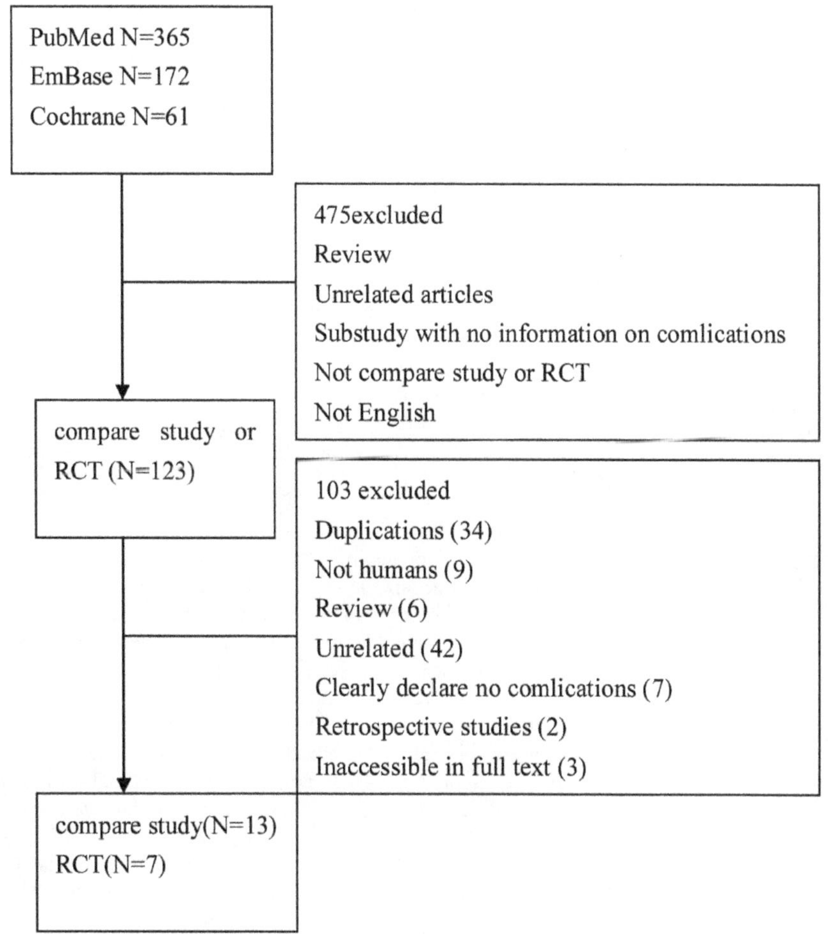

Figure 1. Study flow diagram.

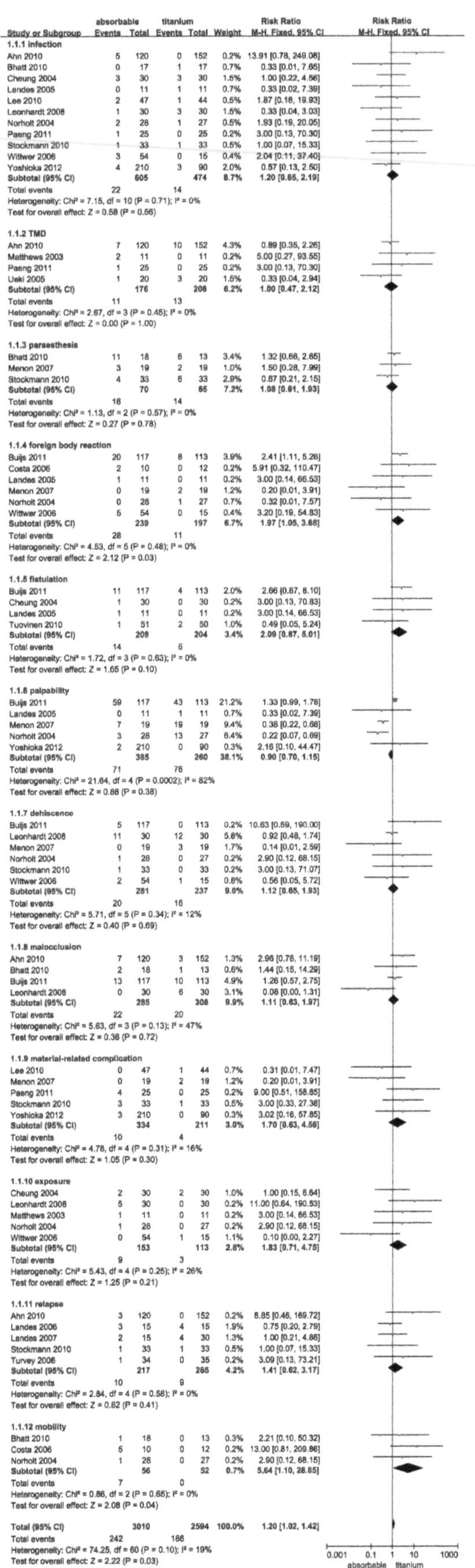

Figure 2. Forest plot of trials of absorbable fixation versus titanium examining the effect on relative risk of complications in all enrolled trials. TMD = temporomandibular joint dysfunction; df = degrees of freedom; M-H = Mantel-Haenszel.

considered for further analysis; and (5) Type of study: studies had to be compared studies or RCTs comparing absorbable with non-absorbable (titanium) plates and/or screws. Exclusion criteria were the use of an alveolar bone implant, maxillofacial model, cadaver, or animals.

Data Extraction and Quality Assessment

Data concerning the type and number of interferences were extracted and entered onto specially developed forms by two reviewers, and then the verified data were entered into a Microsoft Excel spreadsheet (XP professional edition; Microsoft Corp, Redmond, WA, USA). Trial characteristics, including the disease, mean age of included patients, operation, follow-up period, and absorbable and non-absorbable materials, were collected in detail. Unpublished data were not included. We assessed the methodological quality using the Jadad score, which assigns points (maximum of 7 points) for the following parameters: randomization (2 points), method of randomization generation (2 points), double blinding (2 points) and loss to follow-up (1 point) [10].

Data Synthesis and Analysis

All statistical analyses were performed using Review Manager 5.0.24 statistical software (Cochrane Collaboration, Oxford, United Kingdom) for the meta-analysis. As dichotomous outcomes, the 95% confidence intervals (CI) at the end of treatment were calculated for individual trials, and the relative risk (RR) was used as a summary estimator. The fixed-effect model weighted by the Mantel-Haenszel method was used, and the random effect model was used in the case of significant heterogeneity (P value of x^2 test <0.05 and $I^2>50\%$). A funnel plot test was used to assess for evidence of publication bias. Forest plots were used for graphic representation of data. The surface area of the blue square represents the relative quantitative contribution of the trial to the analysis (weight) and the horizontal line indicates the 95% CI. The diamond-shaped symbol is the summary estimate of effect expressed as a RR with 95% CIs, which is an average of the pooled treatment effects across all trials. A $P<0.05$ was considered statistically significant.

Results

Study Identification

The process of identifying eligible studies is summarized in Figure 1. After title and abstract evaluation, 123 articles were identified for further assessment. After a full-text review, 27 met the criteria for inclusion. Complications were reported in 20 of the 27 studies and included 7 RCTs and 13 comparative studies, published between 2002 and 2012.

The characteristics of the included studies are summarized in the Table S1. The 20 studies enrolled a total of 1673 participants (898 in the absorbable group and 775 in the non-absorbable group). According to the operations, three studies described multiple operations termed bimaxillary operation [11,12,13], which consisted of SSRO plus Le Fort I. Six studies were related to BSSRO [14,15,16,17,8,18]. The Le Fort I subgroup included two studies [19,20] and five studies belonged to the fracture fixation subgroup [21,22,23,24,25]. The remaining four studies can't be classified as they included different kinds of maxillofacial surgeries [26,27,28,29]. The absorbable materials were referred to

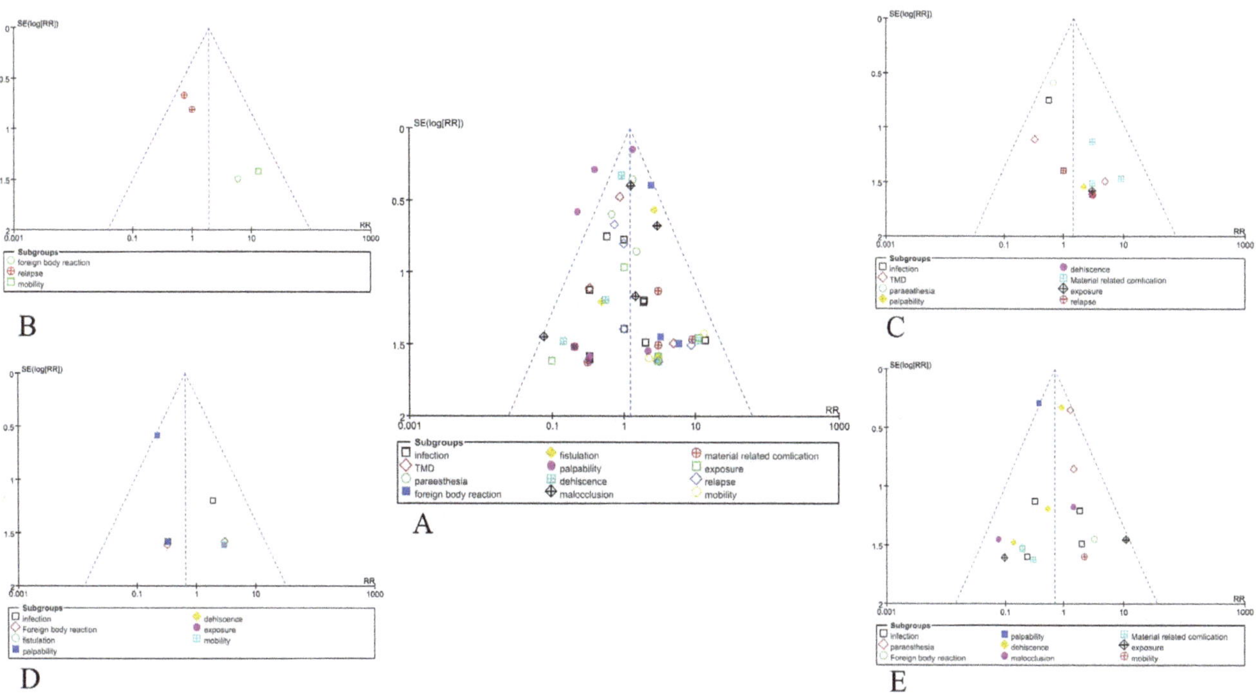

Figure 3. Funnel plot to assess for evidence of publication bias. 3a. Funnel plot for the complication in all studies; 3b. Funnel plot for the complication in bimaxillary operations; 3c. Funnel plot for the complication in BSSRO; 3d. Funnel plot for the complication in Le Fort I; 3e. Funnel plot for the complication in fracture fixation.

poly(L-lactide-co-D/L-lactide (P (L/DL) LA), poly(L-lactic-co-glycolic acid) (PLGA), polyglycolic acid (PGA), PLLA, LactoSorb, Delta and INION, while the non-absorbable materials were titanium. The number of participants in each study ranged from 10 to 210 individuals and the age of individuals ranged from 11 to 71 y.

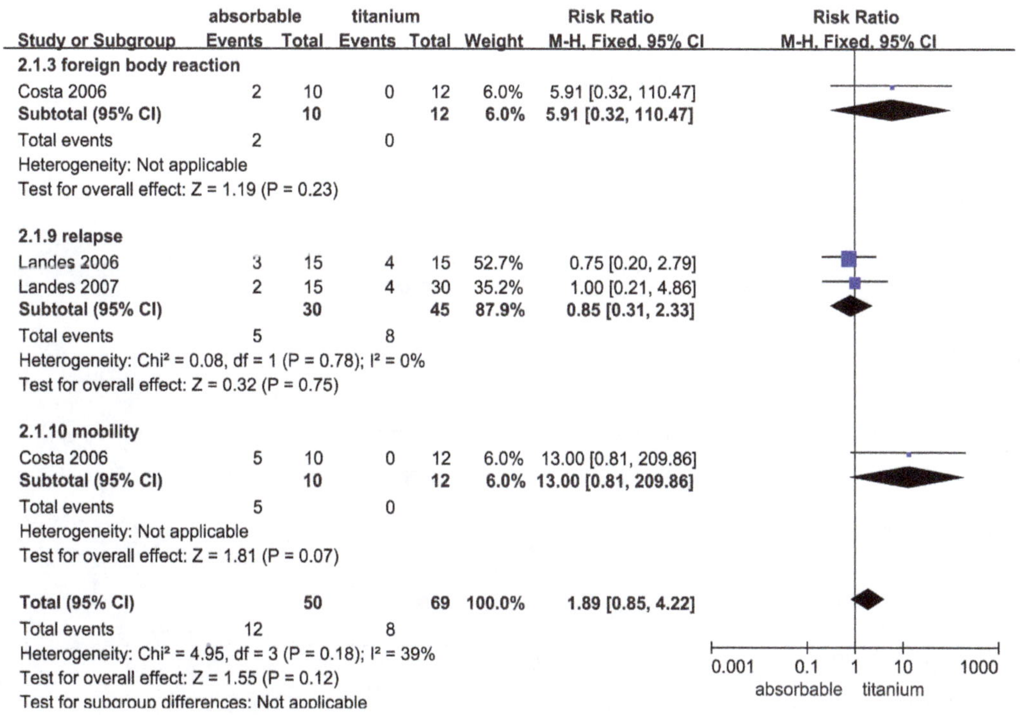

Study or Subgroup	absorbable Events	absorbable Total	titanium Events	titanium Total	Weight	Risk Ratio M-H, Fixed, 95% CI
2.1.3 foreign body reaction						
Costa 2006	2	10	0	12	6.0%	5.91 [0.32, 110.47]
Subtotal (95% CI)		**10**		**12**	**6.0%**	**5.91 [0.32, 110.47]**
Total events	2		0			
Heterogeneity: Not applicable						
Test for overall effect: Z = 1.19 (P = 0.23)						
2.1.9 relapse						
Landes 2006	3	15	4	15	52.7%	0.75 [0.20, 2.79]
Landes 2007	2	15	4	30	35.2%	1.00 [0.21, 4.86]
Subtotal (95% CI)		**30**		**45**	**87.9%**	**0.85 [0.31, 2.33]**
Total events	5		8			
Heterogeneity: Chi² = 0.08, df = 1 (P = 0.78); I² = 0%						
Test for overall effect: Z = 0.32 (P = 0.75)						
2.1.10 mobility						
Costa 2006	5	10	0	12	6.0%	13.00 [0.81, 209.86]
Subtotal (95% CI)		**10**		**12**	**6.0%**	**13.00 [0.81, 209.86]**
Total events	5		0			
Heterogeneity: Not applicable						
Test for overall effect: Z = 1.81 (P = 0.07)						
Total (95% CI)		**50**		**69**	**100.0%**	**1.89 [0.85, 4.22]**
Total events	12		8			
Heterogeneity: Chi² = 4.95, df = 3 (P = 0.18); I² = 39%						
Test for overall effect: Z = 1.55 (P = 0.12)						
Test for subgroup differences: Not applicable						

Risk Ratio M-H, Fixed, 95% CI: 0.001 0.1 1 10 1000; absorbable titanium

Figure 4. Forest plot of trials of absorbable fixation versus titanium examining the effect on relative risk of complications in bimaxillary operation. See Figure 2 legend for expansion of abbreviations.

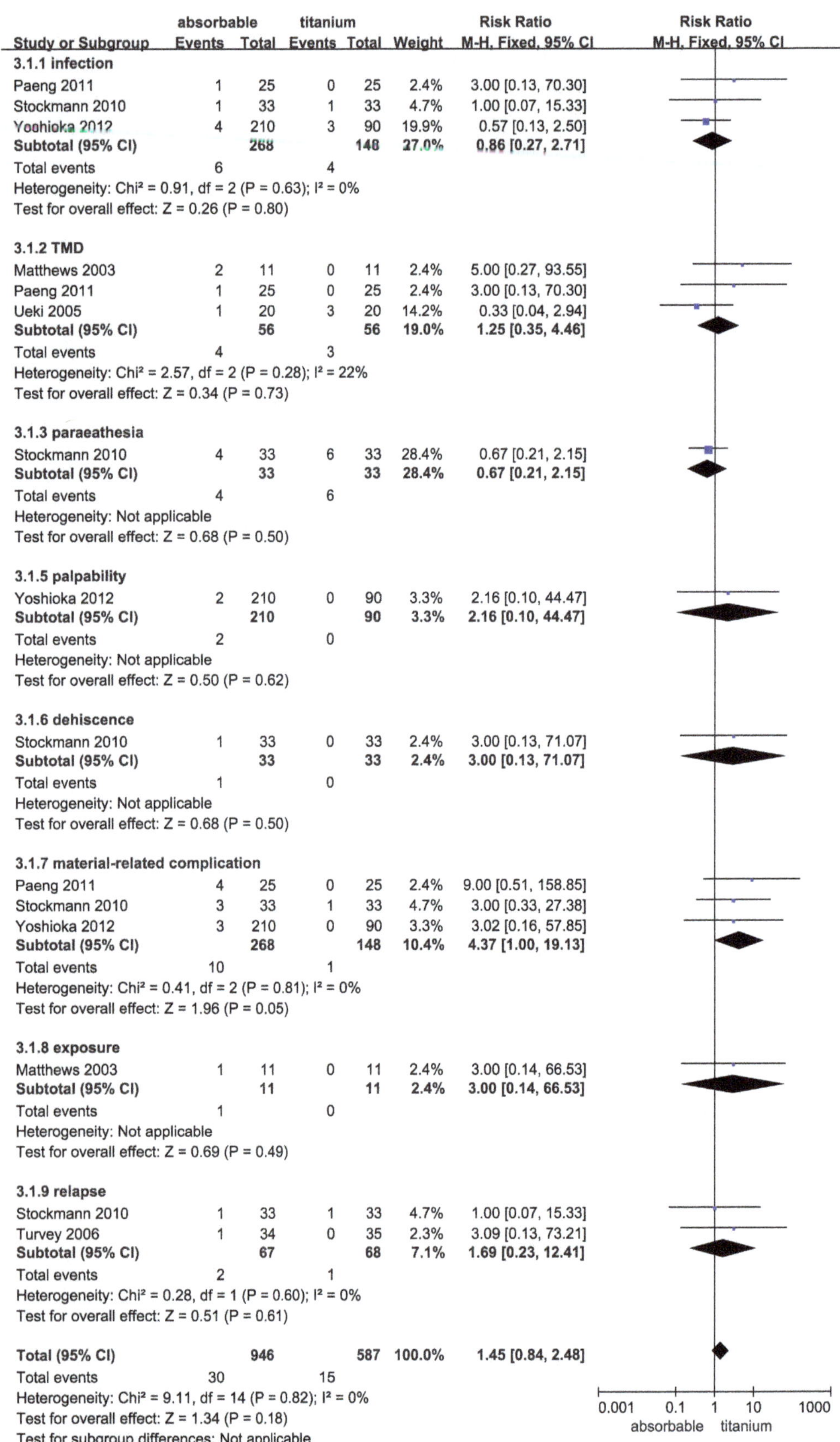

Study or Subgroup	absorbable Events	absorbable Total	titanium Events	titanium Total	Weight	Risk Ratio M-H, Fixed, 95% CI
3.1.1 infection						
Paeng 2011	1	25	0	25	2.4%	3.00 [0.13, 70.30]
Stockmann 2010	1	33	1	33	4.7%	1.00 [0.07, 15.33]
Yoshioka 2012	4	210	3	90	19.9%	0.57 [0.13, 2.50]
Subtotal (95% CI)		**268**		**148**	**27.0%**	**0.86 [0.27, 2.71]**
Total events	6		4			
Heterogeneity: Chi² = 0.91, df = 2 (P = 0.63); I² = 0%						
Test for overall effect: Z = 0.26 (P = 0.80)						
3.1.2 TMD						
Matthews 2003	2	11	0	11	2.4%	5.00 [0.27, 93.55]
Paeng 2011	1	25	0	25	2.4%	3.00 [0.13, 70.30]
Ueki 2005	1	20	3	20	14.2%	0.33 [0.04, 2.94]
Subtotal (95% CI)		**56**		**56**	**19.0%**	**1.25 [0.35, 4.46]**
Total events	4		3			
Heterogeneity: Chi² = 2.57, df = 2 (P = 0.28); I² = 22%						
Test for overall effect: Z = 0.34 (P = 0.73)						
3.1.3 paraeathesia						
Stockmann 2010	4	33	6	33	28.4%	0.67 [0.21, 2.15]
Subtotal (95% CI)		**33**		**33**	**28.4%**	**0.67 [0.21, 2.15]**
Total events	4		6			
Heterogeneity: Not applicable						
Test for overall effect: Z = 0.68 (P = 0.50)						
3.1.5 palpability						
Yoshioka 2012	2	210	0	90	3.3%	2.16 [0.10, 44.47]
Subtotal (95% CI)		**210**		**90**	**3.3%**	**2.16 [0.10, 44.47]**
Total events	2		0			
Heterogeneity: Not applicable						
Test for overall effect: Z = 0.50 (P = 0.62)						
3.1.6 dehiscence						
Stockmann 2010	1	33	0	33	2.4%	3.00 [0.13, 71.07]
Subtotal (95% CI)		**33**		**33**	**2.4%**	**3.00 [0.13, 71.07]**
Total events	1		0			
Heterogeneity: Not applicable						
Test for overall effect: Z = 0.68 (P = 0.50)						
3.1.7 material-related complication						
Paeng 2011	4	25	0	25	2.4%	9.00 [0.51, 158.85]
Stockmann 2010	3	33	1	33	4.7%	3.00 [0.33, 27.38]
Yoshioka 2012	3	210	0	90	3.3%	3.02 [0.16, 57.85]
Subtotal (95% CI)		**268**		**148**	**10.4%**	**4.37 [1.00, 19.13]**
Total events	10		1			
Heterogeneity: Chi² = 0.41, df = 2 (P = 0.81); I² = 0%						
Test for overall effect: Z = 1.96 (P = 0.05)						
3.1.8 exposure						
Matthews 2003	1	11	0	11	2.4%	3.00 [0.14, 66.53]
Subtotal (95% CI)		**11**		**11**	**2.4%**	**3.00 [0.14, 66.53]**
Total events	1		0			
Heterogeneity: Not applicable						
Test for overall effect: Z = 0.69 (P = 0.49)						
3.1.9 relapse						
Stockmann 2010	1	33	1	33	4.7%	1.00 [0.07, 15.33]
Turvey 2006	1	34	0	35	2.3%	3.09 [0.13, 73.21]
Subtotal (95% CI)		**67**		**68**	**7.1%**	**1.69 [0.23, 12.41]**
Total events	2		1			
Heterogeneity: Chi² = 0.28, df = 1 (P = 0.60); I² = 0%						
Test for overall effect: Z = 0.51 (P = 0.61)						
Total (95% CI)		**946**		**587**	**100.0%**	**1.45 [0.84, 2.48]**
Total events	30		15			
Heterogeneity: Chi² = 9.11, df = 14 (P = 0.82); I² = 0%						
Test for overall effect: Z = 1.34 (P = 0.18)						
Test for subgroup differences: Not applicable						

Figure 5. Forest plot of trials of absorbable fixation versus titanium examining the effect on relative risk of complications in BSSRO. See Figure 2 legend for expansion of abbreviations.

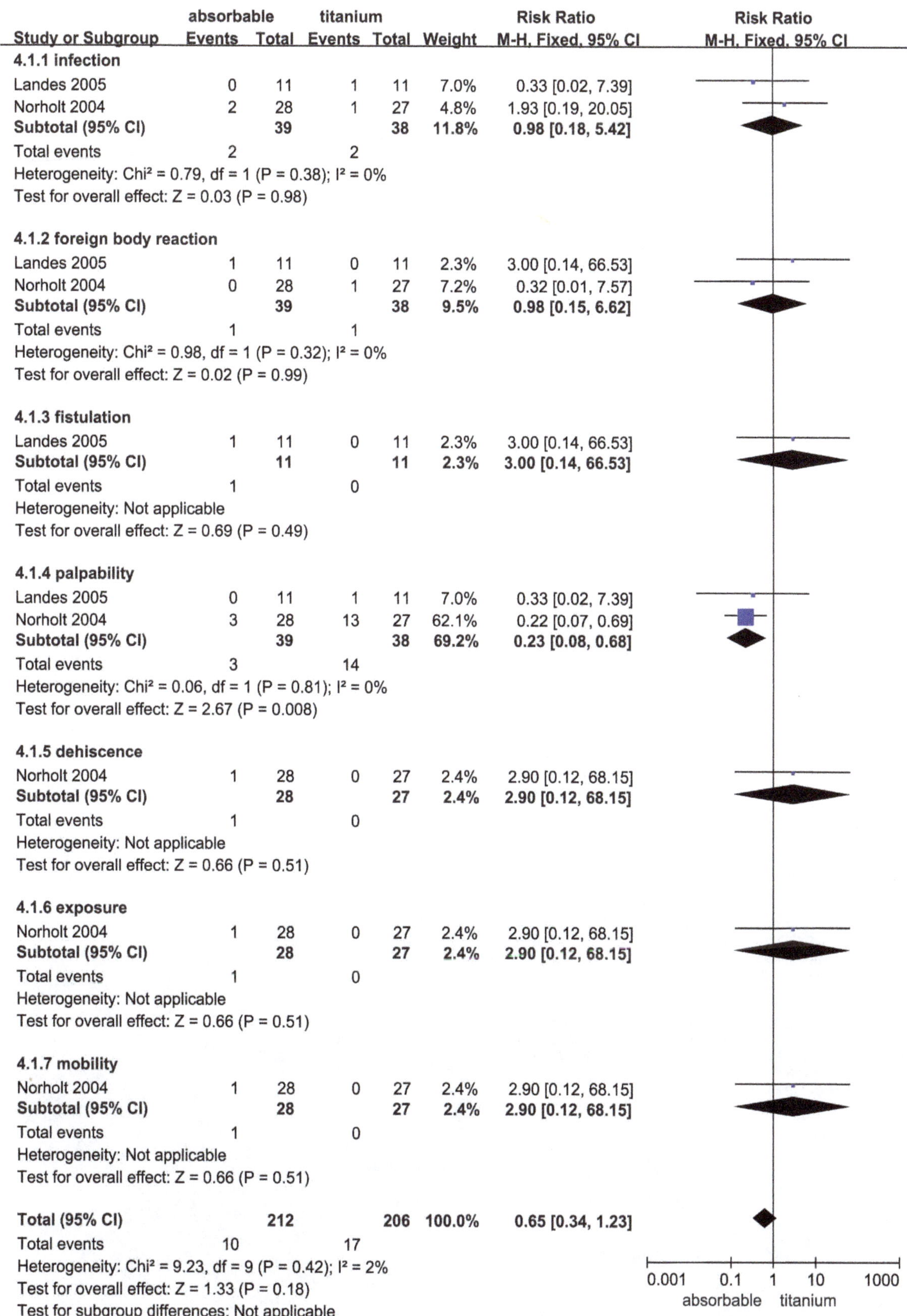

Study or Subgroup	absorbable Events	absorbable Total	titanium Events	titanium Total	Weight	Risk Ratio M-H, Fixed, 95% CI
4.1.1 infection						
Landes 2005	0	11	1	11	7.0%	0.33 [0.02, 7.39]
Norholt 2004	2	28	1	27	4.8%	1.93 [0.19, 20.05]
Subtotal (95% CI)		**39**		**38**	**11.8%**	**0.98 [0.18, 5.42]**
Total events	2		2			
Heterogeneity: Chi² = 0.79, df = 1 (P = 0.38); I² = 0%						
Test for overall effect: Z = 0.03 (P = 0.98)						
4.1.2 foreign body reaction						
Landes 2005	1	11	0	11	2.3%	3.00 [0.14, 66.53]
Norholt 2004	0	28	1	27	7.2%	0.32 [0.01, 7.57]
Subtotal (95% CI)		**39**		**38**	**9.5%**	**0.98 [0.15, 6.62]**
Total events	1		1			
Heterogeneity: Chi² = 0.98, df = 1 (P = 0.32); I² = 0%						
Test for overall effect: Z = 0.02 (P = 0.99)						
4.1.3 fistulation						
Landes 2005	1	11	0	11	2.3%	3.00 [0.14, 66.53]
Subtotal (95% CI)		**11**		**11**	**2.3%**	**3.00 [0.14, 66.53]**
Total events	1		0			
Heterogeneity: Not applicable						
Test for overall effect: Z = 0.69 (P = 0.49)						
4.1.4 palpability						
Landes 2005	0	11	1	11	7.0%	0.33 [0.02, 7.39]
Norholt 2004	3	28	13	27	62.1%	0.22 [0.07, 0.69]
Subtotal (95% CI)		**39**		**38**	**69.2%**	**0.23 [0.08, 0.68]**
Total events	3		14			
Heterogeneity: Chi² = 0.06, df = 1 (P = 0.81); I² = 0%						
Test for overall effect: Z = 2.67 (P = 0.008)						
4.1.5 dehiscence						
Norholt 2004	1	28	0	27	2.4%	2.90 [0.12, 68.15]
Subtotal (95% CI)		**28**		**27**	**2.4%**	**2.90 [0.12, 68.15]**
Total events	1		0			
Heterogeneity: Not applicable						
Test for overall effect: Z = 0.66 (P = 0.51)						
4.1.6 exposure						
Norholt 2004	1	28	0	27	2.4%	2.90 [0.12, 68.15]
Subtotal (95% CI)		**28**		**27**	**2.4%**	**2.90 [0.12, 68.15]**
Total events	1		0			
Heterogeneity: Not applicable						
Test for overall effect: Z = 0.66 (P = 0.51)						
4.1.7 mobility						
Norholt 2004	1	28	0	27	2.4%	2.90 [0.12, 68.15]
Subtotal (95% CI)		**28**		**27**	**2.4%**	**2.90 [0.12, 68.15]**
Total events	1		0			
Heterogeneity: Not applicable						
Test for overall effect: Z = 0.66 (P = 0.51)						
Total (95% CI)		**212**		**206**	**100.0%**	**0.65 [0.34, 1.23]**
Total events	10		17			
Heterogeneity: Chi² = 9.23, df = 9 (P = 0.42); I² = 2%						
Test for overall effect: Z = 1.33 (P = 0.18)						
Test for subgroup differences: Not applicable						

Figure 6. Forest plot of trials of absorbable fixation versus titanium examining the effect on relative risk of complications in Le Fort I. See Figure 2 legend for expansion of abbreviations.

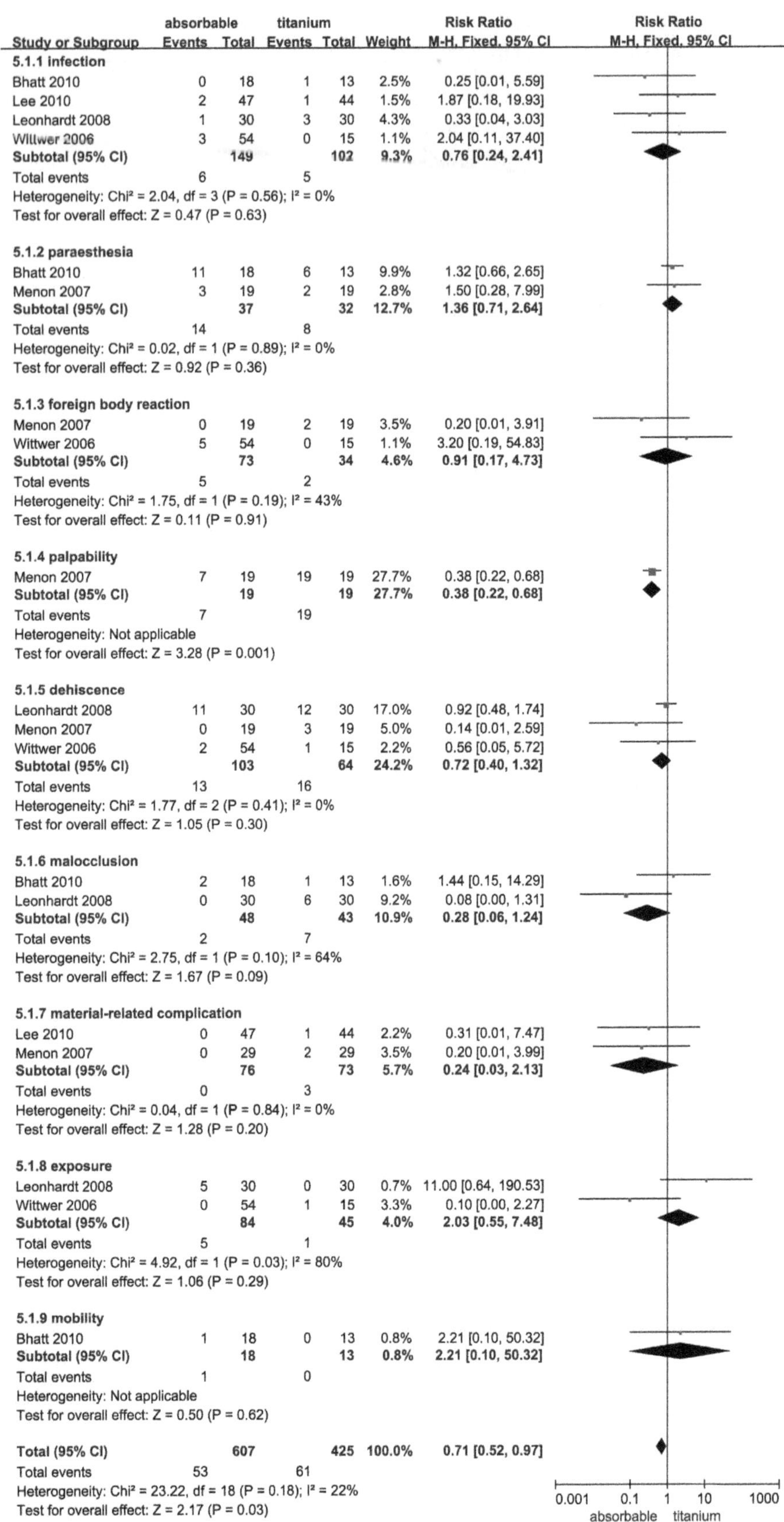

Study or Subgroup	absorbable Events	absorbable Total	titanium Events	titanium Total	Weight	Risk Ratio M-H, Fixed, 95% CI
5.1.1 infection						
Bhatt 2010	0	18	1	13	2.5%	0.25 [0.01, 5.59]
Lee 2010	2	47	1	44	1.5%	1.87 [0.18, 19.93]
Leonhardt 2008	1	30	3	30	4.3%	0.33 [0.04, 3.03]
Wittwer 2006	3	54	0	15	1.1%	2.04 [0.11, 37.40]
Subtotal (95% CI)		**149**		**102**	**9.3%**	**0.76 [0.24, 2.41]**
Total events	6		5			
Heterogeneity: Chi² = 2.04, df = 3 (P = 0.56); I² = 0%						
Test for overall effect: Z = 0.47 (P = 0.63)						
5.1.2 paraesthesia						
Bhatt 2010	11	18	6	13	9.9%	1.32 [0.66, 2.65]
Menon 2007	3	19	2	19	2.8%	1.50 [0.28, 7.99]
Subtotal (95% CI)		**37**		**32**	**12.7%**	**1.36 [0.71, 2.64]**
Total events	14		8			
Heterogeneity: Chi² = 0.02, df = 1 (P = 0.89); I² = 0%						
Test for overall effect: Z = 0.92 (P = 0.36)						
5.1.3 foreign body reaction						
Menon 2007	0	19	2	19	3.5%	0.20 [0.01, 3.91]
Wittwer 2006	5	54	0	15	1.1%	3.20 [0.19, 54.83]
Subtotal (95% CI)		**73**		**34**	**4.6%**	**0.91 [0.17, 4.73]**
Total events	5		2			
Heterogeneity: Chi² = 1.75, df = 1 (P = 0.19); I² = 43%						
Test for overall effect: Z = 0.11 (P = 0.91)						
5.1.4 palpability						
Menon 2007	7	19	19	19	27.7%	0.38 [0.22, 0.68]
Subtotal (95% CI)		**19**		**19**	**27.7%**	**0.38 [0.22, 0.68]**
Total events	7		19			
Heterogeneity: Not applicable						
Test for overall effect: Z = 3.28 (P = 0.001)						
5.1.5 dehiscence						
Leonhardt 2008	11	30	12	30	17.0%	0.92 [0.48, 1.74]
Menon 2007	0	19	3	19	5.0%	0.14 [0.01, 2.59]
Wittwer 2006	2	54	1	15	2.2%	0.56 [0.05, 5.72]
Subtotal (95% CI)		**103**		**64**	**24.2%**	**0.72 [0.40, 1.32]**
Total events	13		16			
Heterogeneity: Chi² = 1.77, df = 2 (P = 0.41); I² = 0%						
Test for overall effect: Z = 1.05 (P = 0.30)						
5.1.6 malocclusion						
Bhatt 2010	2	18	1	13	1.6%	1.44 [0.15, 14.29]
Leonhardt 2008	0	30	6	30	9.2%	0.08 [0.00, 1.31]
Subtotal (95% CI)		**48**		**43**	**10.9%**	**0.28 [0.06, 1.24]**
Total events	2		7			
Heterogeneity: Chi² = 2.75, df = 1 (P = 0.10); I² = 64%						
Test for overall effect: Z = 1.67 (P = 0.09)						
5.1.7 material-related complication						
Lee 2010	0	47	1	44	2.2%	0.31 [0.01, 7.47]
Menon 2007	0	29	2	29	3.5%	0.20 [0.01, 3.99]
Subtotal (95% CI)		**76**		**73**	**5.7%**	**0.24 [0.03, 2.13]**
Total events	0		3			
Heterogeneity: Chi² = 0.04, df = 1 (P = 0.84); I² = 0%						
Test for overall effect: Z = 1.28 (P = 0.20)						
5.1.8 exposure						
Leonhardt 2008	5	30	0	30	0.7%	11.00 [0.64, 190.53]
Wittwer 2006	0	54	1	15	3.3%	0.10 [0.00, 2.27]
Subtotal (95% CI)		**84**		**45**	**4.0%**	**2.03 [0.55, 7.48]**
Total events	5		1			
Heterogeneity: Chi² = 4.92, df = 1 (P = 0.03); I² = 80%						
Test for overall effect: Z = 1.06 (P = 0.29)						
5.1.9 mobility						
Bhatt 2010	1	18	0	13	0.8%	2.21 [0.10, 50.32]
Subtotal (95% CI)		**18**		**13**	**0.8%**	**2.21 [0.10, 50.32]**
Total events	1		0			
Heterogeneity: Not applicable						
Test for overall effect: Z = 0.50 (P = 0.62)						
Total (95% CI)		**607**		**425**	**100.0%**	**0.71 [0.52, 0.97]**
Total events	53		61			
Heterogeneity: Chi² = 23.22, df = 18 (P = 0.18); I² = 22%						
Test for overall effect: Z = 2.17 (P = 0.03)						

Figure 7. Forest plot of trials of absorbable fixation versus titanium examining the effect on relative risk of complications in fracture fixation. See Figure 2 legend for expansion of abbreviations.

Absorbable Versus Non-absorbable Group: Complication in All Enrolled Studies

The combined results of the 20 trials revealed that the absorbable group had significantly more complications when compared with the titanium group (RR = 1.20; 95% CI: 1.02–1.42; P = 0.03). The heterogeneity test was not substantial, as assessed by the I^2 statistics (Q [d.f. = 60] = 74.25; P = 0.10; I^2 = 19%) (Figure 2). A sub-group analysis was performed for complications, including infection, temporomandibular joint dysfunction (TMD), paraesthesia, foreign body reaction (local inflammation and redness), fistulation, palpability, dehiscence, malocclusion, material-related complication (loose screw, screw head fracture and plate fracture), exposure, relapse and mobility. Foreign body reaction (RR = 1.97; 95% CI: 1.05–3.68; P = 0.03) and mobility (RR = 5.64; 95% CI: 1.10–28.85; P = 0.04) occurred significantly more frequently in patients receiving absorbable fixation compared to patients receiving non-absorbable fixation. However, the absorbable group was not associated with a more significant increase in infection (RR = 1.20; 95% CI: 0.65–2.19; P = 0.56), TMD (RR = 1.00; 95% CI: 0.47–2.12; P = 1.00), paraesthesia (RR = 1.08; 95% CI: 0.61–1.93; P = 0.78), fistulation (RR = 2.09; 95% CI: 0.87–5.01; P = 0.10), palpability (RR = 0.90; 95% CI: 0.70–1.15; P = 0.38), dehiscence (RR = 1.12; 95% CI: 0.65–1.93; P = 0.69), malocclusion (RR = 1.11; 95% CI: 0.63–1.97; P = 0.72), material related complication (RR = 1.70; 95% CI: 0.63–4.56; P = 0.30), exposure (RR = 1.83; 95% CI: 0.71–4.75; P = 0.21) and relapse (RR = 1.41; 95% CI: 0.62–3.17; P = 0.41). Publication bias was not evident, as estimated by the funnel plot for the studies on complications (Figure 3a).

Complication Comparison in the Bimaxillary Operation

There were 3 trials comparing the complications of absorbable and titanium fixation in the bimaxillary operation category (BSSRO plus Le Fort I). We found that the application of absorbable fixation did not have a significant increase in complications compared with titanium (RR = 1.89; 95% CI: 0.85–4.22; P = 0.12). The heterogeneity was not evident (Q [d.f. = 3] = 4.95; P = 0.18, I^2 = 39%) (Figure 4). A sub-group analysis of complications was also performed that included foreign body reaction, relapse and mobility. The group receiving absorbable fixation was not associated with a more significant increase in foreign body reaction (RR = 5.91; 95% CI: 0.32–110.47; P = 0.23), relapse (RR = 0.85; 95% CI: 0.31–2.33; P = 0.75) and mobility (RR = 13.00; 95% CI: 0.81–209.86; P = 0.07). Funnel plot for the studies on complications in the bimaxillary operation category was relatively symmetrical, and publication bias was not evident (Figure 3b).

Complication Comparison in the BSSRO Operation

No significant difference was observed between the absorbable and titanium groups (RR = 1.45; 95% CI: 0.84–2.48; P = 0.18). The heterogeneity test was not substantial, as assessed by the I^2 statistics (Q [d.f. = 14] = 9.11; P = 0.82; I^2 = 0%) (Figure 5). A sub-group analysis was performed for complications, including infection, TMD, paraesthesia, palpability, dehiscence, material-related complications, exposure, and relapse. The results showed the same rate for these complications in the absorbable group and the titanium group (P>0.05). There was no evidence to suggest publication bias, as estimated by the funnel plot for the studies on complications in this operation (Figure 3c).

Complication Comparison in the Le Fort I Operation

There were only 2 trials comparing the complications of absorbable and non-absorbable fixation in the Le Fort I operation. There was no significant alteration observed between the absorbable and non-absorbable groups (RR = 0.65; 95% CI: 0.34–1.23; P = 0.18). The heterogeneity test was not substantial, as assessed by the I^2 statistics (Q [d.f. = 9] = 9.23; P = 0.42; I^2 = 2%) (Figure 6). A sub-group analysis was performed for complications, including infection, foreign body reaction, fistulation, palpability, dehiscence, exposure and mobility. Palpability (RR = 0.23; 95% CI: 0.08–0.68; P = 0.008) occurred significantly more frequently in patients fixed with titanium compared to patients receiving absorbable fixation. In addition, patients in the absorbable group were not associated with a more significant increase in infection (RR = 0.98; 95% CI: 0.18–5.42; P = 0.98), foreign body reaction (RR = 0.98; 95% CI: 0.15–6.62; P = 0.99), fistulation (RR = 3.00; 95% CI: 0.14–66.53; P = 0.49), dehiscence (RR = 2.90; 95% CI: 0.12–68.15; P = 0.51), exposure (RR = 2.90; 95% CI: 0.12–68.15; P = 0.51) and mobility (RR = 2.90; 95% CI: 0.12–68.15; P = 0.51). The funnel plot for the studies on complications in Le Fort I operation was relatively symmetrical, and publication bias was not evident (Figure 3d).

Complication Comparison in the Fracture Fixation

Five trials were pooled in the fracture fixation operation. The combined results of the five trials revealed that the absorbable group had a significantly lower rate of complications compared to the titanium group (RR = 0.71; 95% CI: 0.52–0.97; P = 0.03). In addition, the heterogeneity was not observed (Q [d.f. = 18] = 23.22, P = 0.18, I^2 = 22%) (Figure 7). A sub-group analysis was performed for complications, including infection, paraesthesia, foreign body reaction, palpability, dehiscence, malocclusion, material-related complication, exposure and mobility. Palpability (RR = 0.38; 95% CI: 0.22–0.68; P = 0.001) occurred significantly more frequently in patients fixed with titanium compared to patients receiving absorbable fixation. In addition, the absorbable group was not associated with a more significant increase in infection, paraesthesia, foreign body reaction, dehiscence, malocclusion, material-related complication, exposure and mobility (P>0.05). Publication bias was not evident, as estimated by the funnel plot for the studies on complications (Figure 3e).

Discussion

To the best of our knowledge, this is the first meta-analysis to examine the safety profile of absorbable fixation system in maxillofacial surgery which can result in various complications. In addition to the common postoperative complications, including infection and sensory disturbance due to inferior alveolar nerve injury, TMD and relapse can occur [30,31]. Recent developments have led to the introduction of titanium as a fixation material due to its superior qualities. In orthognathic surgery, bone fragments are usually fixed with the use of titanium plates and screws. However, the limitation of titanium fixation is the requirement of a subsequent removal operation, which is highly recommended. Although absorbable fixation systems avoid the need for a second operation, the potential complications that can occur, such as foreign body reaction, deter the wide use of absorbable fixation systems to be widely used. Thus, there is a need to systematically evaluate the safety of absorbable fixation systems in maxillofacial surgery.

Several clinical trials have shown the safety of absorbable fixation system in maxillofacial surgery. Observational studies in maxillofacial surgery have demonstrated that the bioresorbable plate leaves a stable bridge of healed bone or soft tissue after complete degradation with foreign-body reactions. Randomized, prospective controlled trials have shown no statistically significant differences in the incidence of material-related complications between the biodegradable and titanium groups [8,32,24]. However, Buijs et al. reported that biodegradable plates and screws performed inferiorly to titanium plates and screws in non-correct occlusion (11.1% vs. 8.8%), palpability plate/screw (50.4% vs. 38.1%), dehiscence (4.3% vs. 0%), abscess formation (9.4% vs. 3.5%) and inflammatory reactions (17.1% vs. 7.1%), respectively [1]. Most of the previous trials on absorbable fixation systems have systematically included patients receiving partial maxillofacial surgery. In this study, we found that absorbable fixation systems had a significantly higher rate of complications in maxillofacial surgery, especially with foreign body reaction and mobility. Foreign body reactions typically manifest with uniform histopathology, nonspecific inflammation, and abundant polymeric particles surrounded by mononuclear phagocytes and multinucleated foreign-body giant cells [33]. In addition, absorbable fixation systems cost more in clinical use. Therefore, absorbable fixation systems should not be considered as the first selective treatment materials for the management of bone fixation in maxillofacial surgery.

In maxillofacial surgery, the feasibility of applying biodegradable plates and screws for zygomatic fracture fixation was first demonstrated by Bos et al [34]. This technique soon extended to other craniomaxillofacial surgical procedures for fracture and orthognathic surgery. To explore the safety in different maxillofacial surgeries, four subgroups were described. In the bimaxillary operation categories, the application of an absorbable fixation system therapy did not have a significant increase in complications. There was no statistically significant difference in the foreign body reaction, relapse and mobility rates between fixation with titanium or absorbable plates/screws. Absorbable fixation of the single maxillary (Le Fort I) and single mandibular (BSSRO) seem to have a similar safety profile as titanium. A previous study also suggested the use of resorbable copolymer devices as a viable alternative to titanium for fixation of Le Fort I maxillary fixation [35]. In this study, fracture fixation included mandibular and zygomatic operation. Though they have similar stabilities, absorbable fixation is superior for fracture fixation, mainly in palpability. Palpability can be a problem for metallic fixation. In addition, long-term studies on the effects of metal osteosynthesis have identified the presence of metal ions in the vicinity of the site, leading to speculation that metal is gradually leached out by the action of body fluids [36]. Therefore, the application of an absorbable fixation system may be highly recommended for fracture fixation and an alternative option in the case of Le Fort I osteotomy, bimaxillary operation and BSSRO, compared to titanium.

There were several limitations of this study. First, the possibility of publication bias is always of concern. Although the enrolled trials consisted of more than 1500 patients in total, these results may be affected by publication bias. Second, heterogeneities between studies may confuse meta-analysis outcomes, such as with the use of different raw materials and source companies. Third, some of the trials were comparative studies, which are not as convincing. Therefore, more RCTs should be performed in order to obtain more convincing and reliable data to investigate the accuracy of this conclusion.

In conclusion, this meta-analysis found that absorbable fixation systems used for the fixation during maxillofacial surgery do not have adequate safety profiles. Notably, the occurrence of foreign body reactions and mobility were significantly more frequent in patients receiving absorbable fixation systems compared to titanium fixation. Subgroup indicated the safety of absorbable fixation systems was superior during fracture fixation. The absorbable fixation systems tend to have a similar favorable safety profile as titanium fixation during bimaxillary operation, BSSRO and Le Fort I operation, in which the absorbable fixation was superior to titanium fixation with regard to palpability. However, large-scale randomized, prospective trials of absorbable fixation systems used in maxillofacial surgery are needed, which will provide more convincing and reliable data regarding safety.

Author Contributions

Conceived and designed the experiments: LY MX LT. Performed the experiments: LY XJ JX. Analyzed the data: LY JL. Contributed reagents/materials/analysis tools: LY CZ TT. Wrote the paper: LY LT.

References

1. Buijs GJ, van BNB, Jansma J, de Visscher JG, Hoppenreijs TJ, et al. (2012) A randomized clinical trial of biodegradable and titanium fixation systems in maxillofacial surgery. J Dent Res 91: 299–304.
2. Haers PE, Suuronen R, Lindqvist C, Sailer H (1998) Biodegradable polylactide plates and screws in orthognathic surgery: technical note. J Craniomaxillofac Surg 26: 87–91.
3. Ray MS, Matthew IR, Frame JW (1999) Metallic fragments on the surface of miniplates and screws before insertion. Br J Oral Maxillofac Surg 37: 14–18.
4. Siniscalchi EN, Catalfamo L, Allegra A, Musolino C, De Ponte FS (2013) Titanium miniplates: a new risk factor for the development of the bisphosphonate-related osteonecrosis of the jaw. J Craniofac Surg 24: e1–2.
5. Ueki K, Okabe K, Moroi A, Marukawa K, Sotobori M, et al. (2012) Maxillary stability after Le Fort I osteotomy using three different plate systems. Int J Oral Maxillofac Surg 41: 942–948.
6. Shah NM, Shah MA, Chowdhury RI, Menon I (2007) Reasons and correlates of contraceptive discontinuation in Kuwait. Eur J Contracept Reprod Health Care 12: 260–268.
7. Park CH, Kim HS, Lee JH, Hong SM, Ko YG, et al. (2011) Resorbable skeletal fixation systems for treating maxillofacial bone fractures. Arch Otolaryngol Head Neck Surg 137: 125–129.
8. Yoshioka I, Igawa K, Nagata J, Yoshida M, Ogawa Y, et al. (2012) Comparison of material-related complications after bilateral sagittal split mandibular setback surgery: biodegradable versus titanium miniplates. J Oral Maxillofac Surg 70: 919–924.
9. Dorri M, Nasser M, Oliver R (2009) Resorbable versus titanium plates for facial fractures. Cochrane Database Syst Rev: CD007158.
10. Moher D, Jadad AR, Tugwell P (1996) Assessing the quality of randomized controlled trials. Current issues and future directions. Int J Technol Assess Health Care 12: 195–208.
11. Landes CA, Ballon A, Sader R (2007) Segment stability in bimaxillary orthognathic surgery after resorbable Poly(L-lactide-co-glycolide) versus titanium osteosyntheses. J Craniofac Surg 18: 1216–1229.
12. Landes CA, Ballon A (2006) Skeletal stability in bimaxillary orthognathic surgery: P(L/DL)LA-resorbable versus titanium osteofixation. Plast Reconstr Surg 118: 703–721; discussion 722.
13. Costa F, Robiony M, Zorzan E, Zerman N, Politi M (2006) Stability of skeletal Class III malocclusion after combined maxillary and mandibular procedures: titanium versus resorbable plates and screws for maxillary fixation. J Oral Maxillofac Surg 64: 642–651.
14. Ueki K, Nakagawa K, Marukawa K, Takazakura D, Shimada M, et al. (2005) Changes in condylar long axis and skeletal stability after bilateral sagittal split ramus osteotomy with poly-L-lactic acid or titanium plate fixation. Int J Oral Maxillofac Surg 34: 627–634.
15. Stockmann P, Bohm H, Driemel O, Muhling J, Pistner H (2010) Resorbable versus titanium osteosynthesis devices in bilateral sagittal split ramus osteotomy

of the mandible - the results of a two centre randomised clinical study with an eight-year follow-up. J Craniomaxillofac Surg 38: 522–528.
16. Turvey TA, Bell RB, Phillips C, Proffit WR (2006) Self-reinforced biodegradable screw fixation compared with titanium screw fixation in mandibular advancement. J Oral Maxillofac Surg 64: 40–46.
17. Paeng JY, Hong J, Kim CS, Kim MJ (2012) Comparative study of skeletal stability between bicortical resorbable and titanium screw fixation after sagittal split ramus osteotomy for mandibular prognathism. J Craniomaxillofac Surg 40: 660–664.
18. Matthews NS, Khambay BS, Ayoub AF, Koppel D, Wood G (2003) Preliminary assessment of skeletal stability after sagittal split mandibular advancement using a bioresorbable fixation system. Br J Oral Maxillofac Surg 41: 179–184.
19. Norholt SE, Pedersen TK, Jensen J (2004) Le Fort I miniplate osteosynthesis: a randomized, prospective study comparing resorbable PLLA/PGA with titanium. Int J Oral Maxillofac Surg 33: 245–252.
20. Landes CA, Ballon A (2006) Five-year experience comparing resorbable to titanium miniplate osteosynthesis in cleft lip and palate orthognathic surgery. Cleft Palate Craniofac J 43: 67–74.
21. Lee HB, Oh JS, Kim SG, Kim HK, Moon SY, et al. (2010) Comparison of titanium and biodegradable miniplates for fixation of mandibular fractures. J Oral Maxillofac Surg 68: 2065–2069.
22. Bhatt K, Roychoudhury A, Bhutia O, Trikha A, Seith A, et al. (2010) Equivalence randomized controlled trial of bioresorbable versus titanium miniplates in treatment of mandibular fracture: a pilot study. J Oral Maxillofac Surg 68: 1842–1848.
23. Leonhardt H, Demmrich A, Mueller A, Mai R, Loukota R, et al. (2008) INION compared with titanium osteosynthesis: a prospective investigation of the treatment of mandibular fractures. Br J Oral Maxillofac Surg 46: 631–634.
24. Wittwer G, Adeyemo WL, Yerit K, Voracek M, Turhani D, et al. (2006) Complications after zygoma fracture fixation: is there a difference between biodegradable materials and how do they compare with titanium osteosynthesis. Oral Surg Oral Med Oral Pathol Oral Radiol Endod 101: 419–425.
25. Menon S, Chowdhury S (2007) Evaluation of Bioresorbable vis-à-vis Titanium Plates and Screws for Craniofacial Fractures and Osteotomies. MJAFI 63: 331–333.
26. Cheung LK, Chow LK, Chiu WK (2004) A randomized controlled trial of resorbable versus titanium fixation for orthognathic surgery. Oral Surg Oral Med Oral Pathol Oral Radiol Endod 98: 386–397.
27. Ahn YS, Kim SG, Baik SM, Kim BO, Kim HK, et al. (2010) Comparative study between resorbable and nonresorbable plates in orthognathic surgery. J Oral Maxillofac Surg 68: 287–292.
28. Tuovinen V, Suuronen R, Teittinen M, Nurmenniemi P (2010) Comparison of the stability of bioabsorbable and titanium osteosynthesis materials for rigid internal fixation in orthognathic surgery. A prospective randomized controlled study in 101 patients with 192 osteotomies. Int J Oral Maxillofac Surg 39: 1059–1065.
29. Buijs GJ, van Bakelen NB, Jansma J, de Visscher JG, Hoppenreijs TJ, et al. (2011) A randomized clinical trial of biodegradable and titanium fixation systems in maxillofacial surgery. International & American Associations for Dental Research 91.
30. Kim SG, Park SS (2007) Incidence of complications and problems related to orthognathic surgery. J Oral Maxillofac Surg 65: 2438–2444.
31. Lee JG, Kim SG, Lim KJ, Choi KC (2007) Thermographic assessment of inferior alveolar nerve injury in patients with dentofacial deformity. J Oral Maxillofac Surg 65: 74–78.
32. Ueki K, Hashiba Y, Marukawa K, Okabe K, Nakagawa K, et al. (2009) Evaluation of bone formation after sagittal split ramus osteotomy with bent plate fixation using computed tomography. J Oral Maxillofac Surg 67: 1062–1068.
33. Bostman OM (1992) Intense granulomatous inflammatory lesions associated with absorbable internal fixation devices made of polyglycolide in ankle fractures. Clin Orthop Relat Res: 193–199.
34. Bos RR, Boering G, Rozema FR, Leenslag JW (1987) Resorbable poly(L-lactide) plates and screws for the fixation of zygomatic fractures. J Oral Maxillofac Surg 45: 751–753.
35. Dhol WS, Reyneke JP, Tompson B, Sandor GK (2008) Comparison of titanium and resorbable copolymer fixation after Le Fort I maxillary impaction. Am J Orthod Dentofacial Orthop 134: 67–73.
36. Meningaud JP, Poupon J, Bertrand JC, Chenevier C, Galliot-Guilley M, et al. (2001) Dynamic study about metal release from titanium miniplates in maxillofacial surgery. Int J Oral Maxillofac Surg 30: 185–188.

18

Validation of the Surgical Fear Questionnaire in Adult Patients Waiting for Elective Surgery

Maurice Theunissen[1]*, Madelon L. Peters[2], Erik G. W. Schouten[2], Audrey A. A. Fiddelers[1], Mark G. A. Willemsen[1], Patrícia R. Pinto[3], Hans-Fritz Gramke[1], Marco A. E. Marcus[1,4]

1 Department of Anesthesiology and Pain Management, Maastricht University Medical Center+, Maastricht, the Netherlands, **2** Department of Clinical Psychological Science, Maastricht University, Maastricht, the Netherlands, **3** Life and Health Sciences Research Institute (ICVS), School of Health Sciences, University of Minho, Braga, Portugal; ICVS/3B's – PT Government Associate Laboratory, Braga/Guimarães, Portugal, **4** Department of Anesthesia/ICU, Pain and Palliative Care, Hamad Medical Corporation, Doha, Qatar

Abstract

Objectives: Because existing instruments for assessing surgical fear seem either too general or too limited, the Surgical Fear Questionnaire (SFQ) was developed. The aim of this study is to assess the validity and reliability of the SFQ.

Methods: Based on existing literature and expert consultation the ten-item SFQ was composed. Data on the SFQ were obtained from 5 prospective studies (N = 3233) in inpatient or day surgery patients. These data were used for exploratory factor analysis (EFA), confirmatory factor analysis (CFA), reliability analysis and validity analysis.

Results: EFA in Study 1 and 2 revealed a two-factor structure with one factor associated with fear of the short-term consequences of surgery (SFQ-s, item 1–4) and the other factor with fear of the long-term consequences of surgery (SFQ-l, item 5–10). However, in both studies two items of the SFQ-l had low factor loadings. Therefore in Study 3 and 4 the 2-factor structure was tested and confirmed by CFA in an eight-item version of the SFQ. Across all studies significant correlations of the SFQ with pain catastrophizing, state anxiety, and preoperative pain intensity indicated good convergent validity. Internal consistency (Cronbach's alpha) was between 0.765–0.920 (SFQ-total), 0.766–0.877 (SFQ-s), and 0.628–0.899 (SFQ-l). The SFQ proved to be sensitive to detect differences based on age, sex, education level, employment status and preoperative pain intensity.

Discussion: The SFQ is a valid and reliable eight-item index of surgical fear consisting of two subscales: fear of the short-term consequences of surgery and fear of the long-term consequences.

Editor: Jeremy Miles, Research and Development Corporation, United States of America

Funding: This study was conducted with departmental funding and supported by a grant from The Netherlands Organisation for Scientific Research (Zon-MW, http://www.zonmw.nl/en/), grant no. 110000007. The funders had no role in study design, data collection and analysis, decision to publish, or preparation of the manuscript.

Competing Interests: The authors have read the journal's policy and have the following conflicts: The department of Anesthesiology of the MUMC+ receives payments of Grünenthal for consultancy activities of M. Marcus. This does not alter the authors' adherence to PLOS ONE policies on sharing data and materials.

* Email: maurice.theunissen@mumc.nl

Introduction

Preoperative or surgical fear is a well recognizable emotional state for many patients waiting for surgery and is a risk factor for major personal and socio-economic burden. Various studies have found that surgical fear is associated with impaired psychosocial and physical recovery, such as increased levels of acute and chronic postoperative pain [1–3]. Therefore, preoperative assessment of surgical fear could provide essential information for improving perioperative care and could be a first step towards targeted intervention.

Objects of surgical fear can be heterogeneous. Previous studies have listed more than 20 objects of fear, varying from fear of the surgical procedure itself to fear of the anaesthesia, having to undergo blood transfusions, being stung with needles, losing dignity or even dying [4–6]. Some factors that may influence the reported prevalence of surgical fear are type or impact of planned surgery, time span until surgery, previous experience with surgery, provision of preoperative information about surgical procedure, age and sex [3,5,7–9]. Also, the instrument used for assessment of fear may influence the reported prevalence.

Only few instruments are available for assessment of surgical fear and most of these are disease specific, such as the Bypass Grafting Fear Scale (BGFS) [10] and the Surgery Stress Scale (for knee surgery) [11]. Therefore, in many studies, nonspecific instruments have been used such as the Hospital Anxiety and Depression Scale (HADS) [12], State-Trait Anxiety Inventory (STAI) [13], or a Visual Analogue Scale (VAS) assessing anxiety. One generic instrument has been developed for preoperative assessment of surgical fear, the six-item Amsterdam Preoperative Anxiety and Information Scale (APAIS) [14,15]. However, this instrument is relatively limited in scope; it includes two items on fear of the anaesthetic procedure and two items on fear of the surgical procedure. The remaining two items asses the need for information rather than fear.

Because existing instruments for assessing surgical fear are either limited in scope, or too general, or too specific and not broadly generalizable to other surgical populations, we developed the Surgical Fear Questionnaire (SFQ). The SFQ has already been used in several studies [16–22] but formal assessment of its validity and reliability is still lacking. This paper describes the development and psychometric assessment of the SFQ. Similar to the BGFS [10], the SFQ aims to be comprehensive enough to cover the most important targets of fear and at the same time concise enough for general use in clinical practice and research. We present data on the construct, content, convergent, and predictive validity as well as the internal consistency of the SFQ. Data from five different studies in which the SFQ was administered to patients one day to one week prior to undergoing inpatient or day surgery are used. Because patients from different clinical populations and different countries are included, this also allows us to test the stability of the SFQ and its factor structure across different subgroups.

Materials and Methods

Ethics statement

Study 1, 3, 4, and 5 were approved by the Medical Ethics Committee of Maastricht University Medical Center+, Maastricht, the Netherlands. For Study 2 approval was given by the Medical Ethics Committee of the Centro Hospital do Alto Ave, Guimarães, Portugal. All patients gave written informed consent.

Scale development

The SFQ was developed to create a tailor made instrument for the assessment of self-reported surgical fear, suitable for general use among all types of adult surgery patients, and covering a broad range of short-term and long-term surgery-related fears. The composition and phrasing of the SFQ was based on items selected from existing questionnaires [4,6,10,14,23] and expert consultation. The selection of the initial 10 items took place after a consensus meeting of experts in the field of psychology, anaesthesiology, methodology, or epidemiology. All items are scored on an eleven point numeric rating scale (NRS) ranging from 0 (not at all afraid) to 10 (very afraid). This results in a total score of 0 to 100. Selected items are: afraid of operation, anaesthesia, postoperative pain, side effects, health deterioration, failed operation, hospital stay, (worried) about family members, incomplete recovery, long duration of rehabilitation.

Procedure

To establish the factor structure of the SFQ, data of four different studies were used, see table 1. A two stage approach was employed. Exploratory factor analysis (EFA) was performed on the data of the first two studies, followed by confirmatory factor analysis (CFA) on the data of study 3 and 4. EFA is used to explore the underlying factor structure of a set of items without an a priori hypothesis about the number and structure of factors to be identified. CFA is a hypothesis testing technique used to confirm the solution of the EFA in a different sample.

An initial EFA was performed on the SFQ data obtained from a prospective observational cohort study examining predictors of acute and chronic postoperative pain [16,17]. The sample consisted of 1490 Dutch inpatients scheduled to undergo surgery at one of the following departments: general surgery, plastic surgery, orthopedics, ophthalmology, gynaecology, ear-nose-throat, maxillofacial surgery, urology, neurosurgery, or thoracic surgery. Table 1 presents the primary sample characteristics (Study 1). Patients completed the SFQ in the hospital one day before surgery.

To examine the robustness of the factor solution, the EFA was repeated in a second independent sample consisting of 201 women. Data were obtained from a prospective cohort study on predictors of acute and chronic pain after elective hysterectomy carried out in Portugal. The sample characteristics are described in table 1 (Study 2) [18]. In a face to face interview with a trained psychologist the SFQ was completed on the day before surgery in the hospital. For the translation of the SFQ into Portuguese a three stage procedure was performed. The first step was the forward translation of the English version into Portuguese. This was done by a bilingual person, a native speaker of the target language (Portuguese). The second step was a separate back translation. This was performed by a bilingual translator who is a native speaker of the source language (English). The translations coincided. In step three a pilot with the Portuguese version of the SFQ was performed in a sample of 46 women undergoing hysterectomy. Before surgery the SFQ was applied and participants were asked to reflect on the comprehensibility of the scale and asked for additional suggestions. The women agreed with the Portuguese translated version and showed no doubts about the items. After this the Portuguese version of the SFQ was considered ready for use.

Meanwhile a new (Brazilian) Portuguese translation was made from the original Dutch version of the scale (A.C. Mesquita, University of São Paulo at Ribeirão Preto College of Nursing). Back translation to Dutch of this version showed it to be 100% identical to the original version. This new Portuguese translation was compared to the version used in study 2. There were only minor differences in wording which are mostly due to differences between Brazilian and European Portuguese.

On the basis of the results obtained in Study 1 and 2 two items were deleted from the SFQ and a two-factor structure was proposed for the new eight-item SFQ yielding a range of 0–80 (see below). Confirmatory factor analysis (CFA) was used to test the fit of this two-factor model against a one-factor model in a new sample of hysterectomy patients [24]. Data were obtained from the first 192 included patients of an ongoing prospective multicenter study in the Netherlands on predictors of postoperative recovery after hysterectomy. Sample characteristics are presented in table 1 (Study 3). These patients completed the eight-item version of the SFQ at home in the week before surgery.

In the last step we tested the invariance of the factor structure in a mixed male – female sample of patients undergoing various surgical procedures. Data were obtained from a prospective cohort study on the prevalence of postoperative pain in adult patients after elective day surgery performed in the Netherlands [25]. The most frequently performed types of surgery in this study were, among other, general surgery, orthopaedic surgery, ear nose throat surgery, plastic surgery, and gynaecologic surgery. Sample characteristics are presented in table 1 (Study 4). A total of 1275 patients completed the eight-item version of the SFQ at home in the week before surgery.

Convergent validity was tested by comparing the scores on the SFQ with scores on questionnaires assessing general anxiety, or negative cognitions about pain before the operation. All four studies that provided data for the psychometric evaluation of the SFQ included a measure of pain catastrophizing, either the Pain Catastrophizing Scale (PCS) or the catastrophizing subscale of the Coping Strategies Questionnaire-revised (CSQ-R) [26,27]. Both scales measure negative cognitions and worrying about pain. The full thirteen-item PCS was included in Study 1 and 3, a six–item abbreviated version in Study 4 and the catastrophizing subscale of

Table 1. Sociodemographic and surgery characteristics of Study 1–5.

	Study 1 N=1490	Study 2 N=201	Study 3 N=192	Study 4 N=1275	Study 5 N=75
Country					
	NL	P	NL	NL	NL
Surgery					
	Mixed inpatient	Hysterectomy	Hysterectomy	Mixed day surgery	Mixed day surgery
Age					
	55.6±15.5	51.2±9.4	46.2±7.8	51.9±14.7	52.8±15.3
Sex					
Male	702	-	-	722	31
Female	788	201	192	553	44
Education					
Low	392	188	33	396	20
Intermediate & high	788	12	158	864	52
Missing	310	1	1	15	3
Employment					
Occupation	484	99	129	688	34
No occupation	684	102	60	586	37
Missing	322	0	3	1	4
ASA					
I/II	1222	184	180	1196	69
III/IV	268	14	3	53	6
Missing	0	3	9	26	0
Malignancy					
Yes	239	0	0	107	7
No	1251	201	192	1168	68
Preoperative pain					
	3 (0–21)	40 (20–50)	50 (30–60)	20 (0–50)	30 (0–60)
Expected pain					
No/mild	760	48	47	590	28
Moderate/high	679	52	142	651	47
Missing/don't know	51	101	3	34	0

N numbers baseline population; mean ± standard deviation, median (interquartile range).
Country: NL the Netherlands, P Portugal.
- Not applicable. Preoperative pain: VAS/NRS 0–100. Expected pain VAS/NRS 0–100 or Likert scale (Study 2): no/mild pain VAS/NRS <40, moderate/high pain VAS/NRS 40–100. ASA: American Society of Anesthesiologists.

CSQ-R was used in Study 2. Additionally, all studies included a pre-operative assessment of expected pain. Only Study 2 also included a measure of pre-operative general anxiety, namely the anxiety subscale of the HADS. The HADS is a widely used and well validated instrument, developed for assessing self-reported anxiety and depression [28]. For the PCS [29], CSQ-R [30] and HADS [31] validity of the Portuguese and Dutch versions has been established.

Because one of the most frequently used instruments for measuring pre-operative (general) anxiety is the STAI [2], and this instrument was not included in any of the previous studies with the SFQ, we performed an additional study (Study 5) to assess convergent validity of the SFQ with the STAI. The Dutch version of the STAI was has been shown to be valid [32]. Both the state and trait anxiety subscales were included. In addition, patients filled out the PCS and the numerical rating scale to assess expected pain intensity. Study 5 included 75 adult patients scheduled for elective day surgery. Inclusion criteria and types of operation were similar as in study 4. All questionnaires were completed at home in the week before surgery.

Besides construct and convergent validity, also the internal consistency of the SFQ was assessed. Therefore, in all studies Cronbach's alpha was calculated.

The next step in the validation procedure was the assessment of the sensitivity to detect differences in fear between subgroups based on age, sex, employment status, ASA (American Society of Anesthesiologists) classification, surgery because of malignancy (yes/no), preoperative pain status (no/mild or VAS/NRS <40, moderate/high or VAS/NRS 40–100) [33], and education (lower compared to intermediate/higher education). Lower education

Table 2. SFQ scores of Study 1–5.

	Study 1	Study 2	Study 2	Study 3	Study 4	Study 5
	10 items	10 items	8 items	8 items	8 items	8 items
SFQ	23 (0–98)	20 (0–82)	13 (0–62)	22.9 (0–77)	22 (0–80)	25 (0–66)
SFQ-s	12 (0–40)	9 (0–36)	9 (0–36)	14 (0–40)	14 (0–40)	14 (0–38)
SFQ-l	9.5 (0–60)	10 (0–48)	3 (0–35)	7 (0–38)	8 (0–40)	9 (0–32)

Median (minimum-maximum).
SFQ-s: Surgical Fear Questionnaire short-time consequences (item 1–4), SFQ-l: SFQ long-term consequences (10-item version: item 5–10; 8-item version: item 5, 6, 9,10).

was defined as no education, primary education, lower vocational education, or ≤9 years education (Study 2). Intermediate education was defined as secondary education, intermediate vocational education, or 10–12 years of education (Study 2). Higher education was defined as higher vocational education, university, or graduation (Study 2). Finally, predictive validity was assessed on data of Study 1 and 4. Predictor variables were the SFQ and its subscales, dichotomized by median split [16]. Outcome measures were acute postsurgical pain on postoperative day 4 and chronic postsurgical pain, after 6 months in Study 1 and after one year in Study 4. Another outcome measure for predictive validity was self-perceived recovery, assessed by the global surgical recovery index (GSR, range 0–100%, values of 80–100% were considered as good recovery) [16,34].

Statistical analysis

Parametric data were described using mean ± standard deviation, non-parametric data with median and interquartile range (IQR) and minimum-maximum values. EFA (principal component analyses) was performed using oblique factor rotation (oblimin). Factor extraction was based on evaluation of the scree plot and the Kaiser's criterion (factors with eigenvalues >1 were retained). Item selection was based on evaluation of factor loadings (cut-off value >0.40). The factor loadings can be thought of as the Pearson correlation between a factor and a variable. Item selection was further confirmed by reliability analysis (evaluation of Cronbach's alpha, values ≥0.7 are considered fair and ≥0.8 good). For CFA improvement of goodness of fit was assessed by Minimum Fit Function chi square. Other test criteria were the Root Mean Square Error of Approximation (RMSEA), Standardized Root Mean Square Residual (SRMR), Non-Normed Fit Index (NNFI), and the Comparative Fit Index (CFI). The RMSEA and SRMR reflect the deviation of the factor solution from the data (the lower the better, with a minimum of 0) and the NNFI and CFI reflect the deviation of the factor solution with the independence model (the higher the better, with a maximum around 1). Values indicating a good fit are for RMSEA ≤0.06, SRMR ≤0.09, NNFI and CFI ≥0.95 [35]. Convergent validity was assessed using the Pearson correlation coefficient. Sensitivity analysis was performed with the Mann Whitney U-test. For assessing predictive validity of the SFQ, odds ratios (OR) were generated by bivariate logistic regression analyses. For the descriptive statistics, EFA, reliability analysis, validity analysis, and sensitivity analysis the Statistical Package for the Social Sciences was used (SPSS version 18, Chicago, Illinois, USA). The CFA was performed with Lisrel 8.20 (Jöreskog & Sörbom, Scientific Software International, Chicago, Illinois, USA). A p-value <0.05 was considered statistically significant for all analyses except for the convergent and predictive validity analyses. To adjust for multiple testing a Bonferroni correction of 0.05:3 was applied resulting in a p-value <0.017 considered statistically significant for all Pearson correlation coefficients and logistic regression analyses.

Table 3. Exploratory factor analysis.

		Study 1		Study 2	
		SFQ-s	SFQ-l	SFQ-s	SFQ-l
	Eigenvalue	1.211	4.807	3.588	1.440
1	Operation	0.845	0.035	0.889	0.091
2	Anaesthesia	0.907	−0.123	0.756	0.045
3	Pain	0.657	0.200	0.695	−0.073
4	Side effects	0.740	0.054	0.719	0.034
5	Health deterioration	0.040	0.768	0.066	−0.728
6	Failed operation	0.013	0.776	−0.068	−0.761
7	Hospital stay	0.256	0.434	0.393	−0.125
8	Family	0.156	0.464	0.316	−0.008
9	Incomplete recovery	−0.114	0.931	0.094	−0.805
10	Long rehabilitation	−0.057	0.834	−0.028	−0.770

Eigenvalues and factor loadings.

Table 4. Confirmatory factor analysis.

	Study 3		Study 4	
	1 Factor	2 Factors	1 Factor	2 Factors
Minimum Fit Function chi square (df)	251.9179 (20)	88.6924 (19)	1212.1356 (20)	346.5056 (19)
RMSEA	0.2730	0.1357	0.2495	0.1206
Standardized RMR	0.1010	0.0586	0.0838	0.0419
NNFI	0.6435	0.8872	0.7356	0.9236
CFI	0.7476	0.9235	0.8112	0.9481

Minimum Fit Function chi square: improvement of 2 factor model compared to 1 factor model 163.2255 (df 1), $p<0.0001$ (Study 3) and 865.93 (df1) $p<0.0001$ (Study 4). Df: degrees of freedom. RMSEA: Root Mean Square Error of Approximation, Standardized RMR: Standardized Root Mean Square Residual, NNFI: Non-Normed Fit Index, CFI: Comparative Fit Index.

Results

Study 1. Exploratory factor analysis: initial results

The original 10-item version of the SFQ was completed by 1490 patients. A median score of 23 was obtained (IQR 11–38). In table 2 median and minimum-maximum scores are presented. The scores of all items comprised the whole range from 0–10 indicating an appropriate item scaling, although some floor effect cannot be excluded since the distribution is skewed to the right.

The EFA identified two factors together explaining 60.2% of the total variance. All items loaded adequately (defined as >0.40) on one of the two factors (see table 3). Inspection of the items indicated that the items of one of the factors referred to more proximal fears (item 1–4; e.g. fear of pain, fear of anaesthesia) while the items in the other factor referred to more distal fears (item 5–10; e.g. fear of incomplete recovery, fear of long rehabilitation). These factors were labelled "fear of the short-term consequences of surgery" (SFQ-s) and "fear of the long-term consequences of surgery" (SFQ-l) respectively. Cronbach's alpha of the SFQ-s was 0.83, of SFQ-l 0.82 and of the total scale 0.87. The intercorrelation between SFQ-I en SFQ-s was 0.57, $p<0.01$.

This initial EFA thus indicated a two-factor model for the SFQ comprising all ten items. To examine the robustness of this factor structure and the generalizability to a different population, the EFA was repeated using data from a Portuguese study on women undergoing hysterectomy.

Study 2. Exploratory factor analysis: confirmation in an independent sample

The 10-item SFQ was completed by 201 patients. Compared to our previous sample, patients in this sample scored somewhat lower on most items with a median score of 20 (IQR 10–32), see also table 2. All ten items yielded scores ranging the full scale from 0–10. The distribution was skewed to the right.

EFA again revealed a two-factor structure similar to Study 1, explaining 50.3% of the variance. One factor contained items related to fear of short-term consequences of surgery (item 1–4) and one factor contained items related to long-term consequences of surgery (item 5, 6, 9, 10). However, two items (item 7: "I am afraid of staying in the hospital" and item 8 "I worry about my family") did not load above the cut-off of >0.40 on either of the two factors (table 3). These were also the two items that had the lowest factor loading in the previous sample, with loadings well below the other items on the same factor. Moreover, Cronbach's alpha on the SFQ-l subscale indicated only moderate internal consistency (0.63). Deleting these two insufficiently loading items increased the Cronbach's alpha of the SFQ-I subscale to 0.77. Cronbach's alpha of the total scale increased from 0.77 to 0.80; Cronbach's alpha for SFQ-s was 0.77. Intercorrelation between the SFQ-s and SFQ-l subscale was 0.41, $p<0.01$. A post hoc reliability analysis on the SFQ eight-item total scale and four-item SFQ-l subscale of Study 1 revealed a Cronbach's alpha of 0.87 on the total scale (unchanged) and of 0.84 on the SFQ-l.

Based on the factor loadings and internal consistency, the SFQ can best be used as an eight-item scale with two subscales, each consisting of four items. In the next step, we performed a confirmatory factor analysis on the eight-item SFQ in a new sample of women undergoing hysterectomy. We compared the two-factor model with a one-factor model. It may be argued that a one-factor model is equally suitable and more parsimonious for the data because of the high internal consistency of the total scale and the moderate but significant intercorrelation between the subscales.

Study 3. Confirmatory factor analysis

A total of 192 women scheduled for hysterectomy completed the SFQ pre-operatively. Median fear response of this sample was higher than the two previous samples with a score of 22.9 (IQR 11–37) on the eight-item version of the SFQ, which is as high as the score on the ten-item version in our initial sample and even higher than the scores of the Portuguese women on the ten-item version (table 2). Similar as in the previous samples the distribution was skewed to the right, and all item scores covered the full range of 0–10.

CFA was performed to compare a one-factor model with the two-factor model as determined by the previous EFA. Table 4 displays the results of the CFA. All test criteria indicated a poor fit of the one-factor model. The two-factor model revealed a fair model fit, except for the RMSEA. Cronbach's alpha was 0.89 for the total scale and 0.86 and 0.87 for the SFQ-s and SFQ-I respectively. Intercorrelation between the SFQ-s and SFQ-l subscale was 0.61, $p<0.01$.

Thus, based on factor analyses in the first three studies, the two-factor model seems most appropriate for the SFQ. However, the second EFA and the CFA were both performed in an entirely female sample undergoing hysterectomy in an inpatient setting. To exclude that these results are population specific, we repeated the CFA in male and female patients undergoing various procedures in day surgery setting. It may be expected that these procedures are more minor and possibly elicit less fear. Because the SFQ is meant to be generally applicable in all kind of surgical settings, generalizability of the results to another setting is important.

Table 5. Correlations of the SFQ with pain catastrophizing, expected pain, and state anxiety.

		Study 1	Study 2	Study 3	Study 4	Study 5
Pain Catastrophizing	SFQ	0.41[1]	0.44[2]	0.32[1]	0.45[1]	0.60[1]
	SFQ-s	0.34	0.36	0.28	0.41	0.47
	SFQ-l	0.40	0.41	0.31	0.42	0.66
Expected Pain	SFQ	0.33	-	0.39	0.48	0.45
	SFQ-s	0.33	-	0.42	0.46	0.40
	SFQ-l	0.26	-	0.27	0.42	0.42
State anxiety	SFQ	-	0.56[3]	-	-	0.70[4]
	SFQ-s	-	0.53	-	-	0.62
	SFQ-l	-	0.40	-	-	0.66

Pearson correlation, all significant at 0.01 level. - Not applicable.
SFQ: eight items; SFQ-s: Surgical Fear Questionnaire short-time consequences (item 1–4), SFQ-l: SFQ long-term consequences (item 5, 6, 9, and 10).
Catastrophizing: [1]PCS: Pain Catastrophizing Scale, (Study 1, 3 and 5 13 items; Study 4 six items: I feel I can't stand it any more, I become afraid that the pain may get worse, I can't seem to keep it out of my mind, I keep thinking about how badly I want the pain to stop, there is nothing I can do to reduce the intensity of the pain, I wonder whether something serious may happen). Catastrophizing: [2]CSQ-c: Coping Strategies Questionnaire-Revised, subscale pain catastrophizing.
State anxiety: [3]HADS-a: Hospital Anxiety and Depression Scale, anxiety subscale.
State anxiety: [4]STAI: State-Trait Anxiety Inventory, state subscale.

Study 4. Confirmatory factor analysis: generalization to day surgery patients

The eight-item SFQ was completed by 1275 patients at home in the week before surgery. In contrast to our expectation, day surgery patients scored equally high on the SFQ as inpatients, with a median score of 22 (IQR 11–36). This was also true for the subscale fear of long-term consequences, see table 2. All item scores covered the full range of 0–10. Similar to the results in the inpatient sample, the one-factor model did not show adequate fit, whereas the parameters of the two-factor model indicated a fair model, except for the RMSEA. Cronbach's alpha was excellent, i.e. 0.91 for the total scale and 0.88 and 0.89 for the SFQ-s and SFQ-I respectively. Intercorrelation between the SFQ-s and SFQ-l subscale was 0.65, $p<0.01$.

In sum, the SFQ can best be conceived as an eight-item questionnaire consisting of two subscales, with four items measuring fear of the short-term consequences of surgery and four items measuring fear of long-term consequences. The factor structure appears to be robust across different populations and in different languages (Dutch vs. Portuguese). In the next step we assessed the convergent validity of the SFQ with other instruments that have been used to measure pre-operative anxiety or worries, i.e. the PCS, the HADS and the STAI. Also we correlated the SFQ score with pre-operatively assessed expected pain after surgery.

Study 1–5. Convergent validation

Data were obtained from the four studies presented above and from Study 5, which was specifically set-up to further examine convergent validity. Median score on the SFQ in this latter study was 25 (IQR 10–39.3), see table 2. Cronbach's alpha was again excellent with 0.92 for the SFQ, 0.88 for SFQ-s and 0.90 for SFQ-l. Intercorrelation between the SFQ-s and SFQ-l subscale was 0.73, $p<0.01$.

Table 5 shows the Pearson correlation coefficients between the SFQ and its subscales with pain catastrophizing, expected pain, and general anxiety for all five studies. To facilitate comparison of the results across the five studies, correlation coefficients were calculated using the SFQ eight item version. Correlations between the SFQ and the three other scales were significant at 0.01 level. The correlation with pain catastrophizing ranged from 0.32 to 0.60 and with expected pain from 0.33 to 0.48. For the two studies assessing state anxiety (HADS or STAI-state anxiety subscale) correlations with SFQ were 0.56 and 0.70 respectively. In most cases the correlations with the SFQ total score were slightly higher compared to the correlations with the SFQ-s and SFQ-l. In Study 5 also the STAI-trait anxiety subscale was assessed. The correlation between the SFQ and trait anxiety was significant, but the values of 0.45 for the SFQ, 0.40 for the SFQ-s, and 0.42 for the SFQ-l were lower compared to state anxiety.

Thus, the SFQ appeared to be significantly related to other instruments used to assess pre-operative anxiety or worry, in particular to the HADS and the STAI-state anxiety subscale. In the next step we looked at the sensitivity of the SFQ to detect the hypothesized differences in fear in certain subgroups. In accordance with previous studies, we expected that female patients, younger patients, and patients with less education would score higher on surgical fear. The other factors were included exploratory.

Study 1–5. Sensitivity to differences in patient characteristics

To assess the effect of different patient characteristics on the SFQ the following subgroups were defined: age <65 years

Table 6. Sensitivity to differences in patient characteristics.

	Study 1	Study 2	Study 3	Study 4	Study 5
Age					
<65	20 (9–33)	14 (6–25)**	22.9 (11–37)	23 (12–37)	25 (11–40)
≥65	19 (8–33)	6 (0–15)	NA	21 (8–35)	22 (6–35)
Sex					
Male	15 (6–27)***	NA	NA	19 (8–31)***	[a]17 (9–34)
Female	24.5 (12.9–36.7)	13 (5–24)	22.9 (11–37)	26 (13.3–40)	26 (12–44)
Education					
Low	22 (8.8–34.1)	[a]12 (4.3–23.8)	25 (13.5–41)	[b]25 (11.3–39)*	28 (6–44)
Intermediate & high	19 (9–31)	19.5 (11.8–24.5)	21 (10–36)	22 (11–35.7)	25 (10.3–38.8)
Employment					
Occupation	[a]21 (10–34)**	[c]14 (6–28)*	24 (11.3–36)	[b]22 (11–36)	25 (10.8–38.3)
No occupation	18 (8–30)	11.5 (2.8–22)	20 (8–38)	23 (11–38)	22.5 (6.5–39.3)
ASA					
I/II	20 (9–33)	14 (5–24)	24 (11–37)	22 (11–36)	[a]25 (11.3–39.8)
III/IV	20.6 (9.5–33.6)	12 (8–23)	10 (4–NC)	25 (12.5–36)	9.5 (3–25)
Malignancy					
Yes	20 (9–33)	NA	NA	24.5 (13–40)	[a]36 (25–58)*
No	20 (9–33)			22 (11–36)	23 (10–38)
Preoperative pain					
No/mild	19 (8–32)***	14 (6.5–22)	18.5 (7.8–32.3)	18 (9–31)***	17 (6–31)**
Moderate/high	26.1 (13.5–39)	15 (5–25)	26 (14–40)	29 (16–42)	35 (14–43)

SFQ (eight items), median (interquartile range). $*p<0.05$, $**p<0.01$, $***p<0.001$. NA not applicable: hysterectomy patients only, malignancy excluded; in Study 3 age ≥ 65 excluded. NC not calculable. ASA: American Society of Anesthesiologists.

Deviation of SFQ-short term and SFQ-long term subscale from the SFQ results is indicated as: [a]SFQ-s significant difference and SFQ-l non significant difference; [b]SFQ-s non significant difference and SFQ-l significant difference; [c]SFQ-s and SFQ-l non significant difference.

Preoperative pain: no/mild or VAS/NRS <40, moderate/high or VAS/NRS 40–100, Study 1: pain at time of completion questionnaire, Study 2-5: average pain last week.

compared to ≥65 years (in Study 3 patients older than 65 years were excluded), males compared to females, lower compared to intermediate/higher education, employed compared to not employed, ASA classification I/II compared to ASA III/IV, malignancy as indication for surgery yes/no, and preoperative pain <40 compared to ≥40 on 100 mm VAS. In table 6 the

Table 7. Predictive validity of the SFQ, SFQ-s and SFQ-l.

		Study 1		Study 4	
Outcome	Predictor	OR (95 CI)		OR (95 CI)	
APSP	SFQ	2.73	(1.59–4.69)***	2.35	(1.81–3.04)***
APSP	SFQ-s	1.83	(1.08–3.10)	2.12	(1.64–2.73)***
APSP	SGQ-l	3.55	(1.99–6.32)***	2.62	(2.02–3.39)***
CPSP	SFQ	1.77	(1.25–2.51)**	2.28	(1.56–3.34)***
CPSP	SFQ-s	1.66	(1.16–2.37)**	1.66	(1.15–2.39)**
CPSP	SGQ-l	1.77	(1.24–2.51)**	3.05	(2.06–4.51)***
GSR	SFQ	0.44	(0.31–0.62)***	0.56	(0.41–0.77)***
GSR	SFQ-s	0.61	(0.43–0.87)**	0.77	(0.56–1.05)
GSR	SGQ-l	0.44	(0.31–0.63)***	0.40	(0.29–0.55)***

Bivariate logistic regression with median split SFQ, SFQ short term and SFQ long term as predictor. APSP: acute postsurgical pain on day 4. CPSP: chronic postsurgical pain after 6 months in Study 1, after one year in Study 4. Pain scores were dichotomized using a cut of value of 40 for the VAS/NRS. GSR: global surgical recovery on a scale of 0–100%, values of 80–100% were considered as good recovery; long term GSR after 6 months in Study 1, after one year in Study 4.

To adjust for multiple testing a Bonferroni correction was applied: a p-value <0.017 was considered statistically significant. $**p<0.01$, $***p<0.001$.

results of the sensitivity analyses are presented, again using the SFQ eight-item score across all five studies. In general, the results for the SFQ-s and SFQ-l subscales were in line with the SFQ total score. As expected, SFQ scores of the younger participants were higher compared to those reported by older participants although only in the Portuguese sample this difference reached statistical significance. Also in line with our expectations, females appeared to be more fearful about the surgery compared to males (Study 1 and 4 significant, Study 5 non significant (ns)). Concerning the effect of education on surgical fear, a difference between the Portuguese and the Dutch populations occurred: in the Portuguese population lower education level was associated with a lower level of surgical fear (ns) whereas in all four Dutch populations lower educated participants scored higher compared to intermediate or higher educated participants. In two out of five studies participants with an occupation scored significantly higher on the SFQ compared to participants without an occupation. ASA-classification did not affect SFQ scores. SFQ results for the subgroups concerning malignancy or not as indication for surgery revealed no differences in the studies 1 and 4 with large population samples. In the smaller Study 5 malignancy did lead to significantly increased surgical fear. Finally, preoperative pain was associated with increased surgical fear across all five studies.

The final part of this paper presents data on the predictive validity of the SFQ for acute and chronic post-operative pain and for perceived recovery. We also compare the predictive value of the total SFQ score with that of its two subscales.

Study 1 and 4. Predictive validity

Median split was used to identify fearful and non-fearful patients. Using OR's generated by bivariate logistic regression analyses, the predictive value of the SFQ for pain and recovery was assessed. Pain scores were dichotomized using a cut off value of 40 for the VAS/NRS. Values of 80–100% were considered as (near) optimal recovery, on the GSR scale of 0–100%. Results are presented in table 7. Acute pain as well as long-term pain was more strongly predicted by the scores on the SFQ-l subscale than the scores on the SFQ-s subscale. Also for recovery the SFQ-l was the strongest predictor. The predictive value of the SFQ total score was in most cases only slightly lower than that of the SFQ-l score. Predictive value of the two subscales of the SFQ for post-operative pain and perceived recovery using multivariate logistic regression analyses was previously reported in studies of Gramke et al. [36] and Peters et al. [17].

Discussion

The aim of the present study was to establish the reliability and validity of the SFQ. Therefore use was made of data obtained from 5 prospective studies (N = 3233) in inpatient or day surgery patients. Exploratory and confirmatory factor analyses indicated that a two-factor model best describes the structure of the SFQ. Two four-item subscales can be distinguished: fear of immediate consequences of surgery and fear of the long-term consequences. However, the high internal consistency of the SFQ (eight-item total score) and the moderate, but significant intercorrelations between the SFQ short-term and long-term subscales indicate that the SFQ total score may also be suitable for use in studies on surgical fear. This is further attested by the almost comparable predictive value of the SFQ total score compared to the SFQ-l subscale, and both being stronger related to the patient-reported outcomes than the SFQ-s subscale.

Significant intercorrelations with other validated instruments for the measurement of preoperative fear such as pain catastrophizing, expected postoperative pain and state anxiety indicate good convergent validation of the SFQ. As we expected, the SFQ can be used in day surgery as well as in inpatient surgery and has an adequate sensitivity for differences with regard to sex and age, and in the Dutch samples also for education level.

A limitation of this paper is that the SFQ in all five studies was assessed once in the week or evening before surgery. There are no data yet on the effect of preoperative time course on SFQ scores. For coronary surgery patients, Koivula [5] assessed surgical fear during the waiting period at home, at hospital admission, and after surgery. Preoperative fear and anxiety levels were highest during the waiting period at home and dropped after hospital admission. But for other types of surgery most studies only measure preoperative fear or anxiety in the week before surgery [37–41]. However, in the case of undesirable high levels of preoperative fear, treatment will be advocated. Depending on the type of intervention, a certain amount of time may be needed before the intended reduction of surgical fear can be achieved. Therefore, to enable preoperative treatment of surgical fear, as well as to further explore the optimal time point for the assessment of surgical fear, a study measuring the SFQ at different time points, starting from preoperative screening until the day of surgery is necessary. Secondly, the differences in SFQ scores between the Portuguese population and the Dutch population with regard to age, sex, education, and employment status raise the question to what extent sociodemographic factors affect the SFQ. Therefore, the stability of the SFQ across different subgroups needs further exploration. Thirdly, because of the non parametric distribution of the SFQ a median split was used for predictive logistic regression analyses. However, for practical use, e.g. selection of the most fearful patients for preoperative treatment of surgical fear, a more stringent cut-of point seems indicated.

Implications for practice. This paper demonstrated that the SFQ is a concise and generic instrument for the assessment of surgical fear, suitable for most types of elective adult surgery. For further research we suggest additional testing of the convergent validation using biomarkers such as preoperative stress hormone levels. Also the effect of linguistic and cultural influences on the SFQ needs further study. Finally, for diagnostic use optimal cut-of points of the SFQ need to be established. We conclude that the SFQ is a valid and reliable eight-item index of surgical fear, consisting of two subscales: fear of the short-term consequences of surgery and fear of the long-term consequences.

Acknowledgments

We thank Nieke Oversier for the effective patient recruitment and data entry for Study 5 during her scientific traineeship at our department.

Author Contributions

Conceived and designed the experiments: MT MP AF PP HG MM. Performed the experiments: MT AF MW PP. Analyzed the data: MT MP ES AF. Wrote the paper: MT MP ES AF MW PP HG MM.

References

1. Munafo MR, Stevenson J (2001) Anxiety and surgical recovery. Reinterpreting the literature. J Psychosom Res 51: 589–596.
2. Theunissen M, Peters ML, Bruce J, Gramke HF, Marcus MA (2012) Preoperative anxiety and catastrophizing: a systematic review and meta-analysis of the association with chronic postsurgical pain. Clin J Pain 28: 819–841.
3. Zieger M, Schwarz R, Konig HH, Harter M, Riedel-Heller SG (2010) Depression and anxiety in patients undergoing herniated disc surgery: relevant but underresearched - a systematic review. Cent Eur Neurosurg 71: 26–34.
4. Graham LE, Conley EM (1971) Evaluation of anxiety and fear in adult surgical patients. Nurs Res 20: 113–122.
5. Koivula M, Tarkka MT, Tarkka M, Laippala P, Paunonen-Ilmonen M (2002) Fear and anxiety in patients at different time-points in the coronary artery bypass process. Int J Nurs Stud 39: 811–822.
6. Shafer A, Fish MP, Gregg KM, Seavello J, Kosek P (1996) Preoperative anxiety and fear: a comparison of assessments by patients and anesthesia and surgery residents. Anesth Analg 83: 1285–1291.
7. Carr E, Brockbank K, Allen S, Strike P (2006) Patterns and frequency of anxiety in women undergoing gynaecological surgery. J Clin Nurs 15: 341–352.
8. Caumo W, Schmidt AP, Schneider CN, Bergmann J, Iwamoto CW, et al. (2001) Risk factors for preoperative anxiety in adults. Acta Anaesthesiol Scand 45: 298–307.
9. Millar K, Jelicic M, Bonke B, Asbury AJ (1995) Assessment of preoperative anxiety: comparison of measures in patients awaiting surgery for breast cancer. Br J Anaesth 74: 180–183.
10. Koivula M, Tarkka MT, Tarkka M, Laippala P, Paunonen-Ilmonen M (2002) Fear and in-hospital social support for coronary artery bypass grafting patients on the day before surgery. Int J Nurs Stud 39: 415–427.
11. Rosenberger PH, Kerns R, Jokl P, Ickovics JR (2009) Mood and attitude predict pain outcomes following arthroscopic knee surgery. Ann Behav Med 37: 70–76.
12. Zigmond AS, Snaith RP (1983) The hospital anxiety and depression scale. Acta Psychiatr Scand 67: 361–370.
13. Spielberger CD (1985) Assessment of state and trait anxiety: conceptual and methodological issues. South Psychol 2: 6–16.
14. Boker A, Brownell L, Donen N (2002) The Amsterdam preoperative anxiety and information scale provides a simple and reliable measure of preoperative anxiety. Can J Anaesth 49: 792–798.
15. Moerman N, van Dam FS, Muller MJ, Oosting H (1996) The Amsterdam Preoperative Anxiety and Information Scale (APAIS). Anesth Analg 82: 445–451.
16. Peters ML, Sommer M, de Rijke JM, Kessels F, Heineman E, et al. (2007) Somatic and psychologic predictors of long-term unfavorable outcome after surgical intervention. Ann Surg 245: 487–494.
17. Peters ML, Sommer M, van Kleef M, Marcus MA (2010) Predictors of physical and emotional recovery 6 and 12 months after surgery. Br J Surg 97: 1518–1527.
18. Pinto PR, McIntyre T, Almeida A, Araujo-Soares V (2012) The mediating role of pain catastrophizing in the relationship between presurgical anxiety and acute postsurgical pain after hysterectomy. Pain 153: 218–226.
19. Pinto PR, McIntyre T, Fonseca C, Almeida A, Araujo-Soares V (2012) Pre- and post-surgical factors that predict the provision of rescue analgesia following hysterectomy. Eur J Pain.
20. Pinto PR, McIntyre T, Nogueira-Silva C, Almeida A, Araujo-Soares V (2012) Risk factors for persistent postsurgical pain in women undergoing hysterectomy due to benign causes: a prospective predictive study. J Pain 13: 1045–1057.
21. Sommer M, de Rijke JM, van Kleef M, Kessels AG, Peters ML, et al. (2010) Predictors of acute postoperative pain after elective surgery. Clin J Pain 26: 87–94.
22. Sommer M, Geurts JW, Stessel B, Kessels AG, Peters ML, et al. (2009) Prevalence and predictors of postoperative pain after ear, nose, and throat surgery. Arch Otolaryngol Head Neck Surg 135: 124–130.
23. Johnston M (1982) Recognition of patients' worries by nurses and by other patients. Br J Clin Psychol 21 (Pt 4): 255–261.
24. Peters ML, Theunissen HMS, Maas J, Kenis G, Marcus MAE (2011) Recovery after hysterectomy: A study into influencing factors (study protocol). Dutch Trial Register (NTR)
25. Fiddelers A, Hoofwijk D, Gramke H-F, Marcus M (2012) How does persistent postoperative pain correlate with preoperative pain and acute postoperative pain? (Abstract). Eur J Anaesthesiol pp. 198.
26. Riley JL, Robinson ME (1997) CSQ: five factors or fiction? Clin J Pain 13: 156–162.
27. Sullivan MJL, Bishop SR, Pivik J (1995) The Pain Catastrophizing Scale: Development and validation. Psychological Assessment 7: 524–532.
28. Bjelland I, Dahl AA, Haug TT, Neckelmann D (2002) The validity of the Hospital Anxiety and Depression Scale. An updated literature review. J Psychosom Res 52: 69–77.
29. Van Damme S, Crombez G, Bijttebier P, Goubert L, Van Houdenhove B (2002) A confirmatory factor analysis of the Pain Catastrophizing Scale: invariant factor structure across clinical and non-clinical populations. Pain 96: 319–324.
30. Ferreira-Valente MA, Ribeiro JL, Jensen MP, Almeida R (2011) Coping with chronic musculoskeletal pain in Portugal and in the United States: a cross-cultural study. Pain Med 12: 1470–1480.
31. Pais-Ribeiro J, Silva I, Ferreira T, Martins A, Meneses R, et al. (2007) Validation study of a Portuguese version of the Hospital Anxiety and Depression Scale. Psychol Health Med. 12: 225–235; quiz 235–227.
32. Van der Ploeg HM, Defares PB, Spielberger CD (1980) Handleiding bij de Zelf-Beoordelings Vragenlijst ZBV: Een Nederlandstalige bewerking van de Spielberger State-Trait Anxiety Inventory STAI-DY [Manual for the Self-Judgment Questionnaire ZBV: A Dutch adaptation of the SpielbergerState-Trait Anxiety Inventory STAI-DY]. Lisse: Swets & Zeitlinger.
33. Dihle A, Helseth S, Paul SM, Miaskowski C (2006) The exploration of the establishment of cutpoints to categorize the severity of acute postoperative pain. Clin J Pain 22: 617–624.
34. Kleinbeck SV (2000) Self-reported at-home postoperative recovery. Res Nurs Health 23: 461–472.
35. Hu L, Bentler PM (1999) Cutoff criteria for fit indexes in covariance structure analyses: Conventional criteria versus new alternatives. Structural Equation Modeling 6: 1–55.
36. Gramke HF, de Rijke JM, van Kleef M, Kessels AG, Peters ML, et al. (2009) Predictive factors of postoperative pain after day-case surgery. Clin J Pain 25: 455–460.
37. Johnston M (1980) Anxiety in surgical patients. Psychol Med 10: 145–152.
38. de Groot KI, Boeke S, van den Berge HJ, Duivenvoorden HJ, Bonke B, et al. (1997) Assessing short- and long-term recovery from lumbar surgery with pre-operative biographical, medical and psychological variables. Brit J Health Psychol 2: 229–243.
39. Ene KW, Nordberg G, Johansson FG, Sjostrom B (2006) Pain, psychological distress and health-related quality of life at baseline and 3 months after radical prostatectomy. BMC Nurs 5: 8.
40. Graver V, Ljunggren AE, Malt UF, Loeb M, Haaland AK, et al. (1995) Can psychological traits predict the outcome of lumbar disc surgery when anamnestic and physiological risk factors are controlled for? Results of a prospective cohort study. J Psychosom Res 39: 465–476.
41. Poleshuck EL, Katz J, Andrus CH, Hogan LA, Jung BF, et al. (2006) Risk Factors for Chronic Pain Following Breast Cancer Surgery: A Prospective Study. J Pain 7: 626–634.

19

Cruciate Ligament Reconstruction and Risk of Knee Osteoarthritis: The Association between Cruciate Ligament Injury and Post-Traumatic Osteoarthritis. A Population Based Nationwide Study in Sweden, 1987–2009

Richard Nordenvall[1,2]*, Shahram Bahmanyar[3,4,5], Johanna Adami[3], Ville M. Mattila[1,2,6], Li Felländer-Tsai[1,2]

1 Division of Orthopedics and Biotechnology, Department of Clinical Science, Intervention and Technology, Karolinska Institutet, Stockholm, Sweden, **2** Department of Orthopedics, Karolinska University Hospital, Stockholm, Sweden, **3** Clinical Epidemiology Unit, Department of Medicine, Karolinska Institutet, Stockholm, Sweden, **4** Center for Pharmacoepidemiology, Department of Medicine, Karolinska Institutet, Stockholm, Sweden, **5** Faculty of Medicine, Golestan University of Medical Sciences, Gorgan, Iran, **6** Department of Orthopedics and Trauma Surgery, University Hospital of Tampere, Tampere, Finland

Abstract

Objective: To study the association between Cruciate Ligament (CL) injury and development of post-traumatic osteoarthritis in the knee in patients treated operatively with CL reconstruction compared with patients treated non-operatively.

Design: Population based cohort study; level of evidence II-2.

Setting: Sweden, 1987–2009.

Participants: All patients aged between 15–60 years being diagnosed and registered with a CL injury in The National Swedish Patient Register between 1987 and 2009.

Main Outcome Measures: Knee osteoarthritis.

Results: A total of 64,614 patients diagnosed with CL injury during 1987 to 2009 in Sweden were included in the study. Seven percent of the patients were diagnosed with knee OA in specialized healthcare during the follow-up (mean 9 years). Stratified analysis by follow-up showed that while those with shorter follow-up had a non-significant difference in risk (0.99, 95%CI 0.90–1.09 for follow-up less than five years compared with the non-operated cohort), those with longer follow-up had an increased risk of knee OA after CL reconstruction (HR = 1.42, 95%CI 1.27–1.58 for follow-up more than ten years compared with non-operated cohort). The risk to develop OA was not affected by sex.

Conclusion: CL reconstructive surgery does not seem to have a protective effect on long term OA in either men or women.

Editor: Gwendolen Reilly, University of Sheffield, United Kingdom

Funding: This study was fully funded by the Foundation of Martin Rind and by research funds from the Stockholm County Council and Karolinska Institutet, http://ki.se/, http://www.martinrind.nu/. The funders had no role in study design, data collection and analysis, decision to publish, or preparation of the manuscript.

Competing Interests: The authors have declared that no competing interests exist.

* Email: richard.nordenvall@ki.se

Introduction

Musculoskeletal injuries are common worldwide [1]. A predominant location is the knee joint, where the cruciate ligaments play a vital role in both stabilization and kinematics [2].

Injuries to the cruciate ligaments (CL) are common and generally affect the anterior cruciate ligament (ACL) [3]. These injuries occur primarily in activity with knee-pivoting movements such as soccer, basketball and alpine skiing. The mean age at time of diagnosis is 32 years [3]. The incidence of diagnosed CL injury in Sweden is 78 per 100,000 inhabitants and approximately 36% undergo reconstructive surgery [3]. Although men have an increased risk for CL injury in the general population (RR = 1.44) compared with women [3], the risk among women participating in certain sports is between 2–9 times higher than the risk among men participating in the same activities [3–9].

The most important complication after ACL injury is knee osteoarthritis (OA). In the general population OA in the knee has a reported prevalence of 5% in patients over 26 years and 12% in patients over 60 years [10–12]. Known risk factors for OA are age, obesity and knee trauma [13]. CL injury increases the risk for OA and the prevalence of knee OA after CL injury varies in different studies. Results from a meta-analysis and two systematic reviews show a prevalence of OA after CL injury ranging between 0–48% [14–16]. Apart from well-established risk-factors in the CL-sufficient knee the presence of associated injuries such as meniscus and cartilage injuries increase the risk for developing OA after CL-injury. A concomitant meniscal tear occurs in 25–65% of the cases [17].

Optimal treatment of a CL injury is under continuous debate and new inventions range from a multitude of surgical methods, fixation devices and rehabilitation protocols [18,19]. A number of different techniques and grafts have been suggested [20–22]. The purpose of CL reconstruction (CL-R) is to counteract knee instability and to restore kinematics, aiming to facilitate return to a desired activity level (often including pivoting sports) regardless of the risk to develop OA. Although treatment of CL injury varies in different countries reconstructive surgery of the CL is considered as the first line of treatment for specific groups of patients such as elite athletes, while conservative treatment with structured rehabilitation is considered to have a corresponding outcome in the general population [23,24]. Some studies have reported that CL-R decreases the risk of post traumatic OA. However the results are conflicting [14,25,26] and the studies have limitations such as small sample sizes or short follow-up time.

This nationwide cohort study with long follow-up time used data from the National Swedish Patient Register to estimate the risk of OA in the knee after CL injury for patients treated surgically compared to patients treated non-surgically.

Methods

Ethics statement

All registry information was anonymized and de-identified by the Swedish National board of Health and Welfare prior to analysis. This study was approved by the regional Ethics Committee at Karolinska Institutet (Dnr: 2010/1713-32).

Data from the Swedish National Patient Register

The study is a nationwide, open cohort study using data from the Swedish National Patient Register (NPR) [27]. This register was established in 1964 by the Swedish National board of Health and Welfare and has national coverage for all inpatient care since 1987. Information of outpatient care, including information on ambulatory care at hospitals, has been recorded since 2001. Each record in the NPR, corresponding to one hospital-episode, contains the date for hospital admission and discharge, age, sex, hospitals code, clinical ward, surgical procedures and up to eight discharge diagnoses coded according to the International Classification of Disease (ICD-7 until 1968, ICD-8 1969–1986, ICD-9 1987–1996 and ICD-10 thereafter). The national registration number, a unique identifier assigned to all Swedish citizens, allows linkage of data. Visits in primary healthcare, i.e. healthcare by general practitioners, are not included in the Swedish National Patient Register.

Identifying cruciate ligament reconstruction and knee osteoarthritis

We included all patients diagnosed with CL injury (ICD-9: 8442 – Cruciate ligament in knee, ICD-10: S835 – Distortion engaging the cruciate ligament in the knee, S837 – Injury to multiple structures of knee, M235 – Chronic instability in the knee-joint) for the first time between 1987 and 2009 (n = 84,358). We excluded patients younger than 15 years at the time of diagnosis (n = 3,224) since ACL injury among children with open epiphysis differ regarding treatment and outcome from adults. We also excluded patients over 60 years since CL injuries in older patients are relatively rare and we expect many of these cases to be misclassified (n = 1,470).

NPR was also used to identify those who underwent CL reconstructive surgery (the Swedish version of Classification of Surgical Procedures (NOMESCO): NGE41, NGE42, NGE49, NGE51, NGE52). Our main outcome variable was diagnosis of OA (patients with a diagnosis of knee OA (ICD-10 codes M170-M179 and corresponding ICD-9 codes) and those undergoing operations due to knee OA such as osteotomy, prosthesis etc. (surgical procedures code 8191, 8423–8428, NGB09-NGB99, NGC09-NGC99, NGG09-NGG99, NGK59, NGN49; NGU09, NGH2)).

A registered meniscus injury (ICD-10 codes M232, M233, S832, S837 and corresponding ICD-9 codes) or meniscus surgery (surgery code NGD) was classified as an acute meniscus injury if the patient was 35 years old or younger and was included as a confounding factor. By using this age limitation we aimed to exclude the majority of degenerative meniscal injuries which are not confounders but early signs of osteoarthritis and which commonly are miscoded as acute ruptures instead of degenerative meniscal injuries [28]. A meniscal injury was included as a confounding factor independent of the relationship between the date of meniscal injury/surgery and the date of the CL injury diagnosis.

Dates of emigration and death for the entire study period were obtained using the Swedish Total Population Register.

Statistical analysis

Cox proportional hazard model was used to estimate hazard ratios (HR) with 95% confidence intervals (CI) as a measurement for the association between CL-R and development of knee OA where CL-R was treated as time-varying covariate. Follow-up started from the date of registered CL injury until date of diagnosis of knee OA or operation due to knee OA, emigration, death or December 31st 2009, whichever came first. We excluded all patients with a follow-up shorter than two years since OA prevention trials need a follow up time of at least two years (n = 15,050). The models were internally stratified for calendar (year of entry into the cohort) category of age (<20, 20–25, 25–30, 30–35, 35–40, 40–45, 45–50 and >50 years) and sex. In Model 2 we also adjusted for meniscal injury (a registered diagnosis of meniscal injury or meniscal surgery). As the time from CL injury to CL-R might be important, stratified analysis were performed for this covariate (categorized to: <3 months, 3 months to one year, > 1 year). We estimated the follow-up specific relative risks (follow-up 2–4,9 years, 5–9,9 years, >10 years). As information of outpatient care has been recorded since 2001, we also estimated the relative risks for patients being diagnosed before and after 2001.

To check for interaction effects, we added interaction terms of CL-R and meniscal injury (a registered diagnosis of meniscal injury or meniscal surgery) into the full models.

All statistical analyses were performed using SAS (Statistical Analysis Software, version 9.2, SAS Institute Inc).

Results

A total of 64,614 patients diagnosed with CL injury during 1987 to 2009 were included in the analysis. Men represented 63% and the mean age at time of diagnosis was 29 years (range 15–60, SD = 10). In total, 48% went through reconstructive surgery, and 41% of the patients had a traumatic meniscus injury (Table 1). In the group treated surgically the mean age at the time of diagnosis was 26 years (range 15–60, SD = 8) compared with 32 years (range 15–60, SD = 11) in the group treated non-operatively. In total 7% (4,314) of the patients were diagnosed with knee OA. Of those 10% (444) underwent osteotomy or either partial or total knee replacement.

The mean follow-up time for the entire study population was 9 years (range 2–23, SD = 5) and 8 years (range 2–23, SD = 5) for those with an event of OA. The mean delay between CL diagnosis and CL-R was 266 days (range 0–8,346, SD = 598).

There was no statistically significant difference in the risk of OA among males and females (HR 1.03, 95%CI 0.96–1.09). Having a concomitant meniscal injury increased the risk of OA (HR 2.94, 95%CI 2.72–3.17). There was a statistically significant interaction between CL-R and meniscal injury with respect to OA risk (p = 0.01). Stratified analysis by meniscal injury showed no evident difference in risk for those treated surgically compared with those treated non-operatively (HR 1.22 95%CI 1.12–1.33 HR for those with meniscal injury and 1.21 95%CI 1.10–1.33 for those without meniscal injury) when adjusted for sex, age and year of entry in the cohort (Table 2). There was no significant difference in risk to develop OA in patients treated surgically compared with those treated non-surgically when comparing patients being diagnosed before and after 2001.

During the first years of follow-up, the cumulative incidence of OA was higher among those without CL-R and the trend changed after ten years follow-up (Figure 1). Approximately 24% of those with CL-R were diagnosed with OA at the end of follow-up and the corresponding rate was approximately 19% among those who did not undergo CL-R.

In the overall analysis an increased risk for OA in the knee was observed in patients with CL injury who were treated surgically compared with those treated non-surgically (HR = 1,22, 95%CI 1,14–1,30). Stratified analysis by follow-up showed that while those with shorter follow-up showed no significant difference in risk (HR 0.99, 95%CI 0.90–1.09 for follow-up less than five years) those with longer follow-up had an increased risk of knee OA after CL-R (HR = 1.42, 95%CI 1.27–1.58 for follow-up more than ten years). Stratified analysis by time of operation since diagnosis for each strata of follow-up time did not attenuate the relative risks notably (Table 3).

Discussion

To the best of our knowledge this is the first population based nationwide study describing the association between CL injury and the development of knee OA in a large cohort. We observed that surgically reconstructed ACL injured patients were more frequently diagnosed with knee OA in specialized healthcare during follow-up than non-reconstructed patients. This suggests that decreasing the long-term risk for post traumatic OA after CL

Table 1. Characteristics of the study population according to type of treatment and follow-up time.

	Number of subjects	Male (%)	Meniscal-injury (%)	Mean age at CL injury (SD)	Mean age at end of follow-up (SD)
Total	**64614**	**40398 (63%)**	**26797 (41%)**	**29.15 (10,32)**	**38.15 (11.09)**
No CL-R	33695	21036 (62%)	11027 (33%)	32.03 (11.18)	40.75 (11.80)
CL-R	30919	19362 (63%)	15770 (51%)	26.01 (8.22)	35.31 (9.47)
Follow up 2–4,9 years					
No CL-R	10260	6186 (60%)	3371 (33%)	33.04 (11.90)	36.55 (11.93)
CL-R	7644	4516 (59%)	4200 (55%)	26.14 (9.33)	29.63 (9.38)
- CL-R within 3 months	2868	1701 (59%)	1342 (47%)	26.15 (9.28)	29.60 (9.32)
- CL-R between 3 months and 1 year	3328	1962 (59%)	1929 (58%)	25.92 (9.26)	29.38 (9.32)
- CL-R after 1 year	1448	853 (59%)	929 (64%)	26.61 (9.60)	30.26 (9.62)
Follow up 5–9,9 years					
No CL-R	13465	8433 (63%)	4554 (34%)	32.82 (11.14)	40.07 (11.19)
CL-R	11335	7068 (62%)	6283 (55%)	26.51 (8.45)	33.96 (8.59)
- CL-R within 3 months	4905	3052 (62%)	2296 (47%)	26.50 (8.28)	34.26 (8.44)
- CL-R between 3 months and 1 year	3537	2199 (62%)	2065 (58%)	26.35 (8.55)	33.49 (8.66)
- CL-R after 1 year	2893	1817 (63%)	1922 (67%)	26.73 (8.59)	34.04 (8.72)
Follow up >10 years					
No CL-R	9970	6417 (64%)	3102 (31%)	29.93 (10.15)	45.99 (10.43)
CL-R	11940	7778 (65%)	5287 (44%)	25.44 (7.13)	40.23 (7.70)
- CL-R within 3 months	9243	6055 (65%)	3632 (39%)	25.53 (7.10)	40.47 (7.72)
- CL-R between 3 months and 1 year	1105	683 (62%)	658 (60%)	25.42 (7.18)	38.51 (7.38)
- CL-R after 1 year	1592	1040 (65%)	997 (63%)	24.96 (7.24)	40.01 (7.62)

Table 2. Hazard ratio (HR) and 95% confidence interval (CI) for the association between crucial ligament reconstruction and knee osteoarthritis, according to meniscal injury and follow-up.

	Number of events	Adjusted HR (95% CI)*
Overall		
No CL-R	2199	Reference
CL-R	2115	1.26 (1.18–1.34)
- No meniscal injury	780	1.21 (1.10–1.33)
- Meniscal injury	1335	1.22 (1.12–1.33)
- Meniscal injury without surgery	263	1.29 (1,07–1,57)
- Meniscal injury with surgery	1072	1,17 (1,061,29)
Follow up 2–4,9 years		
No CL-R	925	Reference
CL-R	630	1.05 (0.95–1.16)
- No meniscal injury	261	1.04 (0.89–1.22)
- Meniscal injury	369	1,01 (0.85–1.18)
- Meniscal injury without surgery	73	0.94 (0.70–1.26)
- Meniscal injury with surgery	296	0.97 (0.83–1.12)
Follow up 5–9,9 years		
No CL-R	638	Reference
CL-R	731	1.29 (1.16–1.44)
- No meniscal injury	263	1.12 (0.94–1.33)
- Meniscal injury	468	1.10 (0.94–1.29)
- Meniscal injury without surgery	82	1.55 (1.12–2.15)
- Meniscal injury with surgery	386	1.21 (1.04–1.41)
Follow up >10 years		
No CL-R	636	Reference
CL-R	754	1.43 (1.28–1.60)
- No meniscal injury	256	1.42 (1.20–1.70)
- Meniscal injury	498	1.41 (1.22–1.63)
- Meniscal injury without surgery	108	1.63 (1.18–2.23)
- Meniscal injury with surgery	390	1.42 (1.21–1.67)

*The models were internally stratified for sex, age-group and calender.

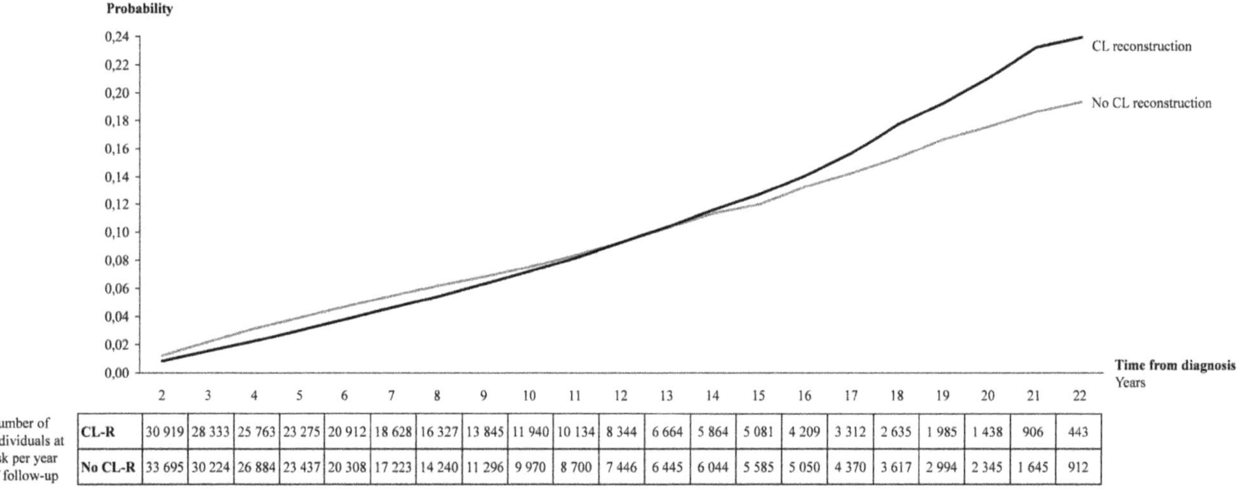

Number of individuals at risk per year of follow-up	2	3	4	5	6	7	8	9	10	11	12	13	14	15	16	17	18	19	20	21	22
CL-R	30 919	28 333	25 763	23 275	20 912	18 628	16 327	13 845	11 940	10 134	8 344	6 664	5 864	5 081	4 209	3 312	2 635	1 985	1 438	906	443
No CL-R	33 695	30 224	26 884	23 437	20 308	17 223	14 240	11 296	9 970	8 700	7 446	6 445	6 044	5 585	5 050	4 370	3 617	2 994	2 345	1 645	912

Figure 1. Cumulative incidence for osteoarthritis in the knee among 33,695 patients with CL diagnosis treated non-operatively and 30,919 patients with CL diagnosis treated surgically in Sweden 1987–2009.

Table 3. Hazard ratio (HR) and 95% confidence interval (CI) for the association between crucial ligament reconstruction and knee osteoarthritis, according to follow-up and time of surgery.

	Number of events	Crude HR (95% CI)	Adjusted HR (95% CI)	
			Model 1*	Model 2**
Overall				
No CL-R	2199	Reference	Reference	Reference
CL-R	2115	1.05 (0.99–1.12)	1.26 (1.18–1.34)	1.22 (1.14–1.30)
- CL-R within 3 months	1419	1.00 (0.94–1.07)	1.21 (1.12–1.29)	1.23 (1.15–1.32)
- CL-R between 3 months and 1 year	364	1.17 (1.04–1.31)	1.40 (1.24–1.57)	1.24 (1.11–1.40)
- CL-R after 1 year	332	1.15 (1.03–1.29)	1.36 (1.21–1.53)	1.13 (1.00–1.27)
Follow up 2–4,9 years				
No CL-R	925	Reference	Reference	Reference
CL-R	630	0.84 (0.77–0.93)	1.05 (0.95–1.16)	0.99 (0.90–1.09)
- CL-R within 3 months	322	0.68 (0.60–0.77)	0.86 (0.75–0.98)	0.88 (0.77–1.01)
- CL-R between 3 months and 1 year	192	1.00 (0.86–1.16)	1.25 (1.07–1.45)	1.15 (0.99–1.34)
- CL-R after 1 year	116	1.04 (0.89–1,20)	1.20 (1.04–1.39)	1.03 (0.89–1.19)
Follow up 5–9,9 years				
No CL-R	638	Reference	Reference	Reference
CL-R	731	1.11 (1.00–1.23)	1.29 (1.16–1.44)	1.26 (1.13–1.40)
- CL-R within 3 months	494	1.07 (0.95–1.19)	1.27 (1.13–1.44)	1.33 (1.18–1.50)
- CL-R between 3 months and 1 year	123	1.23 (1.00–1.50)	1.35 (1.10–1.66)	1.20 (0.98–1.48)
- CL-R after 1 year	114	1.23 (0.98–1.53)	1.33 (1.07–1.66)	1.08 (0.87–1.35)
Follow up >10 years				
No CL-R	636	Reference	Reference	Reference
CL-R	754	1.31 (1.18–1.46)	1.43 (1.28–1.60)	1.42 (1.27–1.58)
- CL-R within 3 months	603	1.30 (1.16–1.45)	1.41 (1.26–1.58)	1.44 (1.29–1.61)
- CL-R between 3 months and 1 year	49	1.52 (1.12–2.07)	1.72 (1.26–2.35)	1.40 (1.02–1.91)
- CL-R after 1 year	102	1.32 (0.99–1.76)	1.49 (1.11–2.00)	1.21 (0.90–1.62)

*The models were internally stratified for sex, age-group and calender.
**Additionally adjusted for meniscal injury.

injury is not an argument for CL reconstruction. The results also demonstrated that the risk to develop OA did not differ between males and females. Concomitant meniscal injury was associated with increased risk for OA irrespective of timing of surgery.

The strengths of this study include the large nationwide patient database with excellent coverage [29], equal access to health care in Sweden and relatively long follow-up allowing for analysis of the development of OA in both patients treated conservatively and surgically. Moreover, since we had the opportunity to control for major confounding factors included in the registry and this is a cohort with prospectively collected outcome data the possibility of bias is limited. However, possible selection bias cannot be completely ruled out since more extensive knee trauma increases the risk for osteoarthritis and might as well be associated with a higher risk to be selected for surgery. The risk for reverse causality is small since the main symptom for osteoarthritis is pain and according to Swedish protocols pain has never been an indication for CL reconstruction. The result of stratified analysis showed that the risk for osteoarthritis increased with increasing time after surgery which also strengthens this argumentation.

The main limitation of this study is potential misclassification of CL-injury, OA and acute meniscus injury since the registry does not include information about criteria or diagnostic methods. CL injury is diagnosed by physical examination, magnetic resonance imaging (MRI), or arthroscopy. Since 2000 there has been a dramatic increase in MRI accessibility and in 2009, around, 50,000 MRI examinations of the knee were undertaken in Sweden, giving an incidence of about 5,5 per 1000 inhabitants [30]. OA, on the other hand, has traditionally been diagnosed mainly by clinical examination and X-ray. In this study knee OA was classified as patients being diagnosed with OA in specialized healthcare. This population is most likely patients with more severe OA then patients being diagnosed with OA in primary healthcare and not included in the study. Detection bias could be a limitation if reconstructed patients have a greater propensity to contact or be referred to specialist healthcare. However this is unlikely since patients treated non-surgically have the same risk to be diagnosed with OA in specialized during the first years of follow-up. Based on the register data, it is not possible to define if the knee diagnosed with OA is the same knee that had previous CL injury, although it has been shown that this is usually the case. For example van der Hart et al. showed that there is an almost 50% higher prevalence of OA in the injured knee [31]. Another limitation is that patients diagnosed or treated in outpatient setting before 2001 are not included in the study. This explains why the descriptive results presented in this study are not coherent with the results presented earlier [3]. This could potentially cause some bias as the inpatient cases might be severe cases. However, restricting the results to those diagnosed after 2001 did not change the results notably. Another limitation is that patients with CL injuries, who never seek medical care for their injury, are not included in this study. However since CL injuries lead to a rapid hemarthrosis of the knee precluding continuation of activity [32], most patients are likely to visit a health-care provider where a correct diagnosis can be established. It is a limitation that bilateral injuries and the type of CL injury cannot be identified, making it impossible to differ between ACL injury and PCL injury. Data from the Swedish Cruciate Ligament Register show that 2% of the patients underwent bilateral reconstruction [33]. Isolated posterior cruciate ligament injuries are uncommon and account for an estimated 3% of all acute knee injuries [34]. Thus, the vast majority of our patients represent patients with ACL injuries and the results can be extrapolated to all ACL injuries. Like most chronic diseases, OA is complex and multifactorial. It cannot be excluded that there might be differences between the patients treated with CL-R and those treated non-operatively that we did not have information on, e.g. level of physical activity.

The increasing number of older people and the changes in lifestyle throughout the world mean that the burden of musculoskeletal injuries and diseases will increase dramatically [1]. Our study reports a prevalence of OA of 10% in patients between 15–60 years 10 years after they were diagnosed with a CL injury. This is less than reported in earlier studies which is most likely explained by the fact that the definition of OA in this study was based on hospital data and concomitant registered diagnosis of OA in specialist care. Patients only diagnosed with OA in primary were not identified in this study.

In this study 41% of the patients had a diagnosed meniscal injury which is to be compared with 25–65% described in earlier studies [17]. Meniscal injury cannot however be assessed as a dichotomy, it is a continuous variable ranging from traumatic lesions to degenerative injuries. Further, meniscal injuries are not always symptomatic [35]. Since we were interested in the acute traumatic injuries, we attempted to exclude degenerative meniscal injuries as well as meniscal injuries in patients older than 35 years. Our results showed that concomitant meniscal injury was the strongest risk factor to develop OA which is coherent with earlier results [14]. Results from cohort studies have shown an association been early CL reconstruction and fewer meniscal surgeries. Reducing the risk of meniscus tear would mean that CL-R might protect a CL injured knee from post-traumatic OA. Although some cohort studies support this hypothesis there are conflicting results reporting no difference or even an increased risk for OA [14,25,36]. A randomized clinical trial by Frobell et al did not show a difference in risk for radiographic OA up to 5 years in patients treated surgically compared to those treated non-surgically [27,37]. Our results suggest that there is an increased long term risk for OA after CL-R. Taking into account the more recent published results together with ours we conclude that decreasing the long-term risk for post-traumatic OA after CL injury is not an argument for CL-reconstruction.

Conclusions

CL reconstructive surgery did not show a protective effect on knee OA in the long term.

Author Contributions

Conceived and designed the experiments: RN LT SB JA VM. Performed the experiments: RN SB. Analyzed the data: RN LT SB. Contributed reagents/materials/analysis tools: RN LT SB JA VM. Wrote the paper: RN LT SB JA VM.

References

1. Woolf AD, Pfleger B (2003) Burden of major musculoskeletal conditions. Bulletin of the World Health Organization 81: 646–656.
2. Andriacchi TP, Mundermann A (2006) The role of ambulatory mechanics in the initiation and progression of knee osteoarthritis. Current opinion in rheumatology 18: 514–518.
3. Nordenvall R, Bahmanyar S, Adami J, Stenros C, Wredmark T, et al. (2012) A population-based nationwide study of cruciate ligament injury in Sweden, 2001–2009: incidence, treatment, and sex differences. The American journal of sports medicine 40: 1808–1813.
4. Arendt E, Dick R (1995) Knee injury patterns among men and women in collegiate basketball and soccer. NCAA data and review of literature. The American journal of sports medicine 23: 694–701.
5. Gwinn DE, Wilckens JH, McDevitt ER, Ross G, Kao TC (2000) The relative incidence of anterior cruciate ligament injury in men and women at the United States Naval Academy. The American journal of sports medicine 28: 98–102.
6. Lindenfeld TN, Schmitt DJ, Hendy MP, Mangine RE, Noyes FR (1994) Incidence of injury in indoor soccer. The American journal of sports medicine 22: 364–371.
7. Messina DF, Farney WC, DeLee JC (1999) The incidence of injury in Texas high school basketball. A prospective study among male and female athletes. The American journal of sports medicine 27: 294–299.
8. Myklebust G, Maehlum S, Holm I, Bahr R (1998) A prospective cohort study of anterior cruciate ligament injuries in elite Norwegian team handball. Scandinavian journal of medicine & science in sports 8: 149–153.
9. Stevenson H, Webster J, Johnson R, Beynnon B (1998) Gender differences in knee injury epidemiology among competitive alpine ski racers. The Iowa orthopaedic journal 18: 64–66.
10. Lawrence RC, Felson DT, Helmick CG, Arnold LM, Choi H, et al. (2008) Estimates of the prevalence of arthritis and other rheumatic conditions in the United States. Part II. Arthritis and rheumatism 58: 26–35.
11. Felson DT, Naimark A, Anderson J, Kazis L, Castelli W, et al. (1987) The prevalence of knee osteoarthritis in the elderly. The Framingham Osteoarthritis Study. Arthritis and rheumatism 30: 914–918.
12. Dillon CF, Rasch EK, Gu Q, Hirsch R (2006) Prevalence of knee osteoarthritis in the United States: arthritis data from the Third National Health and Nutrition Examination Survey 1991–94. The Journal of rheumatology 33: 2271–2279.
13. Niu J, Zhang YQ, Torner J, Nevitt M, Lewis CE, et al. (2009) Is obesity a risk factor for progressive radiographic knee osteoarthritis? Arthritis and rheumatism 61: 329–335.
14. Claes S, Hermie L, Verdonk R, Bellemans J, Verdonk P (2012) Is osteoarthritis an inevitable consequence of anterior cruciate ligament reconstruction? A meta-analysis. Knee surgery, sports traumatology, arthroscopy: official journal of the ESSKA.
15. Oiestad BE, Engebretsen L, Storheim K, Risberg MA (2009) Knee osteoarthritis after anterior cruciate ligament injury: a systematic review. The American journal of sports medicine 37: 1434–1443.
16. Chalmers PN, Mall NA, Moric M, Sherman SL, Paletta GP, et al. (2014) Does ACL reconstruction alter natural history?: A systematic literature review of long-term outcomes. The Journal of bone and joint surgery American volume 96: 292–300.
17. Louboutin H, Debarge R, Richou J, Selmi TA, Donell ST, et al. (2009) Osteoarthritis in patients with anterior cruciate ligament rupture: a review of risk factors. The Knee 16: 239–244.
18. Maffulli N, Longo UG, Denaro V (2009) Anterior cruciate ligament tear. The New England journal of medicine 360: 1463; author reply 1463.
19. Spindler KP, Wright RW (2008) Clinical practice. Anterior cruciate ligament tear. The New England journal of medicine 359: 2135–2142.
20. Bach BR Jr, Tradonsky S, Bojchuk J, Levy ME, Bush-Joseph CA, et al. (1998) Arthroscopically assisted anterior cruciate ligament reconstruction using patellar tendon autograft. Five- to nine-year follow-up evaluation. The American journal of sports medicine 26: 20–29.
21. Reinhardt KR, Hetsroni I, Marx RG (2010) Graft selection for anterior cruciate ligament reconstruction: a level I systematic review comparing failure rates and functional outcomes. The Orthopedic clinics of North America 41: 249–262.
22. van Eck CF, Schreiber VM, Mejia HA, Samuelsson K, van Dijk CN, et al. (2010) "Anatomic" anterior cruciate ligament reconstruction: a systematic review of surgical techniques and reporting of surgical data. Arthroscopy: the journal of arthroscopic & related surgery: official publication of the Arthroscopy Association of North America and the International Arthroscopy Association 26: S2–12.
23. Casteleyn PP, Handelberg F (1996) Non-operative management of anterior cruciate ligament injuries in the general population. The Journal of bone and joint surgery British volume 78: 446–451.
24. Swirtun LR, Eriksson K, Renstrom P (2006) Who chooses anterior cruciate ligament reconstruction and why? A 2-year prospective study. Scandinavian journal of medicine & science in sports 16: 441–446.
25. Friel NA, Chu CR (2013) The Role of ACL Injury in the Development of Posttraumatic Knee Osteoarthritis. Clinics in sports medicine 32: 1–12.

26. Neuman P, Englund M, Kostogiannis I, Friden T, Roos H, et al. (2008) Prevalence of tibiofemoral osteoarthritis 15 years after nonoperative treatment of anterior cruciate ligament injury: a prospective cohort study. The American journal of sports medicine 36: 1717–1725.
27. The National Patient Register.
28. Jones JC, Burks R, Owens BD, Sturdivant RX, Svoboda SJ, et al. (2012) Incidence and risk factors associated with meniscal injuries among active-duty US military service members. Journal of athletic training 47: 67–73.
29. Ludvigsson JF, Andersson E, Ekbom A, Feychting M, Kim JL, et al. (2011) External review and validation of the Swedish national inpatient register. BMC public health 11: 450.
30. Dahlberg LKP, Nilsson K-G, Redlund-Johnell I, Thorstensson C, Wallensten R, et al. (2009) Indikation för magnetkameraundersökning vid knäbesvär.
31. van der Hart CP, van den Bekerom MP, Patt TW (2008) The occurrence of osteoarthritis at a minimum of ten years after reconstruction of the anterior cruciate ligament. Journal of orthopaedic surgery and research 3: 24.
32. Noyes FR, Butler DL, Grood ES, Zernicke RF, Hefzy MS (1984) Biomechanical analysis of human ligament grafts used in knee-ligament repairs and reconstructions. The Journal of bone and joint surgery American volume 66: 344–352.
33. (2010) Annual report 2010. The Swedish National ACL Register.
34. Kim YM, Lee CA, Matava MJ (2011) Clinical results of arthroscopic single-bundle transtibial posterior cruciate ligament reconstruction: a systematic review. The American journal of sports medicine 39: 425–434.
35. Englund M, Guermazi A, Gale D, Hunter DJ, Aliabadi P, et al. (2008) Incidental meniscal findings on knee MRI in middle-aged and elderly persons. The New England journal of medicine 359: 1108–1115.
36. Meuffels DE, Favejee MM, Vissers MM, Heijboer MP, Reijman M, et al. (2009) Ten year follow-up study comparing conservative versus operative treatment of anterior cruciate ligament ruptures. A matched-pair analysis of high level athletes. British journal of sports medicine 43: 347–351.
37. Frobell RB, Roos HP, Roos EM, Roemer FW, Ranstam J, et al. (2013) Treatment for acute anterior cruciate ligament tear: five year outcome of randomised trial. BMJ 346: f232.

20

Factors that Influence Functional Outcome after Total or Subtotal Scapulectomy: Japanese Musculoskeletal Oncology Group (JMOG) Study

Katsuhiro Hayashi[1,6*], Shintaro Iwata[2], Akira Ogose[3], Akira Kawai[4], Takafumi Ueda[5], Takanobu Otsuka[6], Hiroyuki Tsuchiya[1]

1 Department of Orthopaedic Surgery, Graduate School of Medical Science, Kanazawa University, Kanazawa, Japan, **2** Division of Orthopedic Surgery, Chiba Cancer Center, Chiba, Japan, **3** Division of Orthopedic Surgery, Niigata University Graduate School of Medical and Dental Sciences, Niigata, Japan, **4** Department of Orthopaedic Surgery, National Cancer Center Hospital, Kashiwa, Japan, **5** Department of Orthopaedic Surgery, Osaka National Hospital, Osaka, Japan, **6** Department of Orthopaedic Surgery, Nagoya City University Medical School, Nagoya, Japan

Abstract

Background: Scapulectomy requires not only joint resection but also wide resection of the shoulder girdle muscles. Even the significance of reconstruction has not yet been determined because of the difficulties in comparing the different conditions. The purpose of this study was to investigate factors that influence functional outcomes after scapulectomy in a multicenter study.

Methods: This retrospective study comprised 48 patients who underwent total or subtotal scapulectomy and were followed for at least one year after surgery. Patients were registered at the Japanese Musculoskeletal Oncology Group affiliated hospitals. Soft tissue reconstruction for joint stabilization was performed when there was enough remaining tissue for reconstruction of the rotator cuff and tendons. In 23 cases, humeral suspension was performed. The average follow-up period was 61.9 months. Multivariate analysis was performed using the patient's background to determine which factors influence the Enneking functional score or active range of motion.

Results: The average functional score was 21.1 out of 30. Active shoulder range of motion was 42.7 degree in flexion, 39.7 degree in abduction, 49.6 degree of internal rotation and 16.8 degree of external rotation. The amount of remaining bone influenced functional outcome, which means that preserving the glenoid or the acromion lead to better function compared to total scapulectomy ($p<0.01$). Factors that influenced each functional measure include the amount of remaining bone, soft tissue reconstruction, the length of the resected humerus and nerve resection ($p<0.05$).

Conclusion: Although shoulder function was almost eliminated following total or subtotal scapulectomy, minimal resection of bone, and soft tissue reconstruction should lead to better function.

Editor: Robert K. Hills, Cardiff University, United Kingdom

Funding: The authors have no support or funding to report.

Competing Interests: The authors have declared that no competing interests exist.

* Email: hayashikatsu830@aol.com

Introduction

The shoulder girdle is one of the common sites for malignant tumors of bone and soft tissues [1]. When the tumor locates in the scapula, total or partial scapulectomy should be performed. Because of the complexity of the surrounding anatomy and neurovascular structures, scapulectomy with limb salvage is a great challenge for surgeons even today. Moreover, the choice of reconstruction method after bone resection to maintain optimal function is still controversial. There are many procedures, such as humeral suspension, prosthetic replacement, recycled bone grafts, or soft tissue reconstruction. Even though the procedure of scapulectomy has been used for more than 100 years, the optimal reconstruction technique has not yet been determined [2,3]. Humeral suspension is commonly performed, but it is not certain whether it contributes to functional outcomes compared with no reconstruction. We have published seven cases of total scapulectomy in which there was no significant difference in function between the soft tissue reconstruction group and the non-reconstructed group [4].

Prosthetic replacement has been reported, however, the limited availability of the prosthesis has reduced its widespread use [5,6,7]. Few studies of scapulectomy have been published, but these have contained only a small number of cases. Griffin AM et al. reported 24 cases of chondrosarcoma in the scapula and concluded that partial scapulectomy leads to better function than total scapulectomy. Mayil Vahanan *et al.* concluded that retention of the glenohumeral articulation was associated with superior functional results in their series [8]. Sparing bone during tumor resection seems to lead better function, but we do not have clear evidence to explain how much or which part of the scapular resection should influence the functional outcomes. Malawer reported classification of shoulder girdle resections including scapulectomy, but it mainly focuses on joint resection [9,10]. There should be another classification including scapulectomy that relates to clinical outcomes. Another problem is that most of the reports of reconstruction after scapulectomy are from a single institution and each hospital has its own favorite surgical procedure and reconstruction. Thus it is difficult to compare reconstruction methods from these reports.

In the present study, we investigated functional outcomes after total or subtotal scapulectomy in a multicenter study and performed multivariate analysis to identify the factors that influence postoperative limb function.

Patients and Methods

This retrospective study comprised 48 patients (table 1, table S1 in tables S1) who underwent total or subtotal scapulectomy (more than half of the scapula was resected), and who were followed at least one year after surgery. Patients were registered at the Japanese Musculoskeletal Oncology Group (JMOG) affiliated hospitals. This study protocol was approved by the Institutional Review Board of the Kanazawa University Hospital, Kanazawa, Japan. This study complied with ethical standards outlined in the Declaration of Helsinki. Questionnaires were sent and answers obtained from 25 hospitals voluntarily after institutional review-board approval. Written informed consent was obtained from the adult participants and parents on behalf of children enrolled in your study. Surgeries were performed between 1985 and 2010.

The average age of the patients was 46 years (11 to 78 years). Thirty-two were male and sixteen were female. Thirty-one cases were affected on the dominant hand side, 14 on the non-dominant hand side and three were unknown. Eleven patients had chondrosarcomas, eleven had osteosarcomas, seven had metastatic bone tumors, six had Ewing's sarcomas, four had malignant fibrous histiocytomas, two had malignant peripheral nerve sheath tumors, two had synovial sarcomas, one had a fibrosarcoma, one had a rhabdomiosarcoma, one had a dermatofibrosarcoma protuberance, one had a desmoid tumor, and one had an arteriovenous malformation. Using Enneking's surgical stages of 39 sarcomas, four cases were classified as IB, two as IIA, 29 as IIB, one as IIIA, and three as IIIB. Chemotherapy was performed in 22 cases and irradiation was done in 6 cases. The tumor originated in the scapula in 40 cases, in the soft tissue in seven cases and in the proximal humerus in one case.

A total scapulectomy was performed in twenty-six patients because their tumors had either originated in the scapula or originated in the soft tissue around the scapula and invaded into the scapula. Part of the scapula was preserved in twenty-two patients. Seven of these spared the acromion, three spared the glenoid, ten spared both of the acromion and the glenoid, and two resected only the lower half of the scapula. A wide margin was obtained in 42 cases, marginal excision in four cases, and intralesional excision in two cases. An average of 2.6 cm (0 to 12 cm) of the proximal humerus was resected. On average, five (0 to 9) muscles were resected, and the infraspinatus and subscapularis were resected in more than 90% of the cases. Axillary nerve was sacrificed in 12 cases.

Soft tissue reconstruction for joint stabilization was performed when there was enough remaining tissue for reconstruction of the rotator cuff and tendons. In twenty-three cases, soft tissue reconstruction was performed by humeral suspension. One case was reconstructed using a custom-made megaprosthesis, and one was reconstructed by recycled autologous bone grafting. In the remaining twenty-three cases, no soft tissue reconstruction was performed; instead, only the remaining muscles were sutured. The mean operative time was 263 min (70–675) and blood loss was 764 g (10–5700). Complications included two infections and two cases of skin necrosis. Reoperation was performed in eight cases for four recurrences, two skin defects, one protrusion of the clavicle and one infection.

The average follow-up period was 61.9 months (14 to 192 months). The mean upper displacement of the humerus at the final follow-up was −0.2 cm (−4 to 2 cm).

Other parameters are listed in table 1, table S1 in tables S1. Clinical outcome was assessed for all forty-eight cases including the twenty-six total scapulectomy cases. Functional outcome was assessed by the Enneking score, including pain, function, emotional acceptance, hand positioning, manual dexterity and lifting ability, with each having a maximum of five points representing normal or full function (maximum overall score, 30 points). [11]. Univariate analysis was performed for seventeen factors describing the patient's background to determine which influence Enneking's functional score or active range of motion. All the factors that could influence functional outcomes were analyzed, for example, age could contribute physical therapy leading better function.

The univariate analysis was performed using Analysis of Variance (ANOVA) models. A backward elimination method was applied and all variables significant at the $p<0.05$ level in the univariate analysis were entered in the first step of the multivariate model selection procedure. The final models are presented at a 0.05 significance level. SAS version 9.1.2 software was used for statistical analysis.

Results

The average flexion range was 42.7° (0–180°), 39.7° in abduction (0–180°), 49.6° of internal rotation (0–60°) and 16.8° of external rotation (−30–90°). Shoulder range of motion was severely limited in most cases. As for the Enneking functional score, function and hand position, which reflect shoulder ability, had low scores, but pain and dexterity, which reflect usefulness of hand joints, had satisfactory scores. The mean total score was 21.1 out of 30 (12–30), which overall is a satisfactory score following resection of the shoulder girdle.

Multivariate analysis was performed on seventeen factors of the patient's background to determine which influence Enneking's functional score or active range of motion for all cases and total scapulectomy cases, respectively. The amount of remaining bone influenced the Enneking functional score, which means that preserving the glenoid or the acromion leads to better function compared to total scapulectomy (Figure 1). However, soft tissue reconstruction did not improve the total Enneking functional outcome score (table 2, table S2 in tables S1). Factors that influenced the functional data included the amount of remaining bone, soft tissue reconstruction, length of resected humerus and nerve resection ($p<0.05$), listed in table 3, table S3 in tables S1. As for total scapulectomy cases, soft tissue reconstruction did not lead to better total functional score but did improve dexterity of the affected hand (Figure 2). This supports doing soft tissue reconstruction after scapulectomy, which previously had been uncertain to improve functional outcome. Functional outcome would be better overtime. Watanabe et al. reported functional score improved within 2 years after extremity tumor surgery and maintained after that [12]. Our cases are average 5 years follow-up and the functional score should be stabilized in most of the cases.

Table 1. Patient's characteristics and functional outcomes.

		All	Total scapulectomy
	N	48	26
Gender	Male	32 (66.7%)	15 (57.7%)
	Female	16 (33.3%)	11 (42.3%)
Age		46±18.7	44.6±19.4
Type of resection	Total scapulectomy	26 (54.2%)	26 (100.0%)
	Acromion preserved	7 (14.6%)	
	Glenoid preserved	3 (6.3%)	
	Both of acromion and glenoid preserved	10 (20.8%)	
	Resection of lower half	2 (4.2%)	
Length of resected humerus (cm)		2.25±3.15	3.58±3.66
Number of resected muscles		5±2.2	6±1.9
Resected nerve	Axillary	12 (25.0%)	10 (38.5%)
Reconstruction	No	25 (52.1%)	8 (30.8%)
	Humeral suspension	21 (43.8%)	16 (61.5%)
	Others	2 (4.2%)	2 (7.7%)
Material for humeral suspension	Artificial ligament	8 (16.7%)	5 (19.2%)
	Autologous ligament	5 (10.4%)	4 (15.4%)
	Unknown	8 (16.7%)	7 (26.9%)
Blood loss (g)		764.1±1113.4	1034.8±1515.1
Surgical duration (min)		262.5±124.1	277.3±97.4
Follow-up term (mons)		58.8±46.6	69.5±53.1
Upper displacement of humerus (cm)		−0.17±1.23	−0.63±1.46
Enneking functional score	Pain	4.6±0.7	4.4±0.8
	Function	2.8±1.1	2.3±1.1
	Emotional acceptance	3.7±1.2	3.4±1.2
	Hand positioning	2.9±1.4	2.4±1.4
	Dexterity	4.5±1	4.3±1.2
	Lifting ability	2.9±1.2	2.6±0.9
	Total	21.1±4.5	19±3.7
Range of motion	Flexion	42.7±47.2	19.6±25.9
	Abduction	39.7±44.3	17.6±19.6
	Internal rotation	49.6±34.6	46.5±35.5
	External rotation	16.8±30.4	1.8±20.4

This retrospective study comprised 48 patients who underwent total or subtotal scapulectomy (more than half of the scapula was resected) and followed for at least one year after surgery. Patients were registered at the Japanese Musculoskeletal Oncology Group affiliated hospitals. Using the Enneking functional score, function and hand position, which reflect shoulder ability, had low scores, but pain and dexterity, which reflect usefulness of the hand joints, had satisfactory scores. The mean total score was 21.1 out of 30 (12–30), which overall is a satisfactory score following resection of the shoulder girdle. Data are expressed as mean±SD.

Discussion

Since Syme et al. first described total scapulectomy in 1856 as a management for shoulder girdle sarcomas, not only resection techniques but also reconstruction consistently have improved owing to improvements in preoperative imaging evaluation, more effective neoadjuvant chemotherapy, and advances in surgical technique [2,3,13]. In the field of hip or knee joint reconstruction, allograft, recycled bone graft and prosthetic replacement after bone resection has been a well-established strategy. Although those reconstruction procedures already have been introduced in scapular surgery, the choice of reconstruction for the shoulder joint is not as sophisticated as for other sites.

The simple procedure after total or subtotal scapulectomy is resection followed by suturing of the remaining muscles. Next simple procedure comes humeral suspension which the residual humerus is suspended from the clavicle or a proximal rib with the use of biologic or artificial tendon [14].

Biologic reconstruction with massive allogeneic or autogenic bone graft would be an optimal procedure if the grafted bone is regenerated, soft tissue is reattached and bone absorption does not occur. Autologous recycled bone techniques such as irradiated, pasteurized or liquid nitrogen frozen graft is reported to provide remodeling of grafted bone [15]. When the tumor lesion is not osteolytic, recycled scapular grafting could be the option for reconstruction. Allograft is common in Western countries where the bone bank system is well organized. Several surgeons have

Table 2. Statistical analysis of all cases for Enneking functional score.

			Summary statistic		Univariate		Multivariate: initial model P<0.05 in univariate		Multivariate: final model P<0.05 in step-down method	
Factor	**Category**	**N**	**Average**	**SD**	**95% CI**	**P value**	**95% CI**	**P value**	**95% CI**	**P value**
Gender	Male	30	22.1	4.5	–	[0.031*]	–	[0.292]		
	Female	16	19.2	3.8	(−5.616, −0.276)	0.031*	(−3.674, 1.140)	0.292		
Chemotherapy	No	26	22.3	5.0	–	[0.036*]	–	[0.108]		
	Yes	20	19.6	3.1	(−5.330, −0.185)	0.036*	(−4.101, 0.425)	0.108		
Resection range	Total scapulectomy	25	19.0	3.7	–	[0.003**]	–	[0.118]	–	[0.006**]
	Acromion preserved	7	22.6	3.2	(0.245, 6.898)	0.036*	(0.074, 6.279)	0.045*	(0.503, 6.593)	0.024*
	Glenoid preserved	3	21.3	3.1	(−2.420, 7.087)	0.327	(−2.236, 6.409)	0.334	(−1.799, 6.881)	0.243
	Both of acromion and glenoid preserved	9	24.7	4.7	(2.643, 8.691)	<0.001***	(0.517, 6.970)	0.024*	(2.615, 8.137)	<0.001***
	Resection of lower half	2	26.0	5.7	(1.283, 12.717)	0.018*	(−4.650, 9.931)	0.467	(−5.511, 8.696)	0.652
Resected nerve	No	34	22.0	4.3	–	[0.017*]	–	[0.246]		
	Axillary	12	18.5	4.1	(−6.390, −0.669)	0.017*	(−4.061, 1.076)	0.246		
Follow-up term (mons)	<20	13	17.8	3.0	–	[0.002**]	–	[0.039*]	–	[0.005**]
	≥20<70	17	22.8	4.8	(2.038, 7.799)	0.001**	(0.357, 5.804)	0.028*	(1.182, 6.362)	0.005**
	≥70	15	21.5	3.3	(0.658, 6.583)	0.018*	(1.016, 6.463)	0.009**	(1.451, 6.807)	0.003**
	Unknown	1	30.0		(4.040, 20.268)	0.004**	(−2.096, 19.365)	0.111	(2.085, 22.174)	0.019*

Multivariate analysis was performed using seventeen factors of the patient's background to determine which influence Enneking's functional score or active range of motion for all cases and for total scapulectomy cases, separately. The amount of remaining bone influenced the Enneking functional score, which means that preserving the glenoid or the acromion lead to better function compared to total scapulectomy. However, there was no significant evidence that reconstruction improved total functional outcome.

Table 3. Summary of multivariate analysis.

Factor	Category	N	Summary statistic Average	SD	Multivariate: final model P<0.05 in step-down method 95% CI	P value
Total score of Enneking's function (all cases)	Total scapulectomy	25	19.0	3.7	–	[0.006**]
Resection range	Acromion preserved	7	22.6	3.2	(0.503, 6.593)	0.024*
	Glenoid preserved	3	21.3	3.1	(−1.799, 6.881)	0.243
	Both of acromion and glenoid preserved	9	24.7	4.7	(2.615, 8.137)	<0.001***
	Resection of lower half	2	26.0	5.7	(−5.511, 8.696)	0.652
Function score (all cases)	No	34	3.0	1.0	–	[0.018*]
Resected nerve	Axillary	12	2.1	1.2	(−1.490, −0.145)	0.018*
Flexion (all cases)	Total scapulectomy	25	19.6	25.9	–	[<0.001***]
Resection range	Acromion preserved	7	31.4	21.0	(−6.335, 45.634)	0.134
	Glenoid preserved	3	43.3	32.1	(−3.213, 71.266)	0.072
	Both of acromion and glenoid preserved	9	105.0	48.3	(39.562, 92.255)	<0.001***
	Resection of lower half	2	90.0	84.9	(20.023, 107.639)	0.005**
Dexterity score (total scapulectomy cases)	No	8	3.3	1.5	–	[0.016*]
Reconstruction	Humeral suspension: artificial ligament	5	5.0	0.0	(0.606, 2.894)	0.005**
	Humeral suspension: autologous ligament	4	4.5	0.6	(0.021, 2.479)	0.046*
	Humeral suspension: Unknown	6	5.0	0.0	(0.667, 2.833)	0.003**
	Others	2	4.0	1.4	(−0.836, 2.336)	0.336

Factors that influenced functional outcome include the amount of remaining bone, soft tissue reconstruction, length of the resected humerus and nerve resection. As for total scapulectomy cases, soft tissue reconstruction did not lead to better total functional score but did allow better dexterity of affected hand. This result encourages doing soft tissue reconstruction after scapulectomy, which had been uncertain to improve functional outcome.

reported the result of allograft reconstruction with a satisfactory outcome without severe complications. The functional score was assessed at about 80% [16,17]. We need to have long term follow-up to confirm there is no bone resorption, which is known as a late complication after massive bone graft in the upper extremities.

Prosthetic replacement is quite common in other major joints. In the shoulder girdle, it has limited availability, a demanding surgical technique, difficulty of reattaching soft tissue onto the prosthesis, and the risk of postoperative dislocation [5,6,18]. Tang X et al. reported on ten patients who ended up with good functional results (76.7%) following total scapulectomy and reconstruction with a constrained total scapular prosthesis [19]. Their findings suggest that reconstruction using a prosthesis after total scapulectomy is a promising approach to improving postoperative outcome.

However, as shown in present study, most of the hospitals do not have the capacity to do prosthetic replacement at least in Japan, since scapular prosthesis has been introduced. We suggest that humeral suspension should be the primary mode of reconstruction after scapulectomy in many hospitals in the future.

In our previous study, we reported seven cases of total scapulectomy. Even though the soft tissue reconstruction was performed, there were no differences between the humeral suspension group and the non-reconstruction group. Griffin AM et al. reported sixteen patients who underwent partial scapulectomy while eight underwent total scapulectomy. Functional outcome was better in the group undergoing partial scapulectomy with significantly higher score than the total scapulectomy group [20]. Kiss J et al. also found the best results were achieved after partial scapulectomy, and after humeral resection reconstructed with fibular transposition and with preservation of the rotator cuff [21]. Mayil Vahanan N et al. published a study on fifteen patients who underwent total scapulectomy compared to a group who had their glenoid retained. Retention of the glenohumeral articulation gave superior functional results [22].

Comparing humeral suspension and prosthesis, Pritsch T et al. showed that scapular endoprostheses, as compared with humeral suspension, had better functional results, 78.5% and 58.5% respectively, and superior cosmesis. They recommend performing prosthetic reconstructive procedure as long as the rhomboids, latissimus dorsi, deltoid, and trapezius are preserved [23].

Malawer reported classification of shoulder girdle resections including scapulectomy. Six categories included intra-articular proximal humeral resection, partial scapular resection, intra-articular total scapulectomy, extra-articular total scapulectomy and humeral head resection (classical Tikhoff–Linberg resection), extra-articular humeral and glenoid resection, and extra-articular humeral and total scapular resection. Most scapulectomy cases involve just intra-articular total scapulectomy or extra-articular total scapulectomy. More precise scapulectomy classifications would be useful as long as they are related to clinical outcome. Based on the results of the current study and past reports, we have classified scapulectomy into five categories in terms of resection area as follows; 1. Total scapulectomy (include extra-articular resection), 2 Glenoid preserved, 3 Acromion preserved, 4 Both acromion and glenoid preserved, 5 Resection of the lower half of the scapula (Fig. 1). Preserving the glenoid or acromion leads to better function compared to total scapulectomy. Preoperative planning with this classification will contribute to expected postoperative function.

Functional score

30
25
20
15
10
5
0

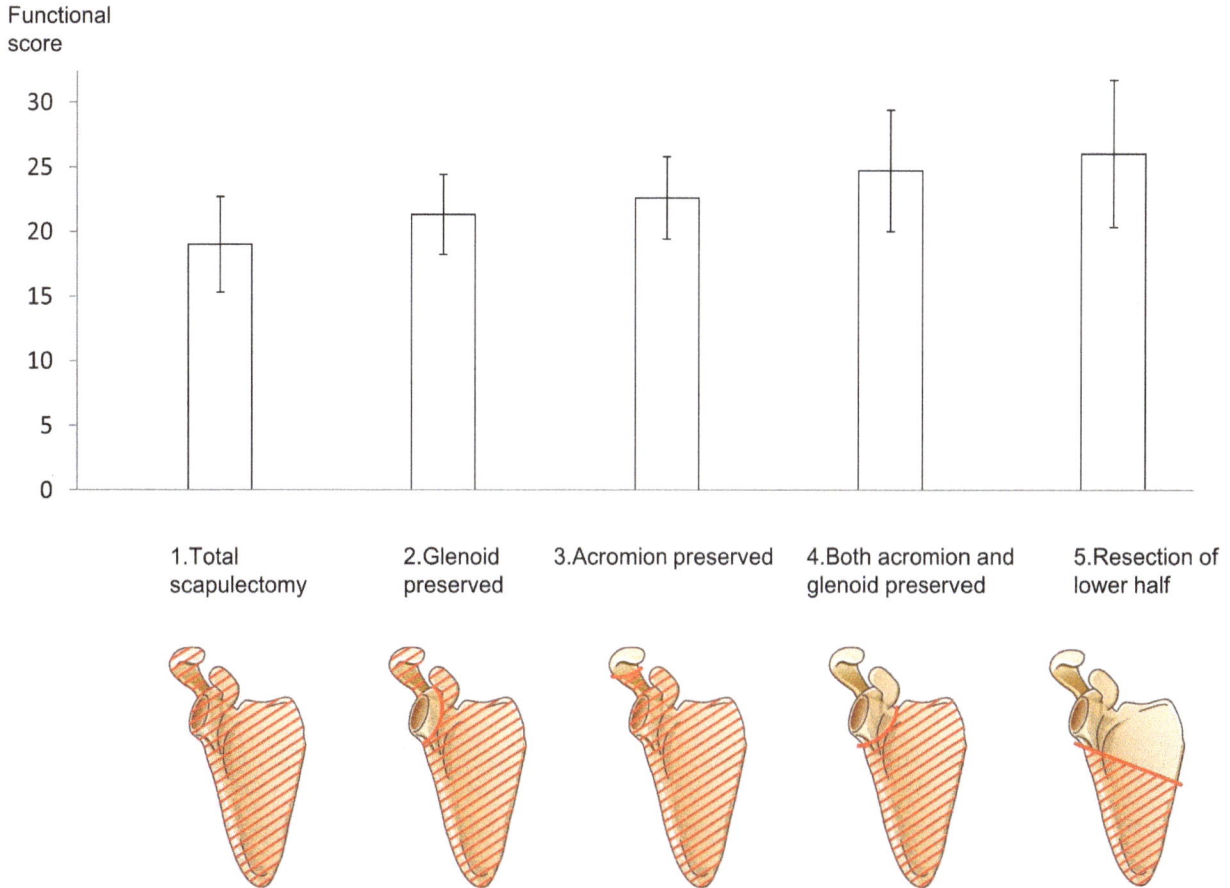

1.Total scapulectomy
2.Glenoid preserved
3.Acromion preserved
4.Both acromion and glenoid preserved
5.Resection of lower half

Figure 1. New classification of scapulectomy. Five categories are created in terms of resection area. Preserving glenoid or acromion lead to better function compared to total scapulectomy. Preoperative planning with this classification will contribute to expected postoperative function.

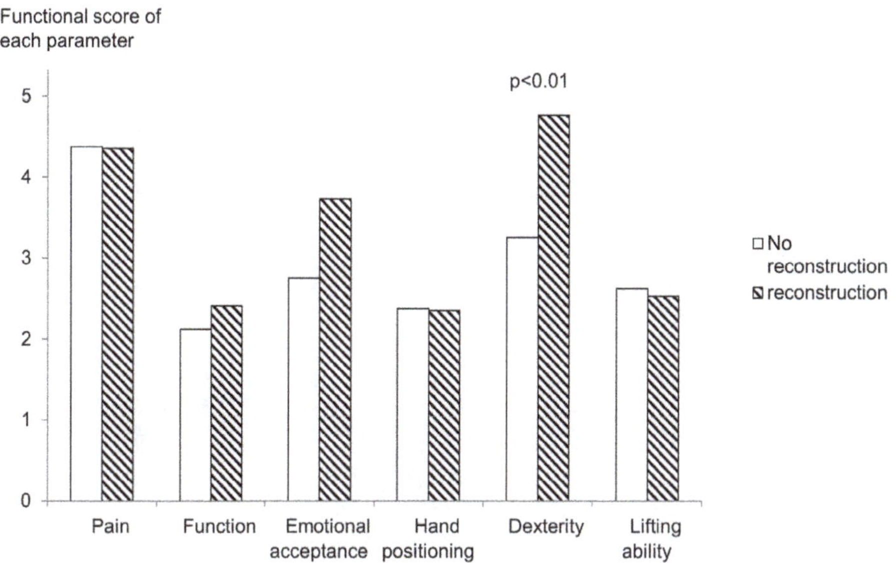

Figure 2. Comparison of soft tissue reconstruction or no reconstruction after total scapulectomy. As for total scapulectomy cases, soft tissue reconstruction does not improve total functional score but does improve dexterity of the affected hand. Previously there was no clear evidence that soft tissue reconstruction after scapulectomy improved functional outcome.

Acknowledgments

The authors wish to acknowledge the following investigators who cooperated with the case questionnaires. : I. Fujita, Hyogo Cancer Center; H Sugiura, Aichi Cancer Center; H. Kakizaki, Hirosaki National Hospital; J Nishida, Iwate Medical University; T Morii, Kyorin University; T Yakushiji, Kumamoto University; K Hiraoka, Kurume University; S Abe, Teikyo University; T Kidani, Ehime University; A Tan, Kinki University; T Nakamura, Mie University; T Akiyama, Jichi Medical University; S Takenaka, Osaka University; T Goto, Tokyo Metropolitan Komagome Hospital; M Emori, Sapporo Medical University.

Author Contributions

Conceived and designed the experiments: KH TU. Performed the experiments: KH SI AO AK TU. Analyzed the data: KH TU. Contributed reagents/materials/analysis tools: KH SI AO AK TU. Wrote the paper: KH TO HT.

References

1. Cleeman E, Auerbach JD, Springfield DS (2013) Tumors of the shoulder girdle: a review of 194 cases. J Shoulder Elbow Surg 14: 460–465.
2. Syme J. (1864) Excision of the Scapula. *Monograph*. Edmonston and Douglas: Edinburgh.
3. De Nancrede CBG. (1909) The original results after total excision of the scapula for sarcoma. Ann Surg 50: 1–22.
4. Hayashi K, Karita M, Yamamoto N, Shirai T, Nishida H, et al. (2011) Functional outcomes after total scapulectomy for malignant bone or soft tissue tumors in the shoulder girdle. Int J Clin Oncol 16: 568–573.
5. Masamed R, Learch TJ, Menendez LR (2008) En bloc shoulder resection with total shoulder prosthetic replacement: indications and imaging findings. AJR Am J Roentgenol 191: 482–489.
6. Mavrogenis AF, Mastorakos DP, Triantafyllopoulos G, Sakellariou VI, Galanis EC, et al. (2009) Total scapulectomy and constrained reverse total shoulder reconstruction for a Ewing's sarcoma. J Surg Oncol 100: 611–615.
7. Villalobos CE, Hayden BL, Silverman A, Choi I, Wittig JC (2009) Limb-sparing resection of the scapula and reconstruction with a constrained total scapula prosthesis: a case of multicentric epithelioid hemangioendothelioma involving the scapula and surrounding soft tissues. Ann Surg Oncol 16: 2321–2322.
8. Mayil Vahanan N, Mohanlal P, Bose JC, Gangadharan R, Karthisundar V. (2007) The functional and oncological results after scapulectomy for scapular tumours: 2-16-year results. Int Orthop 31: 831–6.
9. Malawer MM (1991) Tumors of the shoulder girdle. Technique of resection and description of a surgical classification. Orthop Clin North Am 22: 7–35.
10. Malawer MM, Meller I, Dunham WK (1991) A new surgical classification system for shoulder-girdle resections. Analysis of 38 patients. Clin Orthop Relat Res: 33–44.
11. Enneking WF, Dunham W, Gebhardt MC, Malawar M, Pritchard DJ (1993) A system for the functional evaluation of reconstructive procedures after surgical treatment of tumors of the musculoskeletal system. Clin Orthop Relat Res: 241–246.
12. Watanabe K, Tsuchiya H, Yamamoto N, Shirai T, Nishida H, et al. (2013) Over 10-year follow-up of functional outcome in patients with bone tumors reconstructed using distraction osteogenesis. J Orthop Sci 18: 101–109.
13. Coello AJ (1947) Scapulectomy and thoracoplasty. Br J Tuberc Dis Chest 41: 75–79.
14. Linberg BE (1999) Interscapulo-thoracic resection for malignant tumors of the shoulder joint region. 1928. Clin Orthop Relat Res: 3–7.
15. Tanzawa Y, Tsuchiya H, Shirai T, Hayashi K, Yo Z, et al. (2009) Histological examination of frozen autograft treated by liquid nitrogen removed after implantation. J Orthop Sci 14: 761–768.
16. Mnaymneh WA, Temple HT, Malinin TI (2002) Allograft reconstruction after resection of malignant tumors of the scapula. Clin Orthop Relat Res: 223–229.
17. Zhang K, Duan H, Xiang Z, Tu C (2009) Surgical technique and clinical results for scapular allograft reconstruction following resection of scapular tumors. J Exp Clin Cancer Res 28: 45.
18. Wittig JC, Bickels J, Wodajo F, Kellar-Graney KL, Malawer MM (2002) Constrained total scapula reconstruction after resection of a high-grade sarcoma. Clin Orthop Relat Res: 143–155.
19. Tang X, Guo W, Yang R, Ji T, Sun X (2011) Reconstruction with constrained prosthesis after total scapulectomy. J Shoulder Elbow Surg 20: 1163–1169.
20. Griffin AM, Shaheen M, Bell RS, Wunder JS, Ferguson PC (2008) Oncologic and functional outcome of scapular chondrosarcoma. Ann Surg Oncol 15: 2250–2256.
21. Kiss J, Sztrinkai G, Antal I, Kiss J, Szendroi M (n.d.) Functional results and quality of life after shoulder girdle resections in musculoskeletal tumors. J Shoulder Elbow Surg 16: 273–279.
22. Mayil Vahanan N, Mohanlal P, Bose JC, Gangadharan R, Karthisundar V (2007) The functional and oncological results after scapulectomy for scapular tumours: 2-16-year results. Int Orthop 31: 831–836.
23. Pritsch T, Bickels J, Wu CC, Squires MH, Malawer MM (2007) Is scapular endoprosthesis functionally superior to humeral suspension? Clin Orthop Relat Res 456: 188–195.

21

A Rare Fungal Species, *Quambalaria cyanescens*, Isolated from a Patient after Augmentation Mammoplasty – Environmental Contaminant or Pathogen?

Xin Fan[1]⁹, Meng Xiao[1]⁹, Fanrong Kong[2], Timothy Kudinha[2,3], He Wang[1], Ying-Chun Xu[1]*

1 Department of Clinical Laboratory, Peking Union Medical College Hospital, and Graduate School, Peking Union Medical College, Chinese Academy of Medical Sciences, Beijing, China, **2** Centre for Infectious Diseases and Microbiology Laboratory Services, Westmead Hospital, Westmead, New South Wales, Australia, **3** Charles Sturt University, Orange, New South Wales, Australia

Abstract

Some emerging but less common human fungal pathogens are known environmental species and could be of low virulence. Meanwhile, some species have natural antifungal drug resistance, which may pose significant clinical diagnosis and treatment challenges. Implant breast augmentation is one of the most frequently performed surgical procedures in China, and fungal infection of breast implants is considered rare. Here we report the isolation of a rare human fungal species, *Quambalaria cyanescens*, from a female patient in China. The patient had undergone bilateral augmentation mammoplasty 11 years ago and was admitted to Peking Union Medical College Hospital on 15 September 2011 with primary diagnosis of breast infection. She underwent surgery to remove the implant and fully recovered thereafter. During surgery, implants and surrounding tissues were removed and sent for histopathology and microbiology examination. Our careful review showed that there was no solid histopathologic evidence of infection apart from inflammation. However, a fungal strain, which was initially misidentified as "*Candida tropicalis*" because of the similar appearance on CHROMagar *Candida*, was recovered. The organism was later on re-identified as *Q. cyanescens*, based on sequencing of the rDNA internal transcribed spacer region rather than the D1/D2 domain of 26S rDNA. It exhibited high MICs to 5-flucytosine and all echinocandins, but appeared more susceptible to amphotericin B and azoles tested. The possible pathogenic role of *Q. cyanescens* in breast implants is discussed in this case, and the increased potential for misidentification of the isolate is a cause for concern as it may lead to inappropriate antifungal treatment.

Editor: Zhengguang Zhang, Nanjing Agricultural University, China

Funding: This work was supported by Special Research Foundation for Capital Medical Development: Epidemiology and in vitro Antifungal Susceptibility of Yeast Species Causing Invasive Fungal Infections in Beijing (grant no. 2011-4001-09; URLs: http://www.bjhbkj.com/; identify author: YCX). This work is also supported by Postgraduate Student Innovation Fund in Peking Union Medical College (grant no. S2012001012; URLS: http://graduate.pumc.edu.cn/peiyang/view/86.aspx; identify author: FX). The funders had no role in study design, data collection and analysis, decision to publish, or preparation of the manuscript.

Competing Interests: The authors have declared that no competing interests exist.

* Email: xycpumch@139.com

⁹ These authors contributed equally to this work.

Introduction

Human beings live in a fungal-rich and fungal-diverse environment. Some emerging less common fungal pathogens are known environmental species (from soil, plants, insects, medical facilities, wastes or other outdoor or indoor environments). These fungal organisms are generally of low virulence and some may exhibit natural antifungal drug resistance [1–3], which presents clinical diagnosis and treatment challenges [4–6]. While some of the fungal infections can be diagnosed easily, in particular if isolated from blood, cerebrospinal fluid, etc., and with clear infection clinical signs, others present challenges in understanding their role in certain infections. Here we report an interesting case to highlight the challenges clinical pathologists and medical doctors faced in the decision making process of a case involving a rare fungus.

The *Quambalariaceae* is a family of fungi in the class *Exobasidiomycetes*. The family contains the single genus *Quambalaria*, which contains five species, including *Quambalaria cyanescens*, *Q. coyrecup*, *Q. eucalypti*, *Q. pitereka* and *Q. simpsonii* [7–9]. The first *Q. cyanescens* strain was isolated from human skin (strain no. CBS 357.73, type strain of the species) and reported as *Sporothix cyanescens* by de Hoog *et al.* in 1973 (Table 1) [10]. In 1987, Moore *et al.* erected the genus *Cerinosterus*, reset the previous *S. cyanescens* into this new genus and renamed it as *Cerinosterus cyanescens* [8]. However, a later study by analysis of partial large subunit (LSU)-rDNA sequences and the nutritional profile revealed that *C. cyanescens* was a close relative of *Microstroma juglandis*, but differed from other species within

Table 1. Summary of *Q. cyanescens* isolates from this study, published literatures or GenBank, and genetic comparison within *Q. cyanescens* species and to selected strains of other *Quambalaria* species.

Strain	Country	Origin	ITS		D1/D2		Reference
			GenBank accession no.	Identity (%*)	GenBank accession no.	Identity (%*)	
***Q. cyanescens* Type strain**							
CBS 357.73	Netherlands	Human skin	DQ119135.1; DQ317622.1	Reference sequence	DQ317615.1; AM261925.1	Reference sequence	[8,10,12]
***Q. cyanescens* Human source isolate**							
11PU348	China	Implants	KF953496.1	576/580 (99.3)	KF953497.1	600/600 (100.0)	This study
***Q. cyanescens* Environmental isolates**							
IMI298177	Australia	Plant	AJ535500.1	580/580 (100.0)	NA	NA	Unpublished
IMI178848	Australia	Plant	AJ536610.1	573/575 (99.7)	NA	NA	Unpublished
MK742	Turkey	Beetle	AM261920.1	579/580 (99.8)	AM261920.1	576/576 (100.0)	[12]
MK808	Syria	Beetle	AM261921.2	580/580 (100.0)	NA	NA	[12]
MK1710	Bulgaria	Beetle	AM261922.2	580/580 (100.0)	NA	NA	[12]
CCF3527 = MK617	Hungary	Beetle	AM261923.2	557/559 (99.6)	AM261923.2	576/576 (100.0)	[12]
MK1617	Spain	Beetle	AM261924.2	555/556 (99.8)	NA	NA	[12]
SW326	Unknown	Unknown	NA	NA	AY234900.1	313/313 (100.0)	[38]
CF3526	Czech	Beetle	DQ119134.1	580/580 (100.0)	DQ119136.1	550/552 (99.6)	[12,39]
CBS 876.73	Australia	Plant	DQ317623.1	578/579 (99.8)	DQ317616.1	601/601 (100.0)	[8]
WAC12952	Australia	Beetle	DQ823419.1	579/579 (100.0)	DQ823440.1	561/561 (100.0)	[9]
WAC12954	Australia	Beetle	DQ823420.1	579/579 (100.0)	DQ823442.1	561/561 (100.0)	[9]
WAC129555	Australia	Beetle	DQ823421.1	573/579 (99.0)	DQ823441.1	561/561 (100.0)	[9]
WAC12953	Australia	Beetle	DQ823422.1	574/580 (99.0)	DQ823443.1	560/561 (99.8)	[9]
BRIP48396	Australia	Beetle	EF444874.1	579/580 (99.8)	NA	NA	[39]
BRIP48398	Australia	Beetle	EF444875.1	579/581 (99.7)	NA	NA	[39]
BRIP48403	Australia	Beetle	EF444876.1	579/579 (100.0)	NA	NA	[39]
U16	USA	Beetle	HF569147.1	559/559 (100.0)	NA	NA	Unpublished
U105	USA	Beetle	HF569150.1	556/556 (100.0)	HF569150.1	277/277 (100.0)	Unpublished
U110	USA	Beetle	HF569153.1	559/559 (100.0)	HF569153.1	277/277 (100.0)	Unpublished
U121	USA	Beetle	HF569155.1	577/577 (100.0)	NA	NA	Unpublished
U161	USA	Beetle	HG421947.1	553/556 (99.5)	HG421947.1	277/277 (100.0)	Unpublished
U163	USA	Beetle	HG421948.1	553/556 (99.5)	HG421948.1	277/277 (100.0)	Unpublished
U182	USA	Beetle	HG421949.1	556/559 (99.5)	HG421949.1	277/277 (100.0)	Unpublished
CCF4578	USA	Beetle	HG421950.1	556/556 (100.0)	HG421950.1	277/277 (100.0)	Unpublished
U144a	USA	Beetle	HG421951.1	556/556 (100.0)	HG421951.1	277/277 (100.0)	Unpublished
U100	USA	Beetle	HG421952.1	559/559 (100.0)	HG421952.1	277/277 (100.0)	Unpublished
CCF4580	USA	Beetle	HG421953.1	559/559 (100.0)	HG421953.1	277/277 (100.0)	Unpublished

Table 1. Cont.

Strain	Country	Origin	ITS		D1/D2		Reference
			GenBank accession no.	Identity (%*)	GenBank accession no.	Identity (%*)	
CCF4582	USA	Beetle	HG421954.1	577/577 (100.0)	NA	NA	Unpublished
CCF4583	USA	Beetle	HG421955.1	559/559 (100.0)	NA	NA	Unpublished
QY229	China	Rice	HM013823.1	570/574 (99.3)	NA	NA	[40]
AUMC6293	Egypt	Air	JQ425376.1	576/580 (99.3)	NA	NA	Unpublished
AUMC6294	Egypt	Citrus juice	JQ425382.1	576/580 (99.3)	NA	NA	Unpublished
Other *Quambalaria* species							
CBS124772 (*Q. simpsonii*)	Australia	Plant	GQ303290.1	575/601 (96.3)	GQ303321.1	601/601 (100.0)	[7]
CMW1101 (*Q. eucalypti*)	South Africa	Plant	DQ317625.1	568/601 (94.5)	DQ317618.1	600/601 (99.8)	[8]
CMW6707 (*Q. pitereka*)	Australia	Plant	DQ317627.1	569/598 (95.2)	DQ317620.1	598/601 (99.5)	[8]
WAC12947 (*Q. coyrecup*)	Australia	Plant	DQ823444.1	560/603 (92.9)	DQ823444.1	556/561 (99.1)	[9]

Abbreviations: ITS, ribosomal DNA internal transcribed spacer region; D1/D2, D1/D2 domain of the 26S ribosomal DNA; NA, not available.
*Refers to identity of the ITS region or D1/D2 domain sequences between type strain CBS 357.73 and other isolates.

the genus *Cerinosterus* [11]. To resolve this problem, Sigler *et al.* established the new genus *Fugomyces*, and designated *C. cyanescens* as *Fugomyces cyanescens* [11,12]. Recently, phylogenetic studies conducted by de Beer *et al.* have reassigned this species in the family *Quambalariaceae* as *Q. cyanescens*, based on the analysis of internal transcribed spacer (ITS) region and LSU sequences combined with ultrastructural characteristics [8].

Q. cyanescens is one of the rare clinical basidiomycetous pathogens. Most of *Q. cyanescens* isolated from the humans were reported in the 1990s, including pseudoepidemic nosocomial pneumonia cases reported in a US hospital [13], a possible pulmonary case in a heart transplant patient [14] and potential fungemia in lymphoma patients [11]. However, none of these published human-related cases deposited convincing molecular data.

In this case study, we report the mycology and molecular characteristics of a *Q. cyanescens* isolate from a 43 year-old female who previously received injected augmentation mammoplasty, and discuss the possible pathogenic role of the organism.

Methods

1. Ethics statement

The present case was from China Hospital Invasive Fungal Surveillance Net (CHIF-NET) study. Study protocol was approved by the Human Research Ethics Committee of Peking Union Medical College Hospital (No. S-263), and written consent was obtained from the patient.

2. Clinical case

A 43-year old woman was admitted to the Plastic Surgical Department of Peking Union Medical College Hospital on 15 September 2011 because of left breast pain, with symptoms of redness and swelling. She had previously undergone bilateral injected augmentation mammoplasty around 11 years ago in Fujian Province, China.

The woman was in good health status except for the inflammation of the breast and did not report any other major disease in her clinical history. The blood test results were all within normal values. Clinical examination showed that she was afebrile and no ulceration was present in her left breast. Primary diagnosis was made as left breast infection. Surgical operation was performed to take out the bilateral implants as per patient's request. However, no microbiological examination was done before surgery.

During surgery to remove the implants, it was noted that the yellow-brown semisolid implant had spilled and was mixed with unknown granule, and also there was damage in the mammary tissues. Partial implants and surrounding tissue were sent for histopathologic and microbiological laboratory examination. After surgery, cefmetazole (IV, 1 g bid) was given, combined with metronidazole (IV, 0.915 g, q12h) for 7 days. The patient fully-recovered and was subsequently discharged on 24 September 2011 before the microbiology laboratory results were finalized. She didn't receive any antimicrobial or antifungal treatment since then, nor were any relapses reported at the 12- and 24-month follow-up visits.

3. Initial laboratory examinations

Microbiology and histopathology examinations were immediately performed on the partial implants and surrounding tissue from the left breast (16 September 2011). No other specimens were sent for microbiological testing. On histopathology examination, breast implants were found to be surrounded by fibrous capsules and infiltrated with inflammation cells and phagocytosis by giant cells and capillary hypertrophy was also observed, which indicated foreign-body reaction. However, no solid evidence of bacterial or fungal infection was found.

In the meantime, bacterial culture was performed on the partial implants and tissue by inoculating them on Columbia agar supplemented with 5% sheep blood, China-blue lactose agar and chocolate agar. However, no fungal culture was performed initially as per surgeon's instructions. No bacteria were recovered. However, a notable amount (from the first to the second sector of the streaked plate) of yeast-like colonies were observed on Columbia blood agar on day 4 of incubation. Preliminary microscopic examination of the colonies showed yeast-like cells with a sympodial conidiogenesis. One pure colony of the isolate was then inoculated onto a chromogenic medium (CHROMagar *Candida*, CHROMagar Company, Paris, France) for identification, and was assigned as "*Candida tropicalis*" on day 8 based on the production of dark blue pigments. However, the patient had been discharged before the microbiology results were finalized.

4. Sequence-based identification

The above "*C. tropicalis*" strain was included in the CHIF-NET surveillance study (strain ID no. 11PU348). Genomic DNA was extracted by beating a fungal suspension with glass beads as described before [15]. Amplification of the fungal internal transcribed spacer (ITS) region and the D1/D2 domain of the 26S rRNA gene was performed as previously described with primer pairs ITS1/ITS4 and F63/R635, respectively [15–17]. The PCR products were sequenced in both directions using corresponding PCR amplification primer pairs at Ruibiotech Co. Ltd. (Beijing, China) using the DNA analyzer ABI 3730XL system (Applied Biosystems, Foster City, CA). Species identification was performed by comparing the obtained ITS and D1/D2 sequences against those in the Centraalbureau voor Schimmelcultures (CBS) Fungal Biodiversity Center database and GenBank using the BioloMICSNet and BLASTn software, respectively. A sequence similarity of 97% and 99% was applied as species identification 'cut-off' value for the ITS region and D1/D2 domain, respectively [18].

5. Phylogenetic analysis

All *Q. cyanescens* ITS and D1/D2 nucleotide sequences available in GenBank till 15 November 2013 (34 and 20 sequences for the ITS region and D1/D2 domain, respectively, Table 1) were compiled. Phylogenetic analysis was performed with software MEGA (Molecular Evolutionary Genetic Analysis software, version 6.0) using the Neighbor-Joining (NJ) method [19,20], with all positions containing gaps and missing data eliminated from the data set. The significance of the cluster nodes was determined by bootstrapping with 1,000 randomizations. The evolutionary distances were computed using the Maximum Composite Likelihood method [21] and were in the units of the number of base substitutions per site. In addition, the ITS and D1/D2 sequences of *Q. coyrecup* WAC12947 (GenBank accession no. DQ823444.1 and DQ823431.1) [9], *Q. eucalypti* CMW1101 (DQ317625.1 and DQ317618.1) [8], *Q. pitereka* CMW6707 (DQ317627.1 and DQ317620.1) [8], *Q. simpsonii* CBS124772 (GQ303290.1 and GQ303321.1) [7] and *M. juglandis* KR0015442 (EU069498.1 and EU069497.1) [22] were downloaded for phylogenetic comparison (Table 1).

6. Antifungal susceptibility testing

Minimum inhibitory concentrations (MICs) of *Q. cyanescens* 11PU348 to fluconazole, voriconazole, itraconazole, posaconazole, caspofungin, micafungin, anidulafungin, 5-flucytosine and amphotericin B were determined *in vitro* by broth microdilution methods as per Clinical and Laboratory Standards Institute (CLSI) M38-A2 guidelines [23]. *Candida parapsilosis* ATCC 22019 and *Candida krusei* ATCC 6258 were used as the quality control strains for the test [23].

7. Nucleotide sequence accession numbers

The ITS region and D1/D2 domain sequences of strain 11PU348 were deposited in GenBank with accession numbers KF953496 and KF953497, respectively.

Results

1. Sequence-based identification

By querying ITS region and D1/D2 domain sequences against those in the CBS database, the ITS region and D1/D2 domain sequences of *Q. cyanescens* 11PU348 showed 99.3% (576/580 bp) and 100% (600/600 bp) similarity to the ITS and D1/D2 sequences of *Q. cyanescens* type strain CBS 357.73 (GenBank accession number DQ119135.1 and DQ317615.1, respectively).

2. Phylogenetic analysis

The nucleotide sequence alignments within *Q. cyanescens*, using sequences of *Q. cyanescens* type strain CBS 357.73 as references, showed this species with little inter-species variation within both the ITS region (99.0% to 100%) and D1/D2 domain (99.6% to 100%) (Table 1). Of note, the ITS region can clearly discriminate *Q. cyanescens* and other four *Quambalaria* species, with highest sequence similarity of less than 97.0%. However, the D1/D2 domain was not able to identify the five species within *Quambalaria* genus (sequence similarity >99.0%). The NJ analysis of the ITS region and D1/D2 domain yielded similar results (Figure 1).

3. Phenotypic characteristics on agar

Q. cyanescens isolate 11PU348 grew well at 28°C and 37°C, but failed to grow at 42°C on Sabouraud dextrose agar. By three-sector streaking on Sabouraud dextrose agar, the strain had yeast-like colonies which were initially moist, smooth, of various sizes and white colored within 48 h at 28°C (Figure 2a), and turned to be creamy, butyrous and exuding dark-orange pigment after 72 h incubation (Figure 2b). However, the strain grew slower when incubated at 37°C, and tended to be mold-like, especially in the first sector of the streaked plates (Figure 2d and 2e).

After more than 2 weeks' incubation at either 28°C or 37°C, a pure culture of the organism yielded a typical filamentous fungi phenotype that appeared to be restricted, velvety, furrowed, compact and cerebriform, accompanied by a red pigment and a burgundy reverse color. The production of pigments was more obvious at 28°C than at 37°C (Figure 2c and 2f).

On CHROMagar *Candida*, the colonies of *Q. cyanescens* 11PU348 were dark blue hybridizing with white, which was very similar to the phenotype of *C. tropicalis* when incubated at 37°C for 48 h (Figure 2h), but generating dark-orange pigment when incubated at 28°C (Figure 2g).

4. Microscopic morphology

Yeast-form of *Q. cyanescens* 11PU348 showed the typical sympodial conidiogenesis, and had smooth-walled, obovoidal, solitary or bearing secondary conidia. The filamentous form of the strain showed hyphae which were regular, hyaline, smooth-walled, branched and suberect. The conidia formed by sympodial growth

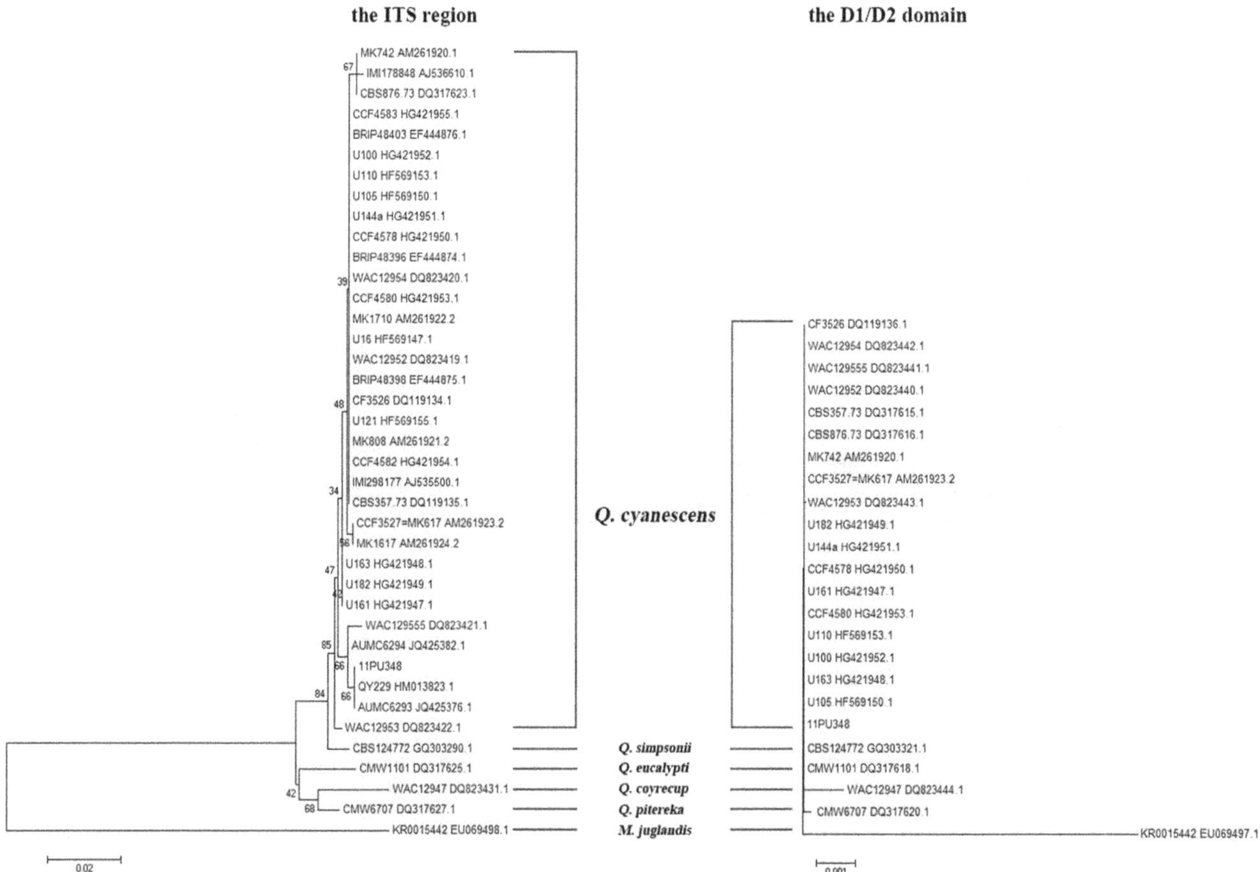

Figure 1. The Neighbor-Joining (NJ) tree of *Q. cyanescens* isolate 11PU348, all *Q. cyanescens* isolates with ITS and/or D1/D2 sequences available in GenBank, and selected isolates of other four *Quambalaria* species and *Microstroma juglandis.*

of the conidiogenous cells (primary conidia) mostly give rise to several secondary conidia.

5. Antifungal susceptibilities

Q. cyanescens isolate 11PU348 exhibited high MICs to 5-flucytosine (MIC >64 μg/ml) and all echinocandins tested, including anidulafungin (MIC >8 μg/ml), micafungin (MIC > 8 μg/ml) and caspofungin (MIC = 8 μg/ml). However, the isolate appeared more susceptible to amphotericin B (MIC = 0.5 μg/ml) and azoles (MICs of fluconazole, voriconazole, itraconazole and posaconazole were 0.5 μg/ml, <0.008 μg/ml, <0.015 μg/ml and 0.015 μg/ml, respectively).

Discussion

Q. cyanescens is rarely identified in the clinical microbiology laboratory, and its pathogenic role is still uncertain. A review of literature shows that this fungus was recovered primarily from individuals who were immunocompromised or debilitated [11,14], including a possible pulmonary case in a heart transplant patient [14], fungemia in lymphoma patients [11]. However, none of the above studies provided unequivocal clinical evidence of infection. In addition, Jackson *et al.* reported a pseudo-epidemic of *Q. cyanescens* pneumonia in a US hospital introduced by contamination of bronchoscopy suites [13], which suggests that the species may be an environmental contaminant in human patients.

Furthermore, fungal infections due to augmentation mammoplasties are rare. To date, only 15 out of 21 cases of breast implant fungal infections have been reported [24–37] (Table 2). *Aspergillus*, *Candida*, *Curvularia*, *Paecilomyces*, *Penicillium*, and *Trichosporon* spp. were potential causative agents. Most of the cases were efficaciously managed with implant removal, but some patients recovered after intravenous antifungal therapies (Table 2).

We note that the pathogenic role of *Q. cyanescens* in this clinical case is questionable. There was no corroborating direct microscopic, histopathologic or serological evidence of fungal infection. Although the isolation was obtained from a specimen which showed histological signs of acute inflammation, this could be due to either real infection or foreign-body reaction. In addition, no samples (except routine bloods) other than the implant and the surrounding tissue removed during surgery were sent for laboratory examination, nor was repeat isolation attempted, as the present study was done retrospectively. The patient fully recovered after removal of implants, without any antifungal therapy administered. Although no other micro-organisms were isolated from this patient, and no fungal organisms were isolated from other patients who underwent plastic surgery during the same time-period, the possibility of environmental contamination cannot be excluded.

If this described case was due to a real infection, the slow progression of the inflammation, and the fact that the patient was both afebrile and asymptomatic with all blood test results within normal values, is consistent with an infection caused by a low

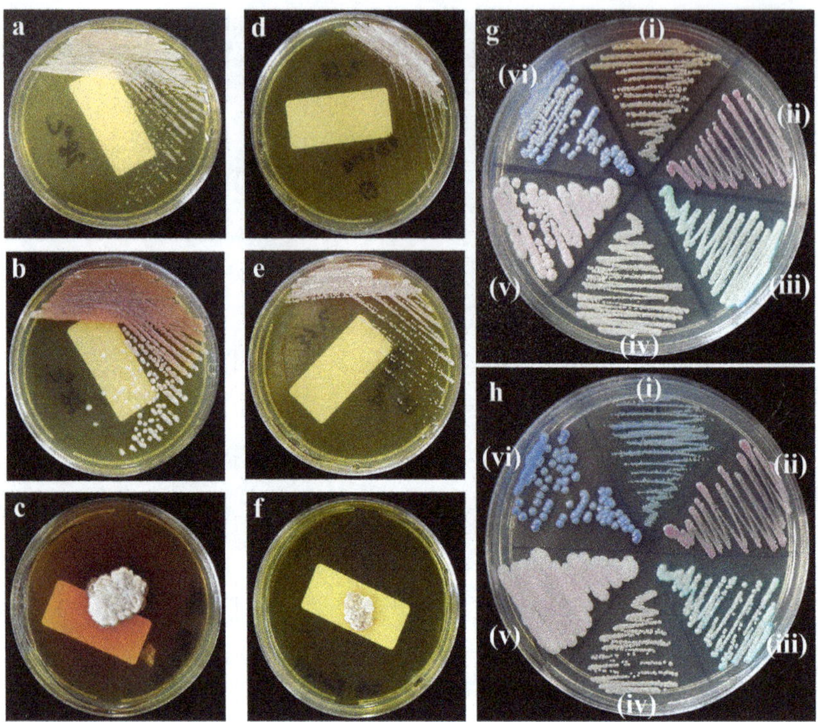

Figure 2. Phenotype of *Quambalaria cyanescens* 11PU348 on Sabouraud dextrose agar (Figure 2a to 2f) and CHROMagar *Candida* (Figure 2g and 2h). Incubation conditions: 2a and 2g, 28°C, 48 h; 2b, 28°C, 72 h; 2c, 28°C, 2 weeks; 2d and 2h, 37°C, 48 h; 2e, 37°C, 72 h; 2f, 37°C, 2 weeks. Strains used in Figure 2g and 2h: (i) *Q. cyanescens* 11PU348; (ii) *C. glabrata* sensu stricto 10H1043; (iii) *C. albicans* ATCC 90028; (iv) *C. parapsilosis* sensu stricto ATCC 22019; (v) *C. krusei* ATCC 6258; (iv) *C. tropicalis* 10H1048. *C. glabrata* sensu stricto 10H1043 and *C. tropicalis* 10H1048 were selected from CHIF-NET study [15].

virulence micro-organism. A previous experimental study in a murine model demonstrated that *Q. cyanescens* does have a low virulence potential [11].

Misidentification of *Q. cyanescens* 11PU348 was noted during confirmative identification process in CHIF-NET study [17]. Initially, two matrix-assisted laser desorption ionization–time of flight mass spectrometry systems (Vitek MS, bioMérieux, Marcy

Table 2. Fungal infections in patients after augmentation mammoplasty previously reported.

Species	No. of cases	Country reported	Duration (mammoplasty to infection)	Implant removal	Antifungal therapy	Reference
Candida albicans	1	Italy	3 years	No	Caspofungin	[25]
Candida albicans	1	Turkey	5 years	Yes	Not specified	[32]
Candida albicans	1	US	4 years	Yes	Fluconazole	[29]
Candida albicans	1	US	10 months	Yes	Not specified	[34]
Candida parapsilosis	1	US	16 days	Yes	Fluconazole	[26]
Trichosporon beigelii	1	US	16 months	No	Fluconazole	[30]
Trichosporon spp.	1	Singapore	17 months	No	Fluconazole	[33]
Aspergillus flavus	1	UK	18 months	Yes	Not specified	[36]
Aspergillus flavus	1	US	4 years	Yes	Not specified	[31]
Aspergillus niger	1	UK	5 years	Yes	Not specified	[24]
Aspergillus niger	1	US	Several months	Yes	Not specified	[35]
Curvularia spp.	5	US	4–12 months	Not specified	Not specified	[27]
Curvularia spp.	1	US	6 months	Yes	Not specified	[34]
Paecilomyces variotii	1	US	14 months	Yes	Not specified	[37]
Penicillium	3	US	Not stated	Not specified	Not specified	[28]

l'Etoile, France; Bruker Biotyper, Bruker Daltonics, Bremen, Germany) failed to identify strain 11PU348. Subsequent ITS sequencing identified the strain as *Q. cyanescens*. The main reason for the misidentification in the initial identification (that reported to clinic) was the yeast-like colonies with dark blue appearance at 48 h on CHROMagar *Candida* at 37°C, which was very similar to the appearance of *C. tropicalis* (Figure 2h). Although the patient in this case was cured by removal of the breast implant, the high MICs to 5-flucytosine and all echinocandins of *Q. cyanescens* were notable. Therefore, accurate identification of *Q. cyanescens* is important to avoid ineffective antifungal treatment. Mass spectra data of *Q. cyanescens* were neither represented in Vitek MS nor in Bruker Biotyper identification databases. Hence both MALDI-TOF MS systems assigned "no identification" to this isolate and importantly, did not misidentify the strain to another species. Although we were not able to identify *Q. cyanescens* against the current commercially available library of spectra, our result will nevertheless contribute to the existing spectral building.

In the most recent study, the ITS and D1/D2 sequences were used to cluster the *Quambalaria* genus and replaced *Q. cyanescens* species from another genus [8]. But in the present study, we found that the D1/D2 domain was not able to distinguish the different species within *Quambalaria* genus (Figure 1; Table 1). Compared with the D1/D2 domain, the ITS region was accurate in the identification of *Q. cyanescens* and other species within this genus (Figure 1; Table 1).

Conclusions

In conclusion, *Q. cyanescens* is a rare clinical basidiomycetous pathogen. Here we report a *Q. cyanescens* strain isolated from a patient after augmentation mammoplasty in China. The possibility of its real pathogenic role was discussed. The high MICs to 5-flucytosine and all echinocandins highlight the importance of accurate identification so that appropriate therapy can be prescribed. To date, ITS sequencing remains the only available method to obtain an accurate identification result on this organism, while the pathogen is potentially misidentified as *C. tropicalis* by CHROMagar *Candida*.

Author Contributions

Conceived and designed the experiments: XF MX FK YCX. Performed the experiments: XF MX. Analyzed the data: XF MX FK. Contributed reagents/materials/analysis tools: HW. Wrote the paper: TK.

References

1. Fleming RV, Walsh TJ, Anaissie EJ (2002) Emerging and less common fungal pathogens. Infect Dis Clin North Am 16: 915–933, vi–vii.
2. Huprikar S, Shoham S, Practice ASTIDCo (2013) Emerging fungal infections in solid organ transplantation. Am J Transplant 13 Suppl 4: 262–271.
3. Shoham S (2013) Emerging fungal infections in solid organ transplant recipients. Infect Dis Clin North Am 27: 305–316.
4. Hsueh PR, Teng LJ, Hsu JH, Liaw YS, Chen YC, et al. (2001) Nosocomial *Exophiala jeanselmei* pseudoinfection after sonography-guided aspiration of thoracic lesions. J Formos Med Assoc 100: 613–619.
5. Purcell J, McKenna J, Critten P, Denning DW, Hassan IA (2011) Mixed mould species in laboratory cultures of respiratory specimens: how should they be reported, and what are the indications for susceptibility testing? J Clin Pathol 64: 543–545.
6. Xiao M, Wang H, Lu J, Chen SC, Kong F, et al. (2014) *Candida quercitrusa* candidemia: investigation of three clustered cases and mycological characteristics of this novel species. J Clin Microbiol. In press.
7. Cheewangkoon R, Groenewald JZ, Summerell BA, Hyde KD, To-Anun C, et al. (2009) Myrtaceae, a cache of fungal biodiversity. Persoonia 23: 55–85.
8. de Beer ZW, Begerow D, Bauer R, Pegg GS, Crous PW, et al. (2006) Phylogeny of the *Quambalariaceae fam.* nov., including important Eucalyptus pathogens in South Africa and Australia. Stud Mycol 55: 289–298.
9. Paap T, Burgess TI, McComb JA, Shearer BL, Hardy GESJ (2008) *Quambalaria* species, including *Q. coyrecup* sp. nov., implicated in canker and shoot blight diseases causing decline of *Corymbia* species in the southwest of Western Australia. Mycol Res 112: 57–69.
10. de Hoog GS, de Vries GA (1973) Two new species of *Sporothrix* and their relation to *Blastobotrys nivea*. Antonie Van Leeuwenhoek 39: 515–520.
11. Sigler L, Harris JL, Dixon DM, Flis AL, Salkin IF, et al. (1990) Microbiology and potential virulence of *Sporothrix cyanescens*, a fungus rarely isolated from blood and skin. J Clin Microbiol 28: 1009–1015.
12. Kolařík M, Slávíková E, Pažoutová S (2006) The taxonomic and ecological characterisation of the clinically important heterobasiodiomycete *Fugomyces cyanescens* and its association with bark beetles. Czech Mycol 58: 81–98.
13. Jackson L, Klotz SA, Normand RE (1990) A pseudoepidemic of *Sporothrix cyanescens* pneumonia occurring during renovation of a bronchoscopy suite. J Med Vet Mycol 28: 455–459.
14. Tambini R, Farina C, Fiocchi R, Dupont B, Gueho E, et al. (1996) Possible pathogenic role for *Sporothrix cyanescens* isolated from a lung lesion in a heart transplant patient. J Med Vet Mycol 34: 195–198.
15. Wang H, Xiao M, Chen SC, Kong F, Sun ZY, et al. (2012) *In vitro* susceptibilities of yeast species to fluconazole and voriconazole as determined by the 2010 National China Hospital Invasive Fungal Surveillance Net (CHIF-NET) study. J Clin Microbiol 50: 3952–3959.
16. Amberg DC, Burke DJ, Strathern JN (2005) Methods in yeast genetics: a Cold Spring Harbor laboratory course manual.
17. Zhang L, Xiao M, Wang H, Gao R, Fan X, et al. (2014) Yeast identification algorithm based on use of the Vitek MS system selectively supplemented with ribosomal DNA sequencing: proposal of a reference assay for invasive fungal surveillance programs in China. J Clin Microbiol 52: 572–577.
18. Taverna CG, Bosco-Borgeat ME, Murisengo OA, Davel G, Boite MC, et al. (2013) Comparative analyses of classical phenotypic method and ribosomal RNA gene sequencing for identification of medically relevant *Candida* species. Mem Inst Oswaldo Cruz 108: 178–185.
19. Saitou N, Nei M (1987) The neighbor-joining method: a new method for reconstructing phylogenetic trees. Mol Biol Evol 4: 406–425.
20. Sohpal VK, Dey A, Singh A (2010) MEGA biocentric software for sequence and phylogenetic analysis: a review. Int J Bioinform Res Appl 6: 230–240.
21. Tamura K, Nei M, Kumar S (2004) Prospects for inferring very large phylogenies by using the neighbor-joining method. Proc Natl Acad Sci USA 101: 11030–11035.
22. Scholler M (2007) Plant parasitic small fungi from the Breitsitter forest near Pirmasens (Rhineland-Palatinate, Germany). Mitt Pollichia 93: 41–44.
23. CLSI (2009) Reference method for broth dilution antifungal susceptibility testing of filamentous fungi; approved standard – second edition.
24. Coady MS, Gaylor J, Knight SL (1995) Fungal growth within a silicone tissue expander: case report. Br J Plast Surg 48: 428–430.
25. Dessy LA, Corrias F, Marchetti F, Marcasciano M, Armenti AF, et al. (2012) Implant infection after augmentation mammaplasty: a review of the literature and report of a multidrug-resistant *Candida albicans* infection. Aesthetic Plast Surg 36: 153–159.
26. Fox PM, Lee GK (2012) Tissue expander with acellular dermal matrix for breast reconstruction infected by an unusual pathogen: *Candida parapsilosis*. J Plast Reconstr Aesthet Surg 65: e286–289.
27. Kainer MA, Keshavarz H, Jensen BJ, Arduino MJ, Brandt ME, et al. (2005) Saline-filled breast implant contamination with *Curvularia* species among women who underwent cosmetic breast augmentation. J Infect Dis 192: 170–177.
28. Netscher DT, Weizer G, Wigoda P, Walker LE, Thornby J, et al. (1995) Clinical relevance of positive breast periprosthetic cultures without overt infection. Plast Reconstr Surg 96: 1125–1129.
29. Niazi ZB, Salzberg CA, Montecalvo M (1996) *Candida albicans* infection of bilateral polyurethane-coated silicone gel breast implants. Ann Plast Surg 37: 91–93.
30. Reddy BT, Torres HA, Kontoyiannis DP (2002) Breast implant infection caused by *Trichosporon beigelii*. Scand J Infect Dis 34: 143–144.
31. Rosenblatt WB, Pollock A (1997) *Aspergillus flavus* cultured from a saline-filled implant. Plast Reconstr Surg 99: 1470–1472.
32. Saray A, Kaygusuz S, Kisa U, Kilic D (2002) *Candida* colonisation within a silicone tissue expander. Br J Plast Surg 55: 257–259.
33. Tian HH, Tan SM, Tay KH (2007) Delayed fungal infection following augmentation mammoplasty in an immunocompetent host. Singapore Med J 48: 256–258.
34. Truppman ES, Ellenby JD, Schwartz BM (1979) Fungi in and around implants after augmentation mammaplasty. Plast Reconstr Surg 64: 804–806.
35. Williams K, Walton RL, Bunkis J (1983) *Aspergillus* colonization associated with bilateral silicone mammary implants. Plast Reconstr Surg 71: 260–261.
36. Wright PK, Raine C, Ragbir M, Macfarlane S, O'Donoghue J (2006) The semi-permeability of silicone: a saline-filled breast implant with intraluminal and pericapsular *Aspergillus flavus*. J Plast Reconstr Aesthet Surg 59: 1118–1121.
37. Young VL, Hertl MC, Murray PR, Lambros VS (1995) *Paecilomyces variotii* contamination in the lumen of a saline-filled breast implant. Plast Reconstr Surg 96: 1430–1434.

38. Hall L, Wohlfiel S, Roberts GD (2003) Experience with the MicroSeq D2 large-subunit ribosomal DNA sequencing kit for identification of commonly encountered, clinically important yeast species. J Clin Microbiol 41: 5099–5102.
39. Pegg GS, O'Dwyer C, Carnegie AJ, Burgess TI, Wingfield MJ, et al. (2008) *Quambalaria* species associated with plantation and native eucalypts in Australia. Plant Pathology 57: 702–714.
40. Zhang Z, Wang C, Yao Z, Zhao J, Lu F, et al. (2011) Isolation and identification of a fungal strain QY229 producing milk-clotting enzyme. European Food Research and Technology 232: 861–866.

Equilibrium-Phase High Spatial Resolution Contrast-Enhanced MR Angiography at 1.5T in Preoperative Imaging for Perforator Flap Breast Reconstruction

Bas Versluis[1,3], Stefania Tuinder[2*], Carla Boetes[1], René Van Der Hulst[2], Arno Lataster[4], Tom Van Mulken[2], Joachim Wildberger[1,3], Michiel de Haan[1,3], Tim Leiner[1,3,5]

1 Department of Radiology, Maastricht University Medical Center, Maastricht, The Netherlands, **2** Department of Plastic and Reconstructive Surgery, Maastricht University Medical Center, Maastricht, The Netherlands, **3** Cardiovascular Research Institute Maastricht, Maastricht University Medical Center, Maastricht, The Netherlands, **4** Department of Anatomy and Embryology, Maastricht University, Maastricht, The Netherlands, **5** Department of Radiology, Utrecht University Medical Center, Utrecht, The Netherlands

Abstract

Objectives: The aim was (i) to evaluate the accuracy of equilibrium-phase high spatial resolution (EP) contrast-enhanced magnetic resonance angiography (CE-MRA) at 1.5T using a blood pool contrast agent for the preoperative evaluation of deep inferior epigastric artery perforator branches (DIEP), and (ii) to compare image quality with conventional first-pass CE-MRA.

Methods: Twenty-three consecutive patients were included. All patients underwent preoperative CE-MRA to determine quality and location of DIEP. First-pass imaging after a single bolus injection of 10 mL gadofosveset trisodium was followed by EP imaging. MRA data were compared to intra-operative findings, which served as the reference standard.

Results: There was 100% agreement between EP CE-MRA and surgical findings in identifying the single best perforator branch. All EP acquisitions were of diagnostic quality, whereas in 10 patients the quality of the first-pass acquisition was qualified as non-diagnostic. Both signal- and contrast-to-noise ratios were significantly higher for EP imaging in comparison with first-pass acquisitions ($p<0.01$).

Conclusions: EP CE-MRA of DIEP in the preoperative evaluation of patients undergoing a breast reconstruction procedure is highly accurate in identifying the single best perforator branch at 1.5Tesla (T). Besides accuracy, image quality of EP imaging proved superior to conventional first-pass CE-MRA.

Editor: Yi Wang, Cornell University, United States of America

Funding: The authors have supporting or funding to report.

Competing Interests: The authors have declared that no competing interests exist.

* E-mail: nervofaciale@yahoo.it

These authors contributed equally to this work.

Introduction

The number of (prophylactic) mastectomies in (the prevention of) breast cancer is increasing, and so is the number of patients that opt for reconstructive breast surgery after mastectomy [1,2,3]. Over the last decade, deep inferior epigastric perforator (DIEP) flap procedures have gained considerable support among plastic surgeons as preferred technique for breast reconstruction [4]. In contrast to the more conventional transverse rectus abdominis musculocutaneous (TRAM) flap procedure, the DIEP flap procedure uses only subcutaneous abdominal fat, centered around the best single large perforator branch of the deep inferior epigastric artery (DIEA) for the blood supply of the flap. Well-known advantages of perforator flaps include less postoperative pain, less donor site complications and less functional impairment compared to TRAM flaps [5,6]. Disadvantages of the DIEP procedure, on the other hand, include difficulties in harvesting the flap, resulting in considerably longer dissection times, and the fact that long-term results depend heavily on the quality of the perforator branch supplying the flap.

Preoperative evaluation of the DIEA perforator branches in the abdomen to identify adequate perforator branches facilitates surgical planning of the procedure and shortens dissection times [6,7,8,9,10]. Currently, the most widely applied techniques in preoperative imaging and planning in DIEP flap procedures are Doppler ultrasound (DUS) and computed tomography angiography (CTA) [5]. Doppler, however, is associated with long imaging times, low accuracy and high interobserver variability [5,11]. CTA, on the other hand, is highly accurate in demonstrating location, size and course of the perforators, but suffers from exposure to ionizing radiation, which is an important drawback in the often (relatively) young patients [12,13,14]. Recently, several authors have demonstrated that MR angiography can also be used in preoperative imaging of the perforator branches of the DIEA [5,6,8,15,16]. Excellent soft-tissue contrast and the absence of ionizing radiation are important advantages of MRI. Nevertheless, experience with contrast-enhanced MR angiography (CE-MRA) in the preoperative workup of patients undergoing DIEP flap procedures is still scarce. Several studies have been performed using state-of-the-art 3T hardware, instead of the more widely available 1.5T magnetic resonance angiography (MRI) systems [5,6,8,15,16], and most of these studies have employed conventional extracellular contrast agents in combination with first-pass imaging to visualize DIEA perforator branches. Considering the small size of DIEA perforator branches we wondered whether it was possible to obtain high spatial resolution equilibrium-phase (EP) images with improved resolution compared to first-pass acquisitions using a recently described new intravascular contrast agent, gadofosveset trisodium [17,18]. Blood pool agents have important benefits over conventional small-sized extracellular agents in CE-MRA, such as the lengthened imaging window and the relatively large R1 [19], both allowing longer acquisition times, enabling data acquisition at a very high resolution and with very high accuracy.

The aims of the current study were (i) to investigate the accuracy of equilibrium-phase high spatial resolution CE-MRA at 1.5T using a blood pool contrast agent in the preoperative evaluation of the DIEA perforator branches, and (ii) to compare image quality of equilibrium-phase high spatial resolution imaging with conventional first-pass CE-MRA.

Material and Methods

Subjects

Twenty-three consecutive patients (all female, 48.1±9.7 years) scheduled to undergo 36 free flap procedures for breast reconstruction were included between January 2008 and September 2009. Exclusion criteria were contra-indications for MRI (i.e. claustrophobia, known gadolinium based contrast agent allergy, and an estimated glomular filtration rate below 30 mL/kg/1.73 m^2). The institutional medical ethics committee of the University Hospital of Maastricht and Maastricht University (METC azM/UM) approved the study and all subjects gave written informed consent before inclusion. All patients underwent preoperative CE-MRA of the abdominal wall and pelvic region to determine the quality and location of the DIEA perforator branches.

MRI protocol

Examinations were performed using a 1.5-T commercially available system (Intera, Philips Medical Systems, Best, The Netherlands). For signal reception we used a 4-element phased-array parallel imaging-capable body coil with craniocaudal coverage of approximately 25 cm (Philips Medical Systems, Best, The Netherlands). Subjects were imaged in the supine position. The entire examination lasted less than 30 minutes. Imaging parameters for all acquisitions are listed in table 1.

Survey. A non-enhanced time-of-flight (TOF) scan was acquired to prescribe the imaging volumes of interest for CE-MRA. A turbo field echo (TFE) pulse sequence with a 180° inversion prepulse was used to suppress stationary tissues. One-hundred axial slices were acquired with 3.0-mm slice thickness and 0-mm interslice gap, and an inferiorly concatenated saturation band. The standard quadrature body coil was used for signal transmission and reception. For positioning of the 3D CE-MRA volume a maximum intensity projection (MIP) was generated in 3 orthogonal directions.

Contrast. For CE-MRA a fixed dose of 10 mL gadofosveset trisodium (Ablavar®, Lantheus Medical Imaging, Billerica, MA), a blood pool contrast agent, was administered intravenously as a single dose at a speed of 1.0 ml/s in the median cubital vein, using a remote controlled injection system (Medrad Spectris, Indianola, PA). Contrast injection was followed by 20 mL saline flush injected at the same rate. Real time bolus monitoring software (BolusTrak, Philips Medical Systems, Best, The Netherlands) was used to visualize the arrival of the bolus in the abdominal aorta with a refresh rate of proximally 1 frame/sec. Upon first sight of contrast arrival in the abdominal aorta, image acquisition for the first-pass CE-MRA sequence was started. Equilibrium-phase imaging commenced approximately 2 minutes after completion of the first-pass sequence, after allowing systemic contrast equilibration in the arterial and venous blood pool.

First-pass CE-MRA

First-pass CE-MRA consisted of single station 3D acquisition of the abdominal wall as previously described [20]. Patients were asked to hold their breath as long as possible (inspiration phase) during the acquisition, which lasted approximately 33 seconds.

Equilibrium-phase high-spatial resolution CE-MRA

A 3D isotropic high spatial resolution equilibrium-phase acquisition of the lower abdomen and pelvic region, comprising both the DIEA and gluteal perforator branches, was performed. As the equilibrium-phase acquisition lasted for approximately 5 minutes, depending on the dimensions of the patient, patients were asked to breathe in a shallow pattern in order to reduce breathing-related motion artifacts as much as possible.

Image analysis

All equilibrium-phase CE-MRA datasets were analyzed in consensus by a radiologist (BV) and the plastic surgeon (ST) scheduled to perform the DIEP flap dissection and breast reconstruction. A dedicated post-processing workstation was used for image analysis (Vitrea release 4.1.2.0, Vital Images, Minnetonka, MN). Using the original source images as well as coronal and sagittal multiplanar reconstructions (MPR) both first-pass (source) images and equilibrium-phase images were evaluated for (i) image quality; (ii) the location of the single best DIEA perforator at each side of the patient; and (iii) the total number of visualized DIEA perforator branches on each side of the patient. Image quality was assessed on a three-point scale (i.e. excellent quality, diagnostic quality and non-diagnostic quality) and by determination of the vessel-to-noise (VNR) and vessel-to-background (fat tissue) (VBR) ratios of the single best perforator branch [21]. The single best perforator branch was located following the criteria used before by Chernyak et al [6]. The location at which these perforators penetrated the rectus fascia with respect to the center of the umbilicus was noted as x,y-coordinates with the center of the umbilicus being the origin (0,0). The total number of perforator branches visualized by both first-pass and equilibrium-phase imaging were determined within a region extending from 5 cm cranial to 10 cm caudal to the umbilicus.

Comparison of CE-MRA and intraoperative findings

DIEP flap dissection was performed by a team of three plastic surgeons. Surgeons noted the location of the single best perforator

Table 1. Acquisition parameters for MRI measurements.

		CE-MRA	
Parameter	**TOF**	**First-pass**	**Equilibrium-phase**
Scan mode	Multi 2D	3D	3D
Technique	TFE	FFE	FFE
TR (ms)	7.20	4.90	12.0
TE (ms)	3.20	1.48	1.90
Flip angle (°)	50	40	20
FOV (mm)	410	400	470
Voxel dimensions (acquired) (mm)	1.60×2.34×3.00	1.00×1.36×2.00	0.84×0.84×1.00
Voxel dimensions (reconstructed) (mm)	1.60×1.60×3.00	0.78×0.78×1.00	0.84×0.84×1.00
Number of slices	100[a]	100[a]	200[a]
Scan direction	Axial	Coronal	Coronal
Parallel imaging acceleration (Factor/direction)	No	Yes (2/R-L)	Yes (2/R-L)
NSA	1	1	1
Scan duration (min:sec)	3:37[a]	0:33[a]	4:39[a]

[a]The number of slices, and therefore scan duration, varied from subject to subject, depending on the dimensions of the abdomen.
TFE, turbo field echo; FFE, fast field echo (gradient echo); FOV, field of view; NSA, number of signal averages.

they found during surgery, within the region that was evaluated with MRA. A handheld device ultrasonography and visual/manual inspection were used to identify perforator branches during surgery. After surgery, CE-MRA and intraoperative findings were compared. Data were considered concordant if differences between MRA and intraoperative findings were less than 1 cm in craniocaudal and/or left-right direction.

Statistical analysis

An independent-samples *t*-test was performed to test the significance of differences in image quality between first-pass and equilibrium-phase CE-MRA and the differences in total number of perforator branches between first-pass and equilibrium-phase CE-MRA and intraoperative findings.

Results

Subjects

All included patients underwent MRA without experiencing side effects or adverse events. In twenty-three patients 36 DIEP flaps were successfully dissected. Ten patients underwent unilateral flap dissection, whereas in 13 patients a bilateral flap dissection was performed.

Diagnostic accuracy of equilibrium-phase high spatial resolution imaging

Equilibrium-phase high spatial resolution acquisitions predicted the location of the single best perforator accurately in all cases, i.e. in 36/36 perforators (100% of the patients). The locations of the perforator branches used for surgery are graphically presented in figure 1. The average location of the single best perforator found during surgery and with equilibrium-phase imaging was located 3.0±1.2 cm (mean ± SD) lateral and 0.6±1.2 cm caudal in respect with the umbilicus (figure 2). There was no significant difference in distance to the umbilicus for left and right sided perforator branches ($p = 0.15$). We consider now the equilibrium-phase versus first-pass CE-MRA.

Image quality

Equilibrium-phase high spatial resolution images were acquired in all patients, whereas because of a timing error first-pass acquisition failed in one patient. Figures 3 and 4 show examples of reconstructed MPR images of an equilibrium-phase acquisition. Image quality results of both equilibrium-phase and first pass acquisitions are presented in table 2. All equilibrium-phase acquisitions were of diagnostic quality, whereas in 10 out of 22 patients the quality of the first-pass images was qualified as non-diagnostic. In those patients it was not possible to identify any perforator branch using the first-pass acquisition. Excellent image quality was obtained in 13 out of 23 patients for equilibrium-phase imaging against only 7 out of 22 in first-pass imaging. Both the signal- and contrast-to-noise ratios were significantly higher for equilibrium-phase imaging in comparison with first-pass acquisitions ($p<0.01$).

Perforator branches

The number of perforator branches identified with equilibrium-phase high spatial resolution imaging was significantly higher compared to first-pass imaging (table 3; $p<0.01$). No significant difference was found in number of perforator branches between the left and right side of patients ($p = 0.31$ and $p = 0.60$ in equilibrium-phase and first-pass imaging respectively).

Single best perforator branch

Because of the large number of non-diagnostic first-pass acquisitions, a direct comparison between equilibrium-phase and first-pass imaging was possible in only 12 patients (19 DIEP flaps) (figure 4). In 8 out of 19 single best perforators, the location in first-pass imaging differed more than 1 cm in any direction as compared to equilibrium-phase imaging and surgery.

Discussion

The accuracy and image quality of contrast-enhanced MR angiography at 1.5T using a blood pool contrast agent in identifying the single best DIEA perforator branch, as desired in

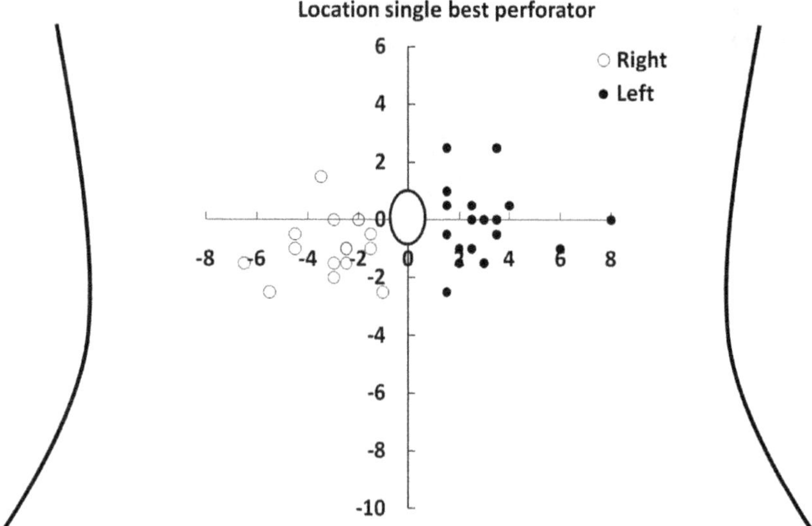

Figure 1. Schematic overview of 36 perforator branches of the deep inferior epigastric artery. Schematic overview of the abdomen and the location of 36 single best perforator branches of the deep inferior epigastric artery found during surgery and with equilibrium-phase high spatial resolution CE-MRA. The x- and y-axis represent the distance (in cm) in respect to the umbilicus.

the preoperative planning of a deep inferior epigastric perforator flap breast reconstruction procedure, was evaluated, both for equilibrium-phase high spatial resolution and first-pass imaging. Equilibrium-phase high spatial resolution imaging proved 100% accurate in identifying the single best perforator branch compared to intraoperative findings, against only 31% (11 out of 36 perforators) in first-pass imaging. Image quality of equilibrium-phase high spatial resolution imaging was significantly higher compared to first pass imaging.

Preoperative identification of suitable perforator branches of the DIEA is highly valuable because it can shorten anesthesia duration and it makes surgery easier to perform and less traumatic compared to surgery based on ultrasonography [10]. Although it is well known that the best perforators usually lie around the umbilicus, the anatomical variation is very high, which is proven by the results presented in figure 1. This also clarifies why preoperative imaging is really a necessity to decrease dissection time, as blindly localizing the perforator branches with a handheld Doppler device per-operative is quite time consuming, whereas MRA in this study proved 100% accurate in identifying the perforator branches. Moreover the MRA gives informations also about the intramuscular course of the perforator and the

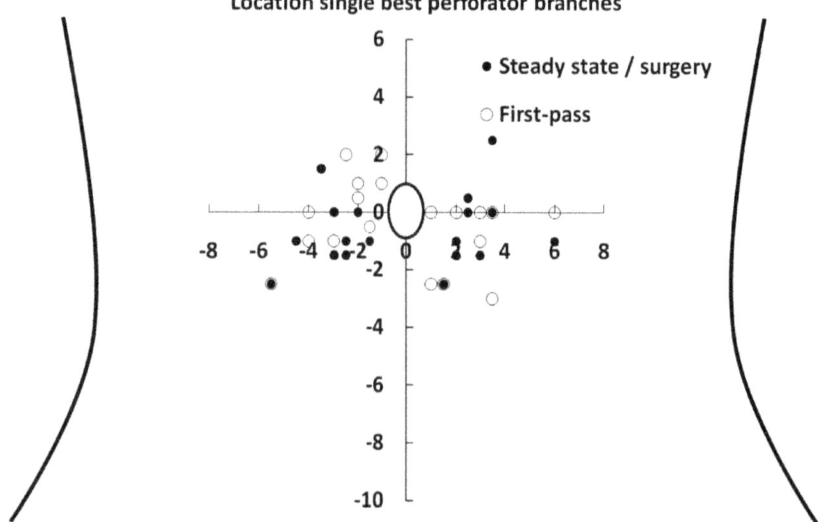

Figure 2. Schematic overview of the best perforator branch of the deep inferior epigastric artery. Schematic overview of the abdomen and the location of the single best perforator branches of the deep inferior epigastric artery found and used during DIEP dissection. The x- and y-axis represent the distance (in cm) in respect to the umbilicus. These perforator branches correlated with equilibrium-phase results for 100%. Only those perforator branches with a first-pass acquisition of diagnostic quality are presented, allowing a 1:1 comparison between equilibrium-phase high spatial resolution and first-pass CE-MRA.

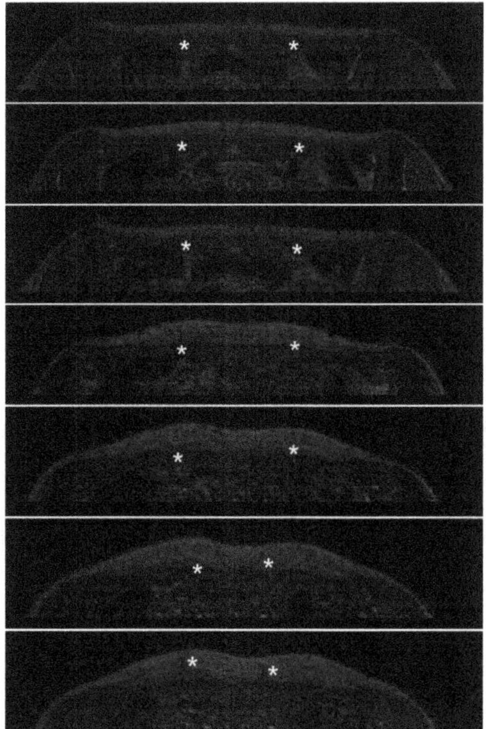

Figure 3. Transverse slices demonstrate the vascular bundle dorsal to the rectus muscle. Transverse source images of equilibrium-phase dataset in the same patient. Images are from caudal (top panel) to cranial (bottom panel), and clearly demonstrate the vascular bundle dorsal to the rectus muscle shortly after branching off the external iliac artery (asterisks in top three panels). The perforating branches can easily be followed when traversing the rectus muscle to the point where they arise in the subcutaneous fat (asterisks in lower 4 panels).

connections between perforator and superficial epigastric system, which is also relevant information from a surgical point of view. However, preoperative imaging with CE-MRA is challenging for a number of reasons. First of all, the relatively small caliber of the perforator branches (0.1 to 1 mm when they emerge from the fascia) makes it difficult to find an adequate balance between spatial resolution and acquisition time, especially as contrast-enhanced MR angiography techniques have a limited temporal imaging window due to the relatively fast passage and subsequent wash-out of the contrast agent from the vessels of interest. Secondly, because perforator branches course through the rectus abdominal muscles and the subcutaneous abdominal fat, it can be difficult to acquire sufficient contrast resolution between the perforator branches and the surrounding static tissues. Also, breathing and bowel motion may lead to seriously compromised image quality due to related image artifacts.

Currently, best results with first-pass CE-MRA of the DIEA perforator branches have been achieved at 3.0T, as this field strength allows to optimally balance spatial resolution, contrast resolution and acquisition time [6]. We sought to investigate whether acquisition of equilibrium phase images with higher spatial resolution compared to imaging during first arterial passage resulted in better image quality and improved diagnostic accuracy in identifying the most suitable perforator branch. Diagnostic accuracy of equilibrium-phase high spatial resolution imaging: in this study, we evaluated the diagnostic accuracy of CE-MRA at

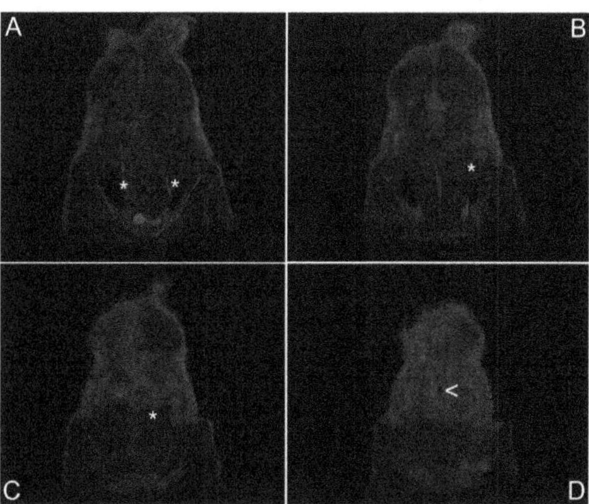

Figure 4. Coronal slices demonstrate the course of perforator branches traversing the rectus muscles. Coronal reformations of equilibrium-phase source images from dorsal (panel A) to ventral (panel D) clearly demonstrate the course of the small perforator branches (asterisks) traversing the rectus muscles. The umbilicus (arrowhead, panel D) is clearly visualized and serves as the reference location for determining the exact point where the perforator branches arise from the muscle. The left side is dominant.

1.5 T with gadofosveset trisodium as contrast agent, both for equilibrium-phase high spatial resolution and first-pass imaging. For both acquisitions a 3D gradient echo (FFE) sequence was used. For equilibrium-phase high spatial resolution imaging, there was 100% agreement between intraoperative and MR findings as far as the location of the single best perforator branch was concerned. In all cases there was no more than 1 cm difference in either craniocaudal or left-right direction between equilibrium-phase high spatial resolution MRA and intraoperative findings. This indicates that equilibrium-phase high spatial resolution MR angiography is a very accurate technique for identifying the location of the single best perforator branch in DIEP-procedures and can be a valuable tool for the surgeon to facilitate preoperative planning of the procedure.

Equilibrium-phase versus first-pass CE-MRA

Whereas equilibrium-phase high spatial resolution imaging was highly accurate, the opposite was true for first-pass imaging. In only 11 out of 36 DIEP flaps, first-pass imaging accurately determined the location of the single best perforator branch. In 10

Table 2. Image quality in CE-MRA.

	CE-MRA	
Image quality	**Equilibrium-phase** *(n = 23)*	**First-pass** *(n = 22)*
Excellent	13 *(57%)*	7 *(32%)*
Diagnostic	10 *(43%)*	5 *(23%)*
Non-diagnostic	0 *(0%)*	10 *(45%)*
VNR (mean ± SD)	16.7±9.1	6.9±4.6[a]
VBR (mean ± SD)	12.0±7.1	3.1±3.5[a]

VNR, vessel-to-noise ratio; VBR, vessel-to-background ratio.
[a]*$p<0.01$.*

Table 3. Number of perforator branches as identified with CE-MRA.

	CE-MRA	
Total number of perforators	**First-pass**	**Equilibrium-phase**
Right	3.3±1.4	7.3±2.0[a]
Left	2.8±1.3	7.9±2.0[a]

[a]$p<0.01$.

patients (17 DIEP flaps), first-pass images were not able to identify any perforator branch (non-diagnostic image quality). Besides low accuracy in identifying the single best perforator branches, the total number of perforator branches determined with first-pass imaging was also significantly lower as compared to equilibrium-phase high spatial resolution imaging. The main reason for these poor results was the poor image quality of first-pass imaging.

First pass imaging was only able to identify half the number perforator branches found with steady state imaging. In many cases, these missed perforator branches with first pass imaging turned out to be the single best perforator branch according to steady state imaging. This explains the large mis-match between first pass and steady state imaging.

Image quality in equilibrium-phase imaging was high on the other hand. All equilibrium-phase high spatial resolution examinations were of diagnostic quality and in 13 out of 23 patients the image quality was qualified as excellent (i.e. there were no disturbing artifacts in the region of the single best perforator branch and high signal intensity was found both in the intramuscular and subcutaneous course of the perforator branch), whereas in 10 patients there were minor motion artifacts that did not interfere with the diagnostic accuracy of the exam. In first-pass acquisitions, however, severe motion artifacts due to the inability of patients to sustain a breath hold during acquisition resulted in 10 non-diagnostic examinations. Another important problem with first-pass imaging was the lack of signal in the intramuscular part of perforator branches. Due to this problem, none of the first-pass acquisitions were of excellent image quality. Besides, signal-to-noise and contrast-to-noise ratios for equilibrium-phase imaging were significantly higher as compared to first-pass imaging.

The superior diagnostic accuracy and image quality of equilibrium-phase imaging is probably the result of the relatively high spatial and contrast resolution compared to first-pass imaging. First-pass imaging was able to identify low signal intensity perforator branches within subcutaneous fat tissue, as the low signal intensity of the vessel fascia ensured a strong contrast with the high signal intensity of surrounding fat tissue. However, the intramuscular course of these perforator branches could not be determined due to the lack of intraluminal signal enhancement. However, the exact length and precise intramuscular course of the perforator branch is important as branches that course through muscle over extended lengths are difficult to dissect and associated with more postoperative pain. Equilibrium-phase imaging with a blood pool contrast agent shows that a longer TR and lower flip angle as well as higher spatial resolution results in better contrast resolution (proven by the significant increase in VNR and VBR for equilibrium-phase imaging) and higher sensitivity for identifying small caliber perforator branches respectively.

Motion artifacts caused by breathing reduced image quality both in equilibrium-phase and first-pass imaging. First-pass imaging was performed during a single breath-hold, while patients were freely breathing during equilibrium-phase imaging, as the acquisition time of the equilibrium-phase sequence was approximately 5 minutes. Yet, image distortion due to breathing turned out to be much less severe in equilibrium-phase imaging as compared to first-pass imaging. This is mainly inherent to the imaging technique and the inability of many patients to hold their breath for the requested 33 seconds in first-pass imaging.

Study limitations

Both equilibrium-phase, but especially first-pass imaging, suffered from motion artifacts, reducing image quality. The influence of breathing may be reduced by imaging patients in prone rather than supine position. Initial findings in our hospital show that abdominal movement is greatly reduced this way, however, drawbacks of this method are distortion of the abdominal wall in prone position and, especially for obese patients, this position is much less comfortable.

Fat suppression might result in an even better contrast resolution and thereby improve image quality. However, use of fat suppression in most cases results in a prolonged acquisition time, which is undesirable for first-pass imaging. For equilibrium-phase imaging image quality already was sufficient, but it is likely that the use of fat suppression will result in even higher VNR and VBR values.

Determining the influence of CE-MRA upon the dissection time of the DIEP flap during surgery was beyond the scope of this study. However, an important next step would be to determine the actual additional value of CE-MRA in both facilitating the preoperative planning of the procedure and the influence upon the dissection time during surgery. This, however, is quite complicated, as many factors are responsible for the dissection time, amongst others the experience and preferences of the surgeon and the between-subject differences in quality and course of the single best perforator branches of the DIEA.

Conclusion

Equilibrium-phase high spatial resolution CE-MRA of the DIEA perforator branches in the preoperative evaluation of patients undergoing a DIEP flap reconstruction procedure is highly accurate in identifying the single best perforator branch at 1.5T, when using a blood pool contrast agent. Besides accuracy, image quality of equilibrium-phase high spatial resolution imaging proved superior to conventional first-pass CE-MRA.

Author Contributions

Conceived and designed the experiments: BV ST CB RVDH TL. Performed the experiments: BV ST CB RVDH TL MdH. Analyzed the data: BV ST TL MdH TVM. Contributed reagents/materials/analysis tools: BV ST TL JW TVM AL. Wrote the paper: BV ST. Revised the manuscript: BV ST CB RVDH AL TVM JW MdH TL.

References

1. Tuttle TM, Abbott A, Arrington A, Rueth N (2010) The increasing use of prophylactic mastectomy in the prevention of breast cancer. Curr Oncol Rep 12: 16–21.
2. Roje Z, Jankovic S, Ninkovic M (2010) Breast reconstruction after mastectomy. Coll Antropol 34 Suppl 1: 113–123.
3. Lee CN, Hultman CS, Sepucha K (2010) Do patients and providers agree about the most important facts and goals for breast reconstruction decisions? Ann Plast Surg 64: 563–566.
4. Selber JC, Serletti JM (2010) The deep inferior epigastric perforator flap: myth and reality. Plast Reconstr Surg 125: 50–58.

5. Mathes DW, Neligan PC (2010) Current techniques in preoperative imaging for abdomen-based perforator flap microsurgical breast reconstruction. J Reconstr Microsurg 26: 3–10.
6. Chernyak V, Rozenblit AM, Greenspun DT, Levine JL, Milikow DL, et al. (2009) Breast reconstruction with deep inferior epigastric artery perforator flap: 3.0-T gadolinium-enhanced MR imaging for preoperative localization of abdominal wall perforators. Radiology 250: 417–424.
7. Rozen WM, Phillips TJ, Ashton MW, Stella DL, Gibson RN, et al. (2008) Preoperative imaging for DIEA perforator flaps: a comparative study of computed tomographic angiography and Doppler ultrasound. Plast Reconstr Surg 121: 9–16.
8. Alonso-Burgos A, Garcia-Tutor E, Bastarrika G, Cano D, Martinez-Cuesta A, et al. (2006) Preoperative planning of deep inferior epigastric artery perforator flap reconstruction with multislice-CT angiography: imaging findings and initial experience. J Plast Reconstr Aesthet Surg 59: 585–593.
9. Masia J, Clavero JA, Larranaga JR, Alomar X, Pons G, et al. (2006) Multidetector-row computed tomography in the planning of abdominal perforator flaps. J Plast Reconstr Aesthet Surg 59: 594–599.
10. Acosta R, Smit JM, Audolfsson T, Darcy CM, Enajat M, et al. (2010) A Clinical Review of 9 Years of Free Perforator Flap Breast Reconstructions: An Analysis of 675 Flaps and the Influence of New Techniques on Clinical Practice. J Reconstr Microsurg.
11. Giunta RE, Geisweid A, Feller AM (2000) The value of preoperative Doppler sonography for planning free perforator flaps. Plast Reconstr Surg 105: 2381–2386.
12. Brenner DJ, Doll R, Goodhead DT, Hall EJ, Land CE, et al. (2003) Cancer risks attributable to low doses of ionizing radiation: assessing what we really know. Proc Natl Acad Sci U S A 100: 13761–13766.
13. Hall EJ, Brenner DJ (2008) Cancer risks from diagnostic radiology. Br J Radiol 81: 362–378.
14. Einstein AJ (2009) Medical imaging: the radiation issue. Nat Rev Cardiol 6: 436–438.
15. Rozen WM, Stella DL, Phillips TJ, Ashton MW, Corlett RJ, et al. (2008) Magnetic resonance angiography in the preoperative planning of DIEA perforator flaps. Plast Reconstr Surg 122: 222e–223e.
16. Fukaya E, Grossman RF, Saloner D, Leon P, Nozaki M, et al. (2007) Magnetic resonance angiography for free fibula flap transfer. J Reconstr Microsurg 23: 205–211.
17. Wang MS, Haynor DR, Wilson GJ, Leiner T, Maki JH (2007) Maximizing contrast-to-noise ratio in ultra-high resolution peripheral MR angiography using a blood pool agent and parallel imaging. J Magn Reson Imaging 26: 580–588.
18. Hartmann M, Wiethoff AJ, Hentrich HR, Rohrer M (2006) Initial imaging recommendations for Vasovist angiography. Eur Radiol 16 Suppl 2: B15–23.
19. Rohrer M, Bauer H, Mintorovitch J, Requardt M, Weinmann HJ (2005) Comparison of magnetic properties of MRI contrast media solutions at different magnetic field strengths. Invest Radiol 40: 715–724.
20. de Vries M, de Koning PJ, de Haan MW, Kessels AG, Nelemans PJ, et al. (2005) Accuracy of semiautomated analysis of 3D contrast-enhanced magnetic resonance angiography for detection and quantification of aortoiliac stenoses. Invest Radiol 40: 495–503.
21. DL P, EM H (1993) Signal-to-noise, contrat-to-noise, and resolution. In: DL P, EM H, JE S, A G, editors. Magnetic resonance angiography: concepts and applications. St. Louis. pp. 56–79.

23

Reconstruction of the Abdominal Vagus Nerve Using Sural Nerve Grafts in Canine Models

Jingbo Liu[1,2,3❾], Jun Wang[4❾], Fen Luo[4*], Zhiming Wang[4*], Yin Wang[5]

1 Department of Hand Surgery, Huashan Hospital, Fudan University, Shanghai, China, **2** Key Laboratory of Hand Reconstruction, Ministry of Health, Shanghai, China, **3** Key Laboratory of Peripheral Nerve and Microsurgery, Shanghai, China, **4** Department of General Surgery, Huashan Hospital, Fudan University, Shanghai, China, **5** Department of Neuropathology, Huashan Hospital, Fudan University, Shanghai, China

Abstract

Background: Recently, vagus nerve preservation or reconstruction of vagus has received increasing attention. The present study aimed to investigate the feasibility of reconstructing the severed vagal trunk using an autologous sural nerve graft.

Methods: Ten adult Beagle dogs were randomly assigned to two groups of five, the nerve grafting group (TG) and the vagal resection group (VG). The gastric secretion and emptying functions in both groups were assessed using Hollander insulin and acetaminophen tests before surgery and three months after surgery. All dogs underwent laparotomy under general anesthesia. In TG group, latency and conduction velocity of the action potential in a vagal trunk were measured, and then nerves of 4 cm long were cut from the abdominal anterior and posterior vagal trunks. Two segments of autologous sural nerve were collected for performing end-to-end anastomoses with the cut ends of vagal trunk (8–0 nylon suture, 3 sutures for each anastomosis). Dogs in VG group only underwent partial resections of the anterior and posterior vagal trunks. Laparotomy was performed in dogs of TG group, and latency and conduction velocity of the action potential in their vagal trunks were measured. The grafted nerve segment was removed, and stained with anti-neurofilament protein and toluidine blue.

Results: Latency of the action potential in the vagal trunk was longer after surgery than before surgery in TG group, while the conduction velocity was lower after surgery. The gastric secretion and emptying functions were weaker after surgery in dogs of both groups, but in TG group they were significantly better than in VG group. Anti-neurofilament protein staining and toluidine blue staining showed there were nerve fibers crossing the anastomosis of the vagus and sural nerves in dogs of TG group.

Conclusion: Reconstruction of the vagus nerve using the sural nerve is technically feasible.

Editor: Robert E. Gross, Emory University, Georgia Institute of Technology, United States of America

Funding: These authors have no support or funding to report.

Competing Interests: The authors have declared that no competing interests exist.

* E-mail: Luofen1025@126.com (FL); Wzhm824@126.com (ZW)

❾ These authors contributed equally to this work.

Introduction

Radical resection of gastric cancer is currently the major procedure for treating of gastric cancer. Generally, the anterior and posterior vagal trunks should be cut off for complete dissection of the first, second and third groups of lymph nodes in the stomach.

Owing to fact that the hepatobiliary and abdominal cavity branches are cut at the same, removal of the anterior and posterior vagal trunks leads to a significant increase in the incidence of post-surgical gallstones [1,2], affects the vagal innervation of the small intestine, parts of the colon, and the pancreas, and affects the post-surgical digestive and absorptive functions of patients. Recently, with increases in the detection of early-stage gastric cancer and improvements in the techniques of radical operation, the overall 5-year survival rate in gastric cancer cases has improved greatly. Radical resection of gastric cancer focuses not only on completion of the resection, but also on preservation of the functions of organs as much as possible. Many experimental and clinical studies have found that radical resection of gastric cancer with vagus nerve preservation reduced the occurrence of post-surgical gallstones, increased gastrointestinal motility and gastric emptying ability, reduced the occurrence of post-surgical gastro-esophageal reflux, accelerated post-operative body weight recovery, and significantly improved post-surgical quality of life [3–5].

In some countries radical resection of gastric cancer with vagus nerve preservation has been performed, which mostly preserves the hepatobiliary and abdominal cavity branches of the nerve. Some are carried out under laparotomy, others under laparoscopy. The procedure has become a very active topic of research of surgical techniques.

However, whichever technique of vagus nerve preservation is employed in radical resection of gastric cancer, its use is mostly limited to early-stage disease. This may be attributed to the following: (1) Progression-stage gastric cancer has many perigastric

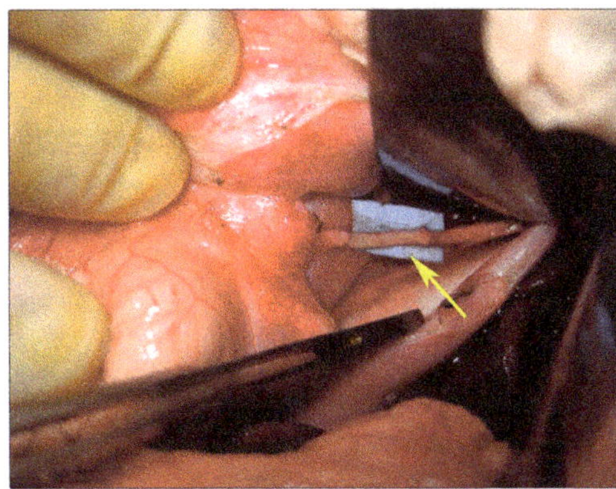

Figure 1. Anastomosis of the vagus nerve with the grafted segment of the sural nerve. The arrow indicates the grafted segment.

metastatic lymph nodes, and preservation of the vagus nerve may affect the removal of the nodes. (2) As progression-stage gastric cancer may directly invade the vagus nerve, preservation of the nerve may lead to incomplete removal of the tumor. Therefore, in order to completely remove the first group of lymph nodes and preserve the function of the hepatobiliary branch of the vagus nerve and the function of pylorus, the removal of the No.1 lymph node with resection of parts of the hepatobiliary branch was performed, followed by *in situ* anastomosis and reconstruction, which achieved good clinical outcomes [6,7]. However, that method cannot ensure removal of the No.3 and No.7 lymph nodes, unless parts of the vagus nerve are removed.

The best known situation in which removal of nerves during radical treatment of a malignant tumor leads to impairment of function is that of prostate cancer. In radical resection of prostate cancer, it is often necessary to remove the cavernous nerve, which causes post-operative erectile dysfunction [8]. Currently, two methods are used to improve post-operative erectile function: (1) unilateral nerve-sparing radical prostatectomy; and (2) unilateral nerve-sparing radical prostatectomy plus a sural nerve graft [5]. It has been reported that post-operative erectile function recovers significantly in patients who have undergone nerve preservation or nerve grafting [9–11].

Based on the success of partial resection of the vagus nerve followed by re-anastomosis and reconstruction for progression-stage gastric cancer (T2, T3) [6,7], the widespread use of cutaneous nerve grafts for repairing nerve defects in plastic surgery, and the fact that the sural nerve is employed to repair parasympathetic nerves in urological surgery, we hypothesized that resection of the vagus followed by re-anastomosis of the anterior and posterior vagal trunks and the hepatobiliary and abdominal cavity branches of the vagus nerve with sections of autologous sural nerve would preserve nerve function and improve quality of life by ensuring complete removal of the No.3 and No.7 lymph nodes.

In order to test this hypothesis, the present study explored the surgical techniques for repairing the hepatobiliary and abdominal cavity branches of the vagus nerve using the sural nerve, seeking experimental evidence for nerve regeneration after graft repair, and for recovery of secretary function of the gastrointestinal tract.

Materials and Methods

Materials

Ten adult Beagle dogs, each weighing 9–12 kg, were purchased from the Laboratory Animal Center of School of Agriculture and Biology, Shanghai Jiantong University. The action potential of the nerve trunk was measured using the Dantec Keypoint® electromyography (EMG)/evoked potentials (EP) system (Alpine Biomed, Denmark). Chitosan was purchased from Shanghai Qisheng Biological Preparation Co., Ltd. (Shanghai, China). Monoclonal mouse anti-human neurofilament protein (NF) was supplied by Dako (clone number: 2F11). The animals were randomly assigned to two groups of five, the nerve grafting group (TG) and the vagal resection group (VG). The protocols in this study were approved by institutional review board and the Animal Care and Use Committee of Huashan Hospital, Fudan University.

Detection of action potential of sural nerve graft and normal vagal trunk

The dogs in the TG group were injected with phenobarbital 25 mg/kg for induction of general anesthesia. Median laparotomy was performed in the middle and upper abdomen; the hepatogastric ligament and the left diaphragmatic angle were opened; and the abdominal esophagus was exposed to gain access to the anterior and posterior vagal trunks. A trunk of about 4.0 cm long was isolated, and stimulation and recording electrodes were placed on both sides 4.0 cm apart. The latency and conduction velocity of the action potential were measured and recorded. Segments of the anterior and posterior trunks were cut off 3 cm anterior to the hepatobiliary branch of the anterior vagal trunk, and the abdominal cavity branch of the posterior vagal trunk, each about 3.5 cm long. Two segments of sural nerve (4 cm) in the left lower limbs of dogs in the TG group were resected. End-to-end anastomosis was performed between the broken ends of the anterior and posterior vagal trunks and the epineurium of the sural nerve, using three sutures of 8–0 proline for each anastomosis (Fig. 1). The anastomosis site was sprayed with chitosan to prevent post-operative adhesion of the site to surrounding tissues.

Anesthesia and nerve isolation in dogs of the VG group were similar to those in the TG group, while the action potential was not measured. After removing parts of the vagal trunk (3.5 cm long), the cut part of the nerve was not anastomosed. When the stomach loses vagal innervation, the emptying and secretion functions are significantly affected. Whether the sural nerve graft led to recovery of the vagal innervation of the stomach could be studied for comparison with the TG group. All dogs received intravenous antibiotics. After two days of surgery, the dogs were given a liquid diet, after which a solid diet was provided.

Assessment of gastric secretion and emptying function

Gastric secretion and emptying function were assessed in dogs of the VG and TG group before surgery and three months after surgery. For gastric secretion function the Hollander insulin test [9] was used. The gastric tube was implanted in all dogs under general anesthesia after fasting for 24 h. After the gastric juice had drained out, it was collected every 10 min for a total of 6 times Dogs were then injected intravenously with insulin 0.2 U/kg, and the gastric juice was collected a further 6 times, again every 10 min. The acidity of gastric acid was titrated with 0.01 M NaOH. The maximal acid output (MAO) was calculated using the following formula:

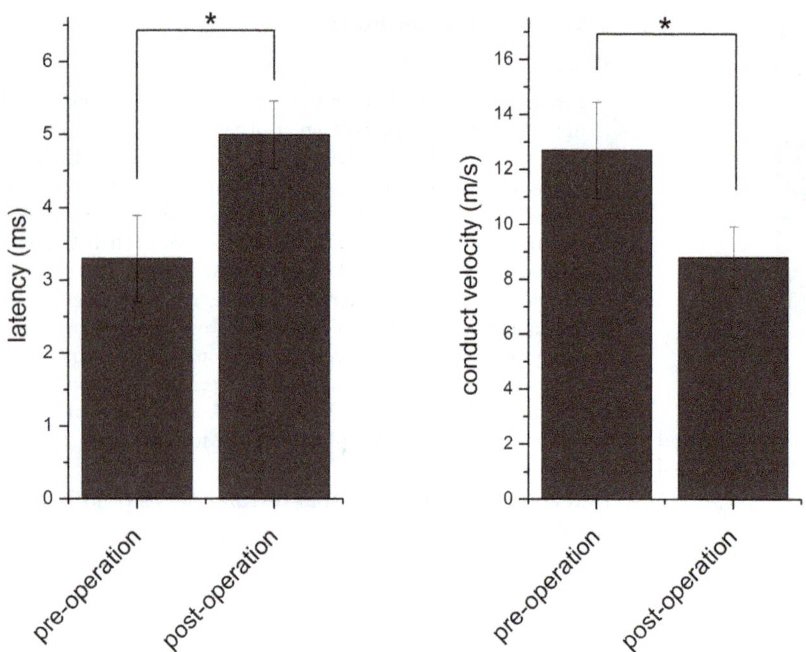

Figure 2. Changes in the latency and conduction velocity of the action potential in the vagal trunk of dogs in the TG group before and after surgery. * The difference before and after surgery was statistically significant ($P<0.05$).

$$\text{Acidity of gastric acid} = 1/10(\text{M}) \times 1000(\text{ml})/5(\text{ml}) \times a(\text{ml}) = 20 \times a(\text{mEq/L})$$

$$\text{MAO} = \text{acidity of gastric acid} \times b(\text{ml})/1000 = 1/50 \times a \times b(\text{mEq/h})$$

Where a indicates the amount of NaOH used for 5 ml of gastric acid

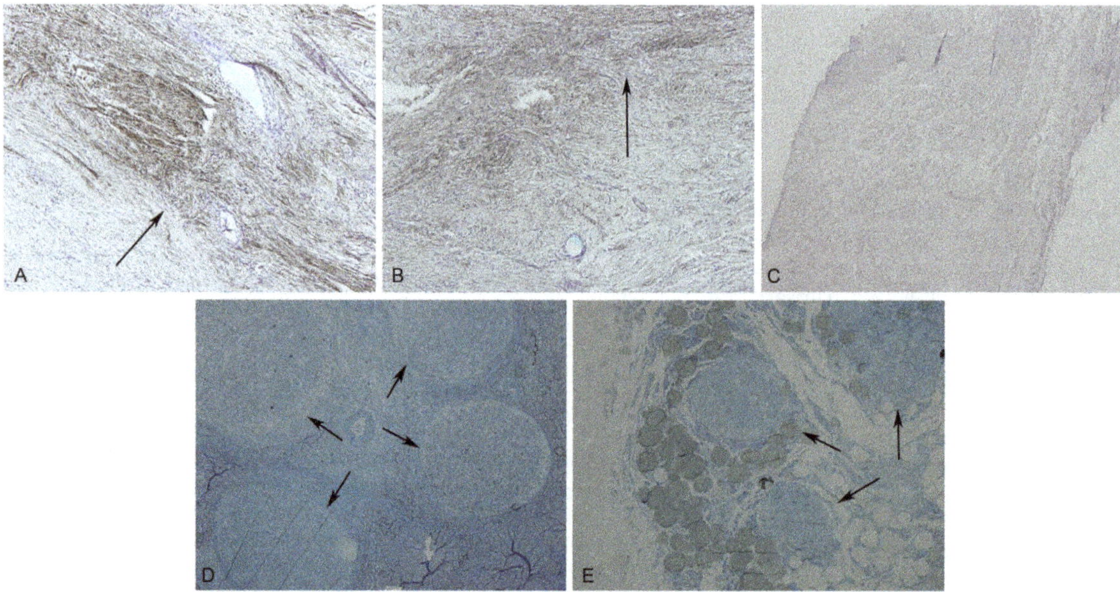

Figure 3. The anastomosis sites of the grafted nerves. A. The anastomosis site on the proximal grafted nerve (NF, ×40). The arrow indicates the anastomosis site. B. The anastomosis site on the distal grafted nerve (NF, ×40). The arrow indicates the anastomosis site. C. Negative control. D. The transverse section of the grafted nerve on the proximal grafted nerve. The arrow indicates the nerve fiber bundle. E. Transverse section of the vagus nerve on the distal grafted nerve. The arrow indicates the nerve fiber bundle.

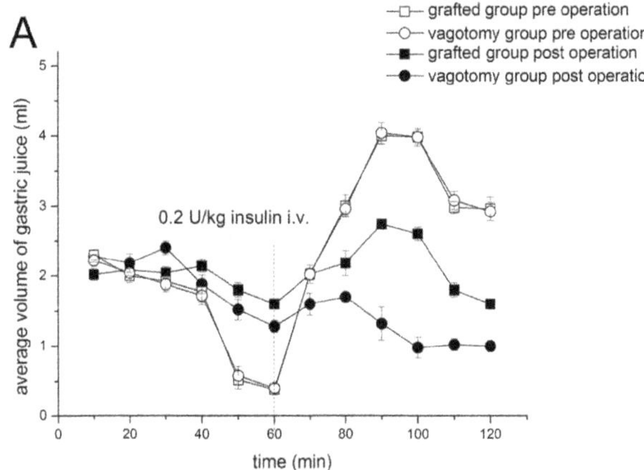

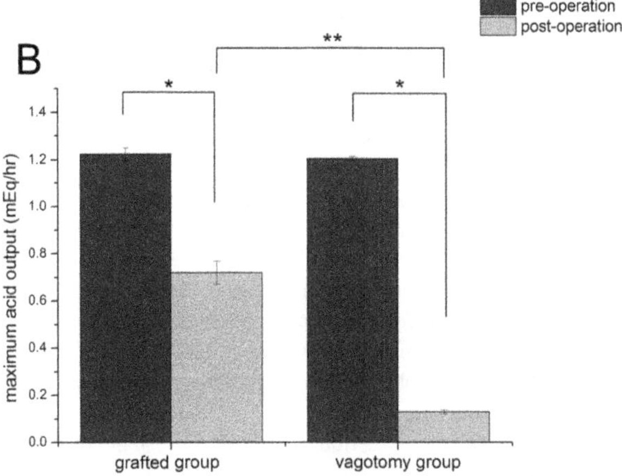

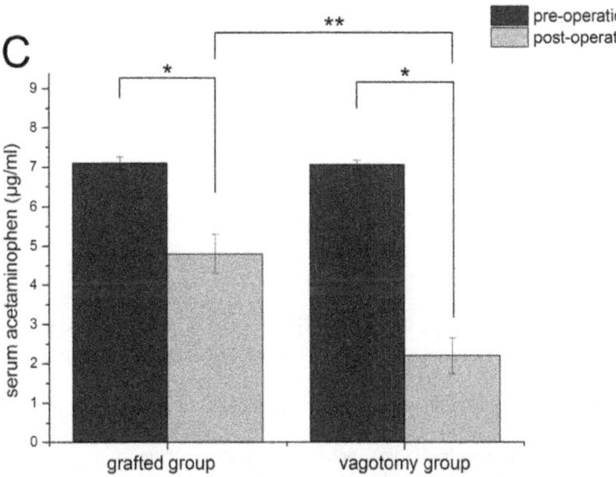

Figure 4. Gastric emptying and secretion function. A. Pre- and post-operation average volume of gastric juice secretion in vagotomy and grafted group. The vertical line indicates the i.v. application of insulin. B. Pre- and post-operation maximum acid output in vagotomy and grafted group. C. Pre- and post-operation serum acetaminophen in vagotomy and grafted group. * shows there are significant difference between pre- and post-operation ($P<0.05$). ** shows there are significant difference between vagotomy and grafted group ($P<0.05$).

titration solution with a pH value of 7, and *b* indicates the amount of gastric juice for 1 h.

Gastric emptying function was assessed using the acetaminophen test. After fasting for 24 h, the dogs were given 20 g bread and 200 ml milk containing acetaminophen at a dose of 0.025 g/kg body weight. After 45 min, blood samples were collected, and the acetaminophen concentration in blood was determined using high performance liquid chromatography (HPLC) [12].

Collection of the grafted nerve samples and detection of action potential in the nerve trunk

Laparotomy was performed in dogs of the TG group; the grafted segment of the vagus nerve was isolated; and the electrode was implanted into the lateral sides of the two anastomosis sites to record the action potential in the nerve trunk again. The grafted nerve and the anastomosis site were removed for examination. After surgery, the dogs in the TG group were sacrificed by injection with air. The dogs in the VG group did not undergo any other treatment, and were not sacrificed. All dogs in the TG group survived till the second surgery, while one dog in the VG group died of diarrhea one month after grafting.

Histology of the grafted nerve

Three grafted nerve samples were collected for examination in the Department of Neuropathology, Huashan Hospital Affiliated to Fudan University. Longitudinal sections were cut in the proximal and distal anastomosis sites, which were then stained with anti-NF. Two samples were collected for examination in the Section of Electron Microscopy, Shanghai Medical College of Fudan University. Semi-thin transverse sections were cut in the upper part of the proximal anastomosis site, lower part of the distal anastomosis site, and the grafted nerve, and then stained with toluidine blue.

Statistical analysis

All data were expressed as mean ± standard deviation (SD), and all statistical analyses were performed using the statistical software SPSS version 13.0 (SPSS, CA, USA). Differences between indices before and after surgery in the same group were tested for statistical significance using paired Student's *t*-test, while Student's *t*-test was used to compare different groups.

Results

Nerve grafting

Fig. 1 shows the anterior vagal trunk. A segment about 4 cm long was removed. The nerve between the two anastomosis sites is the grafted sural nerve.

Determination of action potential of the nerve trunk

The mean latency in the TG group after surgery was 5.0±0.5 ms, compared with 3.3±0.6 ms before surgery ($P<0.05$) (Fig. 2). The mean conduction velocity was 12.7±1.8 m/s before surgery, and 8.8±1.1 m/s after surgery ($P<0.05$). These results suggested that the grafted sural nerve retained some conduction function, although it was reduced.

Histomorphology of the grafted nerve

The NF staining of the grafted nerve with the anastomosis site is shown in Fig. 3A and B. The brown part of the figures indicates NF-positive nerve fibers. NF staining was positive on both sides of the anastomosis site. Toluidine blue staining of the semi-thin sections is shown in Fig. 3D and E. The blue dots in the figures indicate the cross-sections of the nerve fibers. It was found that there were nerve fibers crossing the anterior and posterior parts of the anastomosis site in the distal grafted nerve. After nerve injury, Wallerian degeneration occurred in the distal injured nerve within

2 weeks, and the axon disintegrated and was assimilated. If no regeneration of the grafted nerve occurred, the NF staining in the nerve of the distal anastomosis site appeared negative. Therefore, NF staining revealed that the regenerated nerve fibers had crossed the anastomosis site.

Gastric emptying and secretion function

Fig. 4A shows the average amount of gastric juice collected at each time point before and after surgery in the TG and VG groups. Fig. 4B shows MAO before and after surgery in the two groups. The difference was significantly smaller in the TG group than in the VG group, demonstrating that the recovery of gastric secretion function in the TG group was greater. Fig. 4C shows the results of the acetaminophen tests before and after surgery. In both groups serum acetaminophen concentration was significantly lower after surgery than before surgery. However, the difference in concentration before and after surgery in the TG group was significantly smaller than that in the VG group ($P<0.05$), indicating that the recovery of gastric emptying function was greater in the TG group than in the VG group.

Discussion

Our study has established the feasibility of recovering vagus nerve function by using a graft taken from the sural nerve. Two to three months after the sural nerve was grafted, both nerve staining and the detection of an action potential proved that the grafted nerve crossed the anastomosis site. Determination of gastric secretion and emptying function also showed that the neural innervation of stomach had partially recovered. Although the gastric emptying and secretion functions in the TG group were weaker than in the normal group, they were superior to those in the VG group.

When designing the experiment, there were two key questions: (1) Which autologous nerve should be selected as the graft donor? Or alternatively, should an artificial nerve donor be used? (2) Should both the hepatobiliary and abdominal cavity branches of the vagus nerve be removed and reconstructed, or should one be preserved while the other is reconstructed?

In this study, autologous sural nerve was used for nerve repair, which is widely used in peripheral nerve repair surgery. For instance, in repairing the cavernous nerve with the sural in urological surgery [13]. The problem of prostate cancer treatment is similar to that of treating gastric cancer. To ensure radical resection of tumors, the nerve may be cut, which leads to erectile dysfunction. Sural nerve grafting has been shown to be beneficial to patients with sexual dysfunction after prostate cancer surgery [13]. It has been reported that repair of the cavernous nerve using sural nerve grafts leads to 40%–60% recovery of erectile function [9,11,14]. Both the cavernous and vagus nerves are parasympathetic. Considering that sural nerve grafting can restore the function of the cavernous nerve, it was hoped that it could be used to restore vagus nerve function also. In addition, the sural nerve is easy to collect; the wound in the donor site is small; and its diameter is similar to that of the vagus nerve. Compared with an artificial nerve graft [15], a sural nerve graft provides not only a holder for nerve growth, but also nerve growth factor, which is why it was selected for the present study.

In this study, the two branches of the vagus nerve, hepatobiliary and abdominal cavity branches, were resected together and then reconstructed, which can be explained by two reasons. Firstly, since gastric cancer has a characteristic of submucosal diffusion and growth, and hepatobiliary and abdominal cavity branches both belong to the second station of nodes, these two branches then were generally both removed in a D2 radical resection in the progressive stage of gastric cancer. Secondly, In the present study, if we preserved a branch of the vagus nerve, it was difficult to prove that recovery of the function of the gastrointestinal tract was attributable to nerve reconstruction or nerve preservation, which was the second basis for resection and reconstruction of the hepatobiliary and abdominal cavity branches.

Our study has established the feasibility of improving the recovery of the function of the gastrointestinal tract using nerve grafting during radical resection of progression-stage of gastric cancer. Further studies are merited to investigate the possibility of replacing the autologous nerve with an artificial nerve graft plus nerve growth factor to overcome the problem of numbness and pain in the nerve donor region.

Author Contributions

Conceived and designed the experiments: FL ZMW. Performed the experiments: JBL FL. Analyzed the data: JBL JW. Contributed reagents/materials/analysis tools: YW. Wrote the paper: JBL JW.

References

1. Tomita R, Fujisaki S, Koshinaga T, Kusafuka T (2010) Clinical assessments in patients ten years after pylorus-preserving gastrectomy with or without preserving both pyloric and hepatic branches of the vagal nerve for early gastric cancer. Hepatogastroenterology 57: 984–988.
2. Fukagawa T, Katai H, Saka M, Morita S, Sano T, et al. (2009) Gallstone formation after gastric cancer surgery. J Gastrointest Surg 13: 886–889.
3. Hagiwara A, Imanishi T, Sakakura C, Otsuji E, Kitamura K, et al. (2002) Subtotal gastrectomy for cancer located in the greater curvature of the middle stomach with prevention of the left gastric artery. Am J Surg 183: 692–696.
4. Ando H, Mochiki E, Ohno T, Kogure N, Tanaka N, et al. (2008) Effect of distal subtotal gastrectomy with preservation of the celiac branch of the vagus nerve to gastrointestinal function: an experimental study in conscious dogs. Ann Surg 247: 976–986.
5. Ando S, Tsuji H (2008) Surgical technique of vagus nerve-preserving gastrectomy with D2 lymphadenectomy for gastric cancer. ANZ J Surg 78: 172–176.
6. Nomura E, Isozaki H, Fujii K, Toyoda M, Niki M, et al. (2003) Postoperative evaluation of function-preserving gastrectomy for early gastric cancer. Hepatogastroenterology 50: 2246–2250.
7. Kodama M, Arakawa A, Ito M, Koyama K (1997) The effects of convenient vagorrhaphy on the early recovery of gastric secretion and emptying: an experimental study on function-preserving gastric cancer surgery. Surg Today 27: 741–744.
8. Briganti A, Salonia A, Gallina A, Chun FK, Karakiewicz PI, et al. (2007) Management of erectile dysfunction after radical prostatectomy in 2007. World J Urol 25: 143–148.
9. Hanson GR, Borden LS Jr, Backous DD, Bayles SW, Corman JM (2008) Erectile function following unilateral cavernosal nerve replacement. Can J Urol 15: 3990–3993.
10. Davis JW, Chang DW, Chevray P, Wang R, Shen Y, et al. (2009) Randomized phase II trial evaluation of erectile function after attempted unilateral cavernous nerve-sparing retropubic radical prostatectomy with versus without unilateral sural nerve grafting for clinically localized prostate cancer. European urology 55: 1135–1144.
11. Porpiglia F, Ragni F, Terrone C, Renard J, Musso F, et al. (2005) Is laparoscopic unilateral sural nerve grafting during radical prostatectomy effective in retaining sexual potency? BJU Int 95: 1267–1271.
12. Flores-Pérez C, Chávez-Pacheco JL, Ramírez-Mendiola B, Alemón-Medina R, García-Álvarez R, et al. (2011) A reliable method of liquid chromatography for the quantification of acetaminophen and identification of its toxic metabolite N-acetyl-p-benzoquinoneimine for application in pediatric studies. Biomedical Chromatography 25: 760–766.
13. Burnett AL (2003) Neuroprotection and nerve grafts in the treatment of neurogenic erectile dysfunction. J Urol 170: S31–34; discussion S34.
14. Sim HG, Kliot M, Lange PH, Ellis WJ, Takayama TK, et al. (2006) Two-year outcome of unilateral sural nerve interposition graft after radical prostatectomy. Urology 68: 1290–1294.
15. Wolford LM, Rodrigues DB (2011) Autogenous grafts/allografts/conduits for bridging peripheral trigeminal nerve gaps. Atlas Oral Maxillofac Surg Clin North Am 19: 91–107.

24

Magnetic Resonance Imaging of the Ear for Patient-Specific Reconstructive Surgery

Luc Nimeskern[1], Eva-Maria Feldmann[2], Willy Kuo[1], Silke Schwarz[2], Eva Goldberg-Bockhorn[3], Susanne Dürr[3], Ralph Müller[1], Nicole Rotter[2], Kathryn S. Stok[1]*

1 Institute for Biomechanics, ETH Zurich, Zurich, Switzerland, **2** Department of Otorhinolaryngology, Ulm University Medical Center, Ulm, Germany, **3** Department of Diagnostic and Interventional Radiology, Ulm University Medical Center, Ulm, Germany

Abstract

Introduction: Like a fingerprint, ear shape is a unique personal feature that should be reconstructed with a high fidelity during reconstructive surgery. Ear cartilage tissue engineering (TE) advantageously offers the possibility to use novel 3D manufacturing techniques to reconstruct the ear, thus allowing for a detailed auricular shape. However it also requires detailed patient-specific images of the 3D cartilage structures of the patient's intact contralateral ear (if available). Therefore the aim of this study was to develop and evaluate an imaging strategy for acquiring patient-specific ear cartilage shape, with sufficient precision and accuracy for use in a clinical setting.

Methods and Materials: Magnetic resonance imaging (MRI) was performed on 14 volunteer and six cadaveric auricles and manually segmented. Reproducibility of cartilage volume (Cg.V), surface (Cg.S) and thickness (Cg.Th) was assessed, to determine whether raters could repeatedly define the same volume of interest. Additionally, six cadaveric auricles were harvested, scanned and segmented using the same procedure, then dissected and scanned using high resolution micro-CT. Correlation between MR and micro-CT measurements was assessed to determine accuracy.

Results: Good inter- and intra-rater reproducibility was observed (precision errors <4% for Cg.S and <9% for Cg.V and Cg.Th). Intraclass correlations were good for Cg.V and Cg.S (>0.82), but low for Cg.Th (<0.23) due to similar average Cg.Th between patients. However Pearson's coefficients showed that the ability to detect local cartilage shape variations is unaffected. Good correlation between clinical MRI and micro-CT (r>0.95) demonstrated high accuracy.

Discussion and Conclusion: This study demonstrated that precision and accuracy of the proposed method was high enough to detect patient-specific variation in ear cartilage geometry. The present study provides a clinical strategy to access the necessary information required for the production of 3D ear scaffolds for TE purposes, including detailed patient-specific shape. Furthermore, the protocol is applicable in daily clinical practice with existing infrastructure.

Editor: Joseph Najbauer, University of Pécs Medical School, Hungary

Funding: This study was supported by the Swiss National Science Foundation (NRP63) and ERANET/EuroNanoMed (EAREG-406340-131009/1). The funders had no role in study design, data collection and analysis, decision to publish, or preparation of the manuscript.

Competing Interests: The authors have declared that no competing interests exist.

* Email: kas@ethz.ch

Introduction

A key aspect of tissue-engineering (TE) strategies and reconstructive surgery of the ear, nose and throat (ENT) is the final shape of the reconstructed organ. Since aesthetics and patient satisfaction are critical criteria of success for these procedures [1,2], patient-specific organ shape alongside long-term shape stability must be achieved. Like a fingerprint, ear shape is a unique personal feature [3–5] that should be reconstructed with a high fidelity. This has been recognized as a particularly acute issue for the outer ear [6–9] due to its "*complex architecture and largely unsupported, protruding, three-dimensional structure*" [9].

To repair trauma affecting the outer part of the ear for patients with high comorbidity, epitheses are typically used [10,11] to minimize the risks of complications. Otherwise, surgical solutions are the only other alternatives available today. For this, there are two approaches – autologous reconstruction and synthetic implants [12]. In autologous reconstruction, autologous cartilage is used to create a 3D cartilage framework that mimics the intact contralateral ear which is then implanted subcutaneously at the defect site [10,12–15]. However this procedure presents a significant complication risk, in particular for total ear reconstruction due to donor site morbidity following cartilage harvesting [16]. Additionally the aesthetic outcome is highly dependent on the skill of the surgeon, because the implanted ear framework is made of assembled autologous cartilage pieces carved by hand [17]. Alternatively synthetic implants such as polyethylene implants [18] can be implanted with a better cosmetic outcome but higher risk for infection and extrusion [19,20]. TE applied to reconstructive surgery has gained recently wide attention as a way to alleviate these shortcomings [21]. Ear cartilage TE would potentially obviate the need for hand-carved cartilage frameworks or synthetic implants, by replacing these with a cell-seeded artificial scaffold [21]. Various strategies have been investigated, such as polymeric scaffolds [7], hydrogels [8] or biodegradable scaffolds with a non-biodegradable core [9]. TE advantageously offers also the possibility to use manufacturing techniques for scaffold production [6], which allow more detailed and controlled shapes. However, as such scaffolds are meant to be implanted subcutaneously in order to replace the lost cartilage, these should not be made in the shape of the patient external ear but in the shape of its internal cartilage structure. Hence for an optimal outcome, TE scaffold manufacturing should be combined with 3D imaging techniques so as to obtain detailed and patient-specific scaffolds that mimic the cartilage structure of the patient's intact contralateral ear (if available).

Protocols are already available for the production of 3D scaffolds with customizable shape using computer-aided design and manufacturing techniques [6,22]. For example, Reiffler et al. [22] demonstrated the production of collagen type I scaffolds with patient-specific ear shape. However, imaging techniques such as computed tomography [6] (CT) or digital photogrammetry [22] are limited to the external ear shape. The use of MRI for rapid prototyping of 3D ear epitheses was also reported, although here as well the authors aim at reproducing the external ear shape and not its specific tissue structures [23,24], i.e. skin, fat and cartilage tissues were imaged as one structure, and no information about the unique cartilage structure present in the auricle was obtained. [23,24]Therefore, in this study, the aim is to develop an imaging protocol that allows for segmentation of ear cartilage only and uses resources that are clinically available. Magnetic resonance imaging (MRI), which is a state of the art non-invasive modality for articular cartilage diagnostics, has been identified as a promising technique due to its good soft tissue contrast and widespread availability [25–27].

In order to characterize the quality of an imaging strategy it is necessary to assess its precision and accuracy [28]. Precision is a measure of the error introduced by the operators performing the measurement and analysis. This is important if segmentation of cartilage, whether manual or computer-based, is required. In other words, measures of precision assess whether the 3D ear cartilage shape obtained depends on the operator involved [29]. Accuracy evaluation compares the new method to a standard for high-resolution 3D imaging, such as micro-computed tomography [30] (micro-CT). This indicates how close the 3D ear cartilage shape, obtained with the new strategy, is to true cartilage shape.

The present study aims to identify a potential clinical solution for patient-specific ear shape imaging and to evaluate whether this new strategy can be applied with sufficient accuracy and precision in a clinical setting. It will be assessed whether switching the personnel dedicated to this task (the raters) affects the evaluation of the ear cartilage shape (inter- and intra-rater precision) and whether this method characterizes the true shape of the ear cartilage (accuracy using micro-CT as the standard).

Materials and Methods

Ethics Statement

All subjects gave their written informed consent to the study. The study was approved by the institutional review board of the Ulm University (Ethikantrag 150/12, Ethical Committee, Ulm University).

Identification of an imaging strategy of human ear cartilage

Pilot work was conducted in order to identify the optimal MRI sequences for imaging of human ear cartilage. This sequence must provide resolution and contrast high enough to visually distinguish ear cartilage from the surrounding tissues (perichondrium, skin

Inter-rater repeated measures

Intra-rater repeated measures

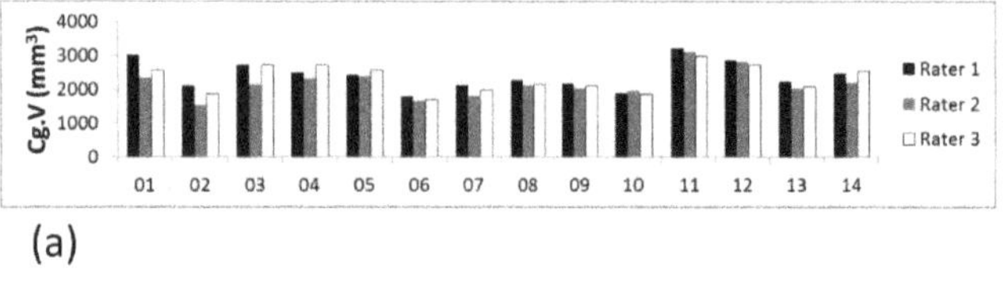

(a)

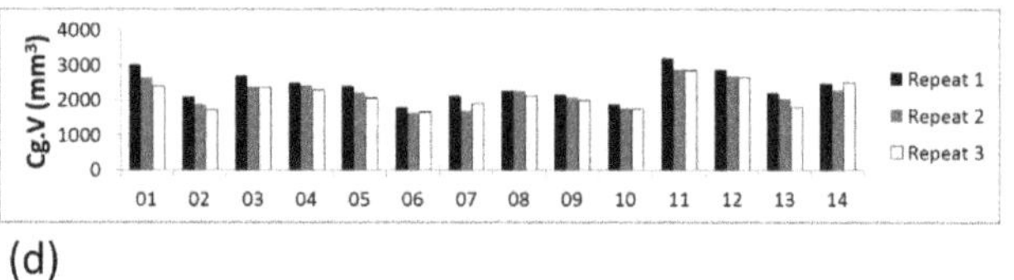

(d)

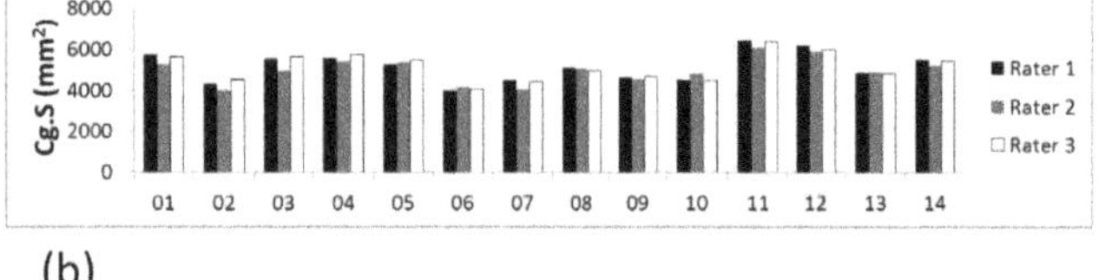

(b)

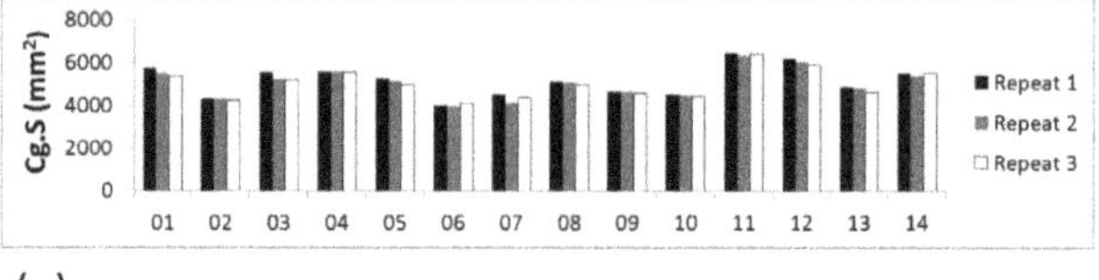

(e)

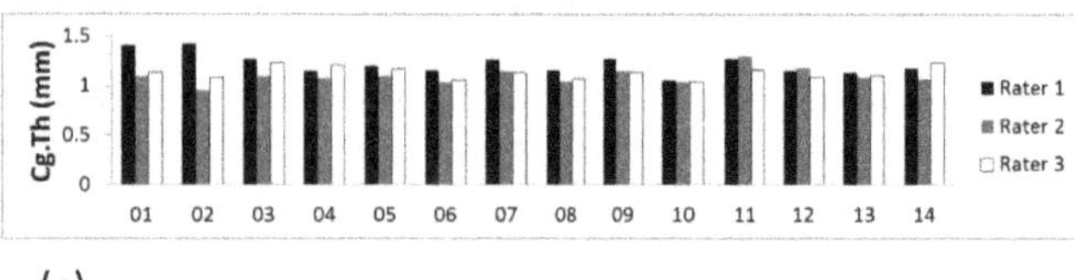

(c)

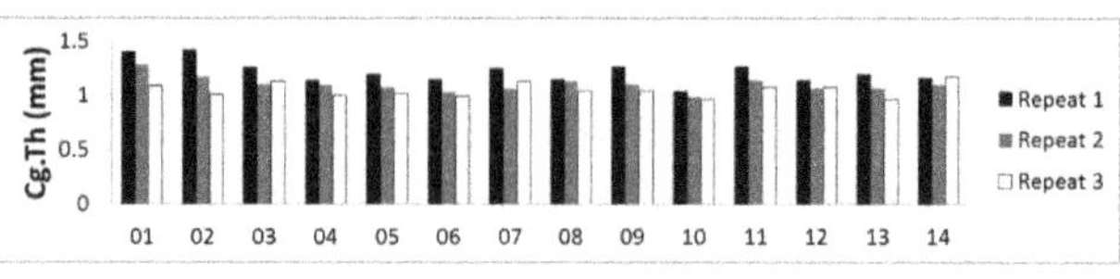

(f)

Figure 1. Inter-rater (a, b c) and intra-rater (d, e, f) repeated measures for cartilage volume (Cg.V), cartilage surface (Cg.S) and mean cartilage thickness (Cg.Th) for all 14 volunteers. Good reproducibility is observed for Cg.V and Cg.S values. Additionally low patient-to-patient variations are observed for Cg.Th, i.e. Cg.Th for all 14 volunteers and all three raters is 1.15±0.10 mm, whereas the average Cg.V and Cg.S are 2295±415 mm^3 and 5102±667 mm^2, respectively.

Table 1. Mean, precision error (PE_{SD}), precision error expressed as a percentage of coefficient of variation of the repeated measurements ($PE_{\%CV}$) and intraclass correlation coefficient (ICC) computed using a two-way model (absolute agreement for single measurements) for inter-rater reproducibility.

Inter-rater reproducibility	Cg.V	Cg.S	Cg.Th
Mean	2295.3 mm^3	5101.8 mm^2	1.15 mm
PE_{SD}	182.6 mm^3	188.6 mm^2	0.10 mm
$PE_{\%CV}$	7.98%	3.74%	8.45%
ICC	0.82	0.92	0.08

and adipose tissue). MRI scans of the ear were performed on healthy volunteers with a clinical MRI (Magnetom Skyra 3T, Siemens AG, Erlangen, Germany) equipped with a head coil (Head/Neck 20, A 3T Tim Coil). Four different sequences were acquired (n = 1, each); spoiled gradient-echo with (FS-SGE) and without (SGE) fat saturation, SPACE (Sampling Perfection with Application optimized Contrasts by using different flip angle Evolutions) and MPRAGE (Magnetization Prepared Rapid Acquisition Gradient Echo). Additionally, FS-SGE sequences at 0.45 mm and 0.30 mm resolution were acquired (n = 3, each). The best visualization of ear cartilage was obtained with the FS-SGE sequences. Comparison between 0.30 mm and 0.45 mm resolution showed that at 0.30 mm resolution, the lower signal to noise ratio limited the ability to visualize ear cartilage despite a smaller voxel size. None of the pilot scans displayed sufficient contrast and resolution to allow for automated computer-based segmentation. Therefore, clinical MRI imaging with a FS-SGE sequence combined with manual segmentation was selected as a potential clinical solution for patient-specific ear shape imaging.

Precision measurement

MRI scanning was performed on the left ear of 14 volunteers with a clinical MRI system (Magnetom Skyra 3T, Siemens AG, Erlangen, Germany) equipped with a head coil (Head/Neck 20, A 3T Tim Coil). All volunteers gave written informed consent for the study. A FS-SGE sequence was used with an in-plane (XY, sagittal plane) resolution of 0.45 mm x 0.45 mm and an out-of-plane (Z, orthogonal to the sagittal plane) resolution of 0.40 mm.

Datasets were scaled up five times in the X and Z directions in order to allow more precise manual contouring in a later step. For each scan, the operators performing manual segmentation were asked to browse the image stack and manually delineate the ear cartilage which would provide a mask of the tissue (micro-CT Evaluation Program 6.5–1 for VMS; Scanco Medical AG, Brüttisellen, Switzerland). Each operator was first trained on three datasets, which were not included in the subsequent analysis. Three different raters (referred to as rater 1, rater 2 and rater 3) independently segmented all 14 scans once (total of 42 masks). Additionally, rater 1 segmented all 14 scans three times. This yielded in one hand, 3 sets of 14 masks created by 3 different raters, which were used to assess whether masks obtained by the different raters were similar (inter-rater reproducibility). On the other hand, the 3 sets of 14 masks created by the same rater (rater 1) were used to assess whether one rater was able to reproduce the same result multiple times (intra-rater reproducibility).

In order to compare the masks obtained by the different raters, morphological characterization was performed. The masks were scaled isotropically, and cartilage volume (Cg.V), surface (Cg.S), and mean thickness (Cg.Th) were computed using in-house scripts, as described previously [28]. Photographs of the left ears of all 14 volunteers were taken for visual comparison with the segmented datasets.

Accuracy measurement

Six cadaveric auricles were harvested by Science Care (Phoenix, Arizona, USA, n = 4) and the Erasmus Medical Center (Rotterdam, The Netherlands, n = 2). In line with the ethical guidelines of the respective institutions (Ethikantrag 150/12, Ethical Committee, Ulm University), harvesting of human material was performed with prior written informed consent of the donor.

The 6 cadaveric auricles were immersed in an agarose gel, in order to enhance the signal to noise ratio, and scanned using the clinical MRI procedure described above. Manual segmentation was performed by rater 1, and Cg.V, Cg.S, and Cg.Th were computed as described above.

After scanning, the auricles were dissected in order to remove all tissue surrounding the cartilage and immersed overnight in a solution of PBS with 40% Hexabrix (Mallinckrodt Inc., St Louis, MO, USA). Hexabrix is a clinical contrast agent used routinely in MRI. In the present setup, Hexabrix increases the X-ray

Table 2. Mean, PE_{SD}, $PE_{\%CV}$ and ICC for intra-rater reproducibility.

Intra-rater reproducibility	Cg.V	Cg.S	Cg.Th
Mean	2253.7 mm^3	5073.4 mm^2	1.13 mm
PE_{SD}	163.6 mm^3	116.2 mm^2	0.10 mm
$PE_{\%CV}$	7.19%	2.33%	8.87%
ICC	0.84	0.97	0.23

$PE_{\%CV}$ values are below 5% for Cg.S and below 10% for Cg.V and Cg.Th which demonstrates good precision. ICC values obtained in both inter-rater and intra-rater measurements are good for Cg.V and Cg.S, but very low for Cg.Th. This indicates that the proposed method is adequate to distinguish patient-specific variations for Cg.V and Cg.S only.

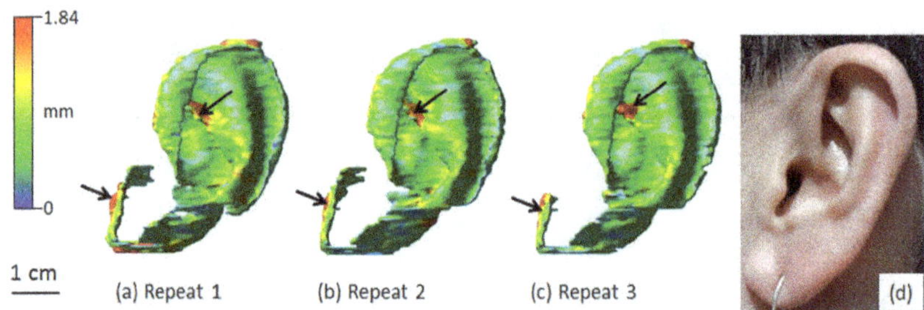

Figure 2. (a,b,c) Thickness maps of a typical set of three ear cartilage masks obtained by clinical MRI imaging combined with manual segmentation, all 3 masks were obtained by rater 1 (intra-rater repeated measures). (d) Corresponding photograph of the volunteer ear. Identical shapes (a, b, c and d) as well as matching regions of higher thickness (a, b and c) can be observed (arrows). Scale bar: 1 cm.

absorption of the cartilage, resulting in improved contrast in the subsequent micro-CT scan. One percent antimycotic-antibiotic (Gibco, Life Technologies, Carlsbad, CA, USA) was added to the solution to prevent tissue degradation. The dissected ear cartilage was scanned in air using micro-CT (µCT100, Scanco Medical AG, Brüttisellen, Switzerland) with an isotropic voxel size of 36.8 µm, 45 kVp energy, 88 µA intensity and 200 ms integration time. Threefold frame averaging was selected to improve the signal-to-noise ratio. A Gaussian filter ($\sigma = 1.2$, support = 1) and a threshold (linear attenuation between 0.9 cm^{-1} and 2.2 cm^{-1}) were then applied to segment the dissected cartilage from the background noise. Cg.V, Cg.S, and Cg.Th were computed as described above.

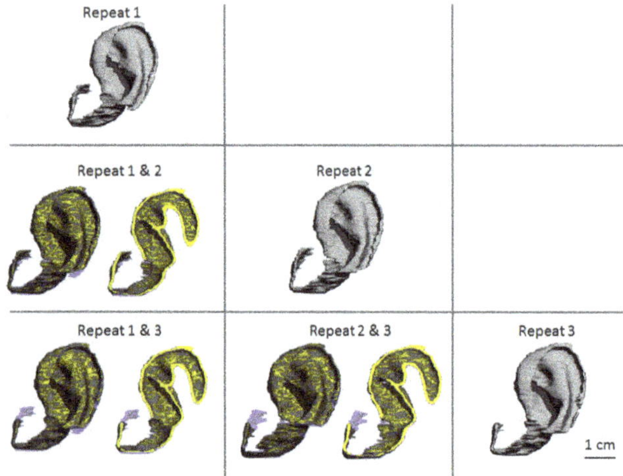

Figure 3. Pairwise comparisons of the three repeated masks obtained by rater 1 for a typical volunteer. The three masks obtained by segmentation are display in the diagonal. These masks are superimposed two-by-two, each overlapped pair of masks (left-hand side) and a corresponding cross-section (right-hand side) are displayed. Common regions are represented in yellow. The areas that belong to only one of the two masks are semi-transparent. Large common regions are observed in all three overlapped pairs of masks, i.e. the overall integrity of shape is maintained, with minor surface variations. This demonstrates that the inability to detect patient-specific variation for mean Cg.Th (low ICC) does not adversely affect the capacity of the proposed clinical method to detect local shape variations within a volunteer auricle. Scale bar: 1 cm.

Statistical analysis

Precision error (PE) calculation in imaging technology was introduced by Glüer et al. to characterize the reproducibility of a given measurement technique [29]. For inter-rater and intra-rater precision studies, PE was calculated for Cg.V, Cg.S, and Cg.Th and expressed as a percentage of the coefficient of variation of the repeated measurements [31] ($PE_{\%CV}$). A set of 14 measurements with three raters ensures 27 degrees of freedom as recommended [29]. The intraclass correlation coefficient (ICC, ranging from 0 to 1) was computed using a two-way model (absolute agreement for single measurements) as described previously [32]. For both inter-rater and intra-rater reproducibility, PEs describe the variations between the three masks obtained for any patient, and ICCs whether the precision is high enough to detect differences between patients. Additionally Pearson's correlation coefficient (r) was used for pairwise comparisons of the masks obtained in both reproducibility studies [33]. Pearson's correlation coefficient indicates whether raters consistently identify local variations in the contoured shape.

All statistics were performed with the SPSS software package (SPSS 20.0 for Windows; SPSS Inc., Chicago, IL, USA). All results are displayed as mean ± standard deviation.

Results

Identification of an imaging strategy of human ear cartilage

In a preliminary study a potential clinical solution for patient-specific ear shape imaging was identified. This solution combines clinical MRI (FS-SGE sequence) with an in-plane (XY, sagittal plane) resolution of 0.45 mm x 0.45 mm and an out-of-plane (Z, orthogonal to the sagittal plane) resolution of 0.40 mm, with manual segmentation to acquire the ear cartilage image.

Precision measurement

Each operator demonstrated a steep learning curve while working on the three training datasets, being able to identify cartilage after the third training dataset. Cg.V, Cg.S, and Cg.Th measured on all 14 volunteers are displayed in Figure 1. Figure 1 a, b, c shows values obtained by the three different raters (inter-rater reproducibility), while Figure 1 d, e, f displays the three repeated measurements performed by rater 1 (intra-rater reproducibility). High similarity between the three repeated measurements obtained for all patients were observed. Additionally, average Cg.V and Cg.S are 2295±415 mm^3 and 5102±667 mm^2 for all 14 volunteers and all three raters, respectively, while, small patient-to-patient variations (i.e. low standard deviation) were

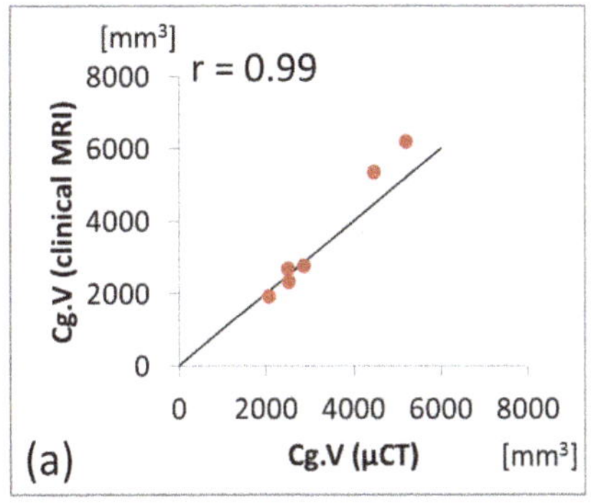

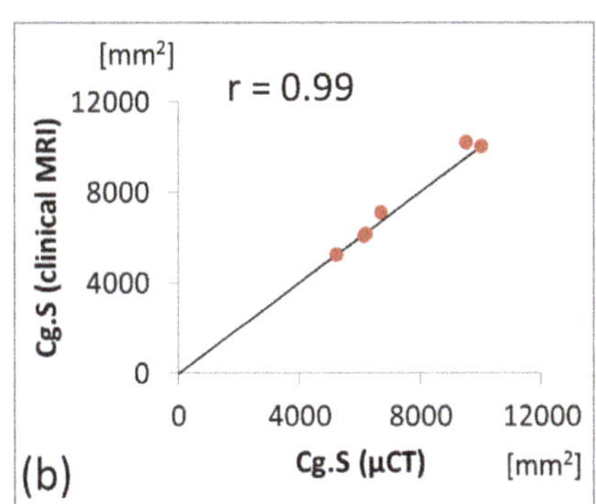

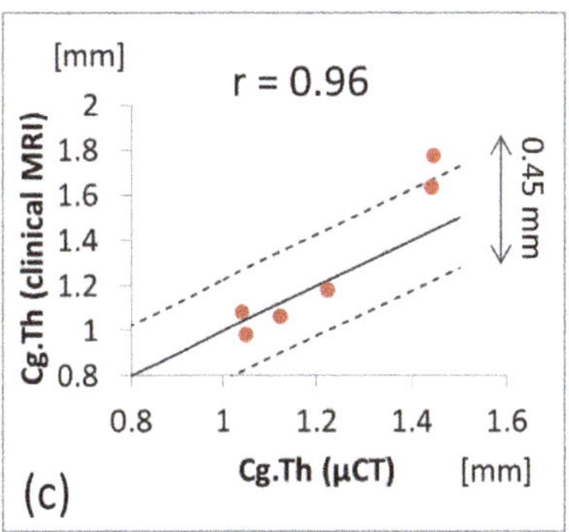

Figure 4. Correlation between values measured with contrast-enhanced micro-CT (after dissection) and values obtained by clinical MRI imaging combined with manual segmentation. Solid line represents y = x. (a) A correlation of r = 0.99 is observed for cartilage surface (Cg.S), (b) r = 0.99 for cartilage volume (Cg.V), (c) r = 0.96 for mean cartilage thickness (Cg.Th), dotted lines represented a 1-voxel error (0.45 mm) on the MRI datasets.

observed for cartilage thickness, i.e. average Cg.Th was 1.15±0.10 mm.

Corresponding $PE_{\%CV}$ and ICC values are displayed in Tables 1 and 2. For both the inter-rater and the intra-rater reproducibility $PE_{\%CV}$ were below 4% for Cg.S and below 9% for Cg.V and Cg.Th. Higher precision in Cg.V and Cg.S was observed for intra-rater when compared to inter-rater reproducibility (e.g. inter-rater vs. intra-rater $PE_{\%CV}$ is 7.98% vs. 7.19% for Cg.V, and 3.74% vs. 2.33% for Cg.S). ICC values obtained in both inter-rater and intra-rater measurements were satisfying for Cg.V (0.82 and 0.84 respectively), very good for Cg.S (0.92 and 0.97 respectively), but very low for Cg.Th (0.08 and 0.23 respectively).

Figure 2 (a, b and c) shows thickness maps of a set of three repeated ear cartilage masks obtained by rater 1 for a typical volunteer, additionally Figure 2 (d) displays a photograph of the corresponding volunteer ear. Identical gross shape (a, b, c and d) as well as matching regions of thickness variation (a, b and c) can be observed.

Good Pearson's coefficients for pairwise comparison within inter-rater reproducibility study (average r value for 42 pairwise combinations: 0.75±0.03) and the intra-rater (average r value for 42 pairwise combinations: 0.81±0.03) were obtained. Figure 3 displays the pairwise comparisons of the three repeated masks obtained by rater 1 for a typical volunteer, where it can be seen that the overall integrity of shape was maintained, with minor surface variations.

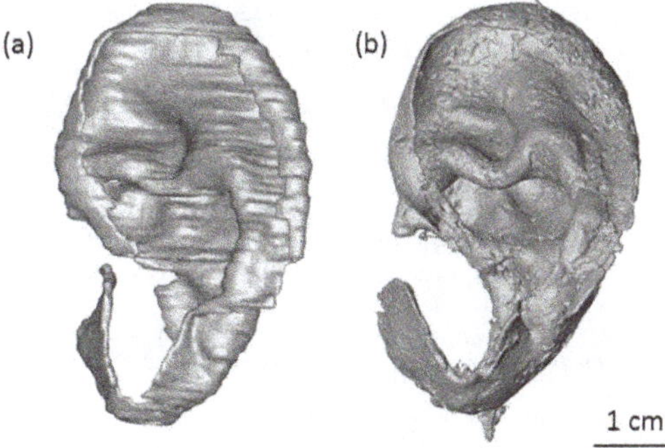

Figure 5. Visual comparison between ear cartilage masks used for accuracy measurement. (a) Cartilage mask obtained by clinical MRI imaging combined with manual segmentation, (b) mask obtained on the same cadaveric sample with contrast-enhanced micro-CT (after ear dissection). Scale bar: 1 cm.

Accuracy measurement

Figure 4 displays the values of Cg.V, Cg.S, and Cg.Th obtained by segmentation of the MRI datasets against the corresponding values obtained with micro-CT. Good correlation was observed between clinical MRI and micro-CT measurements of Cg.V (r = 0.99), Cg.S (r = 0.99), and Cg.Th (r = 0.96), see figure 4 and 5.

Discussion

The $PE_{\%CV}$ values (≤10%) observed for both inter- and intra-rater reproducibility demonstrated good precision (see Tables 1 and 2), i.e. the raters were able to repeatedly define the same volume of interest. Higher precision in Cg.V and Cg.S was observed for intra-rater when compared to inter-rater reproducibility (see Tables 1 and 2) which indicates that variations were smaller when only one rater was involved in the segmentation task. Additionally, whether inter- or intra-rater reproducibility measurements were considered, precision for Cg.S was the highest, followed by Cg.V and finally Cg.Th. To explain this ranking, two observations are necessary. Firstly, the limited spatial resolution of the MRI datasets (0.45 mm), compared to the measured mean cartilage thickness (1.13±0.11 mm), explains the low precision of the mean thickness measurements. Secondly, as ear cartilage shape can - in a first approximation - be considered as a layer-like structure (i.e. a curved sheet of cartilage with homogeneous thickness), Cg.V can be approximated as the product of Cg.S by Cg.Th. This implies that the measurement error on Cg.Th will propagate to Cg.V leading to a lower precision for Cg.V than for Cg.S.

From the measured $PE_{\%CV}$ it can be concluded that using the proposed technique all three parameters of interest can be measured with satisfying precision. As the gain in precision observed between intra- and inter-rater measurements is limited (see Tables 1 and 2), in a clinical set-up different personnel could be involved in this task without adversely influencing the outcome. Nevertheless, initial training will be very important to reduce error and increase consistency.

Similarly, better ICC was obtained for intra-rater repeated measures than for inter-rater repeated measures, which is a direct consequence of the better $PE_{\%CV}$ observed for intra-rater measurements. ICC values obtained in both inter- and intra-rater measurements were good for Cg.V (≥0.8) and for Cg.S (≥0.9), but very low for Cg.Th (≤0.3). ICC characterizes whether the precision of a measurement (i.e. its $PE_{\%CV}$ value) is good enough to detect variations between patients. Therefore the proposed clinical method is adequate to distinguish patient specific variations for Cg.V and Cg.S. However the precision of Cg.Th is too low for the detection of variations in mean cartilage thickness between patients. This is a combined effect of the low precision of Cg.Th (due to low MRI resolution, as explained earlier) and of the small patient to patient variation in mean cartilage thickness, see Figure 1 (a). However, despite low ICC for Cg.Th, satisfying pairwise correlations were observed for both inter- and intra-rater measurements, see Figure 3. This indicates that the inability to detect patient-specific variation of mean cartilage thickness does not affect the capacity of the proposed clinical method to detect local shape variations within an auricle.

In order to assess whether the proposed method for ear shape imaging is applicable in a clinical procedure for ear TE, its accuracy must also be evaluated. In other words, the masks produced with this MRI protocol have to be compared with the actual ear cartilage shape. There are no standard methods for quantitative imaging of ear cartilage. In literature the use of techniques such as clinical CT [6], digital photogrammetry [22] or MRI was limited to the acquisition of external ear shape only [23,24], As opposed to MRI, high resolution micro-CT imaging provides high spatial resolution down to the micrometer range [34], but on the other hand, soft-tissue contrast is low when compared to MRI. The use of contrast agents such as Hexabrix makes micro-CT imaging of soft-tissues possible [35]. Thanks to its greater spatial resolution, contrast enhanced high resolution micro-CT combined with dissection was used as a standard to assess the accuracy of the method. After dissection only the cartilage remains, therefore there is no need to segment it. Using contrast-enhanced micro-CT, cartilage is then readily imaged with a resolution more than ten times higher than MRI (36.8 μm for micro-CT vs. 450 μm for MRI), see figure 5. The good correlation observed between clinical MRI and micro-CT measurements of Cg.V, Cg.S, and Cg.Th show that the values obtained by the proposed clinical method can accurately predict ear cartilage thickness, surface and volume. As seen in Figure 4, Cg.Th values measured with the proposed clinical method differ by less than 0.4 mm (the spatial resolution of the MRI datasets) from their micro-CT counter parts. These values are very satisfying considering the resolution limitation inherent to clinical MRI. These results show that the new imaging strategy proposed is able to characterize the patient-specific ear cartilage shape.

In conclusion, clinical MRI imaging combined with manual segmentation of ear cartilage was demonstrated to be accurate. The precision of this new strategy was high enough to detect patient-specific variation in ear cartilage surface and volume, as well as local shape variations within a volunteer auricle. Precision was additionally shown to be independent of the personnel dedicated to the manual segmentation. Therefore, in a clinical set-up, different personnel could be involved in this task without adversely influencing the outcome. Finally, as the only requirements for this strategy are the access to clinical MRI and personnel for ear cartilage segmentation, this method is applicable in daily clinical practice with existing infrastructures. Alongside novel TE strategies currently under development [7–9], the resulting 3D ear masks have the potential to improve aesthetic outcomes of surgical reconstruction; and in turn give the patient their unique ear shape.

Acknowledgments

The authors would like to thank the donors and their families who enabled this research; as well as Stefan Klein (MD), Arthur Wunderlich (PhD), Birgit Köstler, Heike Wiedelbach and Brigitte Hiller for MRI support; Mieke Pleumeekers (MD) and Gerjo van Osch (PhD) for providing cadaveric samples; Duncan Pawson for support with illustrations.

Author Contributions

Conceived and designed the experiments: LN SS SD RM NR KSS. Performed the experiments: LN EF WK SS EG SD. Analyzed the data: LN RM NR KSS. Contributed reagents/materials/analysis tools: RM NR. Contributed to the writing of the manuscript: LN EF WK SS RM NR KSS.

References

1. Steffen A, Klaiber S, Katzbach R, Nitsch S, Konig IR, et al. (2008) The psychosocial consequences of reconstruction of severe ear defects or third-degree microtia with rib cartilage. Aesthet Surg J 28: 404–411.
2. Dinis PB, Dinis M, Gomes A (1998) Psychosocial consequences of nasal aesthetic and functional surgery: a controlled prospective study in an ENT setting. Rhinology 36: 32–36.
3. Sforza C, Grandi G, Binelli M, Tommasi DG, Rosati R, et al. (2009) Age- and sex-related changes in the normal human ear. Forensic Sci Int 187: 110. e111–117.
4. Meijerman L, van der Lugt C, Maat GJ (2007) Cross-sectional anthropometric study of the external ear. J Forensic Sci 52: 286–293.
5. Cummings AH, Nixon MS, Carter JN (2011) The image ray transform for structural feature detection. Pattern Recogn Lett 32: 2053–2060.
6. Liu Y, Zhang L, Zhou G, Li Q, Liu W, et al. (2010) In vitro engineering of human ear-shaped cartilage assisted with CAD/CAM technology. Biomaterials 31: 2176–2183.
7. Shieh S-J, Terada S, Vacanti JP (2004) Tissue engineering auricular reconstruction: in vitro and in vivo studies. Biomaterials 25: 1545–1557.
8. Kamil SH, Vacanti MP, Aminuddin BS, Jackson MJ, Vacanti CA, et al. (2004) Tissue engineering of a human sized and shaped auricle using a mold. The Laryngoscope 114: 867–870.
9. Zhou L, Pomerantseva I, Bassett EK, Bowley CM, Zhao X, et al. (2011) Engineering ear constructs with a composite scaffold to maintain dimensions. Tissue Eng Part A 17: 1573–1581.
10. Walton RL, Beahm EK (2002) Auricular reconstruction for microtia: part II. surgical techniques. Plast Reconstr Surg 110: 234–251.
11. Ledgerwood LG, Chao J, Tollefson TT (2014) Prosthetic reconstruction of complicated auricular defects: use of a hybrid prosthetic fabrication technique. JAMA Facial Plast Surg 16: 153–154.
12. Storck K, Staudenmaier R, Buchberger M, Strenger T, Kreutzer K, et al. (2014) Total reconstruction of the auricle: our experiences on indications and recent techniques. Biomed Res Int 2014: 373286.
13. Brent B (1992) Auricular repair with autogenous rib cartilage grafts: two decades of experience with 600 cases. Plast Reconstr Surg 90: 355–374.
14. Nagata S (1993) A new method of total reconstruction of the auricle for microtia. Plast Reconstr Surg 92: 187–201.
15. Kasrai L, Snyder-Warwick AK, Fisher DM (2014) Single-stage autologous ear reconstruction for microtia. Plast Reconstr Surg 133: 652–662.
16. Ohara K, Nakamura K, Ohta E (1997) Chest wall deformities and thoracic scoliosis after costal cartilage graft harvesting. Plast Reconstr Surg 99: 1030–1036.
17. Firmin F (1998) Ear reconstruction in cases of typical microtia. Personal experience based on 352 microtic ear corrections. Scand J Plast Reconstr Surg Hand Surg 32: 35–47.
18. Kludt NA, Vu H (2014) Auricular reconstruction with prolonged tissue expansion and porous polyethylene implants. Ann Plast Surg 72 Suppl 1: S14–17.
19. Constantine KK, Gilmore J, Lee K, Leach J, Jr. (2014) Comparison of Microtia Reconstruction Outcomes Using Rib Cartilage vs Porous Polyethylene Implant. JAMA Facial Plast Surg 75235.
20. Cenzi R, Farina A, Zuccarino L, Carinci F (2005) Clinical outcome of 285 Medpor grafts used for craniofacial reconstruction. J Craniofac Surg 16: 526–530.
21. Golas AR, Hernandez KA, Spector JA (2014) Tissue engineering for plastic surgeons: a primer. Aesthetic Plast Surg 38: 207–221.
22. Reiffel AJ, Kafka C, Hernandez KA, Popa S, Perez JL, et al. (2013) High-fidelity tissue engineering of patient-specific auricles for reconstruction of pediatric microtia and other auricular deformities. PloS one 8: e56506.
23. Turgut G, Sacak B, Kiran K, Bas L (2009) Use of rapid prototyping in prosthetic auricular restoration. J Craniofac Surg 20: 321–325.

24. Coward TJ, Watson RM, Wilkinson IC (1999) Fabrication of a wax ear by rapid-process modeling using stereolithography. Int J Prosthodont 12: 20–27.
25. Trattnig S, Mlynarik V, Huber M, Ba-Ssalamah A, Puig S, et al. (2000) Magnetic resonance imaging of articular cartilage and evaluation of cartilage disease. Invest Radiol 35: 595–601.
26. Bauer JS, Barr C, Henning TD, Malfair D, Ma CB, et al. (2008) Magnetic resonance imaging of the ankle at 3.0 Tesla and 1.5 Tesla in human cadaver specimens with artificially created lesions of cartilage and ligaments. Invest Radiol 43: 604–611.
27. Eckstein F, Cicuttini F, Raynauld JP, Waterton JC, Peterfy C (2006) Magnetic resonance imaging (MRI) of articular cartilage in knee osteoarthritis (OA): morphological assessment. Osteoarthr Cartil 14 Suppl A: A46–75.
28. Stok KS, Muller R (2009) Morphometric characterization of murine articular cartilage–novel application of confocal laser scanning microscopy. Microsc Res Tech 72: 650–658.
29. Glüer CC, Blake G, Lu Y, Blunt BA, Jergas M, et al. (1995) Accurate assessment of precision errors: how to measure the reproducibility of bone densitometry techniques. Osteoporos Int 5: 262–270.
30. Palmer AW, Guldberg RE, Levenston ME (2006) Analysis of cartilage matrix fixed charge density and three-dimensional morphology via contrast-enhanced microcomputed tomography. Proc Natl Acad Sci U S A 103: 19255–19260.
31. Kohler T, Beyeler M, Webster D, Muller R (2005) Compartmental bone morphometry in the mouse femur: reproducibility and resolution dependence of microtomographic measurements. Calcif Tissue Int 77: 281–290.
32. Mueller TL, Stauber M, Kohler T, Eckstein F, Muller R, et al. (2009) Non-invasive bone competence analysis by high-resolution pQCT: an in vitro reproducibility study on structural and mechanical properties at the human radius. Bone 44: 364–371.
33. Adler J, Parmryd I (2010) Quantifying colocalization by correlation: the Pearson correlation coefficient is superior to the Mander's overlap coefficient. Cytometry A 77: 733–742.
34. Bouxsein ML, Boyd SK, Christiansen BA, Guldberg RE, Jepsen KJ, et al. (2010) Guidelines for assessment of bone microstructure in rodents using micro-computed tomography. J Bone Miner Res 25: 1468–1486.
35. Xie L, Lin AS, Levenston ME, Guldberg RE (2009) Quantitative assessment of articular cartilage morphology via EPIC-microCT. Osteoarthritis Cartilage 17: 313–320.

Permissions

All chapters in this book were first published in PLOS ONE, by The Public Library of Science; hereby published with permission under the Creative Commons Attribution License or equivalent. Every chapter published in this book has been scrutinized by our experts. Their significance has been extensively debated. The topics covered herein carry significant findings which will fuel the growth of the discipline. They may even be implemented as practical applications or may be referred to as a beginning point for another development.

The contributors of this book come from diverse backgrounds, making this book a truly international effort. This book will bring forth new frontiers with its revolutionizing research information and detailed analysis of the nascent developments around the world.

We would like to thank all the contributing authors for lending their expertise to make the book truly unique. They have played a crucial role in the development of this book. Without their invaluable contributions this book wouldn't have been possible. They have made vital efforts to compile up to date information on the varied aspects of this subject to make this book a valuable addition to the collection of many professionals and students.

This book was conceptualized with the vision of imparting up-to-date information and advanced data in this field. To ensure the same, a matchless editorial board was set up. Every individual on the board went through rigorous rounds of assessment to prove their worth. After which they invested a large part of their time researching and compiling the most relevant data for our readers.

The editorial board has been involved in producing this book since its inception. They have spent rigorous hours researching and exploring the diverse topics which have resulted in the successful publishing of this book. They have passed on their knowledge of decades through this book. To expedite this challenging task, the publisher supported the team at every step. A small team of assistant editors was also appointed to further simplify the editing procedure and attain best results for the readers.

Apart from the editorial board, the designing team has also invested a significant amount of their time in understanding the subject and creating the most relevant covers. They scrutinized every image to scout for the most suitable representation of the subject and create an appropriate cover for the book.

The publishing team has been an ardent support to the editorial, designing and production team. Their endless efforts to recruit the best for this project, has resulted in the accomplishment of this book. They are a veteran in the field of academics and their pool of knowledge is as vast as their experience in printing. Their expertise and guidance has proved useful at every step. Their uncompromising quality standards have made this book an exceptional effort. Their encouragement from time to time has been an inspiration for everyone.

The publisher and the editorial board hope that this book will prove to be a valuable piece of knowledge for researchers, students, practitioners and scholars across the globe.

List of Contributors

Federica Zilio and Katja C. Meyer
Department of Dermatology, University of Lübeck, Lübeck, Germany

Marta Bertolini
Department of Dermatology, University of Lübeck, Lübeck, Germany
Department of Dermatology, University of Münster, Münster, Germany

Alfredo Rossi
Department of Internal Medicine and Medical Specialties, University "La Sapienza", Rome, Italy

Patrick Kleditzsch
Department of Gynaecology and Obstetrics, University of Rostock, Rostock, Germany

Vladimir E. Emelianov
Department of Pharmacology, Clinical Pharmacology and Biochemistry, Chuvash State University Medical School, Cheboksary, Russia

Amos Gilhar
Laboratory for Skin Research, Rappaport Faculty of Medicine, Technion-Israel Institute of Technology, Haifa, Israel
Flieman Medical Center, Haifa, Israe

Aviad Keren
Laboratory for Skin Research, Rappaport Faculty of Medicine, Technion-Israel Institute of Technology, Haifa, Israel

Eddy Wang and Kevin McElwee
Department of Dermatology and Skin Science, University of British Columbia, Vancouver, British Columbia, Canada

Wolfgang Funk
Klinik Dr. Koslowski, Munich, Germany

Ralf Paus
Department of Dermatology, University of Lübeck, Lübeck, Germany
Department of Dermatology, University of Münster, Münster, Germany
Institute for Inflammation and Repair, University of Manchester, Manchester, United Kingdom

Dolores Wolfram, Nadine Eberhart and Gerhard Pierer
Department of Plastic, Reconstructive and Aesthetic Surgery, Innsbruck Medical University, Innsbruck, Austria

Ravi Starzl
Language Technologies Institute, Carnegie Mellon University, Pittsburgh, Pennsylvania, United States of America

Hubert Hackl
Division of Bioinformatics, Biocenter, Innsbruck Medical University, Innsbruck, Austria

Derek Barclay and Yoram Vodovotz
Department of Immunology, University of Pittsburgh, Pittsburgh, Pennsylvania, United States of America

Theresa Hautz and Johann Pratschke
Department of Visceral, Transplant and Thoracic Surgery, Innsbruck Medical University, Innsbruck, Austria

Bettina Zelger
Department of Pathology, Innsbruck Medical University, Innsbruck, Austria

Gerald Brandacher and W. P. Andrew Lee
Department of Plastic and Reconstructive Surgery, Johns Hopkins University School of Medicine, Baltimore, Maryland, United States of America

Stefan Schneeberger
Department of Visceral, Transplant and Thoracic Surgery, Innsbruck Medical University, Innsbruck, Austria
Department of Plastic and Reconstructive Surgery, Johns Hopkins University School of Medicine, Baltimore, Maryland, United States of America

Yuan Zhang, Zhengxue Quan, Zenghui Zhao, Xiaoji Luo, Ke Tang, Jie Li, Xu Zhou and Dianming Jiang
Department of Orthopedic Surgery, The First Affiliated Hospital of Chongqing Medical

University, Chongqing, China

Weijun Fu, Xu Zhang, Peng Zhang, Jiangping Gao, Jun Dong, Guangfu Chen, Axiang Xu, Xin Ma, Hongzhao Li and Lixin Shi
Department of Urology, PLA General Hospital/ Medical school, Beijing, China

Xiaoyi Zhang
Department of Urology, The Second Artillery General Hospital of PLA, Beijing, China

Catherine Jackson
Department of Medical Biochemistry, Oslo University Hospital, Oslo, Norway
University of Oslo, Oslo, Norway

Torstein Lyberg and Jon R. Eidet
Department of Medical Biochemistry, Oslo University Hospital, Oslo, Norway

Peder Aabel
Ear, Nose and Throat Department, Division of Surgery, Akershus University Hospital, Lørenskog, Norway
Institute of Clinical Medicine, University of Oslo, Oslo, Norway

Magnus von Unge
Ear, Nose and Throat Department, Division of Surgery, Akershus University Hospital, Lørenskog, Norway
Institute of Clinical Medicine, University of Oslo, Oslo, Norway
Centre for Clinical Research, LT Vastmanland, Uppsala University, Uppsala, Sweden

Tor P. Utheim
Department of Medical Biochemistry, Oslo University Hospital, Oslo, Norway
Department of Oral Biology, Faculty of Dentistry, University of Oslo, Oslo, Norway

Edward B. Messelt
Department of Oral Biology, Faculty of Dentistry, University of Oslo, Oslo, Norway

XinYing Tan, JinChao Luo, HuaWei Liu and Min Hu
Department of stomatology, General Hospital of the PLA, Beijing, China

Wen Yue
Department of Stem Cell and Regenerative Medicine Lab, Beijing Institute of Transfusion Medicine, Beijing, China

ChangKui Liu
Department of stomatology, General Hospital of the PLA, Beijing, China
Department of Stomatology, The 451th hospital of the People's Libration Army, Xi'an, China

Javaneh Jahanshahi, Farnaz Hashemian, Sara Pazira, Farhad Farahani and Ruholah Abasi
Department of Ear-Nose-Throat Surgery, School of Medicine, Hamadan University of Medical Sciences, Hamadan, Iran

Mohammad Hossein Bakhshaei
Department of Anesthesiology, School of Medicine, Hamadan University of Medical Sciences, Hamadan, Iran

Jalal Poorolajal
Modeling of Noncommunicable Diseases Research Center, Department of Epidemiology & Biostatistics, School of Public Health, Hamadan University of Medical Sciences, Hamadan, Iran

Yujie Liu
Department of Orthopedic and Traumatic Surgery, General Hospital of Jinan Military Command, Jinan, P. R. China
The Hand Surgery Center of Chinese People's Liberation Army, The 401st Hospital of CPLA, Qingdao, P. R. China

Xuecheng Cao
Department of Orthopedic and Traumatic Surgery, General Hospital of Jinan Military Command, Jinan, P. R. China

Hongsheng Jiao, Xiang Ji, Chunlei Liu, Xiaopen Zhong, Hongxun Zhang and Xiaohen Ding
The Hand Surgery Center of Chinese People's Liberation Army, The 401st Hospital of CPLA, Qingdao, P. R. China

Canhua Jiang, Feng Guo, Ning Li, Wen Liu, Tong Su, Xinqun Chen, Lian Zheng and Xinchun Jian
Department of Oral and Maxillofacial Surgery, Xiangya Hospital, Central South University, Changsha, Hunan, China

Qingxiong Yu, Lingling Sheng, Ming Zhu, Xiaolu Huang and Qingfeng Li
Department of Plastic and Reconstructive Surgery,

Shanghai Ninth People's Hospital, Shanghai Jiao Tong University, School of Medicine, Shanghai, P.R. China

Mei Yang
Division of Plastic Surgery, Southern Illinois University School of Medicine, Springfield, Illinois, United States of America

Bruno Ramos Chrcanovic and Ann Wennerberg
Department of Prosthodontics, Faculty of Odontology, Malmö University, Malmö, Sweden

Tomas Albrektsson
Department of Prosthodontics, Faculty of Odontology, Malmö University, Malmö, Sweden
Department of Biomaterials, Göteborg University, Göteborg, Sweden

Jian-feng Pan, Ning-hua Liu and Hui Sun
Department of Orthopaedics, Shanghai Jiao Tong University Affiliated Sixth People's Hospital, Shanghai, China

Feng Xu
Department of Orthopaedics, Kunshan Traditional Chinese Medical Hospital, Suzhou, Jiangsu, China

Andrés A. Maldonado and Lara Cristóbal
Department of Plastic and Reconstructive Surgery and Burn Unit, University Hospital of Getafe, Madrid, Spain

Javier Martín-López
Department of Pathology, University Hospital of Puerta de Hierro, Madrid, Spain

Mar Mallén
Department of Genetics, University Hospital Central de la Defensa, Madrid, Spain

Natalio García-Honduvilla and Julia Buján
Department of Medical Specialties, Faculty of Medicine, University of Alcalá, Networking Research Centre on Bioengineering, Biomaterials and Nanomedicine (CIBER-BBN), Madrid, Spain

Geon A Kim, Hyun Ju Oh, Min Jung Kim, Young Kwang Jo, Jin Choi, Jung Eun Park, Eun Jung Park, Goo Jang and Byeong Chun Lee
Department of Theriogenology & Biotechnology, College of Veterinary Medicine, Seoul National University, Seoul, Republic of Korea

Sang Hyun Lim and Sung Keun Kang
Central Research Institutes, Kstem cell, Seoul, Republic of Korea

Byung Il Yoon
Laboratory of Histology and Molecular Pathogenesis, College of Veterinary Medicine, Kangwon National University, Chuncheon, Gangwon-do, Republic of Korea

Irene A. Slootweg
Professional Performance Research group, Center of Expertise in Evidence-based Education, Academic Medical Center, University of Amsterdam, Amsterdam, the Netherlands
Department of Educational Development and Research, University of Maastricht, Maastricht, the Netherlands

Kiki M. J. M. H. Lombarts, Benjamin C. M. Boerebach and Maas Jan Heineman
Professional Performance Research group, Center of Expertise in Evidence-based Education, Academic Medical Center, University of Amsterdam, Amsterdam, the Netherlands

Cees P. M. van der Vleuten
Department of Educational Development and Research, University of Maastricht, Maastricht, the Netherlands

Albert J. J. A. Scherpbier
Faculty of Health, Medicine and Life Sciences, University of Maastricht, Maastricht, the Netherlands

Syed Zulqarnain Gilani, Faisal Shafait and Ajmal Mian
School of Computer Science and Software Engineering, The University of Western Australia, Perth, Western Australia

Kathleen Rooney
School of Anatomy, Physiology and Human Biology, The University of Western Australia, Perth, Western Australia

Mark Walters
Cranio-MaxilloFacial Unit, Princess Margaret Hospital for Children, Perth, Western Australia

Lucile Drujont, Laura Carretero-Iglesia, Laurence Bouchet-Delbos, Gaelle Beriou,
Emmanuel Merieau, Marcelo Hill, Maria Cristina Cuturi and Cedric Louvet
ITUN, Inserm UMR_S 1064, Center for Research in Transplantation and Immunology, Nantes, France

Yves Delneste
UMR Inserm 892 CNRS 6299, Université d'Angers, CHU Angers, Laboratoire d'Immunologie et Allergologie, Angers, France

Maurice Theunissen, Audrey A. A. Fiddelers, Mark G. A. Willemsen and Hans-Fritz Gramke
Department of Anesthesiology and Pain Management, Maastricht University Medical Center+, Maastricht, the Netherlands

Madelon L. Peters and Erik G. W. Schouten
Department of Clinical Psychological Science, Maastricht University, Maastricht, the Netherlands

Patrícia R. Pinto
Life and Health Sciences Research Institute (ICVS), School of Health Sciences, University of Minho, Braga, Portugal; ICVS/3B's - PT Government Associate Laboratory, Braga/Guimarães, Portugal

Marco A. E. Marcus
Department of Anesthesiology and Pain Management, Maastricht University Medical Center+, Maastricht, the Netherlands
Department of Anesthesia/ICU, Pain and Palliative Care, Hamad Medical Corporation, Doha, Qatar

Richard Nordenvall and Li Felländer-Tsai
Division of Orthopedics and Biotechnology, Department of Clinical Science, Intervention and Technology, Karolinska Institutet, Stockholm, Sweden
Department of Orthopedics, Karolinska University Hospital, Stockholm, Sweden

Shahram Bahmanyar
Clinical Epidemiology Unit, Department of Medicine, Karolinska Institutet, Stockholm, Sweden
Center for Pharmacoepidemiology, Department of Medicine, Karolinska Institutet, Stockholm, Sweden
Faculty of Medicine, Golestan University of Medical Sciences, Gorgan, Iran

Johanna Adami
Clinical Epidemiology Unit, Department of Medicine, Karolinska Institutet, Stockholm, Sweden

Ville M. Mattila
Division of Orthopedics and Biotechnology, Department of Clinical Science, Intervention and Technology, Karolinska Institutet, Stockholm, Sweden
Department of Orthopedics, Karolinska University Hospital, Stockholm, Sweden
Department of Orthopedics and Trauma Surgery, University Hospital of Tampere, Tampere, Finland

Hiroyuki Tsuchiya
Department of Orthopaedic Surgery, Graduate School of Medical Science, Kanazawa University, Kanazawa, Japan

Katsuhiro Hayashi
Department of Orthopaedic Surgery, Graduate School of Medical Science, Kanazawa University, Kanazawa, Japan
Department of Orthopaedic Surgery, Nagoya City University Medical School, Nagoya, Japan

Shintaro Iwata
Division of Orthopedic Surgery, Chiba Cancer Center, Chiba, Japan

Akira Ogose
Division of Orthopedic Surgery, Niigata University Graduate School of Medical and Dental Sciences, Niigata, Japan

Akira Kawai
Department of Orthopaedic Surgery, National Cancer Center Hospital, Kashiwa, Japan

Takafumi Ueda
Department of Orthopaedic Surgery, Osaka National Hospital, Osaka, Japan

Takanobu Otsuka
Department of Orthopaedic Surgery, Nagoya City University Medical School, Nagoya, Japan

Xin Fan, Meng Xiao, He Wang and Ying-Chun Xu
Department of Clinical Laboratory, Peking Union Medical College Hospital, and Graduate School, Peking Union Medical College, Chinese Academy of Medical Sciences, Beijing, China

Fanrong Kong
Centre for Infectious Diseases and Microbiology Laboratory Services, Westmead Hospital, Westmead, New South Wales, Australia

Timothy Kudinha
Centre for Infectious Diseases and Microbiology Laboratory Services, Westmead Hospital, Westmead, New South Wales, Australia
Charles Sturt University, Orange, New South Wales, Australia

Dongdong Xiao, Juan Zhou, Ming Zhang, Zhe Zhou, Yang Zhao, Meng Gu, Zhong Wang and Mujun Lu
Department of Urology, Shanghai Ninth People's Hospital, Shanghai Jiao Tong University, School of Medicine, Shanghai, People's Republic of China

Xin Nie and Wenyue Wang
Department of General Surgery, Shanghai Ninth People's Hospital, Shanghai Jiao Tong University, School of Medicine, Shanghai, People's Republic of China

Åsa Holmner
Department of Radiation Sciences, Umeå University, Umeå, Sweden

Lutfan Lazuardi
Department of Public Health, Faculty of Medicine, Gadjah Mada University, Yogyakarta, Indonesia

Kristie L. Ebi
ClimAdapt, LLC, Seattle, Washington, United States of America
Department of public health and clinical medicine, epidemiology and global health, Umeå University, Umeå, Sweden

Maria Nilsson
Department of public health and clinical medicine, epidemiology and global health, Umeå University, Umeå, Sweden

Luc Nimeskern, Willy Kuo, Ralph Müller and Kathryn S. Stok
Institute for Biomechanics, ETH Zurich, Zurich, Switzerland

Eva-Maria Feldmann, Silke Schwarz and Nicole Rotter
Department of Otorhinolaryngology, Ulm University Medical Center, Ulm, Germany

Eva Goldberg-Bockhorn and Susanne Dürr
Department of Diagnostic and Interventional Radiology, Ulm University Medical Center, Ulm, Germany

Index

www.ingramcontent.com/pod-product-compliance
Lightning Source LLC
Chambersburg PA
CBHW061242190326
41458CB00011B/3556
* 9 7 8 1 6 3 2 4 1 4 3 2 8 *